Dictionary of
Biotechnology

RS Sengar
Associate Professor

Reshu Chaudhary
SRF

Department of Biotechnology
SV Patel University of Agriculture and Technology
Meerut, UP

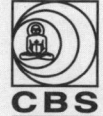

CBS

CBS Publishers & Distributors Pvt Ltd

New Delhi • Bengaluru • Chennai • Kochi • Kolkata • Mumbai
Hyderabad • Jharkhand • Nagpur • Patna • Pune • Uttarakhand

Dictionary of
Biotechnology

RS Sengar PhD
Professor and Head

Reshu Chaudhar y
SRF

Department of Agriculture Biotechnology
College of Agriculture
Sardar Vallabhbhai Patel University of Agriculture and
Technology
Meerut, UP

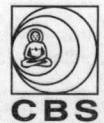

CBS

CBS Publishers & Distributors Pvt Ltd

New Delhi • Bengaluru • Chennai • Kochi • Kolkata • Mumbai
Hyderabad • Jharkhand • Nagpur • Patna • Pune • Uttarakhand

Dictionary of
Biotechnology

ISBN: 978-81-239-2450-2

Copyright © Authors and Publisher

First Edition: 2015
Reprint: 2018

Published by Satish Kumar Jain and produced by Varun Jain for

CBS Publishers & Distributors Pvt Ltd
4819/XI Prahlad Street, 24 Ansari Road, Daryaganj, New Delhi 110 002, India.
Ph: 23289259, 23266861, 23266867   Website: www.cbspd.com
Fax: 011-23243014   e-mail: delhi@cbspd.com; cbspubs@airtelmail.in.
Corporate Office: 204 FIE, Industrial Area, Patparganj, Delhi 110 092
Ph: 4934 4934   Fax: 4934 4935   e-mail: publishing@cbspd.com; publicity@cbspd.com

Branches

- **Bengaluru:** Seema House 2975, 17th Cross, K.R. Road,
  Banasankari 2nd Stage, Bengaluru 560 070, Karnataka
  Ph: +91-80-26771678/79   Fax: +91-80-26771680   e-mail: bangalore@cbspd.com
- **Chennai:** 7, Subbaraya Street, Shenoy Nagar, Chennai 600 030, Tamil Nadu
  Ph: +91-44-26680620, 26681266   Fax: +91-44-42032115   e-mail: chennai@cbspd.com
- **Kochi:** Ashana House, No. 39/1904, AM Thomas Road, Valanjambalam,
  Ernakulam 682 016, Kochi, Kerala
  Ph: +91-484-4059061-65   Fax: +91-484-4059065   e-mail: kochi@cbspd.com
- **Kolkata:** 6/B, Ground Floor, Rameswar Shaw Road, Kolkata-700 014, West Bengal
  Ph: +91-33-22891126, 22891127, 22891128   e-mail: kolkata@cbspd.com
- **Mumbai:** 83-C, Dr E Moses Road, Worli, Mumbai-400018, Maharashtra
  Ph: +91-22-24902340/41   Fax: +91-22-24902342   e-mail: mumbai@cbspd.com

Representatives

- **Hyderabad** 0-9885175004   • **Jharkhand** 0-9811541605   • **Nagpur** 0-9021734563
- **Patna** 0-9334159340   • **Pune** 0-9623451994   • **Uttarakhand** 0-9716462459

Printed At : Goyal Offset Printers

to

_____

our parents
with love and special regards

Preface

Human welfare in all directions had been vastly important with rapid developments in biotechnology. It is essential that students embarking on career in biotechnology should be well versed in nearly all branches of biology.

This book is meant for undergraduate biotechnology and life science students. Many special books on biotechnology are available currently which assumed familiarity with the basic concepts on biotechnology, as these are especially designed for postgraduate students, several universities introduced undergraduate courses in biotechnology. Students are required to develop the conceptual understanding in biotechnology. This book elaborates fundamental concepts and terms which are absolutely necessary for the budding biotechnologist.

It is privilege to acknowledge with praise to God and deep gratitude for the guidance, help and encouragement given during the preparation of the manuscript by my respected teacher and guide late Dr HS Srivastava. I have received generous help from many scientists, senior and fellow teachers for the preparation of *Dictionary of Biotechnology* under reference Dr Shivendra Vikram Sahi, Professor and Head, Department of Biotechnology, Ogden College of Science and Engineering, Western Kentucky University, Bowling Green Ky. 42101, USA. I will ever remain indebted to my respected teacher Prof VP Singh, Head and Dean, Department of Plant Science, MJP Rohilkhnad University, Bareilly; Dr Anil Gupta, Professor and Head, Department of Molecular Biology and Biotechnology, College of Basic Science and Humanities, GB Pant University of Agriculture and Technology, Pantnagar; Prof Vinay Kumar Sharma, Department of Biosciences and Biotechnology, Bansthali University, Rajasthan; Prof RP Singh, Department of Biotechnology, IIT Roorkee; Prof NS Sikhawat, Department of Biotechnology, JNV University, Jodhpur; Dr NK Singh and Dr TR Sharma, Principal Scientist Biotechnology, and Director, National Research Center on Plant Biotechnology, New Delhi; Prof Akhilesh

Tyagi, Director, NIPGR, New Delhi; Rakesh Tuli, NABI Mohali, Chandigarh; Prof BD Singh, BHU, Varanasi; Prof PK Gupta, CCS University, Meerut; Prof RL Singh, Dr RMLA University of Faizabad, Prof KN Singh, ND University of Agriculture and Technology, Kumarganj, Faizabad; Dr Rakesh Singh, Dr Rajesh Singh, Dr Sundeep Kumar Sharma and Dr Amit Singh, NBPGR, New Delhi; Dr AK Sharma, Ramie Research Station (ICAR), Sorbhog Barpeta, Assam; and research scholars for their extraordinary help in shaping the *Dictionary of Biotechnology*. I am thankful to my colleagues for their valuable and constructive suggestions during the course of writing this book.

It is with the deep sense of love and respect, I would like to thank whole-heartedly my reverend mother Smt Kamla Sengar, father Dr SS Sengar, my wife Sarita Sengar, sons Divyanshu Sengar and Kartikey Sengar, my brother Dr Rajesh Singh Sengar and his better half Kalpana Sengar, and their daughters Saumya Singh Sengar and Amripanshi Sengar, my sister Smt Usha Bhadauria and brother-in-law Dr HS Bhadauria, for their persistent, inspiration and encouragement for the preparation of the manuscript.

I would like to thank Mr SK Jain, Mr YN Arjuna, Ms Ritu Chawla, Mr Sunil Dutt, Mr Prasenjit Paul and Mr Vikrant Sharma for their help in bringing out this publication in a presentable form. I would definitely like to await for this opportunity to express my gratitude to all these who have directly or indirectly lent a helping hand in the completion of this book.

RS Sengar

Contents

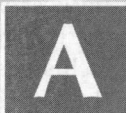

- **A DNA:** One of the many possible double-helical structures of DNA. It is a right-handed double helix, fairly similar to the more common and well-known B-DNA form, but with a shorter, more compact, helical structure. A-DNA is thought to be one of the three biologically active double-helical structures along with B- and Z-DNA (Fig. 1). It appears likely that it occurs only in dehydrated samples of DNA, such as those used in crystallographic experiments and possibly is also assumed by DNA-RNA hybrid helices and by regions of double-stranded RNA.

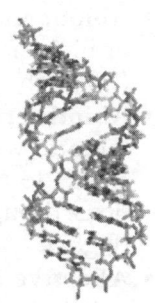

Fig. 1: A-DNA

- **A domain:** The conserved 11 bp sequence of A-T base pairs in the yeast autonomously replicating sequence (ARS) element that comprises the replication origin.
- **A living organism:** An organism whose genetic material has been modified by recombinant DNA technology.
- **A site:** Of ribosome is the site that an aminoacyl-tRNA enters to base with the codon.
- **A:** Adenine residue in either DNA or RNA.
- *ab initio*: A method that derives a three-dimentional (3D) structure from initial physical forces and interactions.
- **ATP-binding cassette (ABC) transporters:** A class of membrane transporter proteins which "transfer" across cell membranes: sugar molecules (i.e. used by cells as "fuel"); inorganic ions (needed to catalyze certain cellular processes); polypeptides (protein molecules); certain anticancer drugs (thereby making it harder to halt certain cancer tumors via use of pharmaceuticals); certain antibiotics (thereby conferring antibiotic resistance to some pathogenic bacteria). ABC transporter molecules are embedded in the plasma membrane (surface "skin") of cells.

A

- **Abduction:** A method of reasoning in which one chooses the hypothesis that would, if true, best explain the relevant evidence. It is also used to just mean the generation of hypothesis to explain observations or conclusions.

- **Abiogenesis:** An early theory that held some organisms originated from nonliving material.

- **Abiotic:** Absence of living organisms.

- **Abiotic elicitor:** An elicitor that is not of biological origin, e.g. ultraviolet (UV) light, salts of heavy metals, etc.

- **Abiotic stress:** Outside (nonliving) factors, which can cause harmful effects to plants, such as soil conditions, drought, extreme temperatures (Fig. 2).

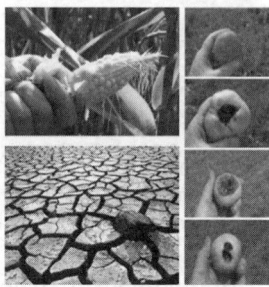

Fig. 2: Abiotic stress

- **Abortive initiation:** Describes a process in which RNA polymerase starts transcription but terminates before it has left the promoter. It then reinitiates. Several cycles may occur before the elongation stage begins.

- **Abortive transduction:** Failure of incorporation of transducing DNA into the recipient chromosome.

- **Abrin:** A toxin derived from the seed of the rosary pea.

- **Abscisic acid:** A phytohormone (plant hormone) utilized to control: the size of stomatal pores, i.e. the openings in leaves through which plants exchange oxygen and carbon dioxide (and water inadvertently) with the atmosphere; abscision (shedding of flowers, fruit, etc.); dormancy (Fig. 3).

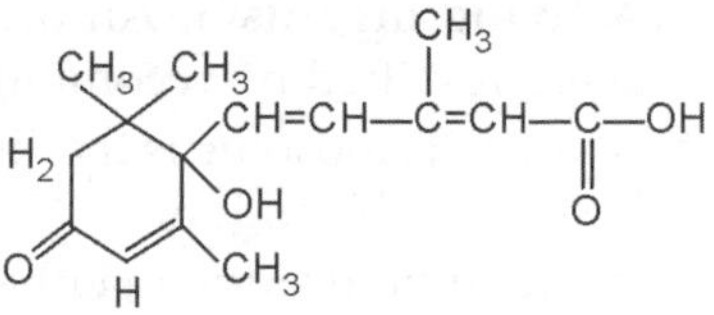

Fig. 3: Abscisic acid (ABA)

- **Absciss abscissa:** The horizontal axis of a graph.

- **Absolute configuration:** The configuration of four different substituent groups around an asymmetric carbon atom, in relation to D- and L-glyceraldehyde.

- **Absorbance (A):** A measure of the amount of light absorbed by a substance suspended in a matrix. The matrix may be gaseous, liquid, or solid in nature. Most biologically active compounds (proteins) absorb light in the UV or visible light portion of the

spectrum. Absorbance is used to quantitate (measure) the **A**
concentration of the substance in question (substance dissolved
in a liquid).

- **Absorbe (1. Ab, away + sorbere, to suck in):** To suck up, or to
take in, in the cell, materials are taken in (absorbed) from a solution.
- **Absorption spectrum:** A graph depicting the ability of a
substance to absorb lights of various wavelengths.
- **Absorption: 1. In general:** The process of absorbing or taking
up of water and nutrients by assimilation or imbibitions. The
taking up by capillary, osmotic, chemical or solvent action, such
as the taking up of a gas by a solid or liquid, or taking up of a
liquid by a solid. **2. In biology:** The movement of a fluid or a
dissolved substance across a cell membrane. In plants: water
and mineral salts are absorbed from the soil by roots. In animals:
soluble food material is absorbed into the circulatory system
through the cells lining the alimentary canal (Fig. 4).

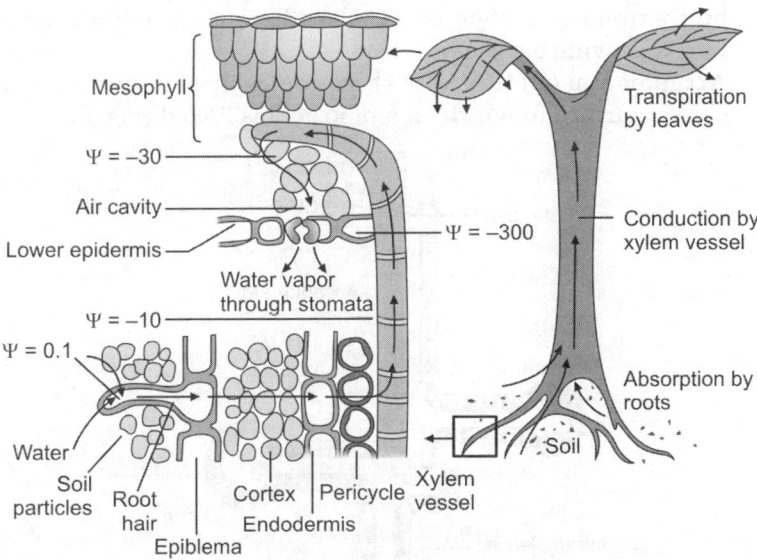

Fig. 4: Absorption

- **Abundance:** Of an mRNA is the average number of molecules
per cell.
- **Abundant mRNAs:** Consist of a small number of individual
species, each present in a large number of copies per cell.

A

- **Abzymes:** Catalytic antibodies that are synthetic constructs. They either stabilize the transition state of a chemical reaction or bind to a specific substrate, thereby increasing the reaction rate of that chemical reaction.
- **Acaricide:** A pesticide used to kill or control mites or ticks.
- **ACC:** Abbreviation/acronym for the compound 1-amino-cyclopropane-1-carboxylic acid, which is produced from S-adenosylmethionine (SAM) in the fruit of certain plants. When the "sam-k" gene is inserted into the genome of those plants, the level of SAM is greatly reduced in their fruit, which inhibits (slows) ripening/softening of that fruit via a reduction/slowdown in production of ethylene (hormone that causes fruit to ripen/soften).
- **ACC synthase:** Aminocyclopropane carboxylic acid synthase/ deaminase; it is one of the most critical enzymes in the metabolic pathway that creates the hormone ethylene inside fruit. Because ethylene causes certain fruit (tomatoes) to ripen (soften), it is possible to significantly delay the softening (i.e. spoilage) process by controlling creation of ACC synthase via manipulation of the ACC synthase gene.
- **Acceptor arm (Of tRNA):** A short duplex that terminates in the CCA sequence to which an amino acid is linked (Fig. 5).

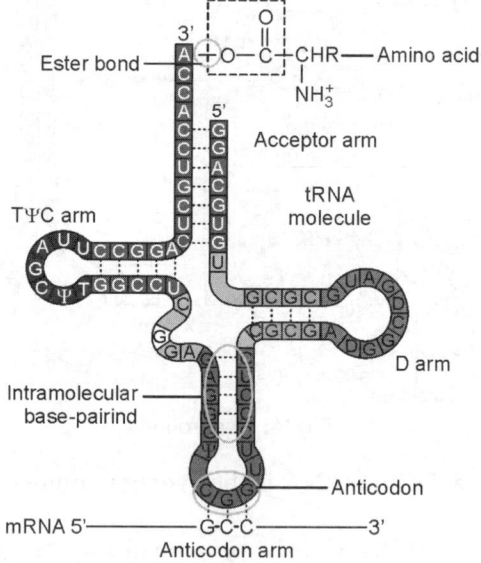

Fig. 5: tRNA structure

- **Acceptor control:** The regulation of the rate of respiration by the availability of ADP as phosphate acceptor.
- **Acceptor junction site:** The junction between the right 3' end of an intron and the left 5' end of an exon.
- **Acceptor site:** The splice site at the 3'end of an intron.
- **Accessible surface:** The surface that is traced by the centre of a probe molecule (usually water) as it rolls on the Vander Walls surface of a molecule.
- **Accession number:** An identifier supplied by the curators of the major biological databases upon submission of a novel entry that uniquely identifies that sequence (or other) entry.
- **Accession:** The addition of germ-plasm deposits to existing germ-plasm storage bands.
- **Accessory bud:** Lateral bud occurring at the base of a terminal bud or at the side of an axillary bud.
- **Acclimatization:** The adaptation of a living organism (plant, animal or microorganism) to a changed environment that subjects it to physiological stress.
- **Acetyl-coenzyme A (Ac-CoA):** It is a chemical synthesized in cell mitochondria by combining the thiol (molecular group) of coenzyme A with an acetyl group (from breakdown/digestion of fats, carbohydrates or proteins) (Fig. 6).

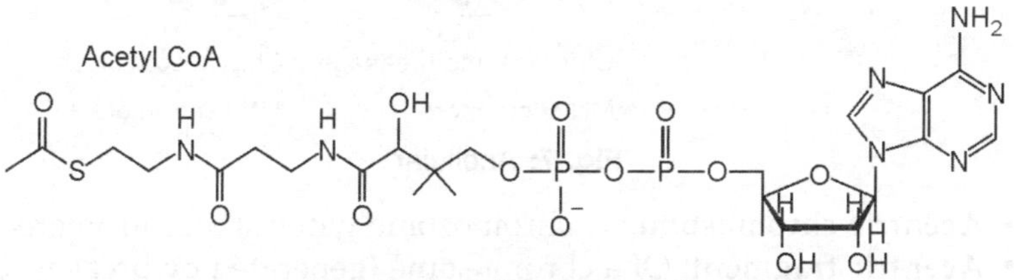

Fig. 6: Acetyl-coenzyme A

- **Angiotensin-converting enzyme (ACE):** A crucial enzyme (within the human vascular system) for catalyzing the formation of angiotensin, a hormone that causes narrowing/restriction of blood vessels, thus increasing the body's blood pressure as the blood is squeezed through those narrowed blood vessels. The action of ACE can be inhibited by the pharmaceuticals known as ACE inhibitors. Research indicates that consumption of whey protein can also result in inhibition of ACE.
- **ACE inhibitors:** A family of chemically-similar pharmaceuticals utilized to lower blood pressure in humans, by blocking

A

formation of a hormone (angiotensin) that narrows/restricts blood vessels. (*See* also ACE).

- **Acellular:** Describing tissues or organisms that are not made up of separate cells but often have more than one nucleus (Fig. 7).

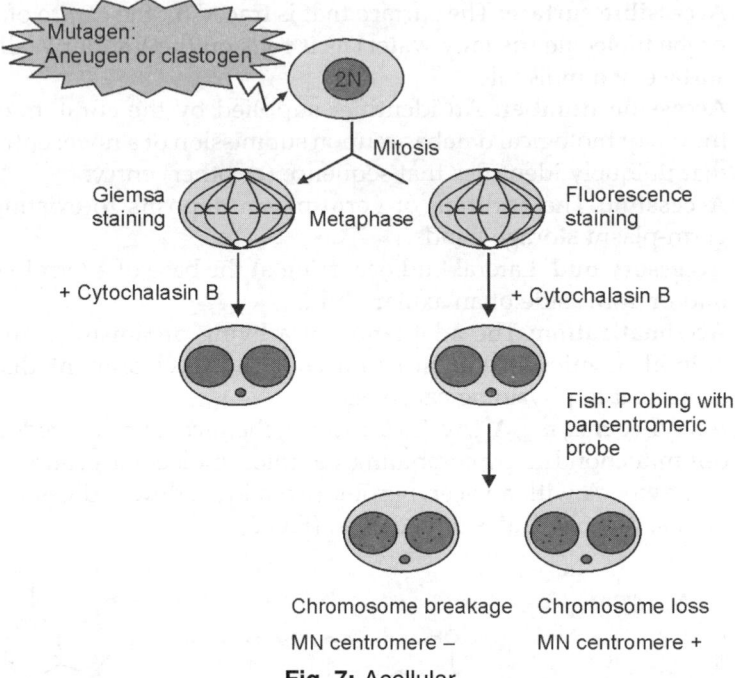

Fig. 7: Acellular

- **Acentric chromosome:** A chromosome without a centromere.
- **Acentric fragment:** Of a chromosome (generated by breakage) lacks a centromere and is lost at cell division.
- **Acetosyringone:** A phenolic compound produced by dicot plant cells at wound sites; acts as signal molecule for the expression of vir regulon of *Agrobacterium tumefaciens*.
- **Acetylation:** Addition of an acetyl (CH_3CO) group.
- **Acetyl carnitine:** One of the metabolites of mitochondria, it is a substrate (substance that is acted upon) for acylcarnitine transferase (which converts the acetyl carnitine to carnitine). Research indicates that consumption of acetyl carnitine helps increase the levels of acetylcholine and nerve growth factor (NGF) in the brain (Fig. 8).

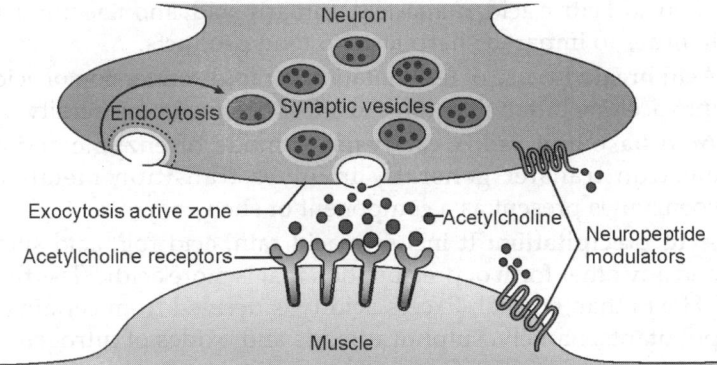

Fig. 8: Acetyl carnitine

- **Acetylcholine:** A neurotransmitter (i.e. one of several relatively small, diffusible molecules utilized by the human body to "transmit" nerve impulses) that is synthesized (manufactured) near the ends of axons (i.e. one type of neuron). That synthesis is accomplished by the "transfer" of an acetyl group (portion of molecule) from Ac-CoA to a choline molecule (available in the body via consumption of soybean lecithin or certain other foods), in a chemical reaction catalyzed by cholinesterase. An increased amount of acetylcholine in the (human) brain has been shown to reduce the symptoms of Alzheimer's disease.

- **Acetylcholinesterase:** An enzyme that hydrolyzes (cuts into smaller pieces) molecules of the neurotransmitter acetylcholine, after the acetylcholine molecules have accomplished "transmission" of a nerve impulse. That hydrolysis (cutting into pieces) of acetylcholine molecules thus serves to prepare the neurons (cells of the body's nervous system) to be able to transmit other, later nerve impulses.

- **Acetyl-CoA:** Acetyl-coenzyme A.

- **Acetyl-CoA carboxylase:** An enzyme that catalyzes the chemical reaction (i.e. conversion of Ac-CoA to malonyl CoA via carboxylation) which is the first step in the series of chemical reactions through which some plants manufacture oils (soybean oil, canola oil, etc.).

- **Acid:** A substance that contains hydrogen atom(s) in its molecular structure, with a pH in the range from 0 to 6, which will react with a base to form a salt. Acids normally taste sour and feel slippery. For example, food product manufacturers often add citric acid, malic acid, fumaric acid, and itaconic acid in order to impart a sharp taste to food products.

- **Acid break:** In case of fermentation, a rapid conversion of acids into acetone butanol leading to a fast decline in the acidity.
- **Acid-base and redox catalysis:** A mode of enzyme action; electron transfer generally involves transition metals or coenzymes present as a component of such enzymes.
- **Acid precipitation:** It includes acid rain, acid fog, acid snow and any other form of precipitation that is more acidic (less than pH 5.6) than normal. Excess acidity is derived from certain air pollutants, namely, sulphur dioxide and oxides of nitrogen.
- **Acidic domain:** A type of activation domain.
- **Acidosis:** A metabolic condition in which the capacity of the body to buffer changes in pH is diminished. Hence, acidosis is accompanied by decreased blood pH (the blood becomes more acidic than is normal) (Fig. 9).

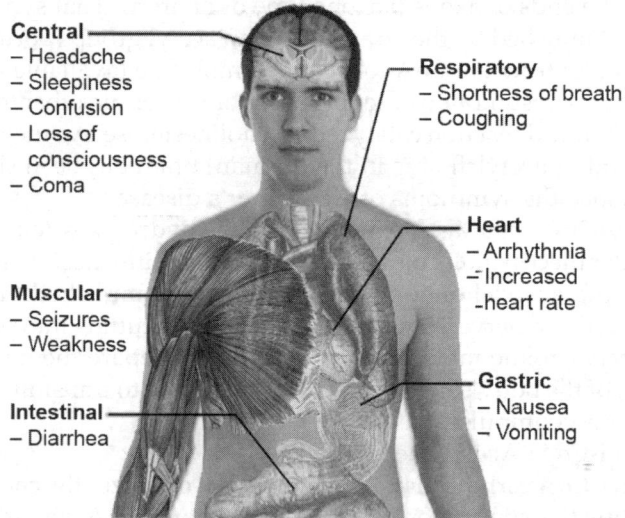

Central
- Headache
- Sleepiness
- Confusion
- Loss of consciousness
- Coma

Respiratory
- Shortness of breath
- Coughing

Heart
- Arrhythmia
- Increased heart rate

Muscular
- Seizures
- Weakness

Intestinal
- Diarrhea

Gastric
- Nausea
- Vomiting

Fig. 9: Acidosis

- **Aconitase:** An enzyme of the Kreb's cycle that, in animals, also acts as an iron regulatory protein.
- **Acoustic wave biosensor:** These devices detect a change in the mass of the biological component of the biosensor.
- **Acyl carrier protein (ACP):** A protein that binds acyl intermediates during the formation of long-chain fatty acids. ACP is

important in that it is involved in every step of fatty acid synthesis.

- **Ac-P:** Acetylphosphate.
- **Acquired:** Developed in response to the environment, not inherited, such as a character trait (acquired characteristic) resulting from environmental effect(s). (acclimatization).
- **Acquired immunity:** Another term for adaptive immunity.
- **Acquired immunodeficiency syndrome (AIDS):** A syndrome caused by infection by the human immunodeficiency virus (HIV).
- **Acquision of totipotency:** Formation of proembryogenic cell masses in cultured cells/tissues, usually in response to a high auxin concentration.
- **Acridine dye:** A chemical compound that intercalates between adjacent base pairs of the double helix, which causes a frameshift mutation.
- **Acridines:** Mutagens that act on DNA to cause the insertion or deletion of a single base pair. They were useful in defining the triplet nature of the genetic code.
- **Acrocentric:** A chromosome in which the centromere lies very near to one end (Fig. 10).

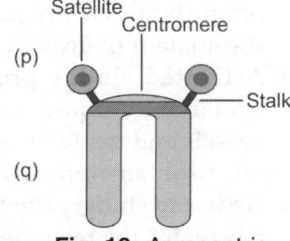

Fig. 10: Acrocentric

- **Acropetal:** 1. Developing or blooming in succession towards the apex, such as leaves or flowers developing acropetally. 2. Transport or movement of substances towards the apex, such as the movement of water through the plant. The opposite tendency is termed basipetal.
- **Acrosome:** An optical organelle in the head of a apermatozoon.
- **Adrenocorticotropic hormone (corticotropin) (ACTH):** A polypeptide secreted by the anterior lobe of the pituitary gland. This is an example of a protein hormone.
- **Actin:** One of the two contractile proteins in muscle (the other being myosin). Actin is also found in the microfilament that form part of the cytoskeleton of all cells (Fig. 11).
- **Actin letter:** An official communication that informs a sponsor of a decision by the agency. An approval letter allows commercial marketing of the product.
- **Action spectrum:** A graph relating the degree of physiological response caused by different wavelengths of light.

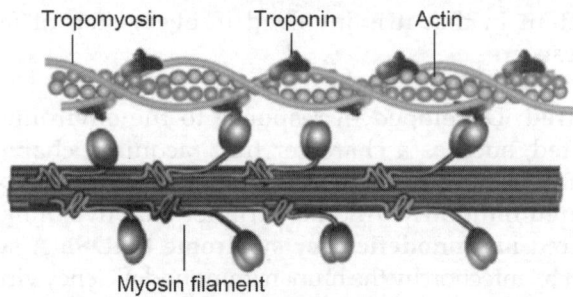

Fig. 11: Actin

- **Activated charcoal; activated carbon:** Charcoal that has been treated to remove hydrocarbons to increase its adsorptive properties. The inhibitory substances in nutrient medium get adsorbed to charcoal when present in the medium. Sometimes, phenolamines present as contaminants in charcoal may stimulate root growth *in vitro*.
- **Activated sludge process:** It uses large aerated vessels for oxidation of liquid waste, which continuously flows into the vessels and treated water flows out of them at a predetermined rate to obtain optimal digestion of the dissolved organic matter.
- **Activated sludge:** The sediment from biologically treated sewage; it contains the microbes for anaerobic digestion of sewage.
- **Activation domain:** The part of a transcription factor that makes contact with the initiation complex (Fig. 12).

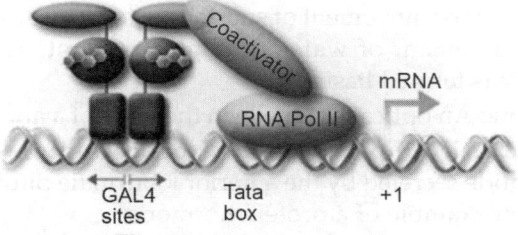

Fig. 12: Activation domain

- **Activation energy:** The free energy needed to elevate a molecule from its stable ground state to the unstable transition state.
- **Activation function:** A function that translates a neuron's net input to an activation value.
- **Activation:** The time-varying value that is the output of a neuron.
- **Activator:** A protein that stimulates the expression of a gene, typically by acting at a promoter to stimulate RNA polymerase.

In eukaryotes, the sequence to which it binds in the promoter is A called a response element.

- **Active collection:** A collection which complements a base collection from which seed samples are drawn for distribution, exchange and other purposes such as multiplication and evaluation.
- **Active immunity: 1.** A type of acquired immunity whereby resistance to a disease is built up by either having a vaccine to it. **2.** Immunity acquired after stimulation with an antigen by natural infection or other exposure (Fig. 13).

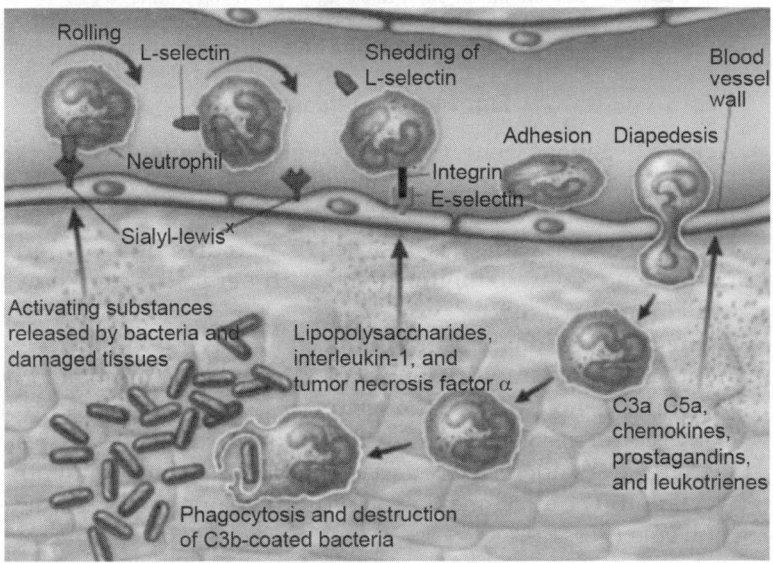

Fig. 13: Active immunity

- **Active initiation:** Describes a process in which RNA polymerase starts transcription but terminates before it has left the promoter. It then reinitiates. Several cycles may occur before the elongation stage begins.
- **Active site:** The restricted part of an enzyme to which a substrate binds.
- **Active transport (Fig. 14):** An energy-consuming process that moves molecules against an electrochemical gradient. Energy for the movement is provided by hydrolysis of ATP.
- **Activity coefficient:** The factor by which the concentration of a solute must be multiplied to give its true thermodynamic activity.

Passive transport systems involve motion from high concentration lower concentrations of the object being transported, and the energy that drives them is just random thermal energy

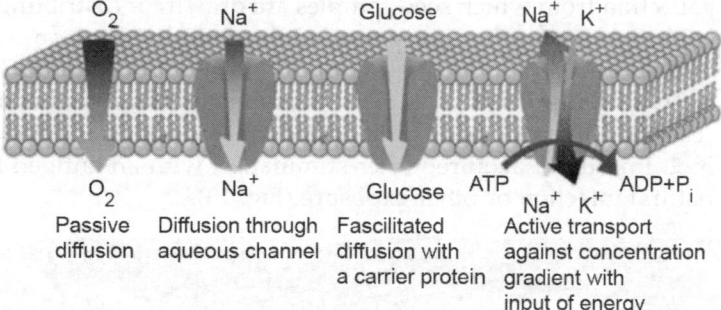

Fig. 14: Active transport

- **Acuron™ gene:** A gene, trademarked by syngenta AG, that can be inserted into plants via genetic engineering techniques. Inserted into the genome (DNA) of a plant, the gene confers tolerance to herbicide(s) whose active ingredient is protoporphyrinogen oxidase inhibitor (thus, such herbicides are known as PPO inhibitors).
- **Acute transfection:** Short-term infection of cells with DNA.
- **Acute transforming virus:** Carries a gene(s) that originated in a cellular genome. Its transforming capacity is the result of expression of that gene. Because the gene replaced viral sequences, the virus does not have the capacity to replicate independently.
- **Acylation:** The attachment of a lipid side chain to a polypeptide molecule (Fig. 15).

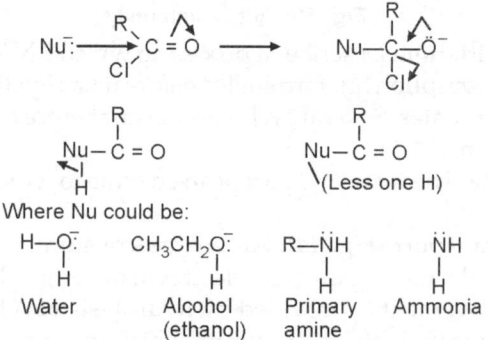

Fig. 15: Acylation

- **Acylcarnitine transferase:** An enzyme that converts the mitochondrial metabolite acetyl carnitine into carnitine.
- **Acyl-CoA:** Acyl derivatives of coenzyme A (acyl-S-CoA).
- **AD:** An acronym referring to the group of diseases known collectively as autoimmune disorders. These include diseases such as multiple sclerosis, lupus, rheumatoid arthritis, etc.
- **Ada enzyme:** An enzyme in *Escherichia coli* that is involved in the direct repair of alkylation mutations.
- **Adaptability:** The potential or ability of a population to adapt to changes in the environmental condition through changes of its genetic structure.
- **Adaptation:** An internal change in a system in response to an external event in the system's environment (Fig. 16).

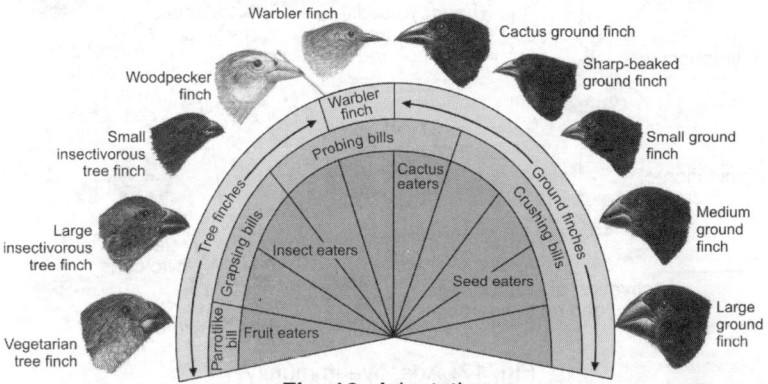

Fig. 16: Adaptation

- **Adaptation traits:** The complex of traits related to reproduction and survival of the individual in a particular production environment. Adaptation traits contribute to individual fitness. They are the traits subjected to selection during the evolution of animal genetic resources. By definition, these traits are also important to the ability of the animal genetic resource to be sustained in the production environment.
- **Adaptin:** A subunit of the cytosolic adaptor proteins that mediate formation of clathrin-coated vesicles. There are several types of adaptin subunits.
- **Adaptive genetic variance:** The proportion of genetic variation that is the summation of the effect of all individual genes influencing a trait. It is the average effect of substituting one allele for another.

A • **Adaptive immunity:** The response mediated by lymphocytes that are activated by their specific interaction with antigen. The adaptive immune response develops over several days as lymphocytes with antigen-specific receptors are stimulated to proliferate and become effectors cells. It is responsible for immunological memory (Fig. 17).

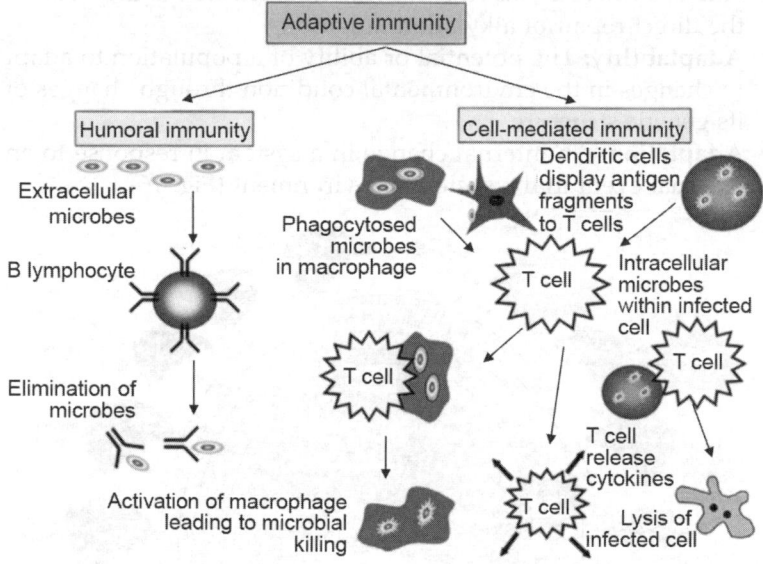

Fig. 17: Adaptive immunity

• **Adaptive radiation:** Evolutionary diversification of a generalized ancestral from with the production of a number of specialized forms by adaptation.

• **Adaptive surface:** A surface plotted in three dimensions with all possible combinations of allele frequencies for different loci plotted along the plane, and the mean fitness for each combination plotted as the height of the surface.

• **Adaptive:** Subject to adaptation, i.e. able to change over time to improve fitness.

• **Adaptor:** A synthetic single-stranded oligonucleotides that, after self-hybridization, produces a molecule with cohesive ends and an internal restriction endonuclease site. When the adaptor is inserted into a cloning vector by means of cohesive ends, the internal sequence provides a new restriction endonuclease site.

- **Adaptor:** Proteins bind to signals in the cytoplasmic tails of transmembrane cargo proteins and recruit clathrin molecules in the assembly of clathrin-coated pits and vesicles. Different types of adaptor proteins function at different compartments. Each adaptor protein contains four different subunits (Fig. 18).

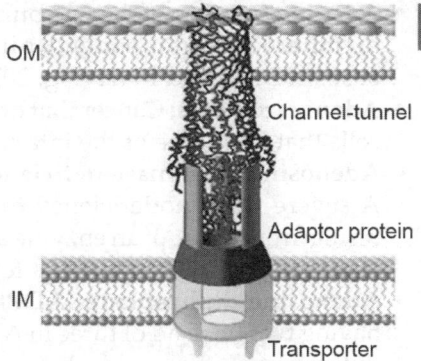

Fig. 18: Adaptor

- **Addendum (plural: addenda):** In formulation of tissue culture media—an item or a constituent substance to be added.
- **Addiction system:** A survival mechanism used by plasmids. The mechanism kills the bacterium upon loss of the plasmid.
- **Additive allelic effects:** Effects of alleles at a locus, where the heterozygote is exactly intermediate between the two homozygotes.
- **Additive gene effects:** Additive allelic effects summed across all the loci that contribute to genetic variation in a quantitative trait.
- **Additive genes:** Genes that interact but do not show dominance (in the case of alleles) or epistasis (if they are not alleles) (Fig. 19).

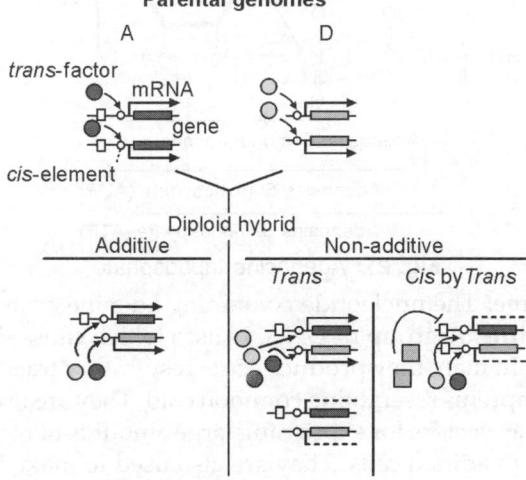

Fig. 19: Additive gene effects

A

- **Adenine (A):** One of the two purines (nine-membered double-ringed nitrogenous base) in DNA and RNA (Fig. 20).

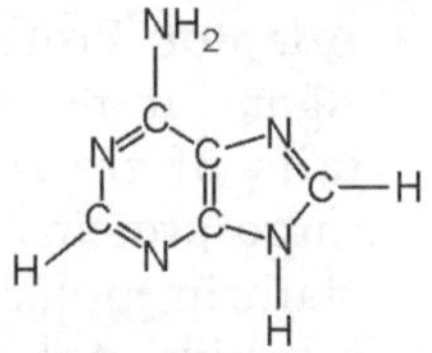

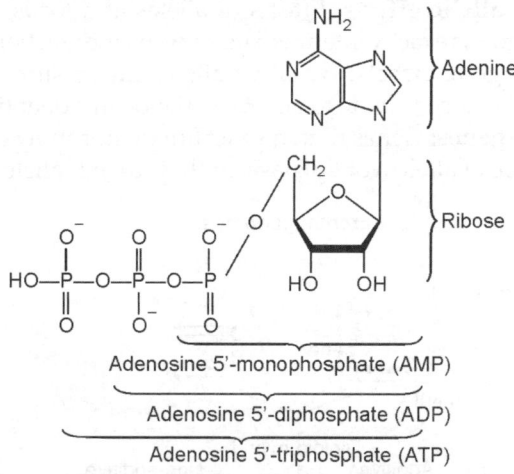

Fig. 20: Adenine

- **Adenocarcinoma:** Cancer that originates in cells that line some of the internal organs.
- **Adenosine deaminase deficiency (ADA):** A severe immunodeficiency disease that results from a lack of an enzyme adenosine deaminase. It usually leads to death within the first few months of life.
- **Adenosine diphosphate (ADP):** Lower energy form of ATP, having two (instead of three in ATP) phosphate groups attached to the adenine base and ribose sugar.
- **Adenosine monophosphate (AMP):** A ribonucleoside 5'-monophosphate that is formed by hydrolysis of ATP or ADP.
- **Adenosine triphosphate (ATP):** A common form in which energy is stored in living systems. It consists of a nucleotide (with ribose sugar) with three phosphate groups (Fig. 21).

Fig. 21: Adenosine triphosphate

- **Adenosine:** The nucleotide containing adenine as its base.
- **Adenovirus:** A group of DNA viruses which cause diseases in animals. In man, they produce acute respiratory tract infections with symptoms resembling common cold. They are used in gene cloning, as vectors for expressing large amounts of recombinant proteins in animal cells. They are also used to make live- virus vaccines against more dangerous pathogens (Fig. 22).

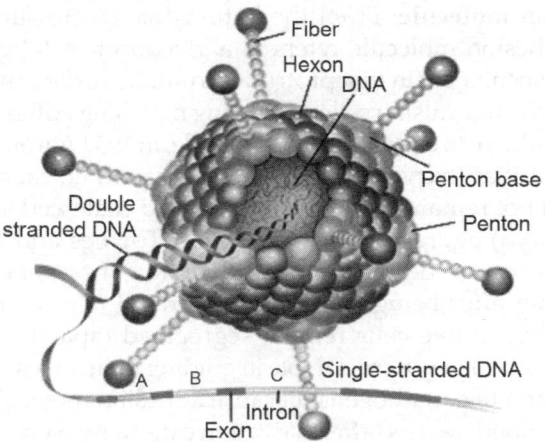

Fig. 22: Adenovirus

- **Adenovirus-associated virus:** A small virus that requires adenovirus for growth. This virus causes no known human disease, and hence recombinant AAV is used as a gene therapy vector.
- **Adenylate cyclase:** An enzyme that uses ATP as a substrate to generate cyclic AMP, in which 5′ and 3′ positions of the sugar ring are connected via a phosphate group.
- **Adept (antibody-directed enzyme prodrug therapy):** A way to target a drug to a specific tissue. The drug is administered as an inactive prodrug, and then converted into an active drug by an enzyme administered with a second infection. The enzyme is coupled to an antibody that concentrates it in the target tissue. When the enzyme arrives at the target tissue, the prodrug is activated to form the active drug, while elsewhere it remains inactive.
- **Adherent cells:** Immune cells (such as dendritic cells and macrophages) with the property of adhering to tissue culture, flasks. This property allows the cells to be separated and purified.

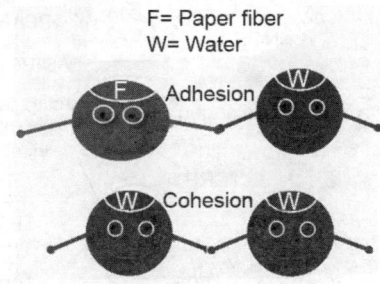

Fig. 23: Adhesion

- **Adhesion (1. adhere, to stick to):** The attraction of dissimilar for each other. A sticking together of unlike substances, such as soil and water (Fig. 23).

A • **Adhesion molecule:** From the Latin *adhaērere*, to stick to, the term adhesion molecule refers to a glycoprotein (oligosaccharide) molecular chain that protrudes from the surface membrane of certain cells, causing cells possessing matching adhesion molecules to adhere to each other. For example, in 1952 Aaron Moscona observed that (harvesting enzyme-separated) chicken embryo cells did not remain separated, but instead coalesced again into an (embryo) aggregate. In 1955, Philip Townes and Johannes Holtfreter showed that like amphibian (e.g. frog) neuron cells will rejoin after being physically separated (e.g. with a knife blade); but unlike cells remain segregated (apart). Adhesion molecules also play a crucial role in guiding monocytes to sources of infection (e.g. pathogens) because adhesion molecules in the walls of blood vessels (after activation caused by pathogen invasion of adjacent tissue) adhere to like adhesion molecules in the membranes of monocytes in the blood. The monocytes pass through the blood vessel walls, become macrophages, and fight the pathogen infection (e.g. triggering tissue inflammation, etc.).

• **Adipocytes:** Specialized cells within an organism's lymphatic system that store the triacylglycerols (also sometimes called triglycerides) after digestion of those fats, later releasing fatty acids and glycerol into the bloodstream when needed by the organism (Fig. 24).

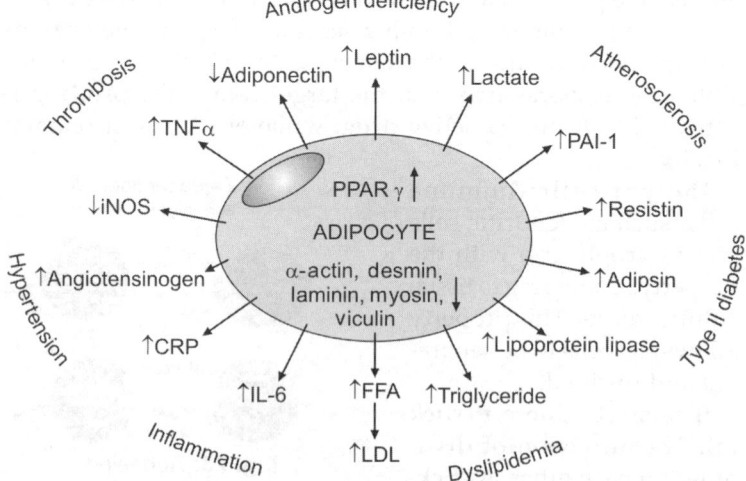

Fig. 24: Adipocyte

- **Adipose:** Refers to energy storage tissues consisting of fat molecules within some animals. Adipose tissue tends to increase if an animal consumes more energy-containing food than needed for its level of energy expenditure (e.g. via exercise). In humans older than 40 years, an increase in the body's adipose tissue is correlated with an increased risk of premature death (e.g. from coronary heart disease).

- **Adjacent segregation:** Segregation of a heterozygous reciprocal translation in which a translocated chromosome and a normal chromosome segregate together, producing an aneuploid gamete.

- **Adjacent-1 segregation:** Segregation from a heterozygous reciprocal translocation in which homologous centromeres go to opposite pole of the first-division spindle.

- **Adjacent-2 segregation:** Segregation from a heterozygous reciprocal translocation in which homologous centromeres go to same pole of the first-division spindle.

- **Adjuncts:** Starch rich materials like wheat, rice, maize, etc. that are added to barley malt during beer production (Fig. 25).

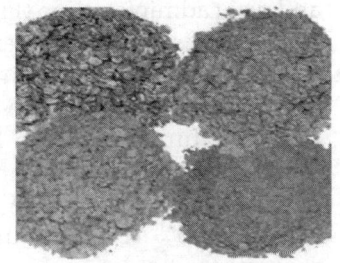

Fig. 25: Adjuncts

- **Adjuvant (to a herbicide):** Any compound that enhances the effectiveness (i.e. weed killing ability) of a given herbicide. For example, adjuvants such as surfactants can be mixed (prior to application to weeds) with herbicide (in water), in order to hasten transport of the herbicide's active ingredient into the weed plant. That is because the herbicide must move from an aqueous (water) environment into one (i.e. the weed plant's cuticle or "skin") comprised of lipids/lipophilic molecules, before it can accomplish its task.

- **Adjuvant (to a pharmaceutical):** Any compound that enhances the desired response by the body to that pharmaceutical. For example, adjuvants such as certain polysaccharides or surface-modified diamond nano particles, can be injected along with (vaccine) antigen in order to increase the immune response (e.g. production of antibodies) to a given antigen. Another example is that consumption of grapefruit juice by humans will increase

A

the impact of certain pharmaceuticals. Those pharmaceuticals include some sedatives, antihypertensives, the antihistamine terfenadine, and the immunosuppressant cyclosporine. The adjuvant effect of grapefruit juice is thought to be caused via inhibition of the enzyme cytochrome P4503A4, which catalyzes reactions involved in the metabolism (breakdown) of those pharmaceuticals. Another example is that consumption of the pharmaceutical known as clopidogrel (commercial name plavix) by people immediately following a mild heart attack (severe chest pain)—along with aspirin—greatly reduces the risk of death, strokes, and (new, additional) heart attacks, versus taking aspirin alone after a mild heart attack.

- **ADME:** Acronym for absorption, distribution (within the body), metabolism and elimination of pharmaceuticals.
- **ADME tests:** Refers to absorption, distribution (within the body), metabolism and elimination tests required by the US food and drug administration (FDA) for approval of new pharmaceuticals or new food ingredients.
- **A-DNA:** A particular right-handed helical form of DNA (possessing 11 base pairs per turn), in which DNA molecules exist when they are partially dehydrated. A-form DNA is found in fibers at 75% relative humidity and requires the presence of sodium, potassium, or cesium as the counterion. Instead of lying flat, the bases are tilted with regard to the helical axis and there are more base pairs per turn. The A-form is biologically interesting because it is probably very close to the conformation adopted by DNA-RNA hybrids or by RNA-RNA double-stranded regions. The reason is that the presence of the 2'2 hydroxyl group prevents RNA from lying in the B-form (Fig. 26).

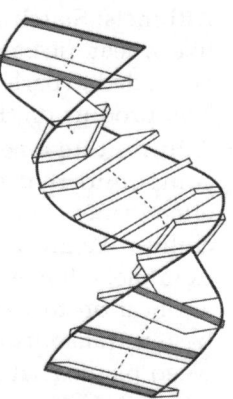

Fig. 26: A-DNA

- **Adoptive cellular therapy:** The increase in immune response that is achieved by selectively removing certain immune system cells from a (patient's) body, multiplying them *in vitro* outside the body to increase their number greatly, then reinserting those (more numerous) immune system cells into the same body.

- **Adoptive immunization:** The transfer of an immune state from one animal to another by means of lymphocyte transfusions.
- **Adoptive transfer:** The transfer of immune cells from a primed donor to an unprimed recipient.
- **Adsorbent:** A substance to which compounds adhere, e.g. activated charcoal.
- **Adsorption chromatography:** Separation of molecules due to their differential adsorption onto the solid matrix surface.
- **Adsorption:** The formation of a layer of gas, liquid or solid on the surface of a solid (Fig. 27).

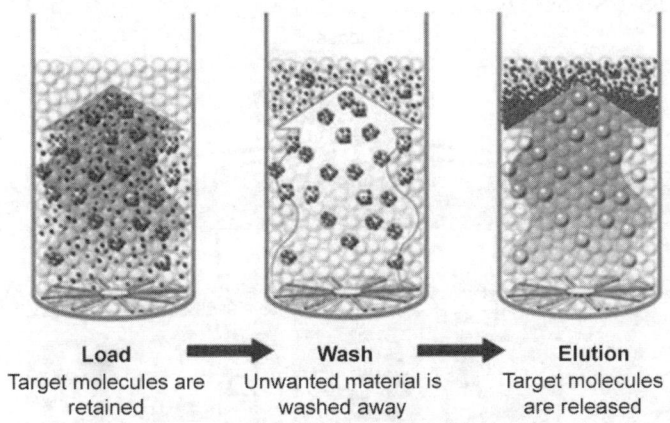

Load	Wash	Elution
Target molecules are retained	Unwanted material is washed away	Target molecules are released

Fig. 27: Adsorption

- **Adult cloning:** The creation of identical copies of an adult animal by nuclear transfer from differentiated adult tissue.
- **Advanced:** Applied to an organism or a part thereof, implying considerable development from the ancestral stage or from the explants stage.
- **Advantageous mutation:** A mutation that increases the fitness of the organism carrying it.
- **Adventitious:** Adjective used to describes organs developing from positions on the plant from which they would not normally be derived, e.g. shoots from leaf root, petiole, cotyledon, or embryos, etc. from any cell other than a zygote (Fig. 28).

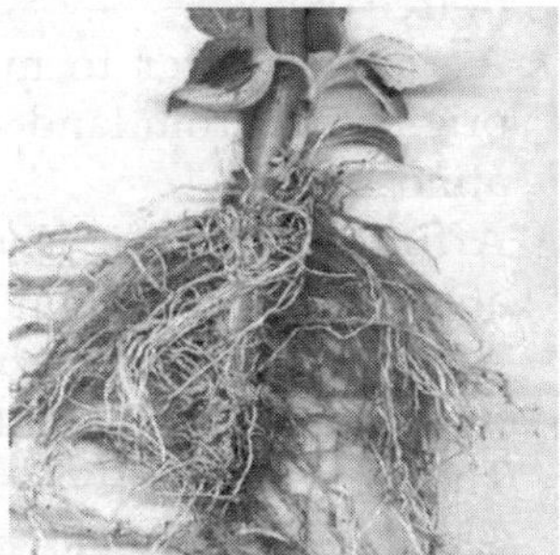

Fig. 28: Adventitious

- **Aerate:** To supply with or mix with air or gas. The process is aeration.
- **Aerobe:** A microorganism that grows in the presence of oxygen.
- **Aerobic bacteria:** Bacteria that can live in the presence of oxygen.
- **Aerobic fermentation:** It requires an efficient air supply, usually by sparging and stirring; two types: stirred tank and air lift type.
- **Aerobic respiration:** A type of respiration in which food stuffs are completely oxidized to carbon dioxide and water, with the release of chemical energy, in a process requiring atmospheric oxygen (Fig. 29).

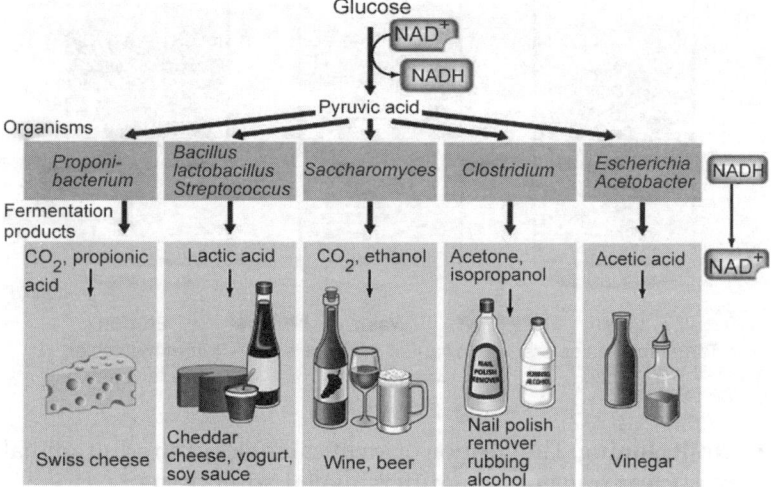

Fig. 29: Aerobic fermentation

- **Aerobic:** 1. needing oxygen for growth. 2. active in the presence of free oxygen.
- **Aerosols:** Refer to microscopic liquid and solid particles originating from land and water surfaces and carried into the atmosphere.
- **Affinity biosensor:** The biological material simply binds to the analyte molecules that leads to a change in its mass.
- **Affinity chromatography:** A method for separating molecules by exploiting their ability to bind specifically to other molecules. There are several types of biological affinity chromatography. A biological molecule can be immobilized and a smaller molecule to which it is to bind can be stuck to it, or the smaller ligand can

be immobilized and the macromolecule stuck to it. A variant is to use an antibody as the immobilized molecule and use it to 'capture' its antigen, this is often called immune-affinity chromatography. A variation is pseudoaffinity chromatography, in which a compound which is like a biological ligand is immobilized on a solid material, and enzymes or other proteins are bound to it. Other techniques include metal affinity chromatography, where a metal ion is immobilized on a solid support; metal ions bind tightly and specifically to many bio-molecules. The metal ion is bound to a chelator or chelating group, a chemical group that binds specifically and extremely tightly to that metal (Fig. 30).

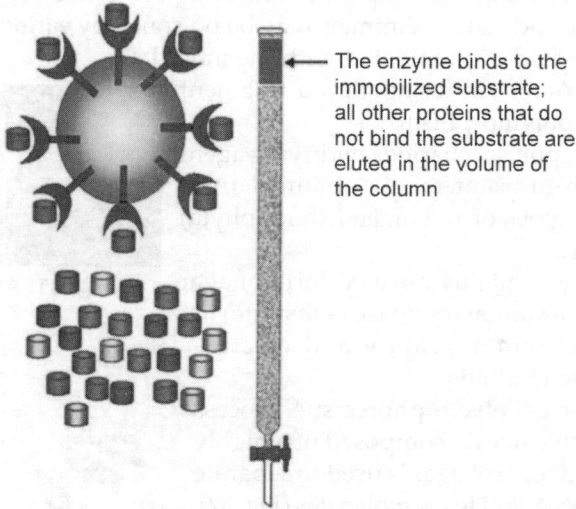

The enzyme binds to the immobilized substrate; all other proteins that do not bind the substrate are eluted in the volume of the column

Fig. 30: Affinity chromatography

- **Affinity tag purification tag:** An amino acid sequence that has been engineered into a protein to make its purification easier. These can work in a number of ways. The tag could be another protein, which binds to some other material very tightly thus allowing the protein to be purified by affinity chromatography. The tag could be a short amino acid sequence, which is recognized by an antibody. The antibody would then bind to the protein whereas it would not have done so before. One such short peptide, called FLAG, has been designed so that it is particularly easy to make antibodies against it. The tag could be a few amino

A

acids, which are then used as a chemical tag on the protein. For example, a string of positively charged amino acids will bind very strongly to a negatively charged filter. This could be used as the basis of a separation system. Some amino acids bind metals very strongly, especially in pairs; this chemical property can be exploited by using a filter with metal atoms chemically linked onto it to pull a protein out of a mixture of proteins.

- **Affinity:** A measure of the strength of binding of one molecule to another, e.g. of a ligand to a receptor or a substrate to an enzyme.

- **Afflatoxin:** Toxic compounds, produced by moulds (fungi) of the *Aspergillus flavus* group, that bind to DNA and prevent replication and transcription. Aflatoxins can cause acute liver damage and cancer. Animals may be poisoned by eating stored food or feed contaminated with the mould.

- **AFLP:** Acronym for amplified fragment length polymorphism.

- **Agar:** A polysaccharide solidifying agent used in nutrient media obtained from certain types of red algae (Rhodophyta) (Fig. 31).

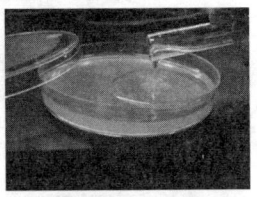

Fig. 31: Agar

- **Agarose:** A highly purified form of agar used as a stationary phase (substrate) in some chromatography and electro-phoretic methods.

- **Agarose gel electrophoresis:** A process in which a matrix composed of a highly purified form of agar is used to separate large DNA and RNA molecules (Fig. 32).

- **Agents:** Independent, autonomous, software modules that can search the

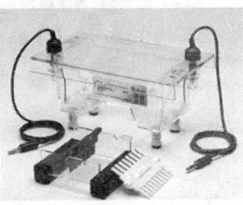

Fig. 32: Agarose gel electrophoresis

internet for data or content pertinent to a particular application, such as a gene, protein, or biological system.

- **Agglutinogen:** An antigen carried by red blood cells that reacts with a specific agglutinin in the plasma and causes clumping of the cells. When a specific antigen is injected into an animal body, it stimulates the production of a corresponding antibody.

- **Aggregate:** 1. A clump or mass formed by gathering or collecting units. 2. A body of loosely associated cells, such as a friable callus or cell suspension. 3. Coarse inert material, such as gravel, that is mixed with soil to increase its porosity. 4. A serological reaction (aggregation) in which the antibody and antigen react and precipitate out of solution.

- **Aging:** The process, affecting organisms and most cells, whereby each cell division (mitosis) brings that cell (or organism composed of such cells) closer to its final cell division (i.e. death). Notable exceptions to this aging process include cancerous cells (e.g. myelomas) and the single-celled organism; both of which are "immortal."

- **Aglycon:** A nonsugar component of a glycoside.

- **Aglycone:** The biologically active (molecular) form of molecules of isoflavones.

- **Agonist:** A drug, hormone or transmitter substance that forms a complex with a receptor site that is capable of triggering an active response from a cell.

- **Agonists:** Small protein or organic molecules that bind to certain cell proteins (i.e. receptors) at a site that is adjacent to the cell's docking site of protein hormones, neurotransmitters, etc. (i.e. receptor) to induce a conformational change in that cell protein, thereby enhancing its activity (i.e. effect upon the cell).

- **Agricultural biotechnology:** The application of rDNA technology to agriculturally important plants and organisms (Fig. 33).

- *Agrobacterium tumefaciens* – **mediated transformation:** A naturally occurring process of DNA transfer from the bacterium. A tumefaciens to plants (Fig. 34).

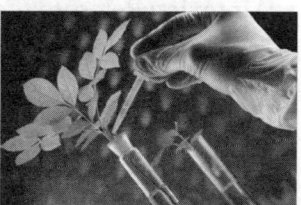

Fig. 33: Agricultural biotecnology

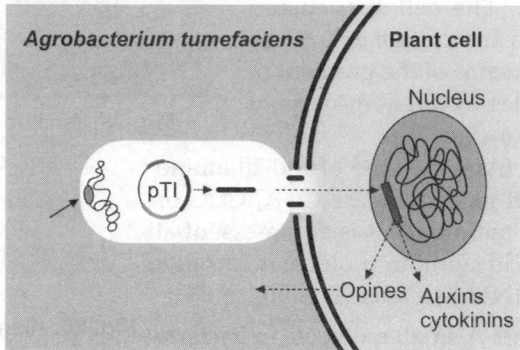

Fig. 34: *Agrobacterium tumefaciens*–mediated transformation

A

- *Agrobacterium tumefaciens*: *Agrobacterium* that cause crown gall disease. The cells form a crown gall due to Ti plasmid present in these bacteria.

- *Agrobacterium*: A genius of bacteria that includes several plant pathogenic species causing tumor like symptoms.

- **Agrobiodiversity:** That component of biodiversity which is relevant to food and agriculture production. The term agrobiodiversity encompasses within-species, species and ecosystem diversity.

- **Agroinfection:** Introduction of a viral genome into plant cells using *Agrobacterium*; usually, a tandem dimer of viral genome is placed within the T-DNA of *Agrobacterium*.

- **Agropine:** Plasmids carry genes coding for the synthesis of opines of the agropine type. The tumors usually die early.

- **Air pollution disaster:** A short-term situation in industrial cities in which intense industrial smog brings about a significant increase in human mortality.

- **Air toxics:** Refers to the category of air pollutants that includes radioactive materials and other toxic chemicals, which are present at low concentrations but are of concern because they often are carcinogenic.

- **Airlift fermenter:** A cylindrical fermentation vessel in which the cells are mixed by air introduced at the base of the vessel and that rises through column of culture medium. The cell suspension circulates around the column as a consequence of the gradient of air bubbles in different parts of the reactor (Fig. 35).

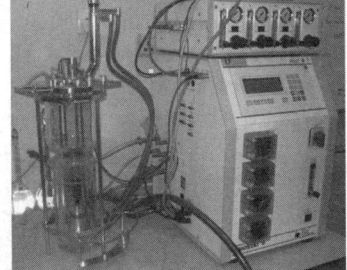

Fig. 35: Airlift fermenter

- **Alanine (Ala, A):** One of the 20 amino acids and its codons are GCA, GCC or GCU. In mammals, it is a non-essential amino acid with an molecular formula CH_3-$CH(NH_2)$-COOH (Fig. 36).

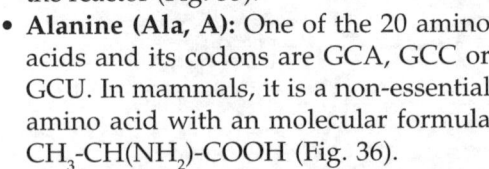

Alanine

Fig. 36: Alanine (Ala, A)

- **Alarmone:** A small molecule in bacteria that is produced as a result of stress and which acts to alter the state of gene expression. The unusual nucleotides ppGpp and pppGpp are examples.

- **Albinism:** Hereditary absence of pigment in an organism. Albino animals have no color in their skin, hair and eyes. The term is also used for absence of chlorophyll in plants.
- **Albino:** 1. An organism lacking pigmentation, due to genetic factors. The condition is albinism. 2. A conspicuous plastome (plastid) mutant involving loss of chlorophyll (Fig. 37).
- **Albumin:** A protein that the liver synthesizes (manufactures). Most minerals and hormones utilized by

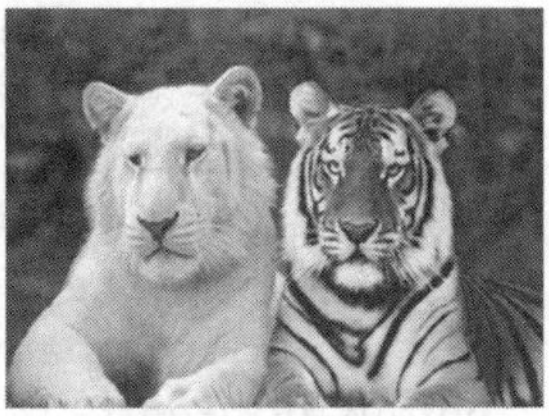

Fig. 37: Albino

the human body are first "attached" to a molecule of albumin before they are transported in the bloodstream to where they are needed in the body.
- **ALCAR:** Acronym for acetyl-L-carnitine.
- **Aldose:** A simple sugar in which the carbonyl carbon atom is at one end of the carbon chain. A class of monosaccharide sugars; the molecule contains an aldehyde group.
- **Aleurone:** The outermost layer of the endosperm in a seed.
- **AlfAFP:** Acronym for alfalfa antifungal peptide.
- **Algae:** A heterogeneous (widely varying) group of photosynthetic plants, ranging from microscopic single-cell forms to multicellular, very large forms such as seaweed. All of them contain chlorophyll and hence most are green, but some may be different colours due to the presence of other, overshadowing pigments (Fig. 38).

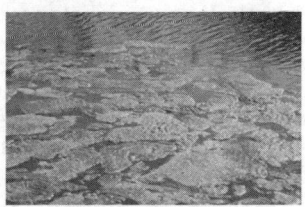

Fig. 38: Algae

- **Algal biomass:** Single-celled plants, such as *Chlorella* spp. And *Spirulina* spp., are grown commercially in ponds to make feed materials. *Chlorella* is grown commercially to make into fish food; it fed to zooplankton, and these in turn are harvested as feed for fish farms. This is a means of converting sunlight into food in a way convenient and controllable than normal farming.
- **Algal bloom:** Sudden heavy growth of algae; generally occurs due to addition of nutrients, whose scarcity is normally limiting.

A

- **Algalization:** The process of application of blue-green algae (cyanobacteria) in fields as biofertilizer.
- **Alginate:** A polysaccharide gelling agent.
- **Algorithm:** A series of steps defining a procedure or formula for solving a problem that can be coded into a programming language and executed. Bioinformatics algorithms typically are used to process, store, analyze, visualize and make predictions from biological data.
- **Alicin:** A compound that is produced naturally by the garlic plant when the cells within garlic bulbs are broken open (e.g. during food preparation or consumption). Enzymes present within those garlic cells convert (precursor compound) to alicin. Research indicates that human consumption of alicin confers some specific health benefits (antithrombotic, reduce blood cholesterol levels, reduce/avoid coronary heart disease, enhance the immune system, etc.).
- **Alignment:** The result of a comparison of two or more gene or protein sequences in order to determine their degree of base or amino acid similarity. Sequence alignments are used to determine the similarity, homology, function or other degree of relatedness between two or more genes or gene products.
- **Alkaline hydrolysis:** A chemical method of liberating DNA from a DNA-RNA hybrid.
- **Alkaline:** A substance that releases hydroxyl ions or uses up hydrogen ions.
- **Alkaloids:** A class of toxic compounds that are naturally produced by some organisms (e.g. ants, certain plants such as lupines, and certain fungi such as ergot). For example, certain species of ants naturally produce alkaloids, as a self-defense mechanism. Poison- dart frogs (*Dendrobates azureus*) and two species of New Guinea songbirds (*Pitohui dichrous* and *Ifrita kowaldi*) can tolerate those ant-produced alkaloids, so they also acquire that self-defense (toxin) by eating those particular ants. Another example is the moth *Utetheisa ornatrix*, whose larvae (caterpillars) feed on certain plants that contain pyrrolizidine alkaloids. Because those alkaloids are extremely bitter tasting and toxic, spiders that normally prey on them refuse to eat those *Utetheisa ornatrix*; even after they later become adult moths. If those moths (who consumed those pyrrolizidine alkaloids as larvae) get caught in the spider's web, the spider will cut it out

of the web and release that particular (toxic) moth. Vinca alkaloids, isolated from the specific plants that produce them, have been utilized as cancer-treating (antitumor) drugs (Fig. 39).

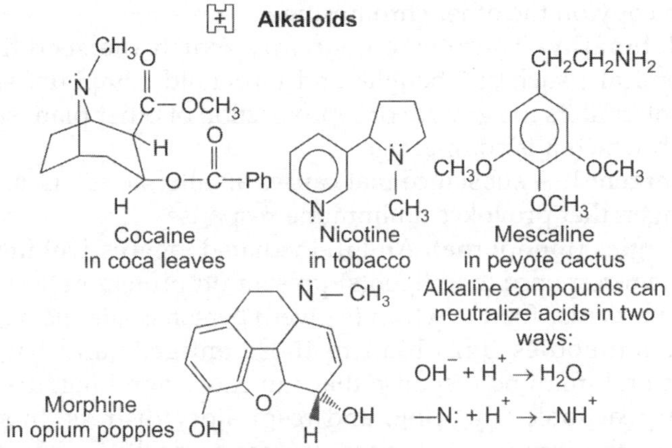

Fig. 39: Alkaloids

- **Alkylating agents:** Chemical mutagens (acridine orange, proflavin) which wedge between nitrogenous bases and cause frameshift mutations.
- **All-beta:** A class that includes two major fold groups: sandwiches and barrels.
- **Allele frequency:** The number of copies of an allele in a population, expressed as a proportion of the total number of copies of all alleles at a locus in a population.
- **Allele:** (Gr. Allelon, of one another, mutually each other); allelomorph (adjallelic, allelomorphic). One of a pair, or series, of variant forms of a gene that occur at a given locus in a chromosome.
- **Allele-specific ligation:** Two short synthetic oligonucleotides that base-pair adjacent to each other on a DNA fragment, and are ligated by DNA ligase. If one of the alleles contains a mutation overlapped by the 3'-end of one oligonucleotide, ligation with the other oligonucleotide will be prevented.
- **Allele-specific oligonucleotide hybridization (ASO hybridization):** The use of an oligonucleotide probe to determine which of two alternative nucleotide sequences is contained in a DNA molecule.

A

- **Allelic exclusion:** Describes the expression in any particular lymphocyte of only one allele coding for the expressed immunoglobulin. This is caused by feedback from the first immunoglobulin allele to be expressed that prevents activation of a copy on the other chromosome.
- **Allelopathy:** The phenomenon by which the secretion of chemicals, such as phenolic and terpenoid compounds, by a plant inhibits the growth or reproduction of other plant species with which it is competing.
- **Allergen:** 1. A substance that causes an allergic reaction. 2. An antigen that provokes an immune response.
- **Allergies (foodborne):** An IgE-mediated (aggressive) immune system response to antigen(s) present on protein molecules in the particular food to which (a given) person is allergic (Fig. 40). The antibodies (IgE) bind to those antigens and trigger a humoral immune response that can cause vomiting, diarrhea, skin reactions, wheezing, and respiratory distress. In severe cases, the immune response can cause death. In some rare instances, the allergic reaction is mediated by sensitized T cells. In some rare instances, the onset of a food allergy incident is induced by exercise (before or after eating that particular food). The US Food and Drug Administration (US–FDA) requires testing in advance to determine if a genetically engineered foodstuff has the potential to cause allergic reactions in humans,

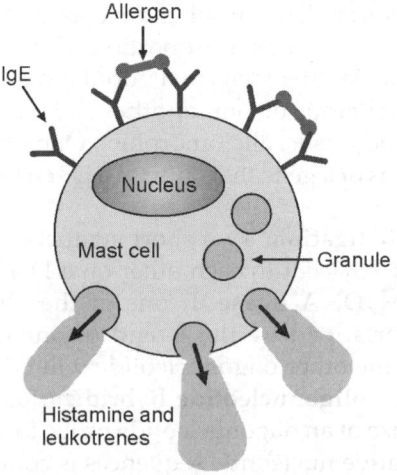

Fig. 40: Allergies

before that genetically engineered foodstuff (e.g. a modified crop plant) is approved by the FDA. In general, known food allergens (e.g. peanuts, Brazil nuts, wheat, etc.) are protein molecules that are resistant to rapid digestion (because those protein molecules are too tightly "folded together" for digestive enzymes to access their chemical bonds to break down). One potential way to genetically engineer currently allergenic crops (e.g. wheat) to make them less allergenic, is to insert gene(s) for extra production of thioredoxin. Found in all living organisms, thioredoxin is a protein that targets and breaks down the chemical bonds holding together a tightly folded together protein molecule (thereby making those protein molecules easier to digest). Future crops engineered to contain more thioredoxin than the traditional average level may be nonallergenic.

- **Allergy:** An unusual sensitivity to certain foods, pollens, insect bites, etc; appears on skin.
- **Allogamy:** Cross fertilization in plants.
- **Allogenic:** Of the same species, but with a different genotype.
- **Allograft:** Graft obtained from genetically different individuals of the same species.
- **Allohaploid:** A haploid obtained from an allopolyploid.
- **Allometric:** When the growth rate of one part of an organism differs from that of another part or of the rest of the body.
- **Allopatric speciation:** Speciation occurring at least in part because of geographic isolation.
- **Alloplasmic line:** A line having nucleus from one species and cytoplasm from a different species.
- **Allopolyploid:** A polyploidy resulting from the union of two separate chromosome sets and their subsequent doubling.
- **Allosteric effect:** Reversible interaction of a small molecule with a protein molecule, causing change in the shape of the protein and a consequent alteration of the interaction of that protein with a third molecule.
- **Allosteric enzyme:** An enzyme that has two structurally distinct forms, one of which is active and the other inactive (Fig. 41). Active forms of allosteric

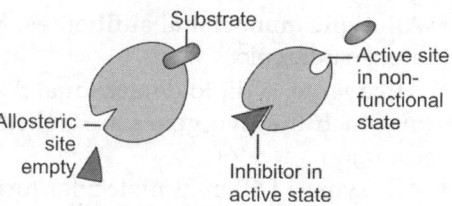

Fig. 41: Allosteric enzyme

A

enzymes tend to catalyze the initial step in a pathway, leading to the synthesis of molecules. The end product of this synthesis can act as a feedback inhibitor, converting the enzyme to the inactive form, thus controlling the amount of product synthesized.

- **Allosteric regulation:** A catalysis-regulating process in which the binding of a small effector molecule to one site on an enzyme affects the activity at another site (Fig. 42).

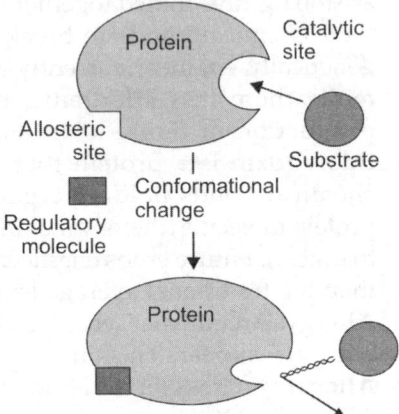

Fig. 42: Allosteric regulation

- **Allosteric site:** The site on an (allosteric) enzyme molecule where, via noncovalent binding to the site, a given effector can increase or decrease that enzyme's catalytic activity. Such an effector is called an allosteric effector because it binds at a site on the enzyme molecule that is other (allo) than the enzyme's catalytic site.

- **Allosteric transition:** A reversible interaction of a small molecule with a protein molecule, resulting in a change in the shape of the protein and a consequent alternation of the interaction of that protein with a third molecule.

- **Allosteric:** Regulation describes the ability of a protein to change its conformation (and therefore activity) at one site as the result of binding a small molecule to a second site located elsewhere on the protein.

- **Allotetraploid:** An organism with four genomes derived from hybridization of different species. Usually, in forms that become established, two of the four genomes are from one species and two are from another species.

- **Allotypic monoclonal antibodies:** Monoclonal antibodies that are isoantigenic.

- **Allozygote:** A diploid individual that is homozygous at a locus in which the two genes are not identical by descent from a common ancestor.

- **Allozymes:** Different molecular forms of an enzyme coded by different allelic forms of a gene.

- *Aloe vera L:* A plant whose sap (juice) contains certain carbohydrates that naturally assist healing of human skin (wounds). Those carbohydrates "activate" macrophages, which cause those macrophages to produce cytokines (that regulate human immune system and inflammatory responses which promote healing) (Fig. 43).

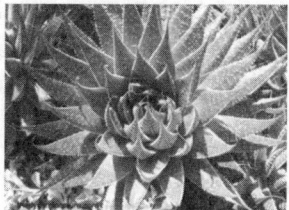

Fig. 43: Aloe vera

- **Alpha-amylase inhibitor-1:** A protein naturally produced in the seeds of the plant known as the common bean *Phaseolus vulgaris* that inhibits the amylase enzyme in the gut of the pest insect known as the pea weevil. Because the amylase enzyme (in its gut) is inhibited (prevented from helping digestion) by the alpha amylase inhibitor-1, the seeds of the *Phaseolus vulgaris* plant are protected from depradation by the pea weevil.

- **Alpha carbon:** Central carbon atom of an amino acid that carries both the amino group and the carboxyl group.

- **Alpha galactosides:** Term referring to a family of poly-saccharides (produced in plant seeds) composed (at the molecular level) of one sucrose unit linked by a 1, 6 molecular bond to several galactose units. Alpha galactosides include raffinose, stachyose, and verbascose.

- **Alpha-helix:** A helical structure formed by polypeptide that is one of the principal secondary structural forms found in proteins (Fig. 44).

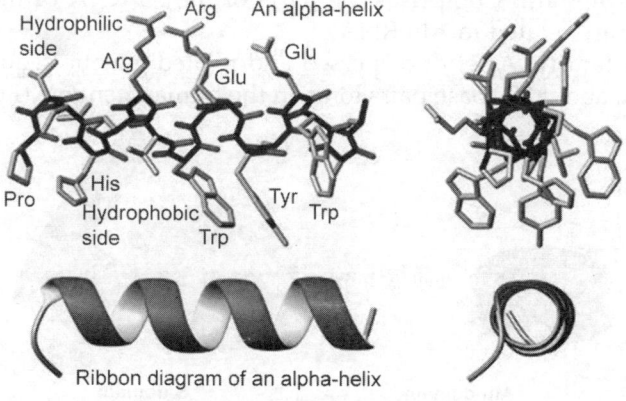

Fig. 44: Alpha-helix

A

- **Alpha interferon:** Also written as α-interferon, it has been shown to prolong life and reduce tumor size in patients suffering from Kaposi's sarcoma (a cancer that affects approximately 10% of people with acquired immune deficiency syndrome). It is also effective against hairy-cell leukemia and may work against other cancers. It has recently been approved by the US-FDA for use against certain types of sarcoma. Recent research indicates that injections of alpha-interferon can limit the liver damage typically caused by hepatitis C, a viral disease.
- **Alphabet:** The set of all possible symbols in an application.
- **Alpha-lactalbumin:** Protein component of milk.
- **Alphoid DNA:** The tandemly repeated nucleotide sequences located in the centromeric regions of human chromosomes.
- **ALS:** A plant enzyme (also present in some microoganisms) known as acetolactate synthase or acetohydroxy acid synthase. ALS catalyzes (enables to occur) one of the early chemical reaction steps in the synthesis (manufacturing) of branched-chain amino acids (isoleucine, leucine, valine) required by plants to sustain life (i.e. to make needed proteins). Herbicides that deactivate/destroy ALS are effective at killing plants (e.g. weeds).
- **ALS gene:** Gene that codes for (i.e. causes to be produced in microorganisms or plants' chloroplasts) the critical-to-plants enzyme acetolactate synthase (ALS).
- **Alternative splicing:** Describes the production of different RNA products from a single product by changes in the usages of splicing junctions.
- **Alu-domain:** Comprises the parts of the 7S RNA of the SRP that are related to Alu RNA.
- **Alu family:** A set of dispersed and related genetic sequences, each about 300 base pairs long, in the human genome (Fig. 45).

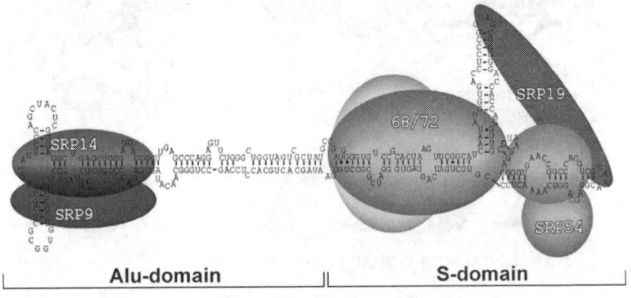

Fig. 45: Alu family

At both ends of these 300 bp segments there is an A-G-C-T sequence. Alu 1 is a restriction enzyme that recognizes this sequence and cleaves (cuts) it between the G (guanine) and the C (cytosine).

- **Alu PCR:** A clone fingerprinting technique that uses PCR (Polymerase chain reaction) to detect the relative positions of Alu sequences in the cloned DNA fragments.
- **Alu sequences:** A family of 300-bp sequences occurring nearly a million times in the human genome.
- **Alu:** A short, repetitive string of about 300 DNA bases that are scattered throughout the genome, often in regions that have many genes.
- **Alzheimer's disease:** A disease characterized by among other things, progressive loss of memory. The development of Alzheimer's disease is thought to be associated, in part, with processing certain alleles of the gene that encodes apolipoprotein E.
- **Amanitin (more fully α-amanitin):** A bicyclic octapeptide derived from the poisonous mushroom *Amanita phalloides*; it inhibits transcription by certain eukaryotic RNA polymerases, especially RNA polymerase II.
- **Amber codon:** UAG-One of the nonsense or stop or chain termination codons that ends protein synthesis.
- **Amber mutation:** Mutation of the UAG termination codon.
- **Amber:** The triplet codon UAG, one of the three termination codons that end protein synthesis.
- **Ambient temperature:** Air temperature at a given time and place, not the radiant temperature.
- **Ambients standards:** It is a air-quality standard, set by the environmental protection agency (EPA) delimits certain levels of pollutants that should not be exceeded in order to maintain environmental and human health.
- **AMD:** Acronym for age-related macular degeneration.
- **American Society for Biotechnology (ASB):** A society founded for the purpose of "providing a multi- and interdisciplinary forum for those persons from academia, industry, and government who are interested in any and all aspects of biotechnology, and will achieve its aims by cooperation with existing organizations active in the field." To join, write to ASB, P.O. Box 2820, Sausalito, California, 94966–2820.

A

- **American type culture collection (ATCC):** An independent, nonprofit organization established in 1925 for the preservation and distribution of reference cultures.
- **Ames test:** A simple bacterial-based carcinogens test that was developed by Bruce Ames in 1961. Although this test evaluates mutagenesis (causation of mutations) in the DNA of bacteria, its results have been utilized to approve or not approve certain compounds for consumption by humans.
- **Amino acid alphabet:** A twenty character alphabet (A, C, D, E, F, G, H, I, K, L, M, N, P, Q, R, S, T, V, W, Y), each representing one of the twenty amino acids coded by DNA.
- **Amino acid profile:** Also known as "protein quality," this refers to a quantitative delineation of how much of each amino acid is contained in a given source of (livestock feed or food) protein. For example, the amino acid profile of soybean meal is matched closest to the profile of amino acids needed for human nutrition, of all protein meals.
- **Amino acid:** An organic compound containing an amino (–NH$_2$) and an acid carboxyl group (–COOH) (Fig. 46).
- **Amino group:** One of the 20 chemical building blocks that are joined by amide (peptide) linkages to form a polypeptide chain of a protein.

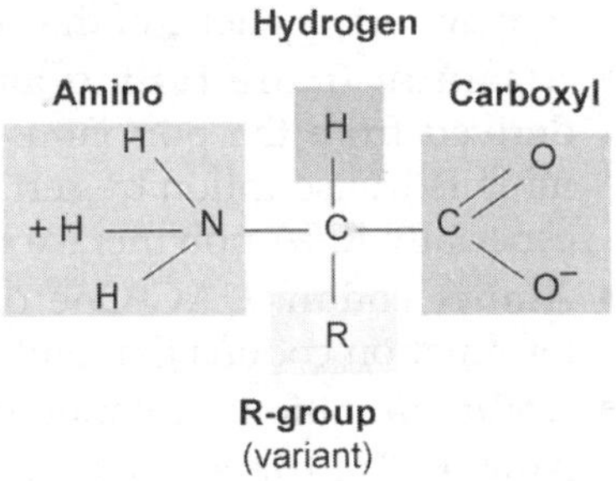

Fig. 46: Amino acid

- **Amino terminal domain:** The end of a polypeptide chain containing a free amino group.
- **Amino terminus:** The –NH$_2$ (amino) end of a polypeptide.
- **Aminoacyl site (a-site):** One of two sites on ribosome to which the incoming aminoacyl-tRNA binds.
- **Aminoacylation:** Attachment of an amino acid to the acceptor arm of a tRNA molecule.
- **Aminoacyl-tRNA synthetases:** Enzymes responsible for covalently linking amino acids to the 2'- or 3'-OH position of tRNA.
- **Aminoacyl-tRNA:** A tRNA linked to an amino acid. The COOH group of the amino acid is linked to the 3'- or 2'-OH group of the terminal base of the tRNA.

- **Amitosis:** Cell division (cytokinesis), including nuclear division through constriction of the nucleus, without chromosome differentiation as in mitosis (Fig. 47). The maintenance of genetic integrity and diploidy during amitosis is uncertain. This process occurs in the endosperm of flowering plants.

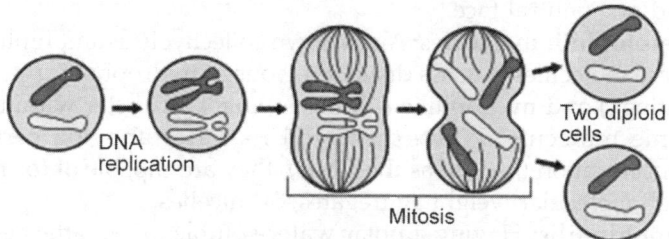

DNA replication

Two diploid cells

Mitosis

Fig. 47: Stages of Amitosis

- **Amniocentesis:** A procedure used to test for fetal defects. Fluid and fetal cells are withdrawn from the amniotic layer surrounding the fetus.
- **Amniocyte:** A fetal cell suspended within the amniotic fluid surrounding the fetus.
- **Amnion:** The thin membrane that lines the fluid-filled sac in which the embryo develops in higher vertebrates, reptiles and birds.
- **Amniotic fluid:** Liquid contents of the amniotic sac of higher vertebrates, containing cells of the embryo (not of the mother). Both fluid and cells are used for diagnosis of genetic abnormalities in the embryo or fetus.
- **Amorph null mutation:** A mutation that obliterates gene function.
- **Amperometric biosensor:** It measures the transfer of electrons to O_2 (present in the biosensor) due to redox reactions.
- **Amphibolic pathway:** A metabolic pathway used in both catabolism and anabolism.
- **Amphidiploid:** A species derived by doubling of chromosomes in the F_1 hybrid of two species.
- **Amphimixis:** True sexual reproduction involving the fusion of male and female gametes and the formation of a zygote (Fig. 48).

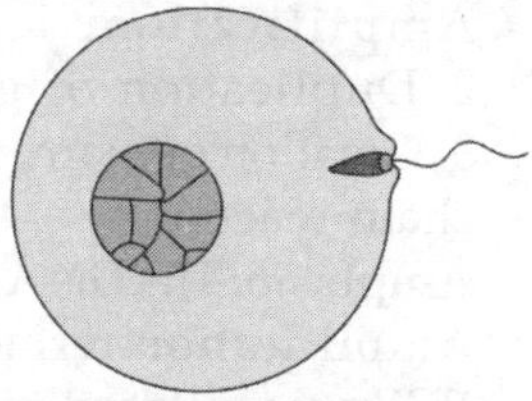

Fig. 48: Amphimixis

- **Amphipathic molecules:** Molecules bearing both polar and nonpolar domains (within the same molecule). Some examples of amphipathic molecules are wetting agents (SDS), and membrane lipids such as lecithin.

- **Amphipathic:** Structures have two surfaces, one hydrophilic and one hydrophobic. Lipids are amphipathic; and some protein regions may form amphipathic helices, with one charged face and one neutral face.
- **Amphiphilic molecules:** Also known collectively as amphiphiles, these molecules possess distinct regions of hydrophobic ("water hating") and hydrophilic ("water loving") character within the same molecule. When dissolved in water above a certain concentration (known as the CMC), they are capable of forming high molecular weight aggregates, or micelles.
- **Amphiphilic:** Having a polar water-soluble group attached to a water-insoluble hydrocarbon chain.
- **Ampholyte:** A trade name for a mixture of substances with a range of isoelectric points that have high buffering capacity at their isoelectric points.
- **Amphoteric compound:** A compound capable of both donating and accepting protons and thus able to act chemically as either an acid or a base.
- **Amphotropic virus:** Recombinant virus that has the capacity to infect a wide variety of mammalian (human) cells.
- **Ampicillin:** A penicillin derived antibiotic that prevents bacterial growth by interfering with synthesis of the cell wall (Fig. 49).

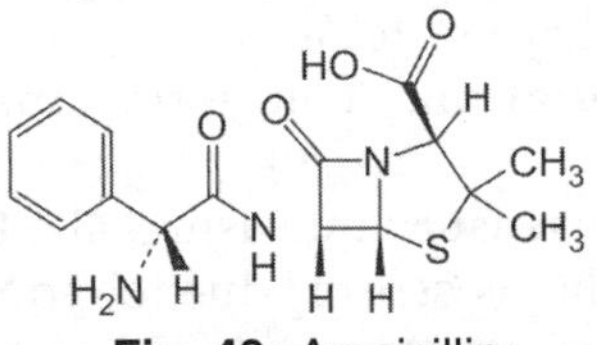

Fig. 49: Ampicillin

- **Amplification:** 1. Replication of a gene library in bulk 2. Duplication of gene(s) within a chromosomal segment 3. Creation of many copies of a segment of DNA by polymerase chain reaction.
- **Amplicon:** The DNA sequence/fragment that is amplified by PCR.
- **Amplification refractive mutation system (ARMS) PCR:** This PCR was devised to achieved sequence-specific amplification.
- **Amplification:** Refers to the production of additional copies of a chromosomal sequence, found as intrachromosomal or extrachromosomal DNA.

- **Amplified fragment length polymorphism (AFLP):** A A combination of RELP and RAPD very sensitive in detecting polymorphism throughout the genome (Fig. 50).

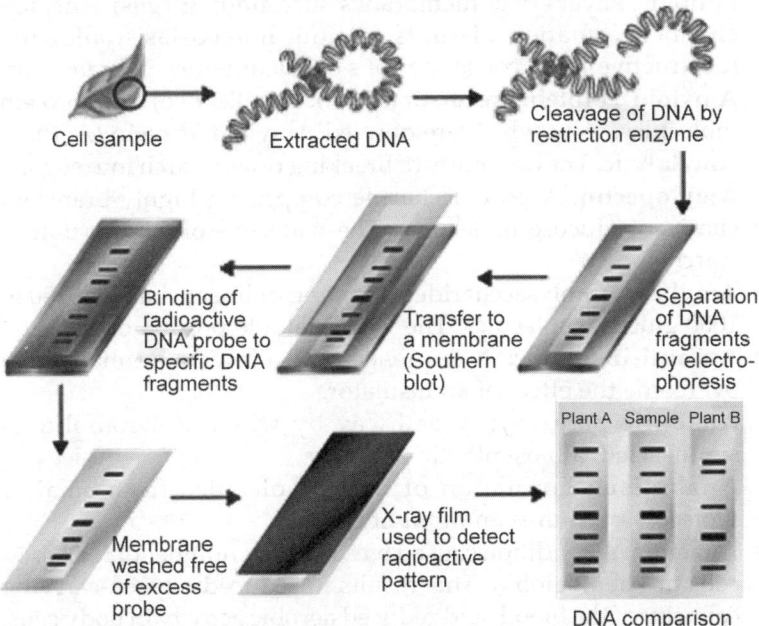

Cell sample   Extracted DNA   Cleavage of DNA by restriction enzyme

Binding of radioactive DNA probe to specific DNA fragments   Transfer to a membrane (Southern blot)   Separation of DNA fragments by electro-phoresis

Membrane washed free of excess probe   X-ray film used to detect radioactive pattern

Plant A   Sample   Plant B

DNA comparison

Fig. 50: Amplified fragment length polymorphism (AFLP)

- **Amplified genomic library:** Refers to the library which consists of recombinant phage lysates or bacterial clones of a genomic library.
- **Amplified ribosomal DNA restriction analysis (ARDRA):** The amplification product of the gene encoding the 16S ribosomal RNA is subjected to restriction fragment length polymorphism; this analysis is important for the bacterial identification/ taxonomy.
- **Amplify:** To increase the number of copies of a DNA sequence, *in vivo* by inserting into a cloning vector that replicates within a host cell, or *in vitro* by polymerase chain reaction (PCR).
- **Amylase:** A group of enzymes that degrade starch, glycogen and other polysaccharides, producing a mixture of glucose and maltose. Plants have both α- and β-amylase and animals have only α-amylase.

A

- **Amyloid_Protein (A_P):** A small protein that forms plaque in the brains and in the brain blood vessels of victims of Alzheimer's disease. A_P forms cation-selective ion channels in lipid bilayers (e.g. membranes surrounding cells). This ion channel formation disrupts calcium homeostasis, allowing (destructive) high concentrations of calcium ions in brain cells.
- **Amyloid_Protein precursor (A_PP):** A (collective) set of protein molecules, from which are derived Amyloid_Protein (A_P).
- **Amylolytic:** The capability of breaking down starch into sugars.
- **Amylopectin:** A polysaccharide comprising highly branched chains of glucose molecules. The water-in-soluble portion of starch.
- **Amylose:** A polysaccharide consisting of linear chains of 100 to 1000 glucose molecules. The water-soluble portion of starch.
- **An anti-insulator:** A sequence that allows an enhancer to overcome the effect of an insulator.
- **Anabolic pathway:** A pathway by which a metabolite is synthesized, a biosynthetic pathway.
- **Anabolism:** Formation of macromolecules from smaller molecules; requires an input of energy.
- **Anaemia:** A condition caused by a reduced number of red blood cells or haemoglobin. This results in reduced oxygen-carrying capacity of the blood, and reduced aerobic activity in body cells.
- **Anaerobe:** An organism that can grow in the absence of oxygen. Opposite: Aerobe.
- **Anaerobic digestion:** Digestion of materials in the absence of oxygen.
- **Anaerobic fermentation:** Fermentation in the absence of O_2, e.g. alcohol fermentation.
- **Anaerobic respiration:** Respiration in which foodstiffs are partially oxidised, with the release of chemical energy, in a process not involving atmospheric oxygen, such as alcoholic fermentation, in which one of the end products is ethanol (Fig. 51).
- **Anaerobic:** 1. Growing in the absence of oxygen. 2. An environment or condition in which molecular oxygen is not available for chemical, physical or biological processes.
- **Anagenesis:** An evolutionary process in which the act of one species evolving into another without a split in the phylogenetic tree.

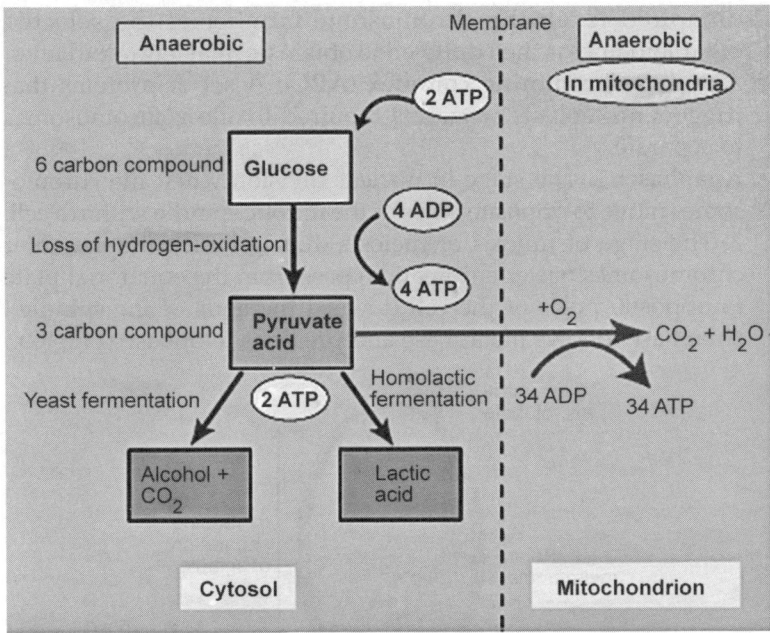

Fig. 51: Anaerobic respiration

- **Analog:** Biological structures which perform similar functions by similar mechanisms but evolved separately, e.g. a chemical so similar to one of the normal bases that it can be incorporated into DNA.
- **Analogous structures:** Body parts that serve the same function in different organisms, but differ in structure and embryological development, e.g. the wings of insects and birds.
- **Analogous:** Feature of organisms which are functionally similar but have evolved in different ways.
- **Analogy:** Reasoning by which the function of a novel gene or protein sequence may be deduced from comparisons with other gene or protein sequences of known function. Identifying analogous or homologous genes via similarity searching and alignment is one of the chief uses of bioinformatics.
- **Analyte:** The substance or component in a sample that is being measured.
- **Analytical breeding:** In this strategy, dihaploids are isolated from autotetraploids, and breeding work is carried out at the

A

dihaploid level; the chromosome number of the selected dihaploid lines is then doubled to obtain normal tetraploid lines.

- **Anaphase promoting complex (APC):** A set of proteins that triggers proteolysis or targets required to allow chromosomes to separate.
- **Anaphase:** 1. The stage in nuclear division when the chromosomes move to opposite poles of the mitotic spindle within a cell. 2. The stage of mitosis or meiosis during which the daughter chromosomes (sister chromatids) pass from the equatorial plate to opposite poles of the cell (toward the ends of the spindle). Anaphase follows metaphase and precedes telophase (Fig. 52).

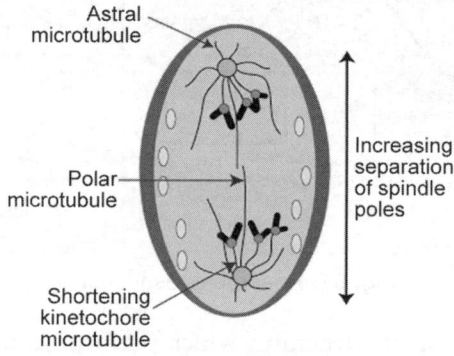

Fig. 52: Anaphase stage

- **Anatomic barriers:** In case of innate immunity; these barriers include skin and surfaces of mucous membranes; they together prevent the entry of most microorganisms.
- **Ancestral character state:** A character state possessed by a remote common ancestor of a group of organisms.
- **Anchor (stop-transfer) (often referred to as a "transmembrane anchor"):** A segment of a transmembrane protein which resides in the membrane.
- **Anchor gene:** A gene that has been positioned on both the physical map and the linkage map of a chromosome.
- **Anchor sequence:** Sequence added to primers or probes that may be used for binding to a support or may incorporate convenient restriction sites, primer bindings sites for subsequent PCR reactions.
- **Anchorage dependence:** Describes the need of normal eukaryotic cells for a surface to attach in order to grow in culture.

- **Anchored PCR:** When sequence of only one end of a DNA **A** segment is known, the primer specific to the known 3′-end is used to obtain copies of this strand; an oligo-G tail is then added at the 3′-ends of the single-strand copies, and oligo-C is used as primer to obtain double-strand copies.
- **Ancient DNA:** DNA preserved in ancient biological material.
- **ANDA FDA:** Abbreviated new drug application (to the US FDA).
- **Androgen:** Any hormone that stimulates the development of male secondary sexual characteristics, and contributes to the control of sexual activity in vertebrate animals. Usually synthesized by the testes.
- **Androgenesis:** Development of haploid plants from the male gametophyte following a developmental pattern resembling embryogenesis, resulting from the culture of anthers or microscopes.
- **Androgenic grains:** Pollen grains, which exhibit androgenesis; believed to be s-grains.
- **Anergy:** The absence of an expected cell-mediated immune reaction in sensitized organisms, caused by inactivated B and T cells. Also used to describe inactivated B or T cells.
- **Aneuploid:** Set of chromosomes differs from the usual diploid constitution by loss or duplication of chromosomes or chromosomal segments.
- **Aneuploidy:** The loss or gain of chromosomes from the normal euploid number by various processes.
- **Aneusomaty:** Presence of aneuploid and euploid cells in the same tissue, especially *in vivo*.
- **Angina pectoris:** The medical term for chest pain caused by inadequate blood supply to parts of the heart generally referred to as coronary heart disease.
- **Angiogenesis:** The process of new blood vessel formation including angiogenesis around the heart, for example, may generate a natural heart bypass without the requirement of invasive surgery. Conversely, the prevention of angiogenesis is a goal for anticancer strategies where tumor death is achieved by cutting off the blood supply to tumors.
- **Angiogenic growth factors:** Proteins that stimulate formation of blood vessels (e.g. in tissue being formed by the body to repair wounds).

A

- **Angiogenin:** One of the human angiogenic growth factors, it possesses potent angiogenic (formation of blood vessels) activity. In addition to stimulating (normal) blood vessel formation, angiogenin levels are correlated with placenta formation and tumor growth (tumors require new blood vessels).
- **Angiostatin:** A protein fragment (derived from plasminogen) that has antiangiogenic properties.
- **Angstrom (Å):** Unit of length equal to 10^{-10} meter.
- **Animal biotechnology:** Use of animal cells, tissues, organs or their components to generate useful products or services; examples, monoclonal antibodies, cell culture-derived vaccines, transgenic animals, etc.
- **Animal cell culture:** Culture of dispersed animal cells either as monolayer or as suspension of cells.
- **Animal cell immobilization:** Entrapment of animal cells in some solid material in order to produce some natural product or genetically engineered protein. Animal cells have the advantage that they already produce many proteins of pharmacological interest, and that genetically engineered proteins are produced by them with the post-translation modifications normal to animals. However, because animal cells are much more fragile than bacterial ones, they cannot tolerate a commercial material are hollow fibre membrane bioreactors, or porous carriers made of polysaccharide, protein, plastic or ceramic materials with microscopic holes inside which the cells grow.
- **Animal cloning:** The process of producing a group of complete normal animals from somatic cells of an adult animal; somatic cell is fused with eunucleate fertilized egg and the egg is implanted in the uterus of surrogate mother.
- **Animal genetic resources databank:** A databank that contains inventories of farm animal genetic resources and their immediate wild relatives, including any information that helps to characterize these resources.
- **Animal genome (gene) bank:** A planned and managed repository containing animal genetic resources. Repositories include the environment in which the genetic resource has developed, or is now normally found (*In situ*) or facilities elsewhere (*Ex situ – in vivo* or *in vitro*). For *in vitro*, *ex situ* genome bank facilities, germplasm is stored in the form of one or more of the following: semen, ova, embryos and tissue samples.

- **Animal model:** A laboratory animal useful for medical research because it has specific characteristics that resemble a human disease or disorder.

- **Animal organ culture:** Whole embryogenic organs or small tissue fragments are cultured *in vitro* in such a manner that they retain their natural tissue architecture.

- **Animal testing:** Procedures used to assess the toxicity of chemical substances using rats, mice and guinea pigs as surrogates for humans.

- **Animal tissue culture:** Culture of aseptically isolated whole organs, tissue fragments as well as dispersed cells of animals in a suitable nutrient medium under controlled environments.

- **Anion:** A negatively charged ion; opposite is cation.

- **Anisometric genes:** Several genes having one-directional and unequal effects. Their expressivity and heritability are intermediate between those of major genes and polygenes.

- **Anneal:** The pairing of complementary DNA or RNA sequences, via hydrogen bonding, to form a double-standard polynucleotide. Most often used to describe the binding of a short primer or probe.

- **Annealing:** The process of heating (denaturing step) and slowly cooling (renaturing step) double-stranded DNA to allow the formation of hybrid DNA or complementary strands of DNA or of DNA and RNA.

- **Annotation:** A combination of comments, notations, references, and citations, either in free format or utilizing a controlled vocabulary, that together describe all the experimental and inferred information about a gene or protein. Annotations can also be applied to the description of other biological systems. Batch, automated annotation of bulk biological sequence is one of the key uses of bioinformatics tools.

- **Annual:** 1. Taking 1 year, or occurring at intervals of 1 year. 2. In botany, a plant that completes its life cycle within 1 year. During this time, the plant germinates, grows, flowers, produces seeds, and dies.

- **Anonymous DNA marker:** A DNA marker detectable by virtue of variation in its sequence, irrespective of whether or not it actually occurs in or near a coding sequence. Microsatellites are typical anonymous DNA markers.

A

- **Antagonism:** Inhibitory relationships between microorganisms by involving amensalism, competition, and predation and parasitism.
- **Antagonist:** A compound that inhibits the effect of an agonist in such a way that the combined biological effect of the two becomes smaller than the sum of their individual effects.
- **Anterior system:** In *Drosophila*, the anterior system is one of the maternal systems that establish the polarity of the oocyte. The set of genes in the anterior system play a role in the proper formation of the head and the thorax.
- **Anterior-posterior axis:** The line running from the head to tail of an animal.
- **Anterograde transport:** The direction of membrane transport specified by the movement of macromolecules through the secretory pathway (from the rough endoplasmic reticulum, through the Golgi complex, and to the plasma membrane). It is also called forward transport.
- **Anther culture:** The aseptic culture of anthers for the production of haploid plants from microspores.
- **Anther walls factors:** Biochemicals/nutrients provided by anther wall to the developing pollen embryos during androgenesis; replaced by a mixture of glutamine, serine and m-inositol in *Datura*, and by only glutamine in tobacco.
- **Anther:** Microsporangium bearing microspores which develop into pollen (microgametophytes) (Fig. 53).

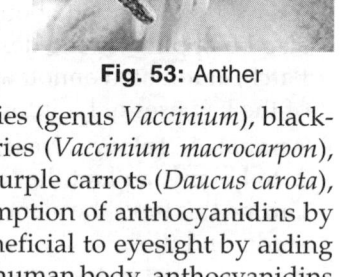

Fig. 53: Anther

- **Anthesis:** Anthesis is the flowering period. It is the time of full bloom, which lasts till fruit set.
- **Anthocyanidins:** Natural pigments (flavonoids) produced in blueberries (genus *Vaccinium*), blackberries (*Rubus fruticosus*), cranberries (*Vaccinium macrocarpon*), cherries (genus *Prunus*), black or purple carrots (*Daucus carota*), and some types of grapes. Consumption of anthocyanidins by humans has been shown to be beneficial to eyesight by aiding the health of the retina. Within the human body, anthocyanidins act as antioxidants (i.e. "quenchers" of free radicals), so consumption apparently reduces the risk of some cancers, coronary heart disease, eyesight loss, and cataracts.

- **Anthocyanin:** Water-soluble blue, purple and red flavonoid pigments found in vacuoles of cells.

- **Anthropogenic:** Arising out of human actions.
- **Antiangiogenesis:** Refers to impact of any compound that prevents angiogenesis (i.e. formation/development of new blood vessels). Because angiogenesis is required for malignant tumors to grow and/or metastasize (spread), antiangiogenesis was proposed by Judah Folkman in 1970 as a means to combat cancer. Because angiogenesis is required for embryonic development, antiangiogenic drugs inhibit proper development/ growth of infants in the womb. Fumagillin, ovalicin, and thalidomide have been found to possess antiangiogenic properties. Also, the human proteins angiostatin and endostatin.
- **Antiauxin:** A chemical that interferes with auxin response. Antiauxin may or may not involve prevention of auxin transport or movement in plants. Some antiauxins are said to promote morphogenesis *in vitro*, such as 2,3,5, tri-iodobenzoic acid (TIBA) or 2,4,5-trichlorophenoxyacetate (2,4,5-T), which stimulate the growth of some cultures.
- **Antibiosis:** Growth inhibition of an organism by a substance of another organism.
- **Antibiotic resistance:** The ability of a microorganism to produce a protein that disables an antibiotic or prevents transport of the antibiotic into the cell.
- **Antibiotic:** Classes of natural and synthetic compounds that inhibit the growth of microorganisms.
- **Antibody affinity chromatography:** A type of chromatography in which antibodies are immobilized onto the column material. The antibodies bind to their target molecules while the other components in the solution are not retained. In this way a separation (purification) is achieved.
- **Antibody engineering:** Refers to the use of recombinant DNA technology to modify or design antibodies.
- **Antibody microarray:** It consists of spots of different antibodies and is used to measure the abundance of thousands of different proteins in the samples.
- **Antibody:** A protein (immunoglobin) molecule, produced by the immune system that recognizes a particular substance (antigen) and bind to it (Fig. 54).

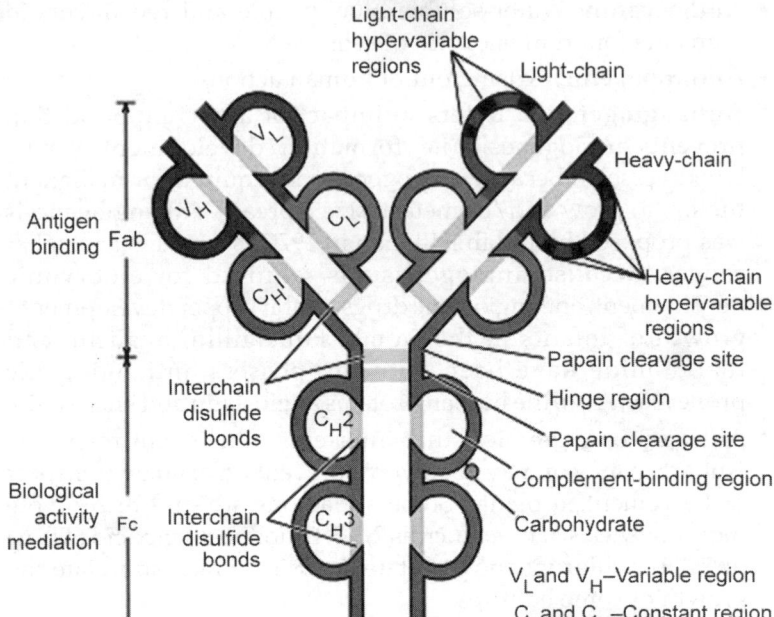

Fig. 54: Antibody

- **Anticaking agents:** Substances which check powders such as milk powder from caking and sticking.
- **Anticipation:** The process whereby some genetic diseases get more severe in each successive generation.
- **Anticoagulant:** Substance that prevents blood from clotting.
- **Anticoding strand:** The strand of DNA double helix that is actually transcribed. Also known as antisense or template strand. The strand has $3' \to 5'$ direction which directs the synthesis of mRNA in $5' \to 3'$ direction.
- **Anticodon:** The trinucleotide sequences in anticodon loop in a tRNA which pairs with a triplet (codon) by complementary base pairing.
- **Anticodon:** Triplet of bases carried by the tRNA molecule which are complementary to the codon in mRNA.
- **Anticodon arm (of tRNA):** A stem loop structure that express the anticodon triplet at one end (Fig. 55).
- **Antifoaming agents:** Substances which reduce or prevent foaming in foods/fermenters.

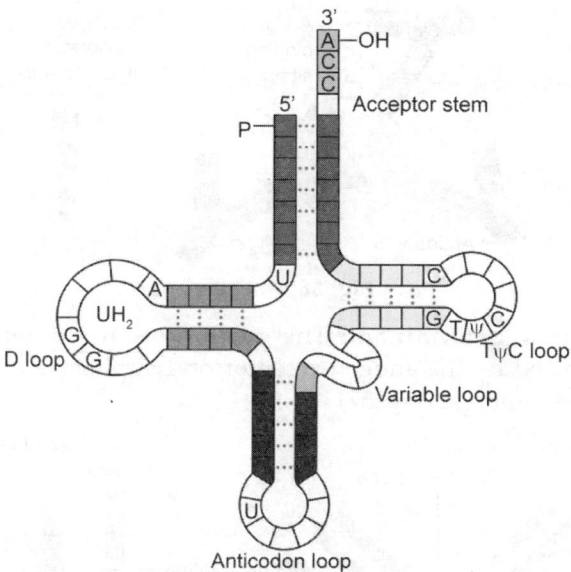

Fig. 55: Anticodon arm

- **Antigen presentation:** The antigenic peptides bind within the cleft of (major histocompatibility complex I) MHC I or MHC II molecules and are displayed on the surface of antigen processing cells (APCs).
- **Antigen presenting cells (APCs):** These cells have on their surfaces class II MHC molecules, which bind to antigen-derived peptides and present them to a group of lymphocytes, which are then activated to mount the immune response.
- **Antigen processing:** A foreign antigen is degraded into short peptides of 8–18 amino acids by antigen processing cells.
- **Antigen:** A molecule that is capable of stimulating the production of neutralizing antibody proteins when injected into an organism. Or any foreign substance whose entry into an organism provokes an immune response by stimulating the synthesis of an antibody (an immunoglobulin protein that can bind to the antigen) (Fig. 56).
- **Antigen-antibody interaction:** Highly specific binding of an antibody to an antigen epitope, which induced its production.
- **Antigen-binding domain:** In antibodies, the area that binds to the antigen-epitope.

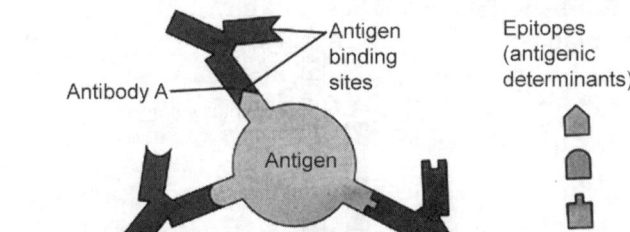

Fig. 56: Antigen

- **Antigenic determinant:** The portion of an antigen that is recognized by the antigen receptor on lymphocytes. It is also called an epitope (Fig. 57).

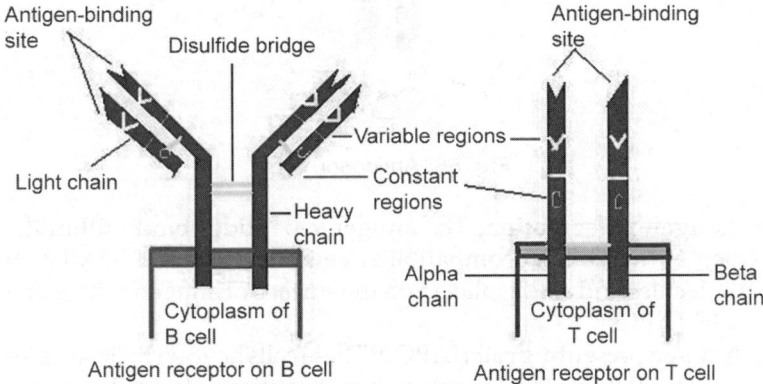

Fig. 57: Antigenic determinant

- **Antigenic index:** A prediction of the antigenicity of a sequence based on its hydrophilicity, predicted side chain flexibility, surface probability, and the predicted turns.
- **Antigenic specificity:** Ability of antibodies to differentiate between antigen molecules differing by a single amino acid.
- **Antigenic variation:** The ability of a trypanosome to change its surface protein, so that the host is challenged with a different antigen.
- **Antigenically committed:** The mature B cell is said to be antigenically committed since it is predetermined in its ability to recognize and respond to a specific antigen.
- **Antigenicity:** Ability of an antigen to interact with an antibody, which is specific to it.

- **Antihemophilic factor VIII:** Also known as factor VIII or antihemophilic globulin (AHG). **A**
- **Antihemophilic globulin:** Also known as factor VIII or antihemophilic factor VIII.
- **Anti-idiotypes:** Antibodies to antibodies. In other words, if a human antibody is injected into rabbits, the rabbit immune systems will recognize the human antibodies as foreign (regardless of the fact that they are antibodies) and produce antibodies against them. To the rabbit, the foreign antibodies represent just another invader or non-self to be targeted and destroyed. Anti-idiotypes mimic antigens in that they are shaped to fit into the antibody's binding site (in lock-and-key fashion). As such, anti-idiotypes can be used to create vaccines that stimulate production of antibodies to the antigen (that the anti-idiotype mimics). This confers disease resistance (to the pathogen associated with that antigen) without the risk that a vaccine using attenuated pathogens entails (i.e. that the pathogen revives to cause the disease).
- **Anti-immunoglobulin:** An antibody specific to another antibody; binds to the constant region of all antibodies of the class.
- **Anti-insulator:** A sequence that allows an enhancer to overcome the effect of an insulator.
- **Anti-interferon:** An antibody to interferon. Used for the purification of interferons.
- **Antimicrobial agent:** Any chemical or biological agent that harms the growth of microorganisms.
- **Antinutrients:** Compounds that inhibit normal uptake of nutrients.
- **Anti-oncogene:** A gene whose product prevents the normal growth of tissue.
- **Antioxidants:** A group of chemicals which prevent oxidation, e.g. ascorbic acid, citric acid. They retard senescence and browning of tissue.
- **Antiparallel:** The two DNA strands are organized in opposite directions, the 5' end of one strand aligns with the 3' end of other strand.
- **Antiporter:** A type of carrier protein that simultaneously moves two different types of solutes in opposite directions across the plasma membrane.

A

- **Antisense DNA:** The sequence of chromosomal DNA that is transcribed.
- **Antisense gene:** A gene that produces a transcript (mRNA) that is complementary to the pre-mRNA or mRNA of a normal gene (unusually constructed by inverting the coding region relative to the promoter).
- **Antisense orientation:** Reverse orientation of a gene in relation to its promoter; the promoter is now located at the 5'-end of the antisense strand so that natural sense strand is now transcribed.
- **Antisense RNA:** RNA produced by transcription of the sense strand; usually, in case of antisense gene constructs; complementary to antisense strand of the gene and to mRNA; pairs with mRNA. RNA with sequence complementary to mRNA.
- **Antisense RNA technology:** An antisense construct of the target gene is integrated into the genome to suppress the concerned endogenous genes (Fig. 58).

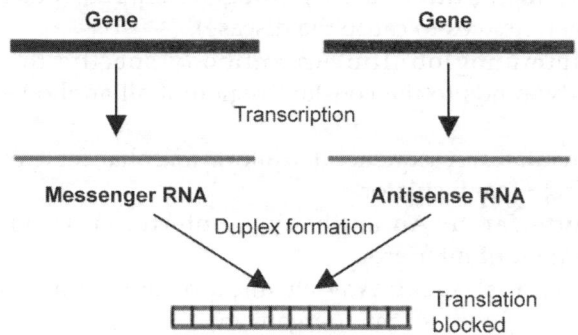

Fig. 58: Antisense RNA technology

- **Antisense strand:** Antisense strand acts as the template for the synthesis of mRNA.
- **Antisense therapy:** *In vivo* treatment of a genetic disease by blocking translation of a protein with a DNA or RNA sequence that is complementary to a specific mRNA.
- **Antiseptic:** Any substance that kills or inhibits the growth of disease-causing microorganism (a microorganism capable of causing sepsis), but is essentially nontoxic to cells of the body.
- **Antiserum:** 1. Blood serum containing specific antibodies against an antigen. Antisera are used to confer passive immunity to many diseases. 2. The fluid portion of the blood of an animal

(after coagulation of the blood), containing antibodies. 3. Serum from an animal that contains antibodies against a particular antigen.

- **Anti-Sm:** An autoimmune antiserum that defines the Sm epitope that is common to a group of proteins found in snRNPs that are involved in RNA splicing.
- **Antitermination:** A mechanism of transcriptional control in which termination is prevented at a specific terminator site, allowing RNA polymerase to read into the genes beyond it.
- **Antitermination proteins:** Proteins allow RNA polymerase to transcribe through certain terminator sites.
- **Antiterminator:** A type of protein which enables RNA polymerase to ignore certain transcriptional stop or certain transcriptional stop or termination signals and read through them to produce longer mRNA transcripts.
- **Antithrombogenous polymers:** Synthetic polymers (i.e. plastics) used to make medical devices that will be in contact with a patient's blood (e.g. catheters), but will not initiate the coagulation process as synthetic polymers usually do. The natural anticoagulant heparin is incorporated into the polymer and is gradually released into the bloodstream by the polymer, thus preventing blood coagulation on the surface of the polymer.
- **Antitranspirant:** A compound designed to reduce transpiration when sprayed or painted on leaves of newly transplanted trees, shrubs or vines, or used as a dip for cuttings in lieu of misting may interfere with photosynthesis and respiration if the coating is too thick or unbroken.
- **Anucleate:** Bacteria lack nuclei, but are of similar shape to wild type bacteria (Fig. 59).

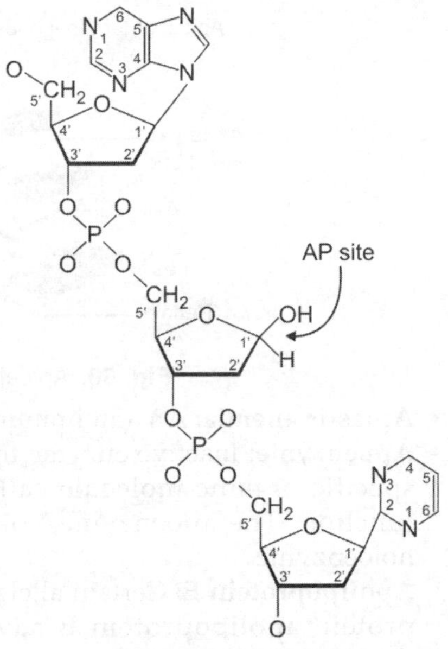

Fig. 59: Anucleate

A

- **AP:** Atrial peptide.
- **AP endonuclease:** An enzyme that is involved in base excision repair.
- **AP site:** A nucleotide position in a DNA molecule where the nitrogenous base component is missing.
- **Apex:** The tip, point or angular summit. The tip of a leaf the portion of a root or shoot containing apical and primary meristems. Usually used to designate the apical tip of the meristem.
- **APHIS:** The animal and plant health inspection service is the agency of the US department of agriculture responsible for regulating the field (outdoor) testing of genetically engineered plants and certain microorganisms.
- **Apical cell:** A meristematic initial in the apical meristem of shoots or roots of plants. As this cell divides, new tissues are formed.
- **Apical dominance:** The phenomenon of suppression of growth of an axillary bud in the presence of the terminal bud on the branch.
- **Apical meristem:** A region of the tip of each shoot and root of a plant in which cell division is continually occurring to produce new stem and root tissues, respectively (Fig. 60).

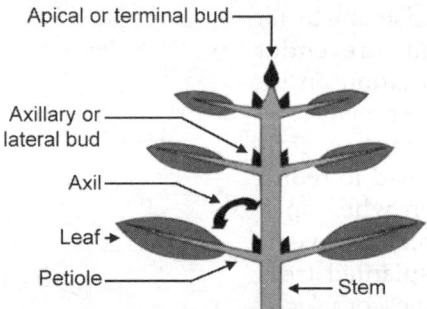

Fig. 60: Apical meristem

- **Aplastic anemia:** An autoimmune disease of the bone marrow.
- **Apoenzyme:** Inactive enzyme that has to be associated with a specific organic molecule called a co-enzyme in order to function. The apoenzyme/co-enzyme complex is called a holoenzyme.
- **Apolipoprotein E:** Certain alleles of the gene that encodes the protein apolipoprotein E have been associated with the development of heart disease and Alzheimer's disease.

- **Apomixis:** The asexual production of diploid offspring without the fusion of gametes. The embryo develops by mitotic division of the maternal or paternal gamete, or in the case of plants, by mitotic division of a diploid cell of the ovule.
- **Apomorphic character state:** A character state that evolved in a recent ansector of a subset of organisms in a group being studied.
- **Apoprotein:** A protein without its coenzymes, cofactors and prosthetic groups that are required for its functionally.
- **Apoptosis:** It is programmed cell death, a genetically controlled program of cell death. For example, the resorption of the tadpole tail at the time of its metamorphosis into a frog; removal of tissue between fingers and toes of the fetus (Fig. 61).

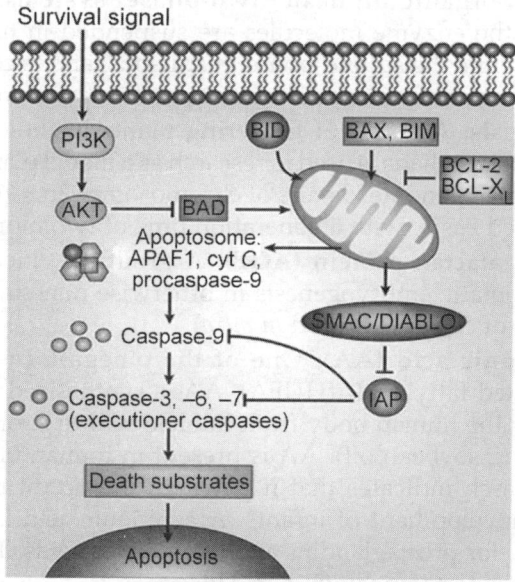

Fig. 61: Apoptosis

- **Aporepressor:** A protein changed into a repressor when a co-repressor binds to it.
- **Approvable letter (from the FDA):** One of the final steps in the US Food and Drug Administration's (US-FDA) review process for new pharmaceuticals. The letter precedes final FDA clearance for marketing of the new compound.
- **Aptamers:** Oligonucleotide molecules that bind (stick to) other, specific molecules (e.g. proteins). Aptamer is from the Latin

A

aptus, to fit. In 1992, Louis Bock and John Toole isolated aptamers that bind and inhibit the blood-coagulation enzyme thrombin. Since thrombin is crucial to the formation of blood clots (coagulation), such aptamers may someday be useful for anticoagulant therapy (e.g. to prevent blood clots following surgery or heart attacks).

- **Aquaculture:** The cultivation of plants using water as the support medium. It can also mean rearing marine life under controlled conditions in water, such as fish farming.
- **Aqueous biphasic (two-phase) systems:** Both phases are aqueous, but they contain different polymers, which do not mix together.
- **Aqueous-organic biphasic (two-phase) systems:** In these systems, the enzyme molecules are suspended in the organic solvent, while the second phase in aqueous, and is constituted by a thin layer of water surrounding each enzyme molecule.
- **Arabidopsis:** A genus of flowering plants in the cruciferae. Arabidopsis thaliana is used in research as a model plant because it has a small genome (5 pairs of chromosomes 2n = 10) and can be cultured easily with a generation time of two months.
- **Arabinogalactan protein (AGP):** A group of glucoproteins; induce somatic embryogenesis in otherwise non-embryogenic cells, e.g. of carrot (cultured *in vitro*).
- **Arachidonic acid (AA):** One of the omega-6 (n-6) highly unsaturated fatty acids (HUFA), AA is synthesized (manufactured) by the human body from linoleic acid (e.g. obtained by consuming soybean oil). AA is present in human breast milk, and research indicates that it plays an important role in the mental development of infants. Arachidonic acid is a crucial precursor for prostaglandins and other eicosanoids. The COX-1 enzyme converts arachidonic acid to constitutive prostaglandins and the COX-2 enzyme converts arachidonic acid to inducible prostaglandins (Fig. 62).

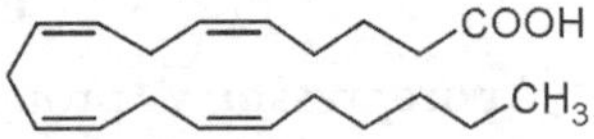

Fig. 62: Arachidonic acid

- *Archaea*: Single-celled life forms that can live at extreme ocean depths (high pressure) and in the absence of oxygen. Enzymes robust (sturdy) enough for industrial process utilization have been isolated by scientists from some strains of *Archaea*. Other *Archaea* strains are sometimes present in the rumen (first

stomach) of cattle and sheep. Those *Archaea* produce methane [A]
gas by breaking down some of the feed consumed by the cattle
and sheep.

* **Archaea:** One of the two main groups
  of prokaryotes, mostly found in
  extreme environments.
* **Arginine (Arg, R):** An amino acid
  (Fig. 63).

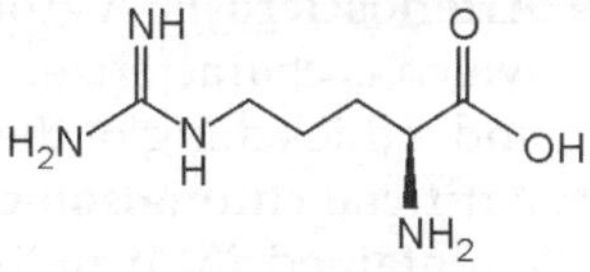

Fig. 63: Arginine

* **Arm:** One of the four arms of tRNA (or in some case five) stem-loop structures that make up the secondary structure. The arms of a lambda phage attachment site are the sequences flanking the core region where the recombination event occurs.
* **ARMD:** Acronym for age-related macular degeneration.
* **ARMG:** Acronym for antibiotic resistance marker gene.
* **Arms race:** A phenomenon of evolution in which two or more species adapt to one another in a coevolutionary manner.
* **Armyworm:** Caterpillars (pupae) of the Lepidopteran insect *Pseudaletia unipuncta* family; most of which are harmful to crops (e.g. wheat, corn/maize, etc.) grown by humans. Armyworms are susceptible to some of the cry proteins (e.g. they are killed if they eat plants genetically engineered to contain Cry1A(b), Cry9C, or Cry1F proteins). Armyworms are preyed upon by some species of ground beetles, sphecid wasps, toads, birds, etc.
* **AroA:** Refers to the transgene (cassette) which was initially isolated/extracted from the genome of the agrobacterium bacteria species (strain CP4) and inserted via genetic engineering techniques into a crop plant (e.g. soybean, *Glycine max* (L) in order to make that (soybean) plant tolerant to glyphosate-based herbicides (and also sulfosate-based herbicides).
* **Array of hairpins:** An assemble of alpha-helices that cannot be described as a bundle or a folded leaf.
* **Arrayed library:** Individual primary recombinant clones (hosted in phage, cosmid, YAC, or other vector) that are placed in two-dimensional arrays in microtitre dishes.
* **ARS (autonomous replication sequence):** An origin for replication in yeast. The common feature among different ARS sequences is a conserved 11 bp sequence called the A-domain.
* **ARS element:** A sequence of DNA that will support autonomous replication (sequence, ARS).

A

- **ARS vector:** A yeast vector having ARS module; it is quickly lost if selection pressure is absent.
- **Arteriosclerosis:** A group of diseases (including atherosclerosis) which is characterized by a decrease in elasticity (stretchiness) and a thickening of the walls of the body's arteries.
- **Artificial chromosome:** A circular or linear vector that is stably maintained in, usually 1 to 2 copies per cell; several types; bacterial artificial chromosome (BAC), PI-derived artificial chromosome (PAC), yeast artificial chromosome (YAC), human artificial chromosome (HAC).
- **Artificial insemination:** The placement of sperm inside the female reproductive tract to improve the chances of fertilization and pregnancy occurring. It is also called intrauterine insemination.
- **Artificial intelligence (AI):** The study or application of techniques to emulate intelligent behaviors, such as planning, vision, or language processing.
- **Artificial intelligence in medicine (AIM):** The application of artificial intelligence methods to solve problems in medicine such as diagnosis or therapy planning.
- **Artificial life:** The study of biological processes within the confines of a computer.
- **Artificial medium:** In plant tissue culture; a chemically defined medium, having inorganic salts, vitamins, sucrose, agar and the required growth regulators. In animal cell and tissue culture; medium having various organic and inorganic nutrients; may or may not contain serum, etc.
- **Artificial neural network (ANN):** A network of neurons that are connected graphically through synapses or weights.
- **Artificial seeds:** A synthetic seed consisting of a somatic embryo surrounded by nutrient medium which is protected by a thin membrane of chemical.
- **Artificial selection:** The practice of choosing individuals from a population for reproduction, usually because these individuals possess one or more desirable traits.
- **Asbestos fibres:** These are crystals of asbestos, a natural mineral, that have the form of minute strands; asbestos is a serious health hazard in indoor spaces.
- **Ascertainment:** In scientific research, ascertainment bias occurs when false results are produced by non-random sampling and conclusions made about an entire group are based on a distorted

or nontypical sample. Ascertainment bias may be easy to recognize or difficult to detect.

- **Ascites:** The fluids that accumulate in the peritoneal cavity due to tumor cells. Hybridomas grown in the peritoneal cavity of mice produce ascites containing high concentrations of the monoclonal antibody chosen for expression in the selection of the hybridoma cell line.

- **Ascorbic acid (vitamin C, $C_6H_8O_6$, F.W. 176.12):** A water-soluble vitamin present naturally in some plants, and also synthetically produced. Aside from its role as a vitamin, it is used as an antioxidant in plant tissue culture and included in disinfections solution (Fig. 64).

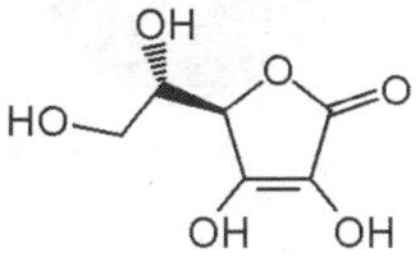

Fig. 64: Ascorbic acid

- **Ascospore:** One of the spores contained in the ascus of certain fungi.

- **Ascus:** Reproductive sac in the sexual stage of a type of fungi (Ascomycetes) in which ascospores are produced.

- **-ase:** The three-letter suffix that is added to a (root) word to denote an enzyme. For example, the stomachs of reindeer contain lichenase, an enzyme that enables reindeer to digest lichen that the reindeer consume as a source of winter food.

- **Aseptic:** Free from contamination by microorganisms.

- **Asexual:** Denotes fertilization and/or reproduction by *in vitro* means. Without sex.

- **Asexual embryogenesis:** The sequence of events whereby embryos develop from somatic cells, also known as somatic embryogenesis.

- **Asexual propagation:** Vegetative, somatic, non-sexual reproduction of a plant, without fertilization.

- **Asexual reproduction:** 1. Reproduction that does not involve the formation and union of gametes from the different sexes or mating types. It occurs mainly in lower animals, microorganisms and plants. In plants asexual reproduction is by vegetative propagation (e.g. bulbs, tubers, corms) and by formation of spores. 2. Nonsexual means of reproduction which can include grafting and budding (Fig. 65).

- **Asian corn borer:** Also known by its Latin name, *Ostrinia furnacalis* is an insect (originally from Asia) whose larvae (caterpillars) eat and bore into the corn/maize (*Zea Mays* L.) plant. In doing so, they can act as vectors (carriers) of the fungi

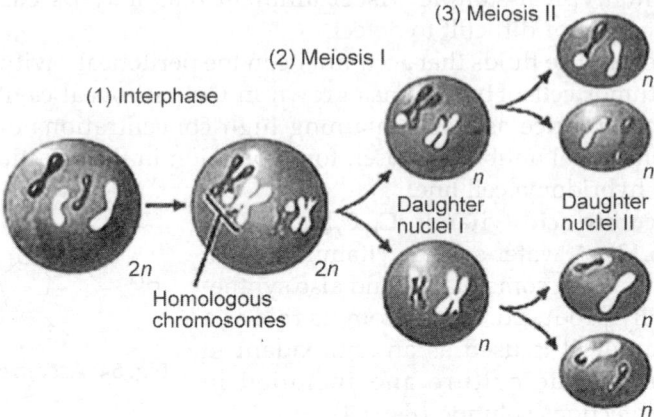

Fig. 65: Anucleate

known as *Aspergillus flavus* (a source of aflatoxin), *Fusarium moniliforme* (a source of fumonisin), or *Aspergillus parasiticus* (a source of aflatoxin).

- **Asparagine (Asn, N):** One of the 20 most common natural amino acids on earth. It has carboxamide as the side chain's functional group. It is not an essential amino acid. Its codons are AAU and AAC (Fig. 66).

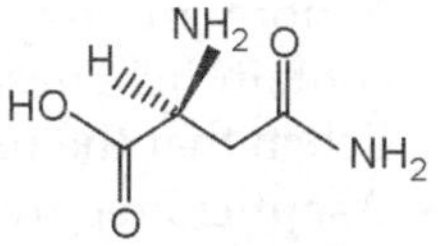

Fig. 66: L-asparagine

- **Aspartic acid (Asp, D):** An α-amino acid with the chemical formula $HO_2CCH(NH_2) CH_2CO_2H$. The carboxylate anion of aspartic acid is known aspartate. The L-isomer of asparatate is one of the 20 proteinogenic amino acids, i.e. the bulding blocks of proteins. Its codons are GAU and GAC.
- **Assay culture:** Microbial culture used for the assay of biological activities of microbial products.
- **Assay:** A test to detect the presence of some substances in small amount in solution.
- **Assembly factor:** A protein that is required for formation of a macromolecular structure but is not itself part of that structure.
- **Assembly:** The process of correctly joining together the DNA sequences from individual sequencing experiments into a contiguous segment.
- **Assimilation:** Transformation of food into protoplasm.

- **Association of biotechnology companies (ABC):** An American Trade Association of Companies involved in biotechnology and services to biotechnology companies (e.g. accounting, law, etc.). Formed in 1984, the ABC tended to consist of the smaller firms involved in biotechnology (and service firms that worked for all biotechnology companies). In 1993, the ABC was merged with the Industrial Biotechnology Association (IBA) to form the Biotechnology Industry Organization (BIO).

- **Assortative mating:** The tendency for mates to be chosen non-randomly.

- **Assortment:** The movement of homologous chromosomes to opposite poles in the first meiotic division and chromatids in the second meiotic division leading to the segregation of alleles.

- **Astaxanthin:** A carotenoid pigment responsible for the characteristic pink coloring of salmon, trout, and shrimp. It is produced by the microorganisms in the natural (wild) diets of those aquatic animals. Research has shown that astaxanthin (an antioxidant) helps boost the immune systems of humans that consume it. Research has also shown that astaxanthin helps to reduce oral cancer in rats and inhibit breast cancer in mice.

- **Astrocytoma:** A type of brain tumor that begins in the astrocyte cells of the brain or signal chord.

- **Asymmetric gap-LCR (AG-LCR):** LCR using reverse transcriptase; specific for detection of RNA.

- **Asymmetric polymerase chain reaction (PCR):** The two PCR primers are used in a 100:1 ratio so that one primer is finished ~10 cycles before the other; yields predominantly single-strand copies that can be used for DNA sequencing (Fig. 67).

- **Asymmetric somatic hybrid:** A somatic hybrid that contains full chromosome complement of one fusion parent plus one or few chromosomes from the other fusion parent.

- **Asymmetric unit:** In a crystal, the level at which there is no symmetry. For example, the alpha-beta dimer can be considered to be the asymmetric unit of the hemoglobin tetramer in solution.

- **Asymmetrical exon:** An exon flanked by introns of different phase classes.

- **Asynapsis:** The failure or partial failure in the pairing of homologous chromosomes during the meiotic prophase.

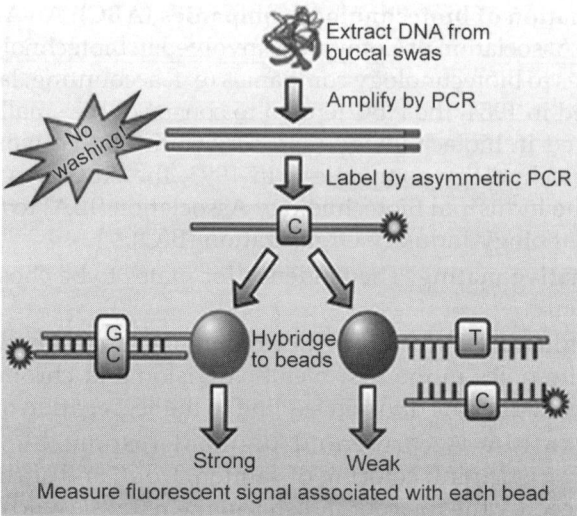

Fig. 67: Asymmetric polymerase chain reaction (PCR)

- **Asynchronous communication:** A mode of communication between two or more parties in which the exchange does not require the parties to participate at the same time.
- **Asynchronous:** Occurring independently, but on a similar timescale.
- **Atavism:** Reappearance of an ancestral trait after several generations because of recessiveness or other masking effects.
- **Ataxia-telangiectasia:** A rare fatal disease involving a damaged immune system, unsteady walk, premature aging, and a strong predisposition to some kinds of cancer.
- **Atherosclerosis:** A form of arteriosclerosis characterized by deposition and buildup of fatty deposits (plaque) on the internal walls of the body's arteries, in addition to the decreased elasticity of artery walls that characterizes all forms of arteriosclerosis. When a piece of plaque breaks off, a blood clot generally forms, and that clot often blocks

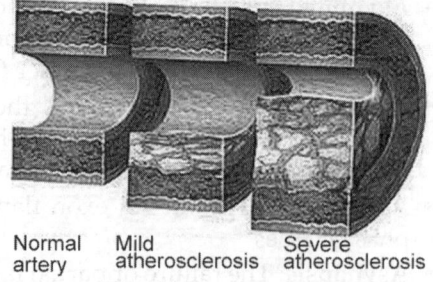

Fig. 68: Atherosclerosis

blood flow through the artery, causing a heart attack or stroke (Fig. 68).

- **AT-III:** A human blood factor that promotes clotting. A deficiency of AT-III can be inherited or can result from certain surgical procedures, certain illnesses, and sometimes use of certain oral contraceptives.

- **Atomic weight:** The total mass of an atom equal to the sum of the isotope's number of protons and neutrons (in the atom's nucleus). The atomic weights of the earth's elements are based on the assignment of exactly 12.000 as the atomic weight of the carbon-12 isotope (variation of atom). The atomic (weight) theory was established as a framework in 1869 by Meyer and Mendeléev, but standard precise values were not adopted internationally until an international commission on atomic weights was formed in 1899 in response to an initiative by the German Chemical Society. An element's atomic weight does not come out to a whole number (with the exception of carbon), because of the existence of isotopes which differ slightly with respect to the number of neutrons each contains.

- **ATP synthase:** A group of polypeptides that converts ADP and inorganic phosphate (Pi) to ATP and H_2O.

- **ATPase:** An enzyme that brings about the hydrolysis of ATP by the cleavage of either one phosphate group with the formation of ADP and inorganic phosphate, or of two phosphate groups, with the formation of AMP and pyrophosphate.

- **Atrial natriuretic factor:** An atrial peptide hormone that may regulate blood pressure and electrolyte balance within the body. An example is a peptide hormone.

- **Atrial peptides:** Endocrine components (proteins) that act to regulate blood pressure, as well as water and electrolyte homeostasis within the body. Atrial peptides are made by the heart in response to elevated blood pressure levels, and they stimulate the kidneys to excrete water and sodium into the urine, thus lowering blood pressure. They also slow the heartbeat. An example is a peptide hormone.

- *Att* **sites:** The loci on a phage and the bacterial chromosome at which recombination integrates the phage into, or excises it from, the bacterial chromosome.

- **Attenuated vaccine:** 1. A virulent organism that has been modified to produce a less virulent form, but nevertheless retains the ability to elicit antibodies against the virulent form. 2. A vaccine composed of infectious organisms (typically whole viruses) that exhibit low virulence or that cannot multiply in their host due to their inactivation or attenuation by exposure to radiation, chemical treatment or genetic manipulation.

- **Attenuated:** Weakened with reference to vaccines, made from pathogenetic organisms that have been treated so as to render them a virulent.

- **Attenuation (of RNA):** Premature termination of an elongating RNA chain.

- **Attenuation:** Regulation of a bacterial operon by termination of transcription at a site which is located before the first structural gene.

- **Attenuator:** A nucleotide sequence in the 5th region of a prokaryotic gene (or in its RNA) that causes premature termination of transcription, possibly by forming a secondary structure.

- **Attractor:** A characterization of the long-term behavior of a dissipative dynamical system.

- **Attribute:** A single data item related to a database object.

- **AU-AC intron:** A type of intron found in eukaryotic nuclear gens. The first-two nucleotides in the intron are 5'-AU-3' and the last two are 5'-AC-3'.

- **Augmentation gene therapy:** The genetically modified cells contain both the defective (endogenous) as well as the functional (introduced) copies of the gene.

- **Aureofacin:** An antifungal antibiotic produced by a strain of *Streptomyces aureofaciens*. At least one company has incorporated the gene for this antibiotic (which acts against wheat take-all disease) into a *Pseudomonas fluorescens* used to confer resistance to wheat take all disease by allowing the bacteria to colonize the wheat's roots. In this way the plant obtains the benefits of the antibiotic because the bacteria become part of the plant.

- **Authentic protein:** A recombinant protein that has all the properties including any post-translational modification of its naturally occurring counterpart.

- **Auto:** Prefix indicating of self-origin or host origin.

- **Autoantibodies:** Antibodies that the immune system erroneously forms against self-antigens.

- **Autoantigen:** A self protein that is the target of an autoimmune response.

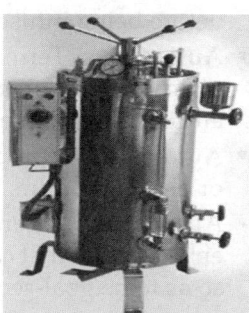

- **Autocatalysis:** Catalysis in which one of the products of the reaction is a catalyst for the reaction. Usually, the catalysis starts slowly and increases as the quantity of the catalyst increase, falling off as the product is used up.
- **Autoclavable:** A substance, which does not deteriorate or undergo alteration due to autoclaving.
- **Autoclave:** An instrument used for sterilization of glassware and culture media (Fig. 69).

Fig. 69: Autoclave

- **Autoclaving:** Sterilization using moist heat at 15 psi (1.06 kg/cm^2) and 121°C for 5–40 min; the duration of autoclaving depends on the nature of liquid and its volume; efficiency of sterilization depends on temperature and not directly on pressure.
- **Autogenous control:** The action of a gene product that either inhibits (negative autogenous control) or activates (positive autogenous control) expression of the gene coding for it.
- **Autograft:** Graft obtained from the body of the recipient itself.
- **Autoimmune disease:** 1. A disease in which the body produces antibodies against its own tissues. 2. Disorder in which the immune systems of affected individuals produce antibodies against molecules that are normally produced by those individuals (called self-antigens).
- **Autoimmune lympho-proliferative syndrome (ALPS):** A human disease caused by failure of lymphocytes to die once they have finished doing their job. As a result, the spleen and lymph nodes grow large, and immune cells may attack the body's own tissues, a condition known as autoimmunity.
- **Autoimmunity:** 1. A situation in which the body produces an immune response against its own organs or tissues. 2. A condition in which the body mounts an immune response against one of its own organs or tissues. 3. An immune response of tissues, cells, or molecular components of the host. The pathological result of this response is an autoimmune disease. 4. A disorder in the body's defense mechanism in which an immune response is elicited against its own (self) tissues.

A

- **Autologous cells:** Cells that are taken from an individual, cultured (or stored), and possibly, genetically manipulated before being infused back into the original donor.

- **Autologous:** Term used to denote derivation from self. Tissue from one person returned to the same person is termed an autologous sample.

- **Autolysis:** The process of self-destruction of a cell, cell organelle, or tissue. It occurs by the action of lysosomic enzymes.

- **Autonomous agent:** An entity with limited perception of its environment that can process information to calculate an action so as to be goal-seeking on a local scale.

- **Autonomous controlling element:** In maize is an active transposon with the ability to transpose (compare with nonautonomous controlling element).

- **Autonomous:** A term applied to any biological unit that can function on its own, i.e. without the help of another unit, such as a transposonable element that encodes an enzyme for its own transposition.

- **Autonomously replicating sequence (ARS):** Any clones DNA sequence that initiates and supports extra-chromosomal replication of a DNA molecule in a host cell. It is often used in yeast cells.

- **Autophosphorylation:** The ability of a species of kinase to phosphorylate itself is referred to as. Autophosphorylation does not necessarily occur on the same polypeptide chain as the catalytic site; for example, in a dimer, each subunit may phosphorylate the other.

- **Autopolyploid:** A polyploidy resulting from the doubling of a single genome.

- **Autoradiograph:** A picture prepared by labeling a substance such as DNA with a radioactive material such as tritiated, thymidine and allowing the image produced by decay radiation to develop on a film over a period of time.

- **Autoradiography:** A technique for the detection of radioactively labeled molecules by overlaying the specimen with photographic film. When the film is developed an image is produced which corresponds to the location of the radioactivity (Fig. 70).

- **Autoregulation:** Product of a gene that controls the level of its own synthesis.

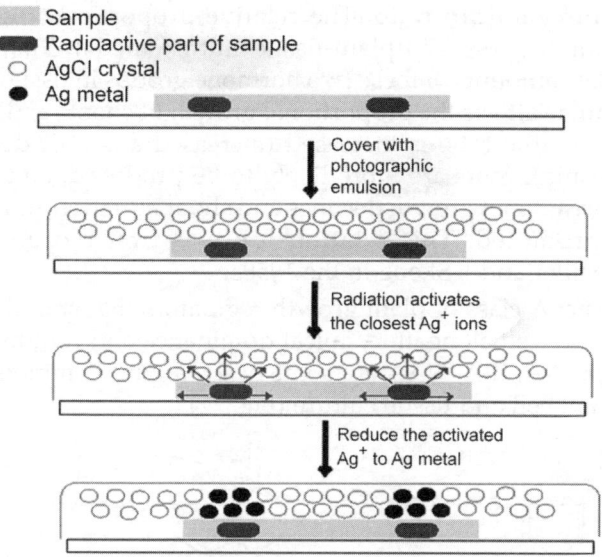

Fig. 70: Autoradiography

- **Autosomal:** A locus on any chromosome other than a sex chromosome. Not sex-linked.
- **Autosome:** A chromosome that is not involved in sex determination.
- **Autosplicing (self-splicing):** The ability of an intron to excise itself from an RNA by a catalytic action that depends only on the sequence of RNA in the intron.
- **Autotroph:** An organism that can live on very simple carbon and nitrogen sources, such as carbon dioxide and ammonia.
- **Autotrophic phase of embryo development:** In ovulo, embryo capable of synthesizing all the biochemical it needs; the specific developmental stage varies with the species, e.g. in Capsella late heart stage and later stages.
- **Autotrophic:** Characteristic of plants that are capable of manufacturing their own food, as in photosynthesis.
- **Autotrophy:** Autotrophy is the capacity of an organism to use light as the sole energy source. In the synthesis of organic material from inorganic elements or compounds. Autotrophic organisms include green photosynthesizing plants and some photosynthetic bacteria.

A

- **Auxin-cytokinin ratio:** The relative proportion of auxin to cytokinin present in plant-tissue-culture media. Varying the relative amounts of these two hormone groups in tissue culture formulae affects the proportional growth of shoots and roots *in vitro*. As the ratio is increased (increased auxin or decreased cytokinin), roots are more likely to be produced, and as it is, decreased root growth declines and shoot initiation and growth are promoted. This relationship was first recognized by CO Miller and F Skoog in the 1950s.

- **Auxins:** A class of plant growth regulators that stimulates cell division, cell elongation, apical dominance and root initiation. 2,4-D, IAA, IBA, NAA are some of the auxins commonly used in plant cell and tissue culture (Fig. 71).

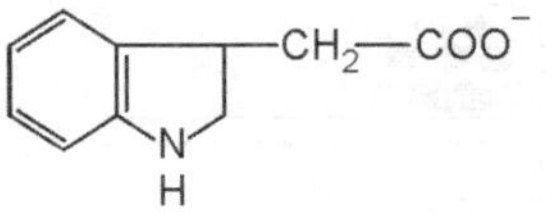

Indol-3-acetic acid (IAA) 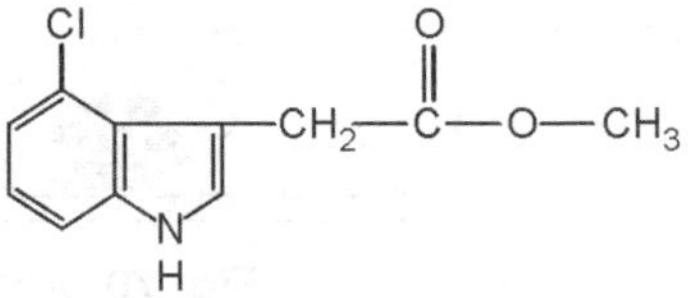   4-Chloroindol-3-acetate

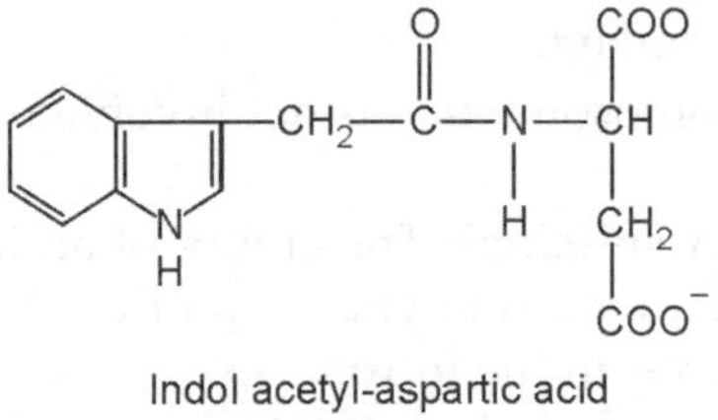

Indol acetyl-aspartic acid

Fig. 71: Auxins

- **Auxotroph:** A mutant microorganism or cell line requiring a substance for growth that can be synthesized by wild-type strains.

- **Auxotrophic mutant:** A mutant requiring a biochemical for its normal growth and development since it cannot synthesize this biochemical due to mutation in a gene.

- **Availability:** A reflection of the form and location of nutritional elements and their suitability for absorption. In tissue culture media, this is related to the abundance of each nutritional element, the osmotic concentration and pH of the medium, the stability and solubility of the item in question, the presence of absorbing agents in the media, and other factors.

- **Avidin:** A protein (derived from egg white) that binds very tightly to biotin. This interaction is exploited in several biological as says, such as ELISA and Western Blots.
- **Avidity model:** According to this model, a low avidity interaction between TCR of double positive ($CD_4^+ CD_8^+$) T-cells and antigen peptide-MHC complex/MHC molecule leads to positive selection; in contrast, negative selection is the consequence if this interaction is of a high avidity.
- **Avidity:** A measurement of the binding of an antiserum to a complex antigen. The avidity of the antiserum depends on the affinities of the various antibodies present in the antiserum to different epitopes on the antigen.
- **Avirulent:** Lacking virulence; a microorganism lacking the properties that normally cause disease.
- **Axenic culture:** Free of external contaminants and internal symbionts, which is generally not possible with surface sterilization alone and incorrectly used to indicate aseptic culture.
- **Axes:** Straight lines passing through an organism, around which the organism is symmetrically arranged.
- **Axial element:** A proteinaceous structure around which the chromosomes condense at the start of synapsis.
- **Axillary bud proliferation:** A technique of micropropagation of plants in culture, which is achieved primarily through hormonal inhibition of apical dominance and stimulation of lateral branching.
- **Axillary bud:** A bud found in the axil of a leaf (synonymous with lateral bud).
- **Axillary:** An adjective describing the relative position of a bud, i.e. axillary bud, in the axils of leaves.
- **Axiom:** A statement that is assumed to be true.
- **Azadirachtin:** The pharmacophore (active ingredient) in secretions of the tropical neem tree, which resists insect depradations.
- **Azoospermia:** A lack of motile sperms in the semen.
- **Azurophil-derived bactericidal factor (ADBF):** Potent antimicrobial protein produced by neutrophils (a type of white blood cell).

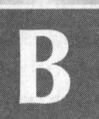

- **B:** An amino acid that is either aspartic acid or glutamic acid.
- **B cells:** An important class of white blood cells that mature in bone marrow and produce antibodies. They are largely responsible for the antibody-mediated of humeral immune response. They give rise to the antibody-producing plasma cells and some other cells of the immune system.
- **B cell memory:** It is responsible for rapid antibody production during a secondary immune response and subsequent responses. Memory B cells produce antibodies of higher affinity than native B cells.
- **B cell receptor (BCR):** It is the antigen receptor complex on the cell surface of B lymphocytes. It consists of membrane-bound immunoglobulin, bound noncovalently to Iga and α, β-chains.
- **B chromosome:** A chromosome possessed by some individuals in a population, but not all.
- **B lymphocytes (B cells):** Lymphocytes derived from bone marrow cells that produce antibodies.
- *Bacillus thuringiensis* **(B.t.)** *israelensis*: One of the approximately 30 subspecies groupings within the approximately 20,000 different strains of the soil bacteria known (collectively) as *B.t.* When eaten (e.g. due to presence on food), the protoxin proteins produced by *B.t. israelensis* are toxic to mosquitoes and black fly (Diptera) larvae.
- *B.t. kurstaki*: One of the approximately 30 subspecies groupings within the approximately 20,000 different strains of the soil bacteria known (collectively) as *B.t.* When eaten (e.g. as part of a genetically engineered plant), the protoxin proteins produced by *B.t. kurstaki* are toxic to certain caterpillars (Lepidoptera larvae), such as the European corn borer (pyralis).
- *B.t. tenebrionis*: One of the approximately 30 subspecies groupings within the approximately 20,000 different strains of

the soil bacteria known (collectively) as *B.t.* When eaten (e.g. as part of a genetically engineered plant), the protoxin proteins produced by *B.t. tenebrionis* are toxic to certain insects.

- **B.t. tolworthi:** One of the approximately 30 subspecies group-ings within the approximately 20,000 different strains of the soil bacteria known (collectively) as *B.t.* When eaten (e.g. as part of a genetically engineered crop plant), the protoxin proteins produced by *B.t. tolworthi* are toxic to certain caterpillars (Lepidoptera larvae), such as the European corn borer (pyralis).
- **BAC:** Acronym for bacterial artificial chromosomes.
- **BAC library:** A resource that identifies a sequence of bacterial artificial chromosomes (BACs).
- **Bacilli Calmette-Guérin (BCG):** An attenuated strain of *Myco-bacterium tuberculosis* that is used as a vaccine for tuberculosis.
- **Bacillus:** Rod-shaped bacteria.
- *Bacillus subtilis:* A (rod-shaped) aerobic bacterium commonly used as a host in recombinant DNA experiments. During the 1990s, research showed that corn (maize) plant tissues infected with the endophyte *Bacillus subtilis* (*B. subtilis*) were less likely to become infected with *Fusarium moniliforme* fungus. Other research has indicated the potential for prior infection of corn (maize) plant tissues to hinder any subsequent aflatoxin production in that plant by *Aspergillus flavus* fungus.
- *Bacillus thuringiensis:* Discovered by bacteriologist Ishiwata Shigetane on a diseased silkworm in 1901. Later discovered on a dead Mediterranean flour moth, and first named *B.t.*, by Ernst Berliner in 1915. Today, *B.t.* refers to a group of rod-shaped soil bacteria found all over the earth, that produce cry proteins which are indigestible by—yet still bind to—specific insects' gut (stomach) lining (epithelium cell) receptors, so those cry proteins are thereby toxic to certain classes of insects (corn borers, corn rootworms, mosquitoes, black flies, some types of beetles, etc.), but are harmless to all mammals. At least 20,000 strains of *B.t.* are known. Genes that code for the production of these cry proteins that are toxic to insects have been inserted by scientists since 1989 into vectors (i.e. viruses, other bacteria, and other microorganisms) in order to confer insect resistance to certain agricultural plants (e.g. via expression of those *B.t.* proteins by one or more tissues of the transgenic plant). For example, the

B.t. strain known as *B.t. kurstaki*, which is fatal when ingested by the European corn borer was first (genetically) inserted into a corn plant (via vector) in 1991. *B.t. kurstaki* kills borers via perforation of that insect's gut by cry (crystal- like) proteins that are coded for by the *B.t. kurstaki* gene. The vectors as listed above are entities that can take up and carry the DNA into plant or other cells. Vectors are DNA-carrying vehicles.

- **Back-bulb propagation:** Procedure, which involves separation of the oldest pseudobulbil to force the development of its dormant bud.
- **Back-bulb:** In sympodial orchids; an old pseudobulb (often without leaves); alive and bears one or more buds behind the actively growing portion.
- **Backcross:** Hybrid is crossed to one of its two parents.
- **Background level** of mutation describes the rate at which sequence changes accumulate in the genome of an organism. It reflects the balance between the occurrence of spontaneous mutations and their removal by repair systems, and is characteristic for any species.
- **Background selection:** Selection for recurrent parent genotype in a backcross program; also used in a pedigree selection scheme to ensure the recovery of a specified level of genome from the desired parent.
- **Backpropagation:** An algorithm for efficiently calculating the error gradient of a neutral network, which can then be used as the basis of learning.
- **Backtracking algorithm:** The process of repeatedly exploring paths until you encounter the solution.
- **Bacteria:** Structurally simple, single-celled organisms that have no nucleus (Fig. 1).
- **Bacterial artificial chromosome (BAC):** A synthetic DNA molecule that contains sequences required for replication and segregation in bacteria, used to amplify 100–200 kb long DNA sequences.
- **Bacterial expressed sequence tags:** These are ESTs (Expressed sequence tags) based on sequenced/mapped bacterial genes instead of the genes of (traditional EST) *C. elegans* nematode. They are utilized to label a given gene (i.e. in terms of that gene's function/protein).
- **Bacterial lawn:** A continuous bacterial growth on an agar plate.

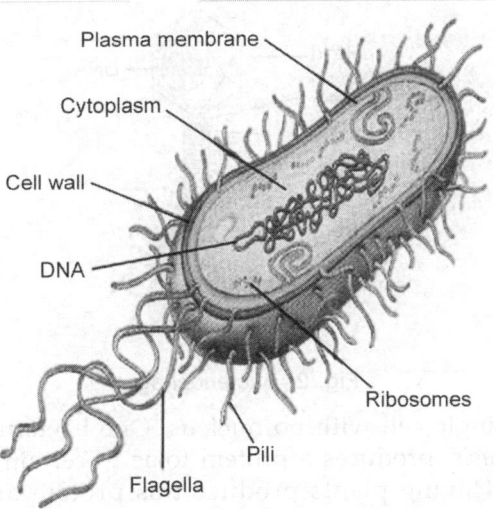

Plasma membrane

Cytoplasm

Cell wall

DNA

Ribosomes

Pili

Flagella

Fig. 1: Bacteria

- **Bacteriocide:** A chemical or drug that kills bacterial cells.
- **Bacteriocin:** A protein produced by bacteria of one strain that is active against those of a closely related strain.
- **Bacteriology:** The science and study of bacteria, a specialized branch of microbiology. The bacteria constitute a useful and essential group in the biological community. Although some bacteria, prey on higher forms of life, relatively few are pathogens (disease-causing organisms). Life on earth depends on the activity of bacteria to mineralize organic compounds and to capture the free nitrogen molecules in the air for use by plants. Also, bacteria are important industrially for the conversion of raw materials into products such as organic chemicals, antibiotics, cheeses, etc. Genetically engineered bacteria are starting to be used to produce high value-added pharmaceuticals and specialty chemicals.
- **Bacteriophage:** A virus that infects and replicates in bacteria. Also called simply phage (Fig. 2).
- **Bacteriostat:** A substance that inhibits or slows down the growth and reproduction of bacteria.
- **Bacteriostatic agent:** An agent that has biostatic effect on bacteria.
- **Bacterium:** 1. A single-celled, microscopic prokaryotic organism: a single cell organism without a distinct nucleus. 2. A structurally

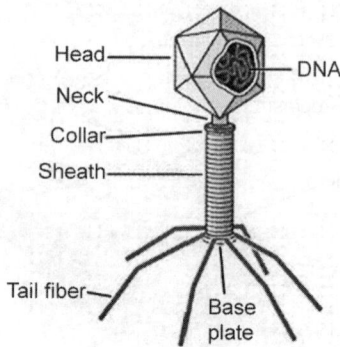

Fig. 2: Bacteriophage

simple single cell with no nucleus. One bacterium, *Bacillus thuringiensis*, produces a protein toxic to certain destructive insects. Having plants produce this protein after genetic engineering is a form of built-in pest-resistance in plants.

- **Bacterization:** A technique of seed-dressing with bacteria as water soluble suspension used for introduction of bacteria in soil.
- **Bacteroids:** The pleomorphic forms of *Rhizobium* present inside root nodules that fix atmospheric nitrogen gas.
- **Baculovirus:** A class of virus that infects lepidopteran insects (e.g. cotton bollworm or gypsy moth larva). Baculoviruses can be modified via genetic engineering to insert new genes into the larva, causing those larva to then produce proteins desired by man (e.g. pharmaceuticals). Baculoviruses are potentially very useful for pharmaceutical production, because the protein molecules produced are glycosylated (i.e. have relevant oligosaccharides attached to them), and baculoviruses cannot infect vertebrate animals. Such pharmaceuticals are thus not even a theoretical risk to humans.
- **Baculovirus expression vectors (BEVs):** Vectors (used by researchers to carry new genes into cells) in which the agent is a baculovirus (a virus that infects certain types of insects only). These could conceivably be used to make a genetically engineered insecticide that is specific to a targeted insect (wouldn't harm anything but that insect). For example, a BEV might be used to cause a cotton bollworm adult protein to be expressed when the bollworm is a juvenile, thus killing the bollworm before it has a chance to damage a cotton crop.

- **Bait:** In yeast two-hybrid (Y2H) system, a protein (say, protein X) expressed as a fusion (a hybrid) protein with the DNA-binding domain of a transcription factor; used to find a protein that interacts with X.
- **Balanced lethal system:** A system for maintaining a recessive lethal allele at each of two loci on the same pair of chromosomes. In a closed population with no crossing-over between the loci, only the double heterozygotes for the lethal mutations survive.
- **Balanced polymorphism:** A polymorphism that is stable over time and is maintained by balanced selection.
- **Balanced selection:** A selection regime that results in the maintenance of two or more alleles at a locus in a population, e.g. over-dominance.
- **Balanced tree:** A common data structure for creating indexes on disk.
- **Balloon angioplasty:** A medical procedure in which a catheter with a balloon at the tip is used to clear or repair damaged blood vessels.
- **Bam Islands:** A series of short, repeated sequences found in the nontranscribed spacer of *Xenopus* rDNA genes. The name reflects their isolation by use of the Bam I restriction enzyme.
- **Band:** A chromatographic zone, that is, a region where the separated substance is concentrated.
- **Bands:** Bands of polytene chromosomes are visible as dense regions that contain the majority of DNA. They include active genes.
- **Bar body:** The highly condensed chromatin formed by an inactivated X chromosome.
- **BAR gene:** A dominant gene from the *Streptomyces hygroscopicus* bacterium, which codes for (causes production of) the enzyme phosphinothricin acetyl transferase (PAT). When the BAR gene is inserted into a plant's genome (its DNA), it imparts resistance to glufosinate-ammonium based herbicides. Because the glufosinate-ammonium herbicides act via inhibition of glutamine synthetase (an enzyme that catalyzes the synthesis of glutamine), this inhibition (of enzyme) kills plants (e.g. weeds). That is because glutamine is crucial for plants to synthesize critically needed amino acids. The BAR gene is often utilized by genetic engineers as a marker gene.
- **Bar:** A unit used for pressure of liquid. 1 bar = 10^5 Pa. 1 bar is approximately equal to 1 atmosphere.

- **Barley malt:** Barley seeds germinated at 17°C to a specific stage and dried at 65°C and, usually, powdered.
- **Barley:** The domesticated plant *Hordeum vulgare*, whose grain is utilized by man for various purposes, such as feed barley varieties (for feeding of livestock). Malting barley varieties (containing beta-amylase in their seeds) were created via mutation breeding (i.e. bombardment of the seeds by ionizing radiation to cause random genetic mutations, followed by selection of the particular mutation in which maltose is produced by that barley plant in its seeds) (Fig. 3).

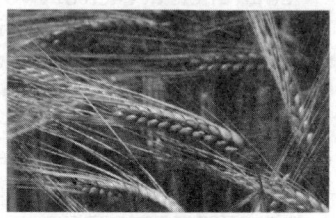

Fig. 3: Barley

- ***Barnase*:** A gene isolate from *Bacillus amyloliquefaciens* that encodes an RNase, which is cytotoxic to the cell expressing it; used to produce male sterility that is restored by *barstar*.
- **Barrier to gene flow:** A factor, such as geographic, mechanical, and behavioral isolating mechanisms that restrict gene flow between populations, leading to populations with differing allele frequencies.
- ***Barstar*:** A gene isolated from *Bacillus amyloliquefaciens* that encodes a specific inhibitor of *barnase* RNase; used for fertility restoration in *barnase* male sterile plants.
- **Basal body:** Small granule to which a cilium or flagellum is attached.
- **Basal factors:** Components of the nucleus that associate with chromosomes and enhance gene transcription.
- **Basal level:** The level of response from a system in the absence of a stimulus is its. The basal level of transcription of a gene is the level that occurs in the absence of any specific activation.
- **Basal medium:** A growth regulator-free medium, i.e. a medium containing inorganic salts, vitamins, sucrose and agar (where needed).
- **Basal promoter:** The position within a eukaryotic promoter where the initiation complex is assembled.
- **Basal rate of transcription:** The number of productive initiations of transcription occurring per unit time at a particular promoter.
- **Basal transcription apparatus** is the complex of transcription factors that assembles at the promoter before RNA polymerase is bound.

- **Basal:** 1. Located at the base of a plant or a plant organ. 2. A fundamental formulation of a tissue culture medium.
- **Base (General):** A substance with a pH in the range 7–14, which will react with an acid to form a salt. Mild bases normally taste bitter and feel slippery to the touch.
- **Base (Nucleotide):** A segment of the DNA (and RNA) molecules. One of the four (repeating) chemical units that comprise DNA/RNA that, according to their order and pairing (on the parallel strands of DNA/RNA molecules), represent the different amino acids (within the protein molecule that each gene in the DNA codes for). The four bases comprising DNA are adenine (A), cytosine (C), guanine (G), and thymine (T).
- **Base analog:** A chemical whose molecular structure mimics that of a DNA base, because of the mimicry, the analog may act as a mutagen.
- **Base collection:** A collection of seed stock or vegetative propagating material (ranging from tissue cultures to whole plants) held for long-term security in order to preserve the genetic variation for scientific purposes and as a basis for plant breeding as multiplication and evaluation.
- **Base excision repair:** A DNA repair process that involves excision and replacement of an abnormal base.
- **Base excision sequence scanning (BESS):** A method that can be utilized to detect a point mutation in DNA (via rapid DNA sequence scanning).
- **Base mispairing:** A coupling between two bases that does not conform to the Watson-Crick rule, e.g. adenine with cytosine, thymine with guanine.
- **Base pair (bp):** It is a partnership of A with T or C with G in a DNA double helix; other pairs can be formed in RNA under certain circumstances.
- **Base pairing:** The specific (complementary) interactions of adenine with thymine or of guanine with cytosine in a DNA double helix (thymine is replaced by uracil in double helical RNA).
- **Base sequence analysis:** A method, sometimes automated, for determining the base sequence of DNA or RNA.
- **Base sequence:** The order of nucleotide bases in a DNA or RNA molecule.
- **Base stacking:** The hydrophobic interactions that occur between adjacent base pairs in a double-stranded DNA molecule.

- **Base substitution:** Replacement of one base by another in a DNA molecule.
- **Base:** One of five molecules which are assembled, along with a ribose and a phosphate, to form nucleotides. Adenine (A), guanine (G), cytosine (C), and thymine (T) are found in DNA while RNA is made from adenine (A), guanine (G), cytosine (C), and uracil (U).
- **Baseless site:** A position in a DNA molecule where the base component of the nucleotide is missing.
- **Basic chromosome number:** Gametic chromosome number of a diploid species of the parental diploid species in case of a polyploidy species.
- **Basic copy:** Each VSG (variable surface glycoprotein) of a trypanosome is coded by a gene.
- **Basic domain:** A type of DNA-binding domain.
- **Basin of attraction:** The subset of states of a dynamical systems' state space that converge into an attractor.
- **Basin portrait:** The set of basins of attraction for a dynamical system.
- **Basophilic:** Staining strongly with basic dye. For example, basophil leukocytes are polymorphonuclear leukocytes which stain strongly with (take up a lot of) basic dyes.
- **Basophils:** Also called basophilic leukocytes. A type of white blood cell (leukocyte) produced by stem cells within the bone marrow that synthesizes and stores histamine and also contains heparin. When two IgE molecules of the same antibody dock at adjacent receptor sites on a basophil cell, the two IgE molecules capture an allergen between them. A chemical signal is sent to the basophil causing the basophil cell to release histamine, serotonin, bradykinin, and slowreacting substance. Release of these chemicals into the body causes the blood vessels to become more permeable, which consequently causes the nose to run. These chemicals also cause smooth muscle contraction, resulting in sneezing, coughing, wheezing, etc.
- **Batch bioreactor:** In such a bioreactor, the medium and inoculum are located into the reactor in the beginning, and the cells are allowed to grow; there is no addition/replacement of medium, and the entire cell mass is harvested at the end of incubation period (Fig. 4).

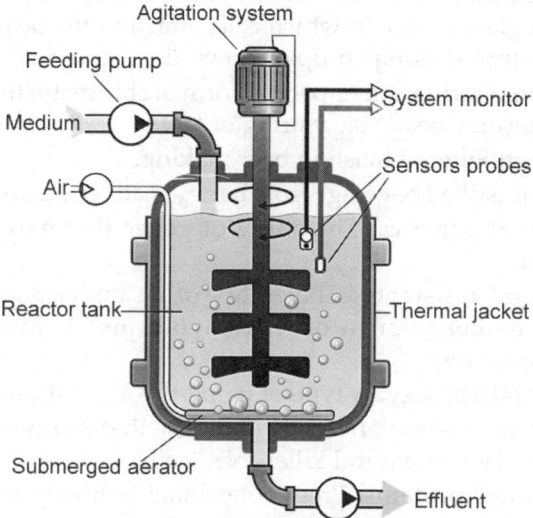

Fig. 4: Batch bioreactor

- **Batch culture:** A cell suspension culture in which cells are grown in a finite volume of nutrient medium and follow a sigmoid pattern of growth.
- **Batch digestors:** These are suited for digestion of solid wastes, where hydrolysis occurs in a solid bed, and the leachate is circulated through a methanogenic digestor and back over the solid waste bed.
- **Batch fermentation:** Fermentation carried out by growing microbes in batch culture.
- **BB rat:** A mutant rat strain that is susceptible to, and therefore acts as a model for insulin-dependent diabetes.
- **Bce4:** The name of a promoter (region of DNA) that controls/ enhances an oilseed plant's gene(s) that code for components (e.g. fatty acids, amino acids, etc.) of that plant's seeds. For example, the Bce4 promoter causes such genes to be expressed during one of the earliest stages of canola plant's seed production.
- **Bcr-Abl gene:** The gene (SNP) that causes the blood cancer chronic myelocytic leukemia (CML) in humans that possess it.
- **B-DNA:** The normal form of DNA found in biological systems. It exists as a right handed helix.

- **Bead bed reactor:** In animal cell culture; column packed with 3–5 mm glass beads, in which cells attach to the bead, surface, and medium is pumped up or down the column.
- **Beads-on-a-string:** An unpacked form of chromatin that consists of nucleosome beads on a string of DNA.
- **Beer wort:** Filtered mash in beer making.
- **Beer:** Undistilled beverage from barley malt fermented by yeast.
- **Behavioral genetics:** The study of genes that may influence behavior.
- **Behavioral resistance:** The ability of an insect population to change its behavior in order to avoid insecticides or other injurious factors.
- **Behavioral strategy:** A type of game-theoretic strategy.
- **Beige mouse:** A mutant strain of mouse that is prone to cancer, due to its lack of natural killer (NK) cells.
- **Bence-Jones proteins:** Free monoclonal antibody light chains found in the urine of patients with multiple myeloma. A source of large quantities of antibodies prior to the development of monoclonal antibody (hybridoma) technology.
- **Bench-scale process:** A small- or laboratory- scale process commonly used in connection with fermentation.
- **Benign tumor:** A non-cancerous growth that does not spread to other parts of the body.
- **Bergmann's cell planting technique:** Cells are suspended in melted agar medium and spread in a 1 mm thick layer, usually in a petri plate.
- **Best linear unbiased prediction (BLUP):** A statistical (data) technique employed by livestock breeders to determine the breeding (genetic trait) value of animals in a breeding program.
- **BEST map:** Map indicating the correlation between bacterial artificial chromosome and expressed sequence tags.
- **Beta carotene:** A phytochemical (vitamin precursor) that is naturally produced in carrots, other orange vegetables, and in the endosperm portion of the corn (maize) kernel. Beta carotene has been found to aid eyesight in people who consume it, and may help to prevent lung cancer and heart disease.
- **Beta cells:** Insulin-producing cells in the pancreas. If these cells are destroyed, childhood (also known as early-onset or Type I) diabetes results.

- **Beta conformation:** An extended, zigzag arrangement of a polypeptide (molecule) chain.
- **Beta DNA:** The normal form of DNA found in biological systems, which exists as a right-handed helix.

B

- **Beta interferon:** One of the interferons, it is a protein that was approved by the US Food and Drug Administration (US-FDA) in 1993 to be used to treat multiple sclerosis (MS).
- **Beta lactamase:** Ampicillin resistance gene.
- **Beta sheet:** A three-dimensional arrangement taken up by polypeptide chains that consists of alternating strands linked by hydrogen bonds. The alternating strands together form a sheet that is frequently twisted. One of the secondary structural elements characteristics of proteins (Fig. 5).

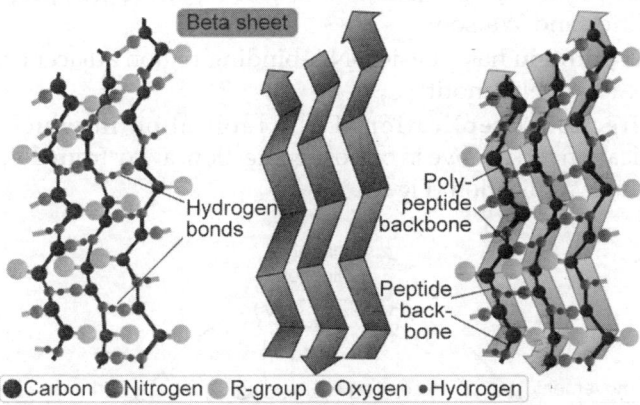

●Carbon ●Nitrogen ●R-group ●Oxygen •Hydrogen

Fig. 5: Beta sheet

- **Beta strand:** A three-dimensional arrangement taken up by polypeptide chains that consists of alternating strands linked by hydrogen bonds. The alternating strands together form a sheet that is frequently twisted. One of the secondary structural elements of proteins, along with the alpha-helix.
- **β-conglycinin:** Abbreviated β-conglycinin. One of the (structural) categories of proteins produced in seeds of legumes. In general, β-conglycinin contains one-quarter to one-third as much cysteine (cys) and methionine (met) per unit of protein as does glycinin. β-conglycinin has greater emulsifying capacity (in water) and emulsion stability than does glycinin, so its presence can assist the manufacture of firmer tofu, and better protein-based (emulsion) drinks.

B

- **Beta-galactosidase:** An enzyme that catalyzes the formation of glucose and galactose from lactose.
- **Beta-lactam antibiotics:** A category of antibiotics (e.g. penicillin G, ampicillin, etc.) that kill targeted bacteria by altering their essential cellular function of enzymatic controls that keep cell wall (peptidoglycan) synthesis (creation/repair) in balance with cell wall degradation. This causes cell wall breakdown and death of those bacteria (pathogens).
- **Beta-secretase:** An enzyme that (in the human brain) is linked to presence of Alzheimer's disease.
- **BFGF:** Basic fibroblast growth factor.
- **B-form:** DNA is a right-handed double helix with 10 base pairs per complete turn (360°) of the helix. This is the form found under physiological conditions whose structure was proposed by Crick and Watson.
- **bHLH protein** has a basic DNA-binding region adjacent to the helix-loop-helix motif.
- **Bidirectional replication:** DNA replication in which two replication forks move in opposite direction, away from the same origin of replication (Fig. 6).

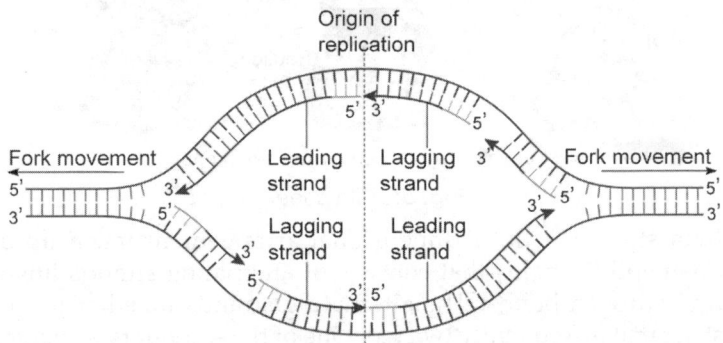

Fig. 6: Bidirectional replication

- **Biennial:** In botany, a plant which completes its life cycle within two years and then dies. For most biennial plants, the two growing seasons have to be separated by a period of cold temperature sufficient to induce flowering and fruit formation.
- *Bifidus:* A family of bacteria species that live within the digestive systems of certain animals (humans, swine, etc.). Examples

include *Bifidobacterium bifidum, Bifidobacterium longum, Bifidobacterium infantis, Bifidobacterium adolescentis,* and *Bifidobacterium acidophilus.*

- **Bifunctional enzyme:** An enzyme, which can catalyze two reactions, encoded by a recombinant gene.
- **Bile:** A liquid (mixture) made by the liver to help digest fats (in the intestine) and facilitate intestinal absorption of certain vitamins and minerals. Bile consists primarily of water, cholesterol, lipids (fat), natural detergents (i.e. salts of bile acids) that help breakup fat globules in the intestines, and bilirubin.
- **Bile acids:** A family of acids derived by the human liver from cholesterol (i.e. from foods), and excreted into the bile by the liver. They help to emulsify (food-source) fats in the small intestine, as part of the crucial first step in the digestion of fats.
- **Bilirubin:** A component (pigment) of red blood cells (i.e. erythrocytes), that is recovered (from old red blood cells) and recycled into making bile (a liquid that aids the digestive process) by the liver.
- **Binary vector system:** A two plasmid system in *Agrobacterium tumefaciens* for gene transfer in plant cells. One plasmid contains the virulence gene for infection which is responsible for transfer of T-DNA present on other plasmid. The other plasmid contains the T-DNA borders, the selectable marker and the DNA to be transferred.
- **Binding affinity:** Measure of the strength of interaction between two molecules.
- **Binding:** The ability of molecules to stick to each other because of the exact shape and chemical nature of parts of their surfaces. Many biological molecules bind extremely tightly and specifically to other molecules—enzymes to their substrates, antibodies to their antigens, DNA strands to their complementary strands and so on. Binding can be characterized by a binding constant or association constant (K_a), or its inverse, the dissociation constant (K_d).
- **Binomial expansion:** The probability that an event will occur 0, 1, 2....n times out of n. It is given by the successive terms of the expression $(p+q)n$, where p is the probability of the event occurring, and $q = 1 - p$.
- **Binomial nomenclature:** In biology, each species is generally identified by two terms, the first is the genus to which it belongs,

and the second is the specific epithet that distinguishes it from others in that genus (e.g. Quercus suber, cork oak).

B

- **Binucleate pollen:** A pollen having two nuclei, produced by the first pollen having two nuclei, produced by the first pollen mitosis; most suitable stage for anther culture.
- **Bio:** A prefix derived from bios and used in scientific words to associate the concept of "living organisms".
- **Bioaccumulation:** Concentration of as chemical agent (e.g. DDT) in the increasing amount in the organism of a food chain.
- **Bioassay:** A procedure for the assessment of a substance by measuring its effect in living cells or an organisms.
- **Bioaugmentation:** Increasing the activity of bacteria that decompose pollutants, a technique used in bioremediation.
- **Biobased products:** Fuels, chemicals, building materials, or electric power or heat produced from biological materials. The term may include any energy, commercial or industrial products, other than food or feed, that uses biological products or renewable domestic agricultural (plant, animal and marine), or forestry materials.
- **Biobutanol:** Butanol produced by microorganisms from biomass.
- **Biocatalysis:** The aim of biocatalysis is to produce a wide variety of chemical substances efficiently in a single step by means of microorganisms or enzymes. Traditional chemical processes are usually more expensive because they require several synthesis steps.
- **Biocatalyst:** Use of enzymes to catalyze chemical reactions.
- **Biochemical pesticides:** These are naturally occurring substances that control pest by nontoxic means. These pesticides include natural insect growth regulators, e.g. neem insecticide and insect pheromones that disrupt mating and reduce reproductive rates.
- **Biochemistry:** The study of chemical processes that comprise living things (systems); the chemistry of life and living matter. Despite the dramatic differences in the appearances of living things, the basic chemistry of all organisms is strikingly similar. Even tiny one-celled creatures carry out essentially the same chemical reactions that each cell of a complex organism (such as man) carries out (Fig. 7).

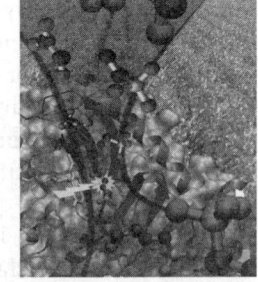

Fig. 7: Biochemistry

- **Biochip:** A term first used with regard to an electronic device that utilizes biological molecules as the framework for other molecules acting as semiconductors and functioning as an integrated circuit. 1. During the 1990s, this term also became commonly used to refer to various laboratories on a chip to: (a) Analyze very small samples of DNA, (b) Assess the impact of pharmaceuticals—or pharmaceutical drug candidate molecules—on specific cells (i.e. attached to the biochip's surface) or on specific cellular receptors (ligand-receptor response of cell), (c) Size and sort DNA fragments (genes) via the (proportional) fluorescence of dyes intercalated in the DNA molecules, (d) Detect presence of specific DNA fragments (genes) via hybridization to a probe (that was fabricated onto the chip), (e) Size and sort protein molecules (via various cells fabricated onto the chip), (f) Assess pharmaceuticals via adhesion molecules attached to the chip, (g) Detect specific pathogens or cancerous cells in a blood sample (e.g. by applying controlled electrical fields to cause those cells to collect at electrodes on the chip), (h) Screen for compounds that act against a disease (e.g. by applying antibodies linked to fluorescent molecules, then measuring electronically the fluorescence triggered by antibody-binding), (i) Conduct gene expression analysis by measuring the fluorescence of messenger RNA (specific to which particular gene is turned on) when that mRNA hybridizes with DNA (from genome) on hybridization surface on the chip. 2. Shortly after the 1990s, several companies manufactured biochips capable of sequencing (determining the sequence of) DNA samples. Such biochips have, attached to their surfaces, all possible DNA probes (short sequences of DNA). The sample (i.e. the unknown DNA molecule) is passed over

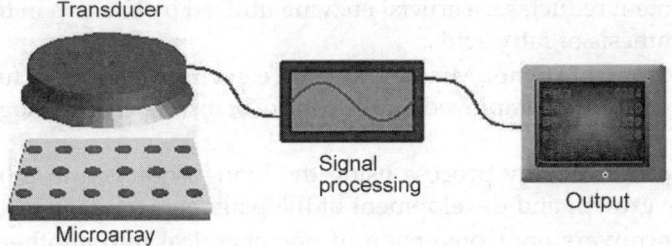

Fig. 8: Biochip

B

the probe-covered surface of the biochip, where each relevant segment (within the large unknown DNA molecule) hybridizes (pairs) with the short DNA probe attached to a known location on the surface of the biochip. Because the sequence of each DNA probe — at each specified location on the biochip — is known, that information (i.e. the probes' sequences to which the unknown DNA molecule hybridized) is then used to assemble the complete sequence of the unknown DNA molecule. 3. Sometimes refers to an electronic device that uses biological molecules as the framework for other molecules that act as semiconductors and function as an integrated circuit. The future working parts of the science of bioelectronics, biochips may consist of two- or three-dimensional arrays of organic molecules used as switching or memory elements. If biochip technology proves to be feasible, one application will be to shrink currently existing biosensors in size. This would enable the biosensors to be implanted in the body or in organs and tissues for the sake of monitoring and controlling certain bodily functions. A future possibility is to try to provide sight for the blind using lightsensitive (e.g. protein-covered electrode) biochips implanted in the eyes to replace a damaged retina. For example, during 2001, Alan Chow implanted such biochips into several men whose retinas had been damaged by the disease retinitis pigmentosa (Fig. 8).

- **Biocidal agents:** Agents that kill the susceptible microorganisms.
- **Biocide:** Any chemical or chemical compound that is toxic to living things (systems). Literally biokiller or killer of biological systems. Includes insecticides, bactericides, fungicides, etc. Most bactericides accomplish their task (killing bacteria) via massive lysis (disintegration) of bacteria cell walls (membranes). However, one (triclosan) kills bacteria by inhibiting enoyl-acyl protein reductase; a crucial enzyme utilized by bacteria in their synthesis of fatty acids.
- **Biocontrol agents:** Microorganisms, e.g. viruses, bacteria, fungi and protozoa employed for the control of insect pests, pathogens or weeds.
- **Biocontrol:** Any process using the living organism to inhibit the growth and development of the pathogenic organisms.
- **Bioconversion:** Conversion of one chemical into another by living organisms, as opposed to their organisms, as opposed to

their conversion (which is biotransformation) or by chemical processes.

- **Biodegradable:** Capable of being biologically decomposed by microorganisms or enzymes.

- **Biodegradation:** The gradual breakdown of a compound to its constituents by a living organism.

- **Biodesulfurization:** The removal of organic and inorganic sulfur (a pollution source) from coal by bacterial and soil micro-organisms.

- **Biodiesel:** Diesel obtained from conversion of hydrocarbons accumulated by certain plants (Fig. 9).

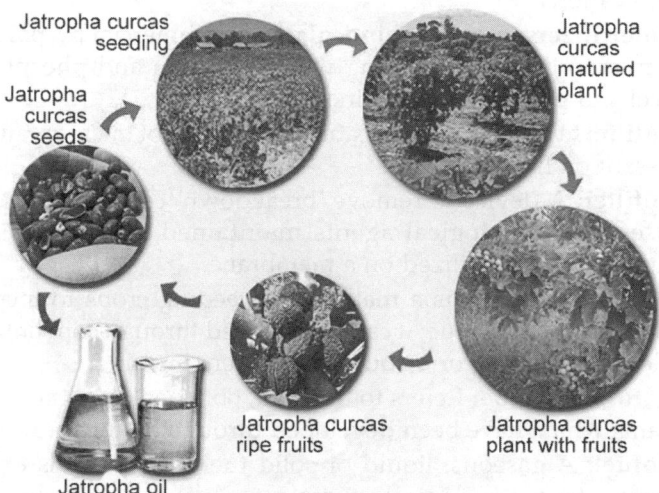

Fig. 9: Biodiesel

- **Biodiversity:** The variability among the living organism from all sources, soil, water, air, extreme habitat or associated with organisms.

- **Bioelectronics:** Also called biomolecular electronics. It is the field where biotechnology is crossed with electronics. The branch of biotechnology that deals with the electroactive properties of biological materials, systems, and processes, together with their exploitation in electronic devices. Bioelectronics will attempt to replace traditional semiconductor materials (e.g. silicon or gallium arsenide) with organic materials such as proteins (biochips).

B

- **Bioenergetics:** The study of the flow and the transformations of energy that occur in living organisms.
- **Bioengineering:** The use of artificial tissues, organs and organ components to replace parts of the body that are damaged, lost or malfunctioning.
- **Bioenrichment:** Adding nutrients or oxygen to increase microbial breakdown of pollutants.
- **Bioethanol:** Ethanol produced from biomass by microorganisms.
- **Bioethics:** 1. The branch of ethics that deals with the life sciences and their potential impact on society. 2. A discipline dealing with the ethical implications of biological research and applications.
- **Biofertilizers (microbial inoculants):** Commercial preparation of microorganisms by using which nitrogen and phosphorus level and growth of plants increased.
- **Biofilm:** In sewage water treatment; the layer of microorganisms present on filter particles.
- **Biofilter:** A device to remove/breakdown/convert hazardous gases using biological agents maintained either in a solid support or immobilized on a membrane.
- **Biofortification:** It is a method of breeding crops to increase their nutritional value; it can be achieved through conventional selective breeding or through genetic engineering.
- **Biofortified food:** Refers to the food, obtained from those crop plants which have been developed through biofortification.
- **Biofuel:** A gaseous, liquid or solid fuel that contains energy derived from a biological source.
- **Biogas:** A mixture of methane and carbon dioxide resulting from the anaerobic decomposition of waste such as domestic, industrial and agricultural sewage, aka gobar.
- **Biogenesis:** The principle that a living organism can only arise from other living organisms similar to itself and can never originate from nonliving material.
- **Biogeochemistry:** A branch of geochemistry that is concerned with biological materials and their relation to earth's chemicals in an area.
- **Bioherbicides:** Biological agents, mainly fungi and insects, used for control of weeds.
- **Biohydrogen:** Hydrogen produced by biological agents.

- **Bioinformatics:** It is a science associated to biomolecular database like activities involving persistent sets of data that are maintained in a consistent state over essentially indefinite periods of time (Fig. 10).

B

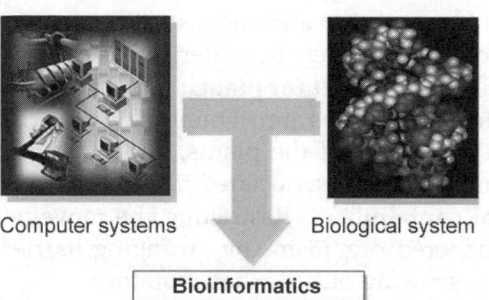

Computer systems   Biological system

Bioinformatics

Fig. 10: Bioinformatics

- **Bioinorganic:** This term refers to the combination of organic (life) materials with inorganic materials to create (useful materials). For example, Abalone shellfish make their shells via a combination of protein and calcium carbonate. Researchers are working on making semiconductor devices (chips) containing peptides, etc. attached to silicon or gallium arsenide.
- **Bioinsecticides:** Use of biocontrol agents of their byproducts including plant extracts to control insect pests.
- **Bioleaching:** Solubilization of metals in the ores by using a solution containing specific microorganisms.
- **Biolistic® Gene Gun:** The word biolistic was coined from the words biological and ballistic (pertaining to a projectile fired from a gun). Used to shoot pellets that are coated with genes (for desired traits) into plant seeds or plant tissues, in order to get those plants to then express the new genes. The gun uses an actual explosive (22 caliber blank) to propel the material. Compressed air or steam may also be used as the propellant. The Biolistic® Gene Gun was invented in 1983–1984 at Cornell University by John Sanford, Edward Wolf, and Nelson Allen. The gun and its registered trademark are now owned by E. I. du Pont de Nemours and company.
- **Biolistics:** A technique to insert DNA into cells. Also known as microprojectile bombardment or particle bombardment.

B

- **Biological activity:** The effect (change in metabolic activity upon living cells) caused by specific compounds or agents. For example, the drug aspirin causes the blood to thin, i.e. to clot less easily.
- **Biological boundaries:** A concept that differentiates one organism from another and suggests that organisms cannot or should not exchange genetic material.
- **Biological containment for plants:** In case of plants, biological containment procedures aim at minimizing the risk of dispersal of pollen and seeds of the plants, and of dissemination and establishment of plant-associated microorganisms and insects.
- **Biological containment:** Restricting the movement of genetically engineered organisms by arranging barriers to prevent them from growing outside the laboratory.
- **Biological control:** Use of biological agents to control insect pests, pathogens, or weeds.
- **Biological diversity:** Biological diversity called biodiversity in short, refers to the diversity present among all living organisms found in natural world; this concept includes diversity among species, ecosystems and genetic diversity within a given species.
- **Biological indicators:** Organisms, whose relative abundance/absence in river water serves as a good indicator of the level of pollution.
- **Biological information:** Refers to the information present in the genome of an organism.
- **Biological invasion:** When exotic species introduced in new areas and native species are subject to competition for food and space and the exotic species eliminate the native species.
- **Biological nutrient removal:** A process employed in sewage treatment to remove nitrogen and phosphorous from the effluent coming from secondary treatment.
- **Biological oxygen demand (BOD):** The oxygen used in meeting the metabolic needs of aerobic organisms in water containing organic compounds. Numerically, it is expressed in terms of the oxygen consumed in water at a temperature of 68°F (20°C) during a 5-day period. The BOD is used as an indication of the degree of water pollution.
- **Biological resistance:** Ability of an insect population to develop enzymes that detoxify an insecticide or other injurious before it can reach its site of action.

- **Biological wealth:** The life sustaining combination of commercial, scientific and esthetic values imparted to a region by its biota.
- **Biologics:** Agents, such as vaccines, that give immunity to diseases or harmful biotic stresses.
- **Biology:** From the two Greek words *bios* (life) and *logos* (word), it is the field of science encompassing the study of life.
- **Bioluminescence:** The enzyme-catalyzed production of light by living organisms, typically during mating or hunting. This word literally means *living light*. First identified/analyzed in 1947 by William McElroy, bioluminescence results when the enzyme luciferase comes into contact with adenosine triphosphate (ATP)/luciferin, inside the photophores (organs which emit the light) of the organism. Such production of light by living organisms is exemplified by fireflies, South America's railroad worm, and by many deep ocean marine organisms. Bioluminescence has been utilized by man as a genetic marker (e.g. to cause a genetically engineered plant to glow as evidence that a gene was successfully transferred into that plant). Another use of bioluminescence by man is for the rapid detection of foodborne pathogenic bacteria (e.g. in a food processing factory).
- **Biomagnification:** Progressive increase in the concentration of a lipid soluble xenobiotic compound as it passes through the food chain.
- **Biomass concentration:** The amount of biological material in a specific volume.
- **Biomass energy:** Energy produced by burning plant related materials such as firewood.
- **Biomass:** 1. The cell mass produced by a population of living organisms. 2. All organic matter grown by the photosynthetic conversion of solar energy (e.g. plants) and organic matter from animals.
- **Biome:** A major ecological community or complex of communities, extending over a large geographical area and characterized by a dominant type of vegetation.
- **BioMEMS:** Refers to MEMS designed to work within biological systems/organisms. Examples include microfluidic cell sorters, or a biochip possessing diverging nanometer scale etched

B

channels and a fluorescence detector. Via an electrical field that would drive electrophoretic separation of DNA (fragments), samples of DNA could be separated/sorted/identified by fluorescence.

- **Biomethane:** Methane produced by biological agents.
- **Biometry:** The application of statistical methods to the analysis of biological problems.
- **Biomimetic materials:** Synthetic (man-made) molecules or systems that are analogues of natural (made by living organisms) materials. For instance, molecules have been synthesized by man that act chemically like natural proteins, but are not as easily degraded by the digestive system (as are those natural protein molecules). Other systems, such as reverse micelles and/or liposomes, exhibit certain properties that mimic certain aspects of living systems.
- **Biomining:** Solubilization and recovery of metals and ores.
- **Biomotors:** Refers to biologically based technologies/techniques used to power nanometer-size machines (e.g. nanobots) in one way or another. For example, during 2000 Bernard Yurke and colleagues created a molecular-machine tweezers (grasper) consisting of three separate strands of DNA (two of them were hybridized separately to small complementary sequences near the two ends of the first DNA strand). The tweezers can then be closed (or opened) by sequentially adding other DNA strands (to the three) which can hybridize to small complementary sequences on second and third strands, or hybridize to the fourth strand, causing it to unhybridize from the second and the third strands.
- **Bionics:** An interscience discipline for constructing artificial systems that resemble or have the characteristics of living systems. Bionics can encompass (in whole, or in part) bioelectronics, biosensors, biomimetic materials, biophysics, biomotors, and self-assembly (of a large molecular structure).
- **Biopesticides:** Commercial preparation of microorganisms by using which insects, termite or nematode pests are killed or their level is minimized and crop yield increased.
- **Biopharmaceuticals:** Biotechnology products having pharmaceutical applications.
- **Biopharming:** The production of biopharmaceuticals in plants or domestic animals.

- **Biophysics:** An area of scientific study in which physical principles, physical methods, and physical instrumentation are used to study living systems or systems related to life. It overlaps with biophysical chemistry, which is more specialized in scope since it is concerned with the physical study of chemically isolated substances found in living organisms.

- **Biopolymer:** A high molecular weight organic compound found in nature, whose structure can be represented by a repeated small unit [i.e. monomer (links)]. Common biopolymers include cellulose (long-chain sugars found in most plants and the main constituent of dried woods, jute, flax, hemp, cotton, etc.) and proteins in general, and specifically collagen and gelatin.

- **Biopolymer:** Any polymer such as protein, nucleic acids, lipids, polysaccharide, produced by a living organism.

- **Bioprocess:** Any process that uses complete living cells or their components (e.g. enzymes, chloroplasts) to effect desired physical or chemical changes.

- **Bioreactor:** A vessel, i.e. fermenter used for fermentation or other processes.

- **Bioreceptors:** Refers to fragments of DNA, antibodies, protein molecules, and cellular probes (e.g. adhesion molecule) when those are attached to a man-made surface (e.g. biochip) for purposes of analyzing biological substances.

- **Biorecovery:** The use of organisms (including bacteria, plants, fungi, and algae) in the recovery (collecting) of various metals and/or organic compounds from ores or garbage (other matrices).

- **Bioremediation:** The process of using organisms to remove contaminants, pollution or unwanted substances from soil or water.

- **Bioseeds:** Plant seeds produced via genetic engineering of existing plants.

- **Biosensors (chemical):** Chemically based devices that are able to detect and/or measure the presence of certain molecules (DNA, antigens, pesticides, etc.). These devices are currently created in the following forms: 1. A two-part diagnostic test that can detect the presence of trace amounts of specific chemicals (e.g. pesticides). The (chemical) biosensor consists of an immobilized enzyme (to bind the trace chemical) combined with a color reagent (to indicate visually the presence of the

B

trace chemical). 2. A one-part test that can detect specific DNA segments in complex (dirty, multiple component) samples. The biosensor consists of 13 nm gold particles onto which are attached numerous nucleotide molecular chains. Each nucleotide chain contains 28 nucleotides. The 13 nucleotides that are closest to each gold particle serve as a spacer, and solutions containing such (spaced) randomly distributed gold particles appear red in color when illuminated by light. The 15 nucleotides that are farthest from each gold particle are chosen to be complementary to, and thus bind to, nucleotide sequences in the target (e.g. DNA) molecule. In the presence of the specific target molecule, a closely linked network of gold particles and double-stranded nucleotide molecular chains forms (overcoming the 13 nucleotide spacer which previously held the gold particles apart). When double-stranded chains form (i.e. target molecule is present), the distance between gold particles becomes less than the size of those particles, making the solution containing (bound) particles appear blue in color when illuminated by light.

- **Biosensors (electronic):** Electronic sensors that are able to detect and measure the presence of biomolecules such as sugars or DNA segments. Currently created by: 1. Fusing organic matter (e.g. enzymes, antibodies, receptors, or nucleic acids) to tiny electrodes; yielding devices that convert natural chemical reactions into electric current to measure blood levels of certain chemicals (e.g. glucose or insulin), control functions in an artificial organ, monitor some industrial processes, act as a robot's nose, etc. 2. Fusing organic matter (segment of DNA, antibody, enzyme, etc.) onto the surfaces of etched silicon wafers; yielding devices that convert supramolecular interactions [e.g. nucleotide hybridization, enzyme-substrate binding, lectin-carbohydrate (sugar) interactions, antibody-antigen binding, host-guest complexation, etc.] into electric current via a charge-coupled device (CCD) detector. The CCD detector measures the shift in interference pattern caused by change in refractive index that results when the (sensed) molecule tightly binds to the fused (electronic) organic matter. For such an etched-silicon-wafer biosensor, the nucleotide hybridization (binding) enables the detection of femtomolar (10–15 mole or 0.000000000000001) concentrations of DNA. If the (sensed) DNA segment is not complementary to the fused DNA segment, there is no significant change in the interference pattern. A major goal is to build future generations of biosensors directly into **B** computer chips. (Researchers have discovered that proteins can replace certain metals in semiconductors.) This would enable low-cost mass production via processes similar to those now used for existing semiconductor chips, with circuits built right into the sensor to process data picked up by the biological matter on the chip.

- **Biosilk:** A biomimetic, man-made fiber produced by: 1. Sequencing the dragline silk protein that is produced by the orb-weaving spider, 2. Synthesizing genes to code for the dragline silk protein (components), 3. Expressing those genes in a suitable host (i.e. yeast, bacteria) to cause production of the protein(s), 4. Dissolving the protein in a solvent, and then spinning the protein into fiber form by passing the liquid (dissolved protein) through a small orifice, followed by drying to remove the solvent.

- **Biosorbents:** Microorganisms which, either by themselves or in conjunction with a support/substrate system (e.g. inert granules) effect the extraction (e.g. from ore) and/or concentration of desired (precious) metals or organic compounds by means of selective retention of those entities. Retention of organic compounds (e.g. gasoline) may be for the purpose of cleaning polluted soil.

- **Biosource:** A patented technology that permits a rapid and effective elucidation of functions of unknown gene/DNA sequences.

- **Biosphere reserves:** Natural areas set aside to protect genetic biodiversity.

- **Biosphere:** The part of the earth and its atmosphere that is inhabited by living organisms.

- **Biostatic agents:** They inhibit growth and multiplication of susceptible microorganisms.

- **Biosurface:** The region on a biological protein, enzyme or receptor that acts as a binding site for ligands or other molecules.

- **Biosynthesis:** Synthesis of compounds by living cells, which is the essential feature of anabolism.

- **Biota:** The sum total of all living organisms of a region.

- **Biotechnology industry organization (BIO):** An American Trade Association composed of companies and individuals involved in biotechnology and in services to biotechnology companies (accounting, law, etc.). Formed in 1993, the BIO was created by the merger of its two predecessor trade associations — the Association of Biotechnology Companies (ABC) and the Industrial Biotechnology Association (IBA). The BIO works with the government and the public to promote safe and rational advancement of genetic engineering and biotechnology.

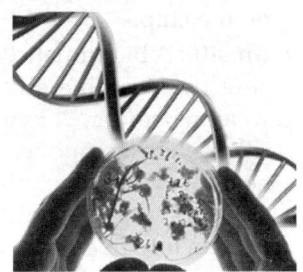

- **Biotechnology:** The scientific manipulation of living organisms, especially at the molecular genetic level, to produce useful products. Gene splicing and use of recombinant DNA (rDNA) are major techniques used (Fig. 11).

Fig. 11: Biotechnology

- **Biotic elicitor:** An elicitor of biological origin; usually, a component of cell wall, e.g. pectin, pectic acid, chitin, chitosan.

- **Biotic factor:** Other living organisms that are a factor of an organism's environment, and form the biotic environment, affecting the organism in many ways.

- **Biotic stress:** 1. Living organisms which can harm plants, such as viruses, fungi, and bacteria, and harmful insects. 2. Stress resulting from living organisms which can harm plants, such as viruses, fungi, bacteria, parasitic weeds and harmful insects.

- **Biotin:** A vitamin of the B-complex. It is a co-enzyme for various enzymes that catalyze the incorporation of carbon dioxide into various compounds (Fig. 12).

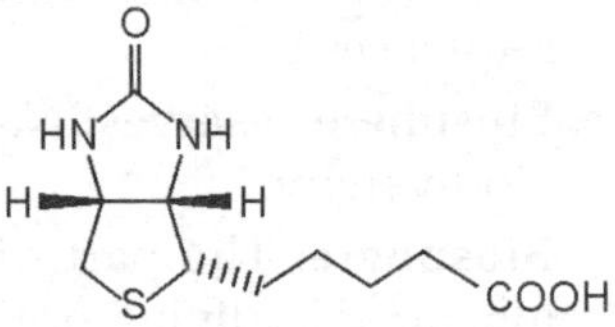

Fig. 12: Biotin

- **Biotope:** A small habitat in a large community.

- **Biotoxin:** A naturally produced toxic compound which shows pronounced biological activity and presumably has some adaptive significance to the organism which produces it.

- **Biotransformation (of an introduced compound):** Biological portion of definition of *persistence*.

- **Biotransformation or bioconversion:** The use of cultured cells to convert substrates into desired organic compounds by the virtue of an endogenous enzyme which catalyzes the reaction.

- **Biphase liquid system:** It consists of two immiscible liquids in which the enzyme is able to function and remains fairly stable; two types: aqueous two-phase systems and aqueous-organic two-phase systems.
- **Bipolar germination:** In most angiosperms; development of roots and shoots from different poles of the embryo.
- **Bispecific monoclonal antibody:** A hybrid antibody specific for two different epitopes; usually, each epitope belong to a different antigen.
- **Bithorax complex:** It is a group of homeotic genes which are responsible for the diversification of the different segments of the fly.
- **Bivalent:** Having two binding sites with two free electrons available for binding (Fig. 13).
- **bla gene:** A gene that confers resistance to β-lactam antibiotics (e.g. ampicillin).
- **Black-layered (corn):** An indicator of a corn plant's maturity. It refers to a distinctive dark line that forms in each corn kernel at maturity.
- **B-lactamase:** An ampicillin resistance gene.
- **Blast cell:** A large, rapidly dividing cell that develops from a B-cell (B lymphocyte) in response to an antigenic stimulus. The blast cell then becomes an antibody-producing plasma cell.

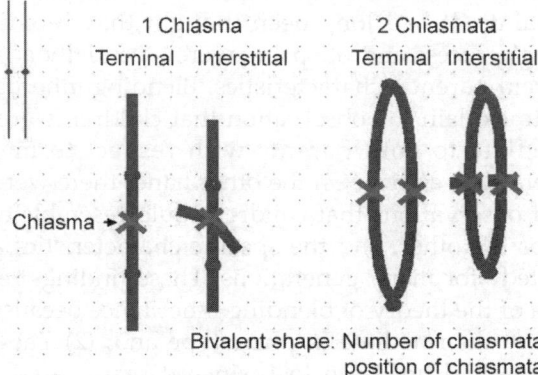

Fig. 13: Bivalent

B

- **Blast transformation:** The process through which a B cell (B lymphocyte) becomes a blast cell.
- **Blastocyst:** A mammalian embryo (fertilized ovum) in the early stages of development, approximately up to the time of implantation. It consists of a hollow ball of cells.
- **Blastomere:** Any one of the cells formed from the first few cleavages in animal embryology. The embryo usually divides into two, then four, then eight blastomeres, and so on.
- **Blastula:** In animals, an early embryo form that follows the morula stage, typically a single-layered sheet (blastoderm) or ball of cells (blastocyst).
- **Bleach:** A fluid, powder or other whitening (bleaching) or cleaning agent, usually with free chlorine ions. Commercial bleach contains calcium hypochlorite or sodium hypochlorite, and is a common disinfectant used for cleaning working surfaces, tools and plant materials in plant tissue culture and grafting.
- **Bleeding:** Used to describe the occasional purplish-black coloration of media due to phenolic products given off by (usually fresh) transfer.
- **Blending theory of inheritance:** According to this view the hereditary material was pictured as some sort of fluid, perhaps even blood. The fluid of two parents would come together and blend in some fashion. If this were true, then all of Mendel's F_1 plants would have exhibited an intermediate expression. It would be impossible to separate these hereditary fluids, just as one would fail in an attempt to separate a mixture of red and white paints. It had long been thought that heredity was a 'blending' process and offspring were essentially a "dilution" of different parental characteristics. Blending inheritance thus helped to explain the observation that children were at times intermediate to both parents with respect to measurable characters such as size. On the other hand, there were also the frequent observations that children could resemble either one parent or the other, and the specific characteristics appeared "undiluted" for many generations. These findings resulted in rejection of the theory of blending inheritance because: (1) The F_1 was not intermediate in phenotype and; (2) The recessive phenotype had not been lost, since it reappeared in the F_2 progeny.

- **Blocked reading frame:** It cannot be translated into protein because of the occurrence of termination codons.
- **Blood derivatives manufacturing association:** A trade organization of firms involved in producing pharmaceuticals from collected blood.
- **Blood-brain barrier:** A network of blood vessels with closely spaced cells that makes it difficult for potentially toxic substances (or therapeutic drugs) to penetrate the blood vessel walls and enter the brain.
- **Blot transfer:** Transfer of blot from a gel to a membrane filter.
- **Blot:** A spot on membrane filter gel made by adopting a solution.
- **Blotting:** The process of transferring DNA, RNA, or protein from a polyacrylamide or agarose gel to a nitrocellulose filter for further analysis (for examples see Southern, Northern and Western blotting).
- **Blunt-end cut:** To cleave phosphodiester bonds in the backbone of duplex DNA between the corresponding nucleotide pairs on opposite strands. This cleavage process results in both strands finishing at the same residue, i.e. there are no nucleotide extensions on either strand, aka flush-end cut.
- **Blunt-end DNA:** A segment of DNA that has both strands terminating at the same basepair location, that is, fully base-paired DNA. No sticky ends.
- **Blunt-end ligation:** A method of joining blunt-ended DNA fragments using the enzyme T4 ligase, which can join fully basepaired, double-stranded DNA.
- **Bone marrow:** The site of origination of stem cells which are the precursors of all blood and immune cells.
- **Bone morphogenetic proteins (BMPs):** A family of protein-aceous growth factors (nine identified as of 1994) for bone tissue formation (e.g. at the site where a bone has been broken). BMPs stimulate a recruitment of bone-forming cells (to the site of bone injury) which first form cartilage, then mineralize that cartilage to form bone.
- **Bonus trait:** When progeny from a somatic hybrid possess some novel feature not present in their fusion parents; such a feature is called bonus trait.
- **Booster (Vaccination):** The secondary immunization sometimes required to 'boost' of increase the weak immune response obtained from the first immunization.

B

- **Boring platform:** Sterile bottom half of a petridish, used for preparing explants with a cork borer.
- **Botanical insecticides:** An insecticides produced from a plant or plant product, e.g. pyrethrum.
- **Bound water:** Water held by the cell and not released if fertilizing occurs in the intracellular space.
- **Boundary:** Edge of a zone; as of macromolecule solution next to the solvent.
- **Bovine somatotrophin (bst):** Bovine growth hormone, this protein is found naturally in cattle, and is the bovine counterpart of human growth hormone, one of the earliest biopharmaceutical products. It has been cloned, using recombinant DNA technology, expressed in large amounts and marketed as an agricultural product to improve the growth rate and protein, fat ratios in farm cattle, and to improve milk yield its use is banned in some countries.
- **Bovine spongiform encephalopathy (BSE):** Mad cow disease. It is hypothesized to be caused by a prion, or small protein, which alters the structure of a normal brain protein, resulting in destruction of brain neural tissue.
- **Bp:** Abbreviation for base pair.
- **Bract:** A modified leaf that subtrands flowers or inflorescences and may appear to be a petal.
- **Bradykinin:** A kinin involved in inflammatory reactions, generated following tissue injury. Bradykinin is involved in vasodilation, smooth muscle contraction, and increased vascular permeability, and is an important target for anti-inflammatory drugs.
- **Branch migration:** It describes the ability of a DNA strand partially paired with its complement in a duplex to extend its pairing by displacing the resident strand with which it is homologous.
- **Branch site:** It is a short sequence just before the end of an intron at which the lariat intermediate is formed in splicing by joining the 5′ nucleotide of the intron to the 2′ position of an adenosine.
- *Brassica*: A fast-growing category of the mustard plant family, which also produces sulfur-based gases (a natural defense against certain fungi, nematodes, and insect pests). For example, Australian CSIRO scientists discovered in 1994 that sulfur-based

isothiocyanates emitted by *Brassica* actively combat Wheat Take-All Disease (a fungal disease that attacks the roots of the wheat plant) (Fig. 14).

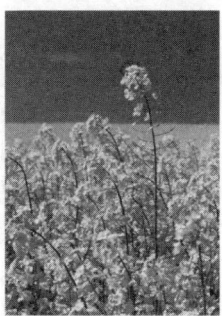

Fig. 14: Brassica

- **BRCA genes:** Oncogenes that, when mutated, can cause development of breast cancer or ovarian cancer. All humans possess BRCA genes of one sort or another (the acronym BRCA stands for breast cancer). However, the two specific BRCA genes most likely to lead to breast cancer (BRCA 1 and BRCA 2) are present in only 2% of women who are of Northern European ancestry, most Caucasian women in the US, and Askenazi Jews whose ancesters are from Central and Eastern Europe. Those women possessing the BRCA 1 gene in their genome (DNA) have a 20–40% chance of developing ovarian cancer (and a 50–85% chance of developing breast cancer) in their lifetime. Those women possessing the BRCA 2 gene in their genome (DNA) have a 15–20% chance of developing ovarian cancer (and a 55–85% chance of developing breast cancer) in their lifetimes.

- **BrdU (5-bromodeoxyuridine):** A mutagenically active analog of thymidine in which the methyl group at 5 positions is replaced by bromine.

- **Breakage and reunion:** Describes the mode of genetic recombination, in which two DNA duplex molecules are broken at corresponding points and then rejoined crosswise (involving formation of a length of heteroduplex DNA around the site of joining).

- **Breakage-fusion-bridge cycle:** A type of chromosomal behavior in which a broken chromatid fuses to its sister, forming a bridge. When the centromeres separate at mitosis, the chromosome breaks again (not necessarily at the bridge), thereby restarting the cycle.

- **Breal:** A gene located on chromosome 17, that in its defective form predisposes some individuals to breast, ovary, and prostate cancer.

- **Breed at risk:** Any breed that may become extinct if the factors causing its decline in numbers are not eliminated or mitigated. Breeds may be in danger to becoming extinct for a variety of reasons. Risk of extinction may result from inter alia, low

B

population size, direct and indirect impacts of policy at the farm, country or international levels, lack of proper breed organization or lack of adaptation to market demands.

- **Breed not at risk:** A breed where the total number of breeding females and males is greater than 1,000 and 20, respectively or the population size approaches 1,000 and the percentage of pure-breed females is close to 100%, and the overall population size is increasing.
- **Breed:** 1. A subspecific group of domestic livestock with definable and identifiable external characteristics that enable it to be separated by visual appraisal from other similarly defined groups within the same species or; 2. A group of domestic livestock for which geographical and/or cultural separation from phenotypically similar groups has led to acceptance of its separate identity breed at risk, breed not at risk critical breed, critical-maintained breed endangered-maintained breed.
- **Breeder's exemption:** Under plant breeder rights (PBR) regime; the use of a protected variety (the initial variety) for the development of new varieties is exempted from protection.
- **Breeding:** 1. In classical plant breeding methods suitable cross breeding partners are selected in an attempt to provide plants with the desired characteristics. The result, however, is dependent on chance. Modern biotechnology is able to produce organisms with specially selected characteristics. 2. The process of sexual reproduction and production of offspring.
- **Brewer's yeast:** Strains of yeast, often *Saccharomyces cerevislae* that are used in the production of beer.
- **Brewing:** The process by which beer is made. In the first stage, the barley grain is soaked in water and allowed to germinate (malting) during which the natural enzymes of the grain convert the seed starch to maltose and then to glucose. Grain is then dried, crushed, and added to water at a specific temperature (steeping) and any remaining starch is converted to sugar. The resulting liquid (wort) is the raw material to which yeast is added to convert sugar to alcohol.
- **Bridge:** A filter paper or other substrate used as a wick and support structure for a plant tissue in culture when a liquid medium is used.
- **Bright greenish-yellow fluorescence (BGYF):** An indication of the presence of fungus (e.g. in a sample of grain), when light of

an appropriate wavelength is shone on sample. For example, when the fungus *Aspergillus flavus* infects cottonseed during boll development on the cotton plant, the resultant seed (when harvested) shows BGYF on its lint and linters. That fungus gains entry into the bolls typically via holes made by the pink bollworm (*Pectinophora gossypiella*).

- **Broad–host – range plasmid:** A plasmid that can replicate in a number of different bacterial species.

- **Broad-sense heritability:** In quantitative genetics, the proportion of the total phenotypic variation due to genetic variation.

- **Bromoxynil:** An active ingredient in some herbicides, it kills certain types of plants (weeds).

- **Broth:** In fermentation; the medium containing both products and microorganism biomass.

- **Brown stem rot (BSR):** A plant disease that can be caused by the soilborne fungus *Phialaphora gregata* in the soybean plant (*Glycine max L. Merrill*). Some soybean varieties are genetically resistant to BSR.

- **Browning:** Discoloration due to phenolic oxidation of freshly cut surfaces of explant tissue. In later stages of culture, such discoloration may indicate a nutritional or pathogenic problem, generally leading to necrosis.

- **Brucellosis:** Disease caused by infection with organisms of the genus *Brucella*.

- **BSE:** Bovine spongiform encephalopathy. A neurodegenerative disease of cattle.

- **Bubble column fermenter:** A fermentation vessel, or bioreactor, in which the cells or microorganisms are kept suspended in a tall cylinder by rising air, which is introduced at the base of the vessel.

- **Bud pollination:** Pollination of flower buds a couple of days, before anthesis, before the stigmas are fully receptive; used to overcome both gametophytic and sporophytic self-incompatibility.

- **Bud scar:** A scar left on a shoot when the bud or bud scales drop.

- **Bud sport:** A somatic mutation arising in a bud and producing a genetically different shoot. Bud sports include changes due to gene mutation, somatic reduction, and chromosome deletion or polyploidy.

B

- **Bud:** A region of meristematic tissue with the potential for developing into leaves, shoots, flowers or combinations, generally protected by modified scale leaves. A terminal or apical bud exists at the tip of a stem or branch, while axillary or lateral bud develops in the axils of leaves.

- **Budding:** A method of asexual reproduction in which a new individual is derived from an outgrowth (bud) that becomes detached from the body of the parent.

- **Buffer:** A solution that maintains the specific pH range needed for a physiological reaction.

- **Buffy coat (cells):** The layer of white blood cells (leukocytes) that separates out when blood is subjected to centrifugation.

- *Bulbosum* **technique:** Production of haploids of wheat or barley by crossing them with *Hordeum bulbosum* ($2n = 4x = 28$); chromosomes of *H. bulbosum* are eliminated during embryo development, and embryo rescue is required specifically for haploid production.

- **Bulked segregant analysis (BSA):** In this method, two bulked DNA samples are drawn from a segregating population originating from a single cross. Each bulk contains DNAs from individuals that are identical for a particular trait but arbitary at all unliked regions. The bulks are screened for DNA polymorphisms; a marker that differs between the two bulks is expected to be linked to the particular trait for which the bulks were created.

- **Bulking agents:** Substances like starch that are added in the food to increase the quantity of a food without affecting its nutritional value.

- **Bundesgesundheitsamt (BGA):** German federal health organization. The German government agency that must approve new pharmaceutical products for sale within Germany, it is the equivalent of the US Food and Drug Administration (US-FDA).

- **Buoyant density:** The intrinsic density, which a molecule, virus or subcellular particle has when suspended in an aqueous solution of a salt, such as CsCl, or a sugar, such as sucrose. DNA from different species has a characteristic buoyant density which reflects the proportion of $G = C$ base pairs. The greater the proportion of $G = C$, the greater the buoyant density of the DNA.

- **Button mushroom:** Fruiting body of *Agaricus bisporus* grown on decomposed horse manure, etc.
- **By stander effect:** The term describing the beneficial therapeutic effects elicited when a primary therapeutic agent triggers events in neighboring cells and tissues via other mediators.
- **Bypass:** A surgical procedure in which a new pathway or the flow of body fluids is created.
- **Bystander effect:** The term describing the beneficial therapeutic effects elicited when a primary therapeutic agent triggers event in neighboring cells and tissues via other mediators.
- **bZIP:** Protein has a basic DNA-binding region adjacent to a leucine zipper dimerization motif.

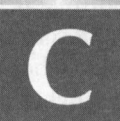

- **C:** Cytosine residue in either DNA or RNA.
- **(Con) cateneted:** (Con) catenated circles of DNA are interlocked like rings on a chain.
- **C genes:** Code for the constant regions of immunoglobulin protein chains.
- **C value:** It is total amount of DNA in a haploid genome.
- **CAAT box:** It is a part of conserved sequence located upstream of the start points of eukaryotic transcription factors. It has the consensus sequence GGCCAATCT; it occurs around 75 bases prior to the transcription initiation site.
- **Cadherins:** A class of (cell surface) adhesion molecules that causes cells (e.g. in the lining of the intestine known as the epithelium) to stick together to form a continuous lining; cadherins sometimes function as cellular adhesion receptors. For example, the (food poisoning) pathogenic bacteria *Listeria monocytogenes* is able to infect humans via its use of the E-cadherin receptor located on the surface of intestinal epithelium cells. That bacteria's key (a bacterial membrane surface protein known as internaulin) is inserted into the E-cadherin (lock), which opens up the otherwise closed-to-bacteria intestinal epithelium. The *L. monocytogenes* bacteria then leave the intestine and infect the human body tissues.
- *Caenorhabditis elegans* **(*C. elegans*):** The name of a nematode (microscopic roundworm) that is commonly utilized by scientists in genetics experiments. Because of this, a large base of knowledge about *C. elegans* genetics has been accumulated by the world's scientific community. For example, of the nearly 300 disease-causing genes in the human genome, more than half of them have an analogous gene within the *C. elegans* genome. *C. elegans* was one of the first animals to have its entire genome sequenced by man. Thus, one of the methodologies utilized by researchers to rapidly screen large numbers of chemical

compounds for their potential use as pharmaceuticals is to—expose large numbers of C. *elegans* to the various chemical compounds that the researcher wants to investigate for potential pharmaceutical activity. Pass those large numbers of previously exposed C. *elegans*, suspended in liquid such as water, through a small transparent chamber where a focused laser beam is shone upon the roundworm's side (for its full length, as the roundworm passes by). Utilize expression-of-fluorescent-protein, autofluorescence, lectin (in the fluid) binding detected via laser reflectance, antibody (in the fluid) binding detected via laser reflectance, etc. as the basis for individual C. *elegans* to be sorted via tiny jets of air that blow into a container those C. *elegans* that show thus visible sign(s) of having been changed by the particular chemical compound to which they were exposed. Evaluate in detail (e.g. via conventional gene expression analysis) the specific impact of that particular chemical compound on those C. *elegans* that had indicated an apparent change, so were sorted into the likely target receptacle.

- **Caffeine:** A chemical naturally produced in some plants (e.g. coffee tree) to repel predatory insects. It also acts as a stimulant (when consumed by humans), so is classified as a phyto-chemical. Research done by Seymour Diamond during 2000 showed that within the human body, caffeine consumption causes interactions with the synthetic chemical painkiller known as Ibuprofen. Consuming both together was shown to be more effective in relieving pain than consuming Ibuprofen alone, and brought pain relief faster than consumption of Ibuprofen alone (Fig. 1).

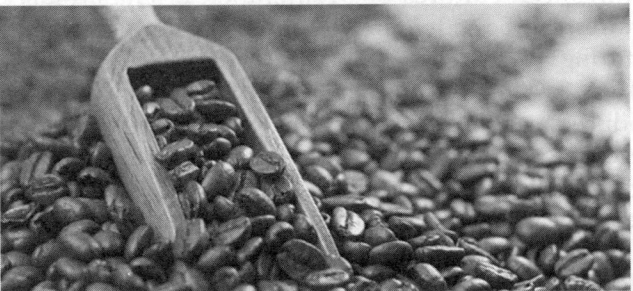

Fig. 1: Caffeine

- **Calcium channel-blockers:** Drugs (e.g. verapamil, amlopidine, diltiazem, nifedipine) used to slow down calcium movement through cell membranes. This leads to dilation of the blood vessels and reduces the heart's workload. Blood vessels need calcium to contract (causing flow constriction and hence an increase in blood pressure), so the drug-induced shortage of available calcium causes the body's blood vessels to remain dilated (which results in lower blood pressure). Research in 1996 indicated the possibility that certain types of calcium channel-blockers might lead to increased rates of some cancers. If so, this is likely due to the drug preventing enough calcium availability for normal apoptosis in body cells.
- **Calcium oxalate:** A crystalline salt normally deposited in the cells of some species of plants. In spinach, the presence of such oxalate inhibits absorption of the calcium (present in spinach) by humans. In many animals, calcium oxalate is excreted in urine or retained by the animal's body in the form of urinary calculi.
- **Calf scours:** A watery diarrhea in calves.
- **Caliclone:** A variant regenerated from a callus culture; *not in common use*.
- **Callipyge:** (Means *beautiful buttocks* in Greek) An inherited trait in livestock (e.g. sheep) that results in thicker, meatier hind quarters. First identified as a genetic trait in 1983, this desirable trait results in a higher meat yield per animal.
- **Callus culture:** A technique of tissue culture. It is usually on solidified medium and initiated by inoculation of small explants or sections from established organ or cultures (the inocula). Callus culture is used as the basis for organogenio (shoot, root) cultures, cell cultures or proliferation of embryoids. Callus cultures can be indefinitely maintained through regular sub-culturing.
- **Callus:** 1. A tissue consisting of differentiated cells generally produced as a result of wounding or of culturing tissues in the presence of an auxin in particular; 2. Actively dividing non-organized masses of undifferentiated and differentiated cells often developing from injury (wounding) or in tissue culture in the presence of growth regulators.
- **Calorie:** Equivalent to the amount of heat required to raise the temperature of 1 gram of water from 14.5°C to 15.5°C (= 4.19J).

- **Calpain-10:** A gene that increases the likelihood for development of diabetes disease in humans whose DNA carries that gene (approximately 80% of humans carry the gene).
- **Calyx:** All the sepal of a flower considered collectively. The outermost whorl of flower parts.
- **Cambial zone:** Region in stems and roots consisting of the cambium and its recent derivatives.
- **Cambium:** A layer, usually regarded as one or two cells thick of persistently meristematic tissue between xylem and phloem tissues, and which gives rise to secondary tissues, thus resulting in an increase in diameter. The two most important cambia are the vascular (fascicular) cambium and the cork cambium (Fig. 2).

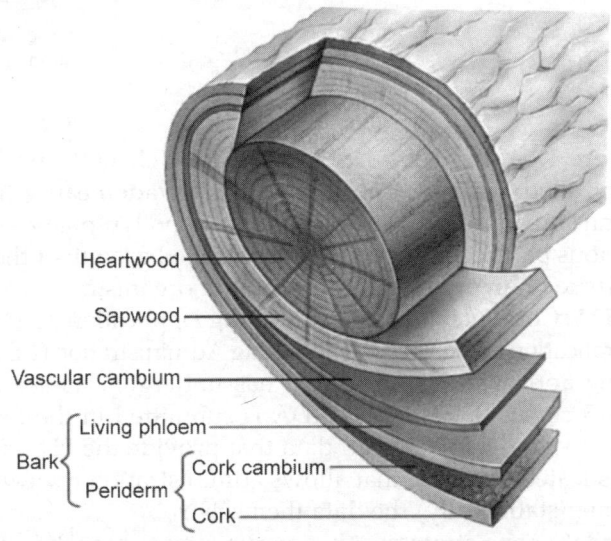

Heartwood
Sapwood
Vascular cambium
Bark { Living phloem
Periderm { Cork cambium
Cork

Fig. 2: Cambium

- **Campesterol:** A phytosterol produced within the seeds of the soybean plant (*Glycine max* L.), among others. Evidence shows human consumption of campesterol helps reduce total serum (blood) cholesterol and low-density lipoproteins (LDLP) levels, thereby lowering risk of coronary heart disease (CHD). Evidence indicates certain phytosterols (including campesterol) interfere with absorption of cholesterol by the intestines, and decrease the body's recovery and reuse of cholesterol-containing bile salts; this causes more (net) cholesterol to be excreted from the body.

- **Canavanine:** An uncommon amino acid. It is used in biology as an arginine (another amino acid) analogue. It is a potent growth inhibitor of many organisms.
- **Cancer cells:** Altered self-cells that do not need to normal growth regulating mechanisms; as a result, they continue to divide and produce a tumor and have the ability for metastasis (Fig. 3).

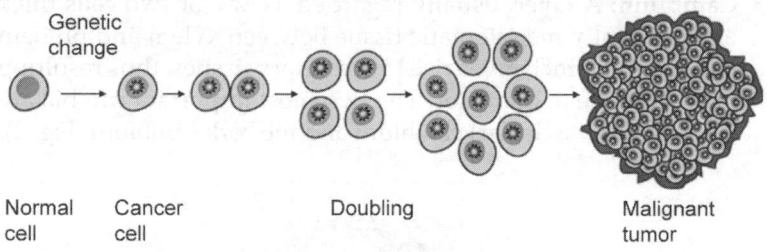

Normal cell   Cancer cell   Doubling   Malignant tumor

Fig. 3: Cancer cells

- **Cancer:** 1. A family of disease in which cells undergo uncontrolled division. Cancer cells can invade nearby tissues and can spread through the bloodstream and lymphatic system to various parts of the body. 2. Uncontrolled growth of the cells of a tissue or an organ in a multicelullar organism.
- **CANDA:** Computer Assisted New Drug Application (CANDA). An application to the US Food and Drug Administration (US-FDA) seeking approval of a drug that has undergone Phase 2 and Phase 3 clinical trials. A CANDA is submitted in the form of computer-readable (clinical) data that provide the FDA with a sophisticated database that allows administration reviewers to evaluate (statistically) the data themselves.
- **Candidate gene strategy:** An experimental approach in which knowledge of the biochemistry and/or physiology of a trait is used to draw up a list of genes whose protein products could be involved in the trait.
- **Candidate gene:** A gene whose function suggests that it may be involved in the genetic variation observed for a particular trait, e.g. the gene for growth hormone is a candidate gene for body weight.
- **Candied fruit:** Fruit impregnated with sugar, drained and dried; it is not sticky, is plump, tender and exceedingly sweet with flavor.

- **Canine:** A pointed tooth between the incisors and premolars of a mammal, often greatly enlarged in carnivores.
- **Canning:** Process of preserving food by the application of heat high enough for destroying essentially all microorganism present together with sealing the food in airtight sterilized cans.
- **Canola:** Any of several cultivars of oil seed rape (more fully canola oil). The vegetable oil high in mono-unsaturated fatty acid obtained from these cultivars (Fig. 4).

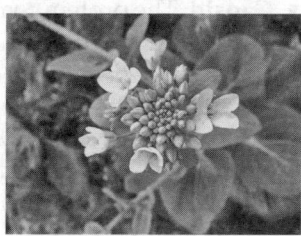

Fig. 4: Canola

- **CAP (Catabolic activator protein):** 1. The structure found on the 5'-end of eukaryotic mRNA, and consisting of an inverted, methylated guanosine residue. 2. A positive control protein that complexes with cAMP and binds to a specific region of a promoter, and which in turn stimulates the binding of RNA polymerase at the start of a gene and hence enables transcription of that gene.
- **Cap 0:** At the 5' end of mRNA has only a methyl group on 7-guanine.
- **Cap 1:** At the 5' end of mRNA has methyl groups on the terminal 7-guanine and the 2'-O position of the next base.
- **Cap 2:** It has three methyl groups (7-guanine, 2'-O position of next base, and N6 adenine) at the 5' end of mRNA.
- **CAP binding site:** The sequence on DNA to which CAP (catabolite activator protein whose presence is necessary for the activation of the lac operon) binds.
- **Cap site:** The site in a gene where translation I initiated, aka translation initiation site.
- **Capacitation:** The final stage in the maturation process of a spermatozoon taking place inside the female genital tract as the sperm penetrates the ovum.
- **Capacity factor:** The ratio of the elution volume of a substance to the void volume in the column.
- **Capillary blotting:** In this approach, gel is placed on top of a buffer-saturated filter paper, the blotting membrane is placed on top of the membrane. The buffer moves from the bottom filter paper through the gel carrying macromolecules along with it; the latter get trapped onto the blotting membrane.

- **Capillary electrophoresis:** In this case, separation by electrophoresis is achieved in 20–30 cm long capillaries of fused silica having internal diameter of 50–100 μm.
- **Capsid:** The protein coat surrounding the genetic material (DNA or RNA) of a virus.
- **Capsule:** An envelope surrounding many types of microorganisms. The capsule is usually composed of polysaccharides, polypeptides, or polysaccharide-protein complexes. These materials are arranged in a compact manner around the cell surface. Capsules are not absolutely essential cellular components.
- **Carbetimer:** An antineoplastic (i.e. anticancer) low molecular weight polymer that acts against several types of cancer tumors, perhaps via stimulation of the patient's immune system. It has minimal toxicity.
- **Carbohydrate engineering:** The selective, deliberate alteration/ creation of carbohydrates (and the oligosaccharide side chains of glycoprotein molecules) by man.
- **Carbohydrate:** An organic compound based on the general formula $C_x(H_2O)_y$ performing many vial roles in living organisms. The simplest carbohydrates are the sugars (saccharine) including glucose and sucrose.
- **Carbon source:** Compound used by cell/tissues as the source of energy as well as carbon for their metabolic needs; usually, sucrose (2–5%).
- **Carboxy terminal domain (CTD):** Carboxy terminal domain of eukaryotic RNA polymerase is phosphorylated at initiation and is involved in coordinating several activities with transcription.
- **Carboxyl group:** The –COOH functional group, acidic in nature, found in all amino acids.
- **Carboxypeptidases:** Two enzymes (A and B) found in pancreatic juice. Their role is to remove the C-terminal amino acid from a peptide. The A form removes any amino acid and the B form removes only lysine or arginine. Used when sequencing peptides.
- **Carcinogen:** A chemical that increases the frequency with which cells are converted to a cancerous condition. A cancer-causing agent.
- **Carcinogenic:** Anything which has property of causing cancer at least in animals and, by implication, in humans.

C

- **Carcinoma:** A malignant tumor derived from epithelial tissue which forms the skin and the outer cell layers of internal organs.
- **Cargo:** Describes any macromolecule (e.g. RNA, soluble or membrane proteins) that is transported from one compartment to another. Cargo may contain sequences or modifications that specify their destination.
- **Carnitine:** A vitamin-like nutrient that occurs naturally in animal cells, and which is needed for the body to convert fatty acids to energy (which can then be used by the body's cells). Carnitine is essential to facilitate the transport of acyl-CoA enzyme (attached to a fatty acid molecule) into the cell's mitochondria, where the beta-oxidation of fatty acids occurs (thereby providing energy to the cell). Before fatty acids can enter the mitochondria, they must be activated by a chemical reaction (which occurs on the outer mitochondrial membrane), in which Acyl-CoA is attached to the fatty acid molecule by a chemical reaction driven by adenosine triphosphate (ATP) and catalyzed by Acyl-CoA synthetase. Adenosine monophosphate (AMP) is a byproduct of that chemical reaction.
- **Carotene:** A reddish-orange plastid pigment involved in light reactions in photosynthesis.
- **Carotenoid:** Red to yellow pigments responsible for the characteristic color of many plant organs or fruits such as tomatoes, carrots, etc. Oxidation products of carotene are called xanthophylls. Carotenoids serve as light-harvesting molecules in photosynthetic assemblies and also play a role in protecting prokaryotes from the deleterious effects of light.
- **Carpel:** Female reproductive organ of flowering plants consisting of sigma, style and ovary. In some plants one or more carpel unite to form the pistil.
- **Carrier:** An individual who possesses a mutant allele but does not express it in the phenotype because of a dominant allelic partner.
- **Carrier DNA:** DNA of undefined sequence content which is added to the transforming (plasmid) DNA used in physical DNA-transfer procedures. This additional DNA increases the efficiency of transformation in electroporation and chemically mediated DNA-delivery systems. The mechanism responsible for this effect is not known.

C

- **Carrier gas:** The gas that carriers the sample in gas chromatography.
- **Carrier matrix:** Materials used for immobilization of cells/enzymes; usually inert polymers or inorganic materials.
- **Carrier molecule:** A molecule that plays a role in transporting electrons through the electron transport chain. Carrier molecules are usually proteins bound to nonprotein groups that are able to undergo oxidation and reduction relatively easy thus, allowing electrons to flow.
- **Carrier protein:** A protein to which a hapten is attached in order to render it more immunogenic.
- **Cartagena protocol:** An international agreement governing trade in genetically modified organisms. This protocol was signed in January, 2000.
- **Cartilage-inducing factors A and B:** Compounds produced by the body which also have immunosuppressive activity.
- **Cascade:** The chain of sequential protein interactions that transmit a signal within a cell or between neighboring cells or tissues.
- **Casein hydrolysate:** A mixture of amino acids and peptides produced by enzymatic or acid hydrolysis of casein. It is an undefined mixture.
- **Casein:** A group of proteins found in the milk.
- **Casing:** Covering of mushroom mycelial growth with a 1.5–2 cm thick layer of sterilized mixture of sand and soil; essential for fruiting bodies to be produced.
- **Caspases:** Comprise a family of proteases some of whose members are involved in apoptosis (programed cell death).
- **Cassette:** A package of genetic material (containing more than one gene) inserted into the genome of a cell via gene splicing techniques. May include promoter(s), leader sequence, termination codon, etc.
- **Catabolic pathway:** A pathway by which an organic molecule is degraded in order to release energy for growth and other cellular processes.
- **Catabolism:** The metabolic breakdown of large molecules in living organism with accompanying release of energy (Fig. 5).
- **Catabolite repression:** The inactivation of an operon caused by the presence of large amounts of the metabolic end product of the operon.

Catabolism

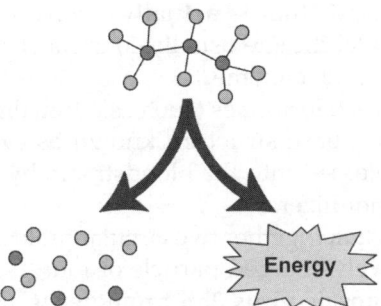

Fig. 5: Catabolism

- **Catalase:** An enzyme that catalyzes very rapid decomposition of hydrogen peroxide to water and oxygen. Catalase is in the group of enzymes known as metalloenzymes because it requires the presence of a metal in order to be catalytically active. The metal (known as a co-factor) is, in the case of catalase, iron round in both plants and animals.

- **Catalysis by approximation:** The substrate bound to an enzyme molecule is held close to another chemical group in the optimal orientation for the reaction to proceed.

- **Catalysis:** The process of changing the rate of a chemical reaction by the use of a catalyst.

- **Catalyst:** A catalyst is a substance that accelerates a (chemical) reaction without being used up itself in the process.

- **Catalytic antibodies:** Antibodies that can act as an enzyme to catalyze a chemical reaction. The antibodies are raised against a transition-state that is analog of the desired substrate.

- **Catalytic biosensor:** Biological component of such a biosensor catalyzes the conversion of analyte into a new compound; this reaction produces a change in temperature, pH, etc.

- **Catalytic converter:** A device used by US automobile manufacturers to reduce the amount of CO and hydrocarbons in a car's exhaust. Converter contains a catalyst that oxidizes these compounds to CO_2 and water as they pass through the exhaust.

- **Catalytic RNA:** An RNA (ribonucleic acid) molecule that acts to cleave (cut) any other RNA.

C

- **Catalytic site:** The site (geometric area) on an enzyme molecule (or other catalyst) that is actually involved in the catalytic process. The catalytic site usually consists of a small portion of the total area of the enzyme.
- **Catecholamines:** Hormones (such as adrenalin) that are amino derivatives of a base structure known as catechol. Catecholamines are released into the bloodstream by exercise, and act as natural tranquilizers.
- **Catenate:** Is to link together two circular molecules as in a chain.
- **Cation:** Positively-charged particle or ion.
- **Cauliflower mosaic virus 35S promoter (CaMV 35S):** A promoter (sequence of DNA) that is often utilized in genetic engineering to control expression of (inserted) gene; i.e. synthesis of desired protein in a plant.
- **Caulogenesis:** Stem organogenesis; induction of shoot development from callus.
- **C-bands:** The bands are generated by staining techniques that react with centromeres. The centromere appears as a darkly-staining dot.
- **CBF1:** A transcription factor (i.e. special protein) that is synthesized (manufactured) within certain plants (*Arabidopsis thaliana*, etc.) when those plants are exposed to cold temperatures. CBF1 then interacts with certain portions of the plants' DNA (i.e. regulatory sequences) to thus switch on the process of cold hardening (via proteins coded for by the plants' genes).
- **CCC DNA:** A covalently linked circular DNA molecule, such as a plasmid.
- **CD molecules (Cluster of differentiation molecules):** Any group of antigens that is associated with a specific subpopulation of T-cells. There are designations for surface molecules on various cells of the immune system, e.g. CD4 is present on the surface of helper T cells.
- **CD region (common docking):** A C-terminal region in a MAP kinase (separate from the active site) that is involved in binding to a target protein.
- **CD3:** A complex of proteins that associates with the T cell antigen receptor's a and p chains. Each complex consists of one each of the 8, 8, 7 chains and two *t* chains.
- **CD4 protein:** An adhesion molecule (protein) imbedded in the outer wall (envelope) of human immune system and brain cells that functions as the receptor (door to entry into the cell) for the

HIV (AIDS) virus. The gp120 envelope glycoprotein of the HIV (i.e. AIDS) virus directly interacts with the CD4 protein on the surface of the helper T cells to enable the virus to invade the helper T cells.

C

- **CD44 protein:** One of the adhesion molecules (embedded in the surface of the linings of blood vessels) that assists the neutrophils on their journey from the bloodstream through the walls of blood vessels (e.g. to combat pathogens into adjacent tissues). Tumor cells also exploit CD44 molecules in order to metastasize (spread throughout the body's tissue from a single beginning tumor) via a similar (tumor cell) through-blood vessel wall adhesion molecule mechanism.

- **CD4-PE40:** An experimental drug discovered in 1988 by Ira Pastan and Bernard Moss that has indicated potential to combat acquired immune deficiency syndrome (AIDS). CD4- PE40 is a conjugated protein consisting of a CD4 protein (molecule) attached to *Pseudomonas* exotoxin (a substance produced by *Pseudomonas* bacteria that is toxic to certain living cells). The gp 120 glycoprotein on the surface of the HIV (i.e. AIDS) virus attaches preferentially to the CD4 portion of this immuno-conjugate, and the virus is inactivated by the *Pseudomonas* exotoxin portion of this immunoconjugate.

- **CD95 protein:** Also called APO-1/Fas, it is a transmembrane protein (embedded within the surface membrane of the cell) that transmits an apoptosis (programmed cell death) signal into cells. Transduction of that apoptosis signal occurs when certain ligands or antigens (i.e. the APO-1/Fas antigen) bind to the extracellular (portion outside of cell membrane) part (i.e. receptor) of the CD95 protein.

- **cdc:** An abbreviation for cell division cycle. It is most frequently used as a part of the names of a large collection of yeast mutants isolated in the 1970s in which the cell cycle arrested at a specific point in each type of mutant.

- **C-DNA:** Also known as copy DNA. A helical form of DNA, it occurs when DNA fibers are maintained in 66% relative humidity in the presence of lithium ions. It has fewer base pairs per turn than B-DNA.

- **cDNA clone:** A double-stranded DNA complement of mRNA synthesized *in vitro* by using reverse tanscriptase and DNA polymerase.

- **cDNA cloning:** A method of cloning the coding sequence of a gene, starting with its mRNA transcript. It is normally used to clone a DNA copy of a eukaryotic mRNA.
- **cDNA:** A single-stranded DNA complementary to an RNA, synthesized from it by reverse transcription *in vitro*.
- **cDNA library:** A collection of cDNA clones that were generated *in vitro* from the mRNA sequences isolated from an organism or a specific tissue or cell type or population of an organism (Fig. 6).

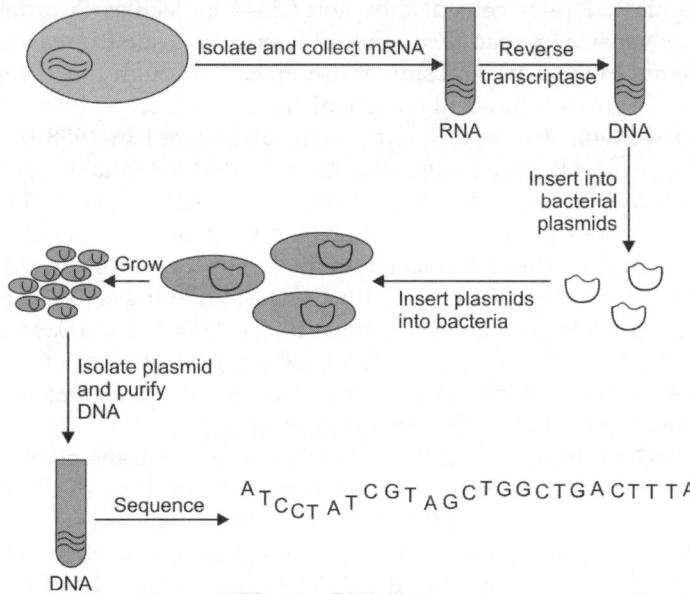

Fig. 6: cDNA library

- **cDNA of satellite RNA-mediated virus resistance:** cDNA copies of such a satellite RNA that reduces disease severity of an RNA virus is transferred into plants; expression of the satellite sequences reduces disease symptoms as well as virus accumulation.
- **cDr (complementarity-determining regions):** These are regions of the variable (V) regions of light and heavy antibody chains that make contact with the antigen. The primary amino acid sequences of these regions are highly variable among antibodies of the same class.
- **Cecrophins:** (lytic proteins) Proteins produced by certain white blood cells [called cytotoxic T lymphocytes (CTL) or killer T-cells].

The proteins allow lysis (i.e. bursting) of infected cells. Cecrophins are amphopathic (i.e. contain both a hydrophobic region and a hydrophilic region); and work by worming the hydrophobic portion into the cell membrane (so the hydrophobic portion of the cecrophin molecule is out of the water). This creates a transmembrane pore (a hole in the membrane) which is lined with the cecrophin's hydrophilic portion. Membranes function simply to separate various components. This separation is required for life to exist. When holes are introduced into cell membranes, water rushes into the targeted cell due to differences in osmotic pressure and the cell ruptures (explodes). The cecrophins are only able to lyse (burst) infected cells because only sick cells have a weakened cytoskeleton (located just inside the cell membrane), which cannot prevent the contents of the cell from spilling out through the pores (created by cecrophins).

- **Cell:** The smallest structural unit of living matter capable of functioning independently. A microscopic mass of protoplasm surrounded by a semi-permeable membrane usually including one or more nuclei and various nonliving products, capable-either alone or by interacting with other cells of performing all the fundamental functions of life (Fig. 7).

- **Cell culture:** The growing of cells *in vitro* derived from

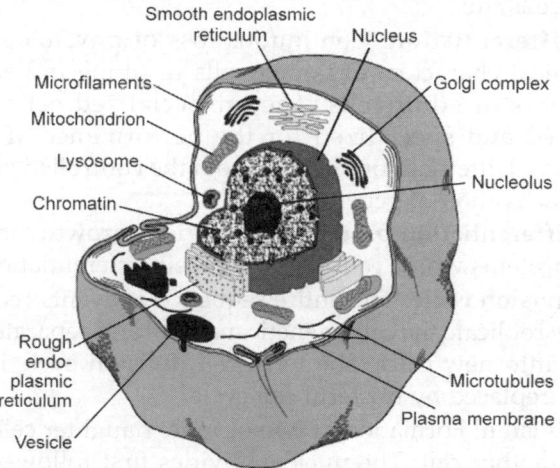

Fig. 7: Cell

multicellular organisms.

C

- **Cell cycle:** Sequence of stages that a cell passes through between one division and the next. The cell cycle oscillates between mitosis and the interphase which is divided into G, S and G2 (Fig. 8).

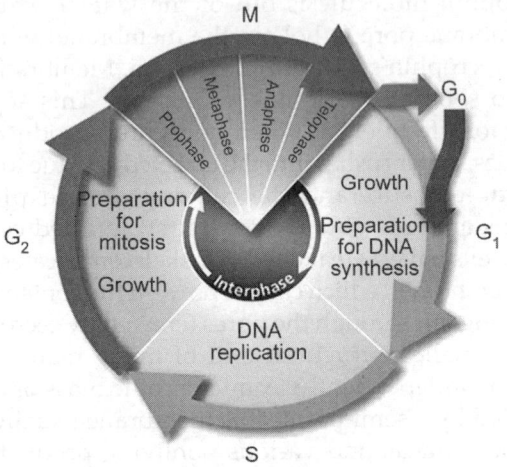

Fig. 8: Cell cycle

- **Cell density:** Number of cells per unit volume; usually, expressed as cells/ml.
- **Cell differentiation:** Continuous loss of physiological and cytological characters of young cells resulting in getting the characters of adult cells. The unspecialized cells become modified and specialized for the performance of specific functions. Differentiation results from the controlled activation and deactivation of genes.
- **Cell-differentiation proteins:** The various growth factors and other proteins which cause/assist in cell differentiation.
- **Cell division cycle:** The entire sequence of events required to reliably replicate the cell's genetic material and separate the two copies into new cells. The term cell division cycle has been largely replaced by the term cell cycle.
- **Cell division:** Formation of two or more daughter cells from a single mother cell. The nucleus divides first followed by the formation of a cell membrane between the daughter nuclei. Division of cytoplasm and nucleus into two or more parts by formation of a cell plate (Fig. 9).

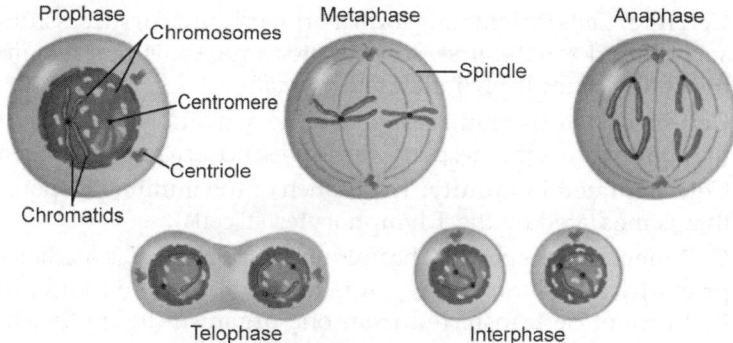

Fig. 9: Cell division

- **Cell fusion:** Formation of a single hybrid cell from two cells of different species cultured *in vitro*. The cells fuse and coalesce but their nuclei may remain separated. During subsequent cell division a single spindle is formed so that each daughter cell has a single nucleus containing sets of chromosomes from each parental line. Subsequent divisions often result in the loss of chromosomes and therefore of genes. The cell fusion technique can be used to determine the control of specific genes and their assignment to chromosomes.

- **Cell generation time:** The interval between the beginnings of consecutive divisions of a cell. The time that it takes for a population of single-celled organisms to double its cell number.

- **Cell hybridization:** The fusion of two or more dissimilar cells leading to the formation of a somatic hybrid (Fig. 10).

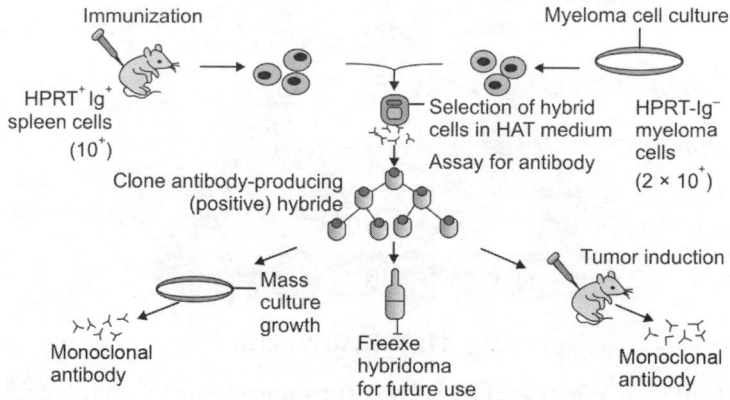

Fig. 10: Cell hybridization

- **Cell line:** Cells (originating form a primary culture) successfully subcultured for the first, second, etc. time. Cells that acquire the ability to multiply indefinetely *in vitro*.
- **Cell-mediated immune response:** The activation of T cells of the immune system in response to the presence of a foreign antigen.
- **Cell-mediated immunity:** The branch of the immune response that is mediated by the T lymphocytes (T cells).
- **Cell-mediated response:** The immune response that is mediated primarily by T lymphocytes. It is defined based on immunity that cannot be transferred from one organism to another by serum antibody.
- **Cell membrane:** The lipid- or fatty- acid based sheath that forms the cell boundary in mammalian and other cells. This layer is hydrophobic and is studded with proteins that allow the transport of nutrients and stimuli into and out of the cell.
- **Cell mobility:** The ability of a cell to move.
- **Cell number:** The number of cells per unit volume of a culture.
- **Cell plate:** The precursor of the cell wall, formed as cytokinesis starts during cell division. The cell plate develops in the region of the equatorial plate and arises from membranes in the cytoplasm.
- **Cell proliferation:** An increase in the number of cells as a result of cell growth and cell division (Fig. 11).

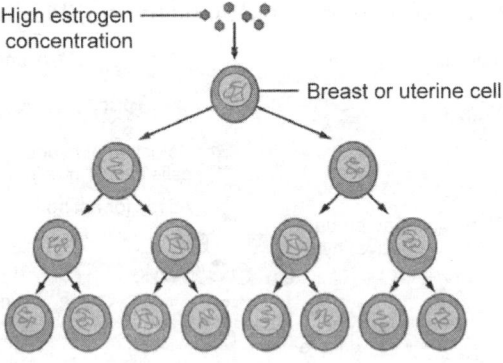

Fig. 11: Cell proliferation

- **Cell sap:** Water and dissolved substances, sugar, amino acids, waste substances, etc. in the plant cell vacuole.

- **Cell selection:** The process of selecting cells within a group of genetically different cells. Selected cells or cell lines are sub-cultured onto fresh medium for continued selection and often are exposed to an increased level of the selection agent. The final objective is to regenerate plants exhibiting the traits selected for at the cellular level.
- **Cell sorting:** A process utilized (e.g. by researchers) to sort/separate different cells (pathogens, cancerous vs normal cells, sperm that are bearing chromosomes for male vs female, etc.). Some automated means of cell sorting include biochips (utilizing controlled electrical fields to collect specific cell types onto electrodes in the biochip), fluorescence-activated cell sorter (FACS) machines, magnetic particles (e.g. attached to antibodies), etc.
- **Cell strain:** A strain of cells having specific properties of makers derived from a primary culture of a cell line by selection or cloning. The selected properties must persist during subsequent cultivation aka single cell line.
- **Cell suspension:** Cells in culture, in moving or shaking liquid medium often used to describe suspension cultures of single cell and cell aggregates.
- **Cell synchronization:** Induction of synchronous cell division in cell cultures; achieved through starvation (of a nutrient or a growth regulator; cells arrested in G_1/G_2, inhibition of DNA synthesis by 5-aminouracil FUdR, etc.), etc.
- **Cell wall:** A rigid external coat which surrounds plant cells. It is formed rounds plant cells. It is formed outside the plasmalemma and consists primarily of cellulose.
- **Cellular affinity:** Tendency of cells to adhere specifically to cells of the same type. This property is lost in some cancer cells.
- **Cellular immune response:** Also called cell-mediated immunity. The immune response that is carried out by specialized cells, in contrast to the response carried out by soluble antibodies. The specialized cells that make-up this group include cytotoxic T-lymphocytes (CTL), helper T-lymphocytes, macrophages, and monocytes. This system works in concert with the humoral immune response.
- **Cellular oncogene (Protooncogene):** A normal mammalian or avian gene that when mutated or improperly expressed, contributes to the development of cancer.

- **Cellulase:** Enzyme that catalyzes the breakdown of cellulose.
- **Cellulose acetate electrophoresis:** Cellulose acetate membranes having large pores are used for separation of molecules entirely on the basis of their charge density; resolution and limit of detection if low.
- **Cellulose:** A complex carbohydrate composed of long, unbranched chains of beta-glucose ((1, 4)-linked-b-d-glucose) molecules which contribute to the structural framework of plant cell walls. It comprises 40–55% by weight of the plant cell wall (Fig. 12).

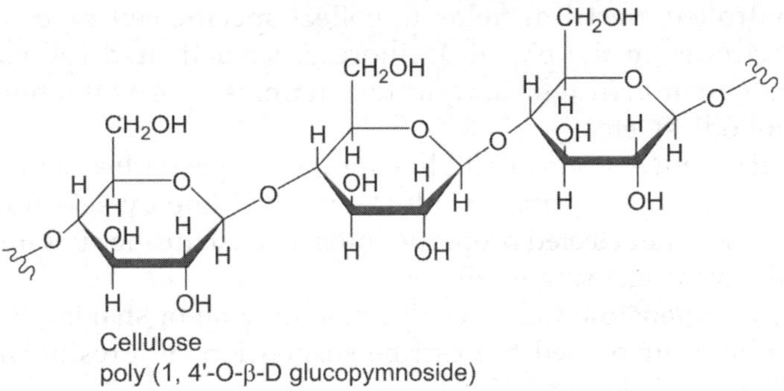

Cellulose
poly (1, 4'-O-β-D glucopymnoside)

Fig. 12: Cellulose

- **Cellulosome:** A multi-protein aggregate that is present in some cellulolytic microorganisms and contains multiple choices of all the enzymes required to completely break down cellulose. This complex is often found on the outer surface of cellulolytic microorganisms.
- **Center for advanced research in biotechnology (CARB):** A protein engineering research consortium established in Rockville, MD, during 1989 by the US government, the University of Maryland, and local government.
- **Centimorgan:** One percent recombination between two loci (cM).
- **Central dogma:** The basic concept that in nature genetic information generally can flow only from DNA to RNA to protein, it is known that information contained in RNA molecules of certain viruses (called retroviruses) can also flow back to DNA.
- **Central element:** A structure that lies in the middle of the synaptonemal complex, along which the lateral elements of homologous chromosomes align.

- **Central mother cell:** A substance of cell located in a plant apical meristem and characterized by a large vacuole.
- **Centers of origin:** Usually, the location in the world where the oldest cultivation of a particular crop has been identified.
- **Centrifugation:** Separating molecules by size or density using centrifugal forces generated by a spinning rotor. G-forces of several hundred thousand times gravity are generated in ultra centrifugation.
- **Centrifuge:** A machine that is used to separate heavier from lighter molecules and cellular components and structures (Fig. 13).
- **Centriole:** It is a small hollow cylinder consisting of microtubules. It occurs in the centrosome (a type of microtubule organizing center) and is thought to play a role in organizing the microtubules.
- **Centromere:** It is a constricted region of a chromosome that includes the site of attachment (the kinetochore) to the mitotic or meiotic spindle (Fig. 14).

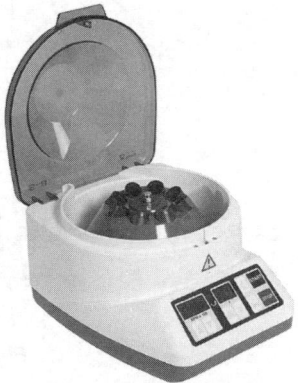

Fig. 13: Centrifuge

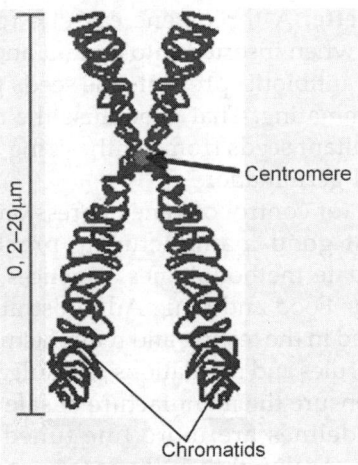

Fig. 14: Centromere

- **Centrosomes:** The regions from which microtubules are organized at the poles of a mitotic cell. In animal cells, each centrosome contains a pair of centrioles surrounded by a dense amorphous region to which the microtubules attach (Fig. 15).

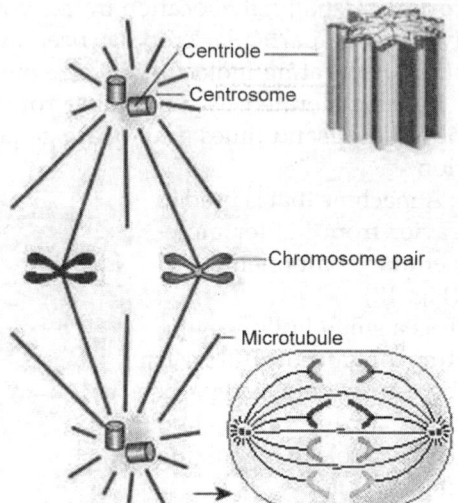

Fig. 15: Centrosome

- **Cephem-type antibiotic:** Antibiotic that shares the basic chemical structure of cephalosporin.
- **Cessation cassette:** A three-gene cassette (genetic sequence construct) that, when inserted into a plant and when activated via tetracycline antibiotic, prevents the seeds produced by that plant from germinating. That is because the cessation cassette stops those resultant seeds from synthesizing a specific protein needed for seed germination.
- **CGE:** Acronym for control of gene expression.
- **cGMP:** Current good manufacturing practices. The set of current, up-to-date methodologies, practices, and procedures mandated by the Food and Drug Administration (FDA) which are to be followed in the testing and manufacture of pharmaceuticals. The set of rules and regulations promulgated and enforced by the FDA to ensure the manufacture of safe clinical supplies. The cGMP guidelines are more fine-tuned and up-to-date (technologically speaking) than the more general GMP.
- **Chaconine:** A neurotoxin that is naturally present at low levels within potatoes. As a result of that, chaconine is present at detectable levels in the bloodstream of humans that consume potatoes.

- **Chain terminator:** Codons which do not code for an amino acid. They are signal ribosomes to terminate protein synthesis. The codona are UAA, UAG and UGA, and have been termed Ochre, Amber and Opal, respectively. Also known as stop codons or termination codons. Often, two of these codons are found together at the end of a coding sequence of RNA.
- **Chakrabarty decision:** Diamond vs Chakrabarty, US Department of Commerce, 1980; a landmark case in which the US Supreme Court held that the inventor of a new microorganism whose invention otherwise met the legal requirements for obtaining a patent, could not be denied a patent solely because the invention was alive. It essentially allowed the patenting of life forms.
- **Changes in chromosomal structure:** Environmental factors including radiation, chemicals, and viruses, can cause chromosomes to break, if the broken ends do not rejoin in the same pattern, this causes a change in chromosomal structure, e.g. deletion, duplication, inversion, translocation.
- **Chaperone:** A protein that binds to other proteins and helps them to fold correctly and also prevents their premature folding (Fig. 16).

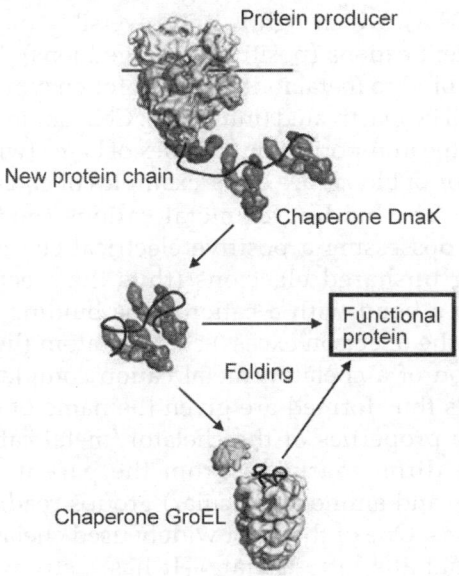

Fig. 16: Chaperone

- **Chaperonins:** Protein molecules inside living cells that facilitate proper folding of the (new) protein molecules that are synthesized (manufactured) in the cell's ribosomes.
- **Character:** An observable/estimable, e.g. morphological, anatomical, biochemical, physiological or behavioral, etc. feature of an organism.
- **Charcoal:** The black porous residue of partly burnt wood, bones, etc. A form of carbon. When treated to purify it and increase its adsorptive power, it is called activated charcoal in which form it is added to nutrient medium in order to prevent or decrease the effect of browning.
- **CHD:** Acronym for coronary heart disease.
- **Checkpoint:** It is an event in the cell cycle that can only proceed if some earlier event has been completed.
- **Chelate:** Complex organic molecule that can combine with cations and does not ionize. Chelates can supply micronutrients to plants at slow, steady rates. Usually used to supply iron to plant cells.
- **Chelating agent:** A molecule capable of binding metal atoms. The chelating agent/metal complex is held together by coordination bonds which have a strong polar character. One example of a common chelating agent is ethylenediamine tetra-acetate (EDTA), which tightly and reversibly binds Mg^{2+} and other divalent cations (positively charged ions). If a chelate is allowed to bind to metal ions required for enzyme activity, the enzyme will be inactivated (inhibited). Cobalamin (vitamin B_{12}), EDTA and the iron-porphyrin complex of heme (which provides the red color of blood) are other examples of chelates.
- **Chelation:** The binding of metal cations (metal atoms or molecules possessing a positive electrical charge) by atoms possessing unshared electrons (thus the electrons can be donated to a bond with a cation). The binding of the metal (cation) to the (electron excess) chelator atom (ligand) results in formation of a chelator/metal cation complex. The intra-atom bonds thus formed are given the name of coordination bonds. The properties of the chelator/metal cation complex frequently differ markedly from the parent cation. Both carboxylate and amino (molecular) groups readily bind with metal cations. One of the most widely used chelators is EDTA (ethylenediamine tetra-acetate). It has a strong affinity for metal cations possessing two (bi) or more positive (electrical)

charges. Each EDTA molecule binds one metal cation. The EDTA molecule can be visualized as a hand (having only four fingers) which grasps the metal cation. Some enzymes (which require metal cations for their activity) are inactivated by EDTA (and other chelators) in that the chelators preferentially remove the metal from the enzyme.

- **Chemical control of organ differentiation:** Hypothesis due to Skoog and Miller (1957); organ differentiation depends on the relative (not absolute) concentrations of auxins and cytokinins; a high auxin to cytokinin ratio favors root regeneration, while the opposite promotes shoot regeneration; in fact, the exogenous need for the two GRs depends on their endogenous levels in the species/tissue.

- **Chemical energy:** The potential energy that is contained in chemicals; most importantly, the energy contained in organic compounds, such as food and fuels, that may be released through respiration or burning.

- **Chemical genetics:** Coined by Rebecca Ward and Tim Mitchison, this term refers to the creation and use of synthetic chemicals that act to either block or enhance the activity of a protein (or gene that codes for protein). This enables scientists to then determine the specific function(s) of specific protein molecules.

- **Chemical mutagen:** A chemical or product capable of causing genetic mutation in living organisms exposed to it.

- **Chemical oxygen demand (COD):** Amount of oxygen required for chemical oxidation of the organic matter present in a water sample; provides an estimate of the total oxidizable organic matter.

- **Chemical proofreading:** Describes a proofreading mechanism in which the correction event occurs after addition of an incorrect subunit to a polymeric chain, by reversing the addition reaction.

- **Chemically-defines medium:** When all of the chemical components of a plant tissue culture medium are fully known and defined.

- **Chemiluminescence:** The emission of light forms a chemical reaction.

- **Chemoautotrophs:** Organisms that derive their energy needs from oxidation of simple inorganic compounds and use CO_2 as carbon source.

- **Chemokines:** A family of cytokines, these small soluble proteins can stimulate and direct leukocyte movement by binding to specific receptors on the cell surface.

C

- **Chemometrics:** An empirical methodology utilized to (inexpensively) infer a chemical quantity/value from (indirect) measurement(s) of other physical/chemical values (which can be obtained inexpensively). The term chemometrics was coined in 1975 by Bruce Kowalski. One example of the use of chemometrics is to infer the TME (N) or true metabolizable energy of high-oil corn from that corn's protein and oil (fat) content.
- **Chemopharmacology:** Therapy (to cure disease) by chemically synthesized drugs.
- **Chemostat:** An open continuous culture in which cell growth rate and cell density; are held constant by a fixed rate of input of growth limiting nutrient.
- **Chemosynthesis:** Process in which microorganisms utilize the chemical energy contained in certain reduced inorganic molecule to produce organic materials.
- **Chemotaxis:** Sensing of, and movement toward or away from, a specific chemical agent by living, freely moving cells (bacteria, macrophages, etc.).
- **Chemotherapy:** Chemical treatment to eradicate viruses from plant cells/tissues; chemicals used: virazole, (ribavirin), actinomycin D, cyclohexamide, etc.
- **Chiasma (Pl. chiasmata):** A site at which two homologous chromosomes appear to have exchanged material during meiosis (Fig. 17).

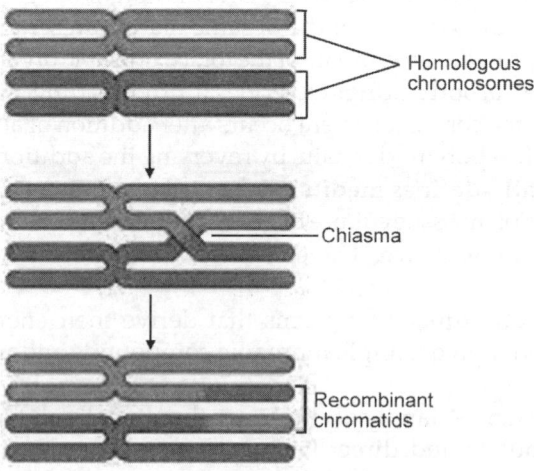

Fig. 17: Chiasma

- **Chimeric DNA:** A recombinant DNA molecule containing unrelated genes.
- **Chimeric gene:** A gene, which contains coding sequence from one organism and regulatory sequence from another organism; all prokaryotic genes expressed in eukaryotes have to be chimeric, and *vice-versa*.
- **Chimera:** Recombinant DNA molecules containing sequences from different organism; a plant or animal that has population of cells with different genotypes.
- **Chimeraplasty:** A method utilized by man to introduce a gene (from the same or another species) into the DNA of a living organism or cell, via gene repair mechanism. Scientists add the desired DNA (gene) to a cell, along with RNA, in a paired-group known as a chimeraplast. The chimeraplast attaches itself to the cell's DNA at the site of the specific gene (to be changed), and repairs it utilizing its (new) chimeraplast-DNA as a template.
- **Chimeric DNA:** (Recombinant) DNA containing spliced genes from two different species.
- **Chimeric gene:** A semisynthetic gene consisting of the coding sequence from one organism fused to promoter and other sequences derived from a different gene. Most genes used in transformation are chimeric.
- **Chimeric proteins:** Fused proteins from different species, produced from the chimeric DNA template.
- **Chimeric selectable marker gene:** A gene that is constructed from parts of two or more different genes and allows the host cell to survive underconditions where it would otherwise die.
- **Chiral compound:** A chemical compound that contains an asymmetrical center and is capable of occurring in two nonsuperimposable mirror images. This phenomenon was first described by Louis Pasteur. Chiral is a word derived from the Greek *cheir* (meaning hand). For example, human hands may be used to illustrate chirality in that when the left and right hands are held one on top of the other, one thumb sticks out on one side while the other thumb sticks out on the other side. The point is that the same number and type of fingers and thumbs exist in both hands, but their arrangement in space may be different. So it is with the arrangement of a given molecule's (e.g. a drug's) atoms in three-dimensional space. Approximately

40% of drugs on the market today, consist of chiral compounds. In many chiral drugs, only one type of the molecule is beneficially biologically active (acts beneficially to control disease, reduce pain, etc.), while the other type of the drug molecule is either inactive or else causes undesired impacts (called side effects of the drug mixture). For example, one enantioner of the drug thalidomide is a potent angiogenesis inhibitor, but the other enantiomer causes birth defects in babies of pregnant women taking it.

- **Chiral products:** Many chemical substances for medicines or crop protection products occur in two forms that are mirror images of each other, as the right hand is of the left hand. The 'image' and 'mirror image' can have completely different effects: one form of the amino acid asparagine, for example, is used as a sweetness enhancer, while the other is perceived as bitter.

- **Chi-squared test (C^2 test):** A significance test used to statistically assess the goodness of observed data to a prediction.

- **Chitin:** A water-insoluble polysaccharide polymer composed of N-acetyl-D-glucosamine molecular units, which forms the exoskeletons of arthropods (insects) and crustacea. Shellac is produced from chitin.

- **Chitinase:** An enzyme that degrades (breaks down) chitin. It is one of the pathogenesis related proteins produced by certain plants as a disease-fighting response to entry-into plant of pathogenic (disease-causing) fungi. Chitinase is also sometimes produced by certain fungi and actinomycetes that destroy the eggs (i.e. chitin-containing shells) of harmful roundworms.

- **Chloramphenicol:** An antibiotic that interferes with protein synthesis.

- **Chlorenchyma:** (Chloros—green; + enchyma—tissue) Tissue containing chloroplasts. Including leaf mesophyll and other parenchyma cells.

- **Chlorinated hydrocarbons:** These are synthetic organic molecules in which one or more hydrogen atoms have been replaced by chlorine atoms. These hydrocarbons are hazardous compounds because they tend to be nonbiodegradable and therefore to bioaccumulate; many have been shown to be carcinogenic.

- **Chlorination:** A disinfection process, in which chlorine is added to drinking water or sewage water to kill pathogenic microorganisms.

- **Chlorofluorocarbons (CFCs):** Synthetic organic molecules that contain one or more of both chlorine and fluorine atoms and that are known to cause ozone destruction.
- **Chlorophyll:** The green pigment in plants responsible for absorbing the light energy required for photosynthesis (Fig. 18).

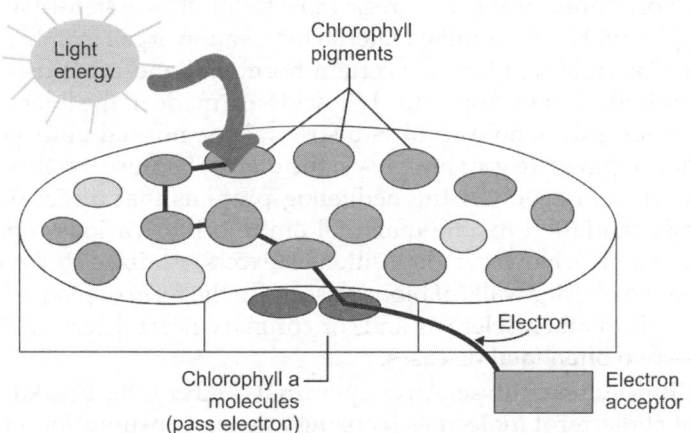

Fig. 18: Chlorophyll

- **Chloroplast DNA (ctDNA):** An independent genome (usually circular) found in a plant chloroplast.
- **Chloroplast transit peptide (CTP):** A transit peptide that, when fused to a protein, acts to transport that protein into chloroplast(s) in a plant. Once both are inside the chloroplast, the transit peptide is cleaved-off the protein and that protein is then free (to do the task it was designed for). For example, the CP4 EPSPS enzyme in genetically engineered glyphosate-resistant soybean [*Glycine max* (L) Merrill] plant is transported into the soybean plant's chloroplasts by the CTP known as N-terminal petunia chloroplast transit peptide. After both reach the chloroplast, the CTP is cleaved and degraded, so the CP4 EPSPS is then free to do its task (i.e. confer resistance to glyphosate).
- **Chloroplast:** Plastids containing chlorophyll; enclosed by two concentric membranes and contain typical stroma and grana organization; contains DNA which contributes to cytoplasmic inheritance.
- **Chlorosis:** Failure of chlorophyll development and appearance of yellow color in plants because of a nutritional disturbance or because an infection by a virus, bacteria or fungus.

- **Cholera toxin:** The toxin produced by the *Vibrio cholerae* (Latin America) bacteria, a source of food/water-borne gastrointestinal disease. The cholera toxin has a strong affinity for certain receptors that are present on the surface of gastrointestinal cells.

- **Cholesterol:** From the Greek *chole* (bile), it is a sterol (sterol-lipid) that is an essential material for creation of cell membranes, and a building block for certain hormones and acids used by the body. For example, the bile acids are made in the liver from cholesterol. Cholesterol is also vital for normal embryonic development (e.g. of humans in the uterus) because it comprises a crucial portion of the hedgehog proteins that direct tissue differentiation (of the mammal embryo into various organs, limbs, etc.). However, deposition of (excess) oxidized cholesterol on the interior walls of blood vessels [in the form of plaque] can result in atherosclerosis and/or coronary heart disease (CHD) — two often fatal diseases.

- **Cholesterol oxidase:** An enzyme that catalyzes the breakdown of cholesterol molecules (causing oxygen consumption in the breakdown process). Because cholesterol molecules are essential for creation and maintenance of cell membranes and some hormones, an excess of cholesterol oxidase can be harmful (e.g. to certain insects). When the gene (that codes) for cholesterol oxidase is inserted into the genome of the corn (maize) plant, it can enable that plant to resist many of the worm pests (corn earworm, European corn borer, corn rootworm, black cutworm, armyworm, etc.) that attack corn (maize) in the field. When the gene (that codes) for cholesterol oxidase is inserted into the cotton plant, it can enable that plant to resist weevils and other sucking insects that attack cotton plants in the field.

- **Choline:** Formerly known as vitamin B_4, choline is a nutrient that takes part in many of the metabolism processes in the human body. Naturally present in egg yolks, organ meats, dairy products, soybean lecithin, spinach, and nuts. Choline promotes fat metabolism in the liver and the synthesis of high-density lipoproteins (HDLP, also known as good cholesterol) by the liver. It is also utilized by the body in order to synthesize (manufacture) acetylcholine, an important neurotransmitter (substance that transmits nerve impulses). Because significant choline deficiency can cause liver carcinogenesis, cirrhosis, and can impair cell signaling, the US government has defined choline to be an essential nutrient. One active metabolite of choline is platelet activating factor (PAF), which is involved in the body's hormonal and reproductive functions. Choline is so important in proper infant development/growth that it is included in manufactured infant formula at the rate of at least 7 mg per 100 kcal.

- **Cholinesterase:** An enzyme that catalyzes the chemical reaction in which the neurotransmitter (substance that transmits nerve impulses) molecule acetylcholine is synthesized (manufactured) from Ac-CoA and choline.

- **Chromatids:** The copies of a chromosome produced by replication. The name is usually used to describe the copies in the period before they separate at the subsequent cell division.

- **Chromatin remodeling:** Describes the energy-dependent displacement or reorganization of nucleosomes that occurs in conjunction with activation of genes for transcription.

- **Chromatin:** Describes the state of nuclear DNA and its associated proteins during the interphase (between mitoses) of the eukaryotic cell cycle.

- **Chromatin fibers:** A basic organizational unit of eukaryotic chromosomes consisting of DNA and associated proteins assembled into strands of 30 nm average diameter.

- **Chromatogram:** A series of separated bands or zones detected either visually, as in chromatographic or thin layer chromatographic separations or indirectly by a detection system. In the latter case, the detection system usually outputs an electrical signal, which is graphically plotted through time, to display the series of separated zones or bands.

- **Chromatography:** Coined by Mikhail S Tswett in 1906, this word refers to a process by which complex mixtures of different molecules may be separated from each other. During the process, the mixture is subjected to many repeated partitionings between a flowing phase and a stationary phase. Chromatography constitutes one of, if not *the* most fundamental, separation techniques used in the biochemistry/biotechnology arena to date (Fig. 19).

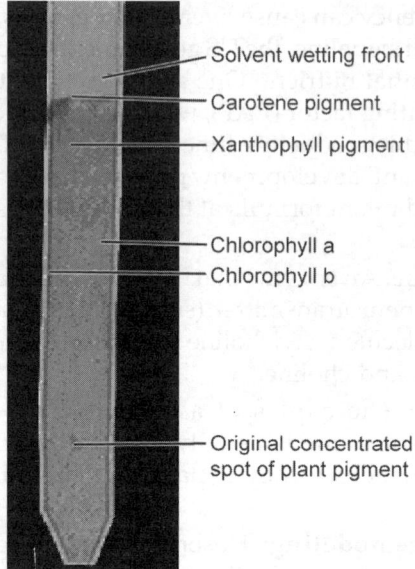

Fig. 19: Chromatography

- **Chromocenter:** An aggregate of heterochromatin from different chromosomes.
- **Chromogenic substrate:** A compound or substance that contains a color-forming group.
- **Chromomeres:** Densely, staining granules visible in chromosomes under certain conditions, especially early in meiosis, when a chromosome may appear to consist of a series of chromomeres. A chromosome is a discrete unit of the genome carrying many genes. Each chromosome consists of a very long molecule of duplex DNA and an approximately equal mass of proteins. It is visible as a morphological entity only during cell division.
- **Chromonema:** An optically single thread forming an axial structure within each chromosome.
- **Chromoplast:** Plastid containing pigments, such as chloroplast or one in which carotenoids predominate.
- **Chromosomal aberration:** Any change in chromosome structure or number. Although it can be a mechanism for enhancing genetic diversity such alterations are usually fatal or ill-adaptive especially in animals.

- **Chromosomal integration site:** A chromosomal location where foreign DNA can be integrated often without impairing any essential function in the host organism.
- **Chromosomal jumping:** A process, analogous to chromosomal walking, in which large segments of intervening DNA sequence are omitted or jumped over in order to locate and sequence a gene or DNA fragment. The basis of this technique is as follows: as in chromosomal walking an array of overlapping clones is needed if some of the clones are too large or difficult to sequence fully, the panel of clones can be looped, and the inverse sequence at one end of the loop will reveal the sequence at the other end. This sequence information can then be used to jump to the next overlapping clone and so on, until the target gene sequence is identified.
- **Chromosomal mutations:** Include changes in chromosome number and structure.
- **Chromosomal polymorphism:** The occurrence of one to several chromosomes in two or more alternative structural forms. Within a population the structurally changed chromosomes are the result of chromosome mutations (i.e. any structural change involving the gain, loss or relocation of chromosome segments).
- **Chromosomal theory of inheritance:** Genes are located on chromosomes; proposed in 1902 by Theodor Boveri and Walter S Sutton, accounts for the similarity of genes and chromosomal behavior during meiosis and fertilization. Both chromosomes and factors (now called alleles) pair in diploid cells, chromosomes and alleles of each pair separate during meiosis, so gametes have one-half chromosomes and alleles that separate independently. Gametes contain all combinations; fertilization restores diploid chromosome number and paired condition for alleles in zygote.
- **Chromosomal translocation:** An aberrant process in which a piece of one chromosome breaks off and attaches to another chromosome. The basis of many diseases including cancer.
- **Chromosomal virulence genes:** In *Agrobacterium*; chromosomal genes involved in infection; most of these genes are concerned with polysaccharide biosynthesis.
- **Chromosome:** A discrete unit of the genome carrying many genes. Each chromosome consists of a very long molecule of duplex

DNA and an approximately equal mass of proteins. It is visible as a morphological entity only during cell division (Fig. 20).

p **arm**-short arm structure

Centromere-Constricted point of the chromosome

q **arm**-long arm structure

DNA molecule-long string like DNA molecule formed into a compact stucture by proteins called histones

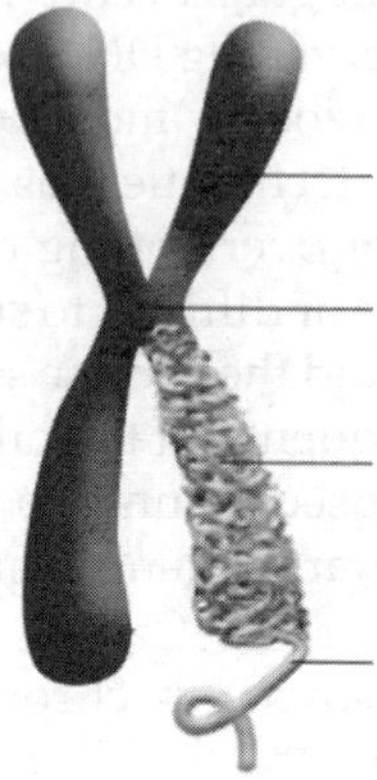

Fig. 20: Chromosome

- **Chromosome aberration:** Abnormal structure or number of chromosomes includes deficiency, duplication, inversion, translocation, aneuploidy, polyploidy or any other change from the normal pattern.
- **Chromosome banding:** Staining of chromosomes in such a way that light and dark areas occur along the length of the chromosomes in repeatable patterns. Lateral comparisons identify paris. Each chromosome can be identified by its banding pattern.
- **Chromosome jumping:** Use of jumping and linking libraries to determine the correct order in a chromosome of the DNA fragments generated by the restriction enzyme used to prepared these libraries.
- **Chromosome mapping:** Percentage of recombinant phenotype measures distance between genes to map the chromosomes, 1% of crossing-over equals one map unit between genes.
- **Chromosome mutation:** A change in the gross structure of a chromosome usually causing severely deleterious effects in the organism. They are often due to an error in pairing during the crossing-over stage of meiosis. The main types of chromosome mutation are translocation, duplication, deletion and inversion.

- **Chromosome pairing:** The coupling of the homologous chromosomes at the start of meiosis (Fig. 21).

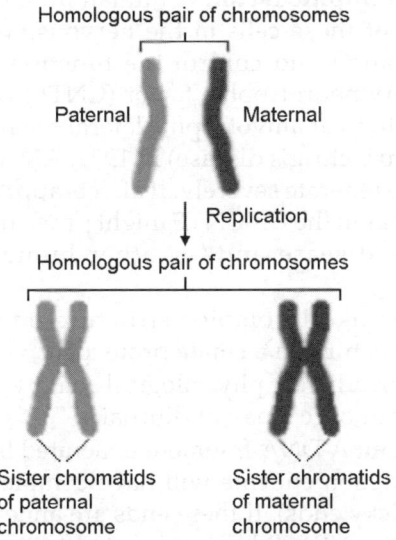

Homologous pair of chromosomes

Paternal　　Maternal

Replication

Homologous pair of chromosomes

Sister chromatids of paternal chromosome

Sister chromatids of maternal chromosome

Fig. 21: Chromosome pairing

- **Chromosome walking:** A technique that identifies overlapping cloned sequences of about 40 kb long that from one continuous segment of a chromosome.
- **Chymosin:** Also known as rennin. It is an enzyme used to make cheeses (from milk). Chymosin occurs naturally in the stomach of calves and is one of the oldest commercially used enzymes. Chymosin (rennin) is chemically similar to renin, an enzyme that plays an important role in regulating blood pressure in humans.
- **Cilia:** Protein-based structures that occur in certain cells of both the plant and animal world. Cilia are very tiny hair-like structure occurring in large numbers on the outside of certain cells. In higher organisms such as man, they usually function to move extracellular material along the cell surface. An example is the sweeping-out-of-foreign matter action of cilia in the bronchial tubes in which very small particles are moved into the throat to be expelled or swallowed. Lower organisms may use cilia for locomotion (swimming). Cilia are used in the swimming motion of bacteria toward sources of nutrients in a process called

chemotaxis. Cilia are shorter and occur in larger numbers per cell than flagella. (singular: cilium).

- **Ciliary neurotrophic factor:** A human protein shown to help the survival of those cells in the nervous system that act to convey sensation and control the function of muscles and organs. Ciliary neurotrophic factor (CNTF) was approved by the US-FDA to treat amyotrophic lateral sclerosis (also known as ALS or Lou Gehrig's disease) in 1992. ALS causes a victim's muscles to degenerate severely. It affects approximately 30,000 people per year in the US-CNTF might prove useful for treating Alzheimer's disease and/or other human neurological diseases.
- **Cilium:** Hair like locomotor structure on certain cells. A locomotor structure on a ciliate protozoan.
- **Circadian:** Circadian of physiological activity, etc. occurring or recurring about once a day of diurnal.
- **Circularization:** A DNA fragment generated by digestion with a single restriction enzyme will have complementary 5' to 3' extension (sticky ends). If these ends are annealed and ligated, the DNA fragment will have converted to a covalently closed circle or circularized.
- *Cis* **acting site:** Affects the activity only of sequences on its own molecule of DNA (or RNA); this property usually implies that the site does not code for protein.
- *Cis* **configuration:** Two sites on the same molecule of DNA.
- *Cis* **dominant site:** Mutation affects the properties of its own molecule of DNA. *cis* dominance is taken to indicate that a site does not code for diffusible project. (A rare exception is that a protein is *cis* dominant when it is constrained to act only on the DNA or RNA from it was synthesized.)
- *Cis* **face:** The side of the Golgi juxtaposed to the nucleus. A cw-acting site affects the activity only of sequences on its own molecule of DNA (or RNA); this property usually implies that the site does not code for protein.
- *Cis* **heterozygote:** A heterozygote that contains two mutations arranged in a *cis*-configuration (e.g. a+b+/ab).
- *Cis/trans* **isomerism:** A type of geometrical isomerism found in alkenic systems in which it is possible for each of the doubly bonded carbons to carry two different atoms or groups. Two similar atoms or groups may be on the same side (*cis*) or on

opposite sides (*trans*) of a plane bisecting the alkenic carbons and perpendicular to the plane of the alkenic systems.

- **Cis/trans test:** Assays (determines) the effect of relative configuration on expression of two (gene) mutations. In a double heterozygote, two mutations in the same gene show mutant phenotype in *trans* configuration, wild (phenotype) in *cis*-configuration. The phenotypic distinction is referred to as the position effect.

- **Cis-acting protein:** A *cis*-acting protein has the exceptional property of acting only on the molecule of DNA from which it was expressed.

- **Cis-acting sequence:** A nucleotide sequence that only affects the expression of genes located on the same chromosome.

- **Cisgenic plants:** Refer to plants which have foreign gene(s) belong to the same species/a related species; risk of transfer of genes through pollen will not be a big issue in this case.

- **Cisplatin:** A drug used in chemotherapy regimens against certain types of cancer tumors. Cisplatin works against (tumor) cells by binding to the cell's DNA and generating intrastrand cross-links (between the two strands of the DNA molecule). These intrastrand cross-links prevent replication and cause cell death.

- **Cisternae:** The successive stacks of the Golgi apparatus, each bounded by a membrane, that makes up individual compartments (Fig. 22).

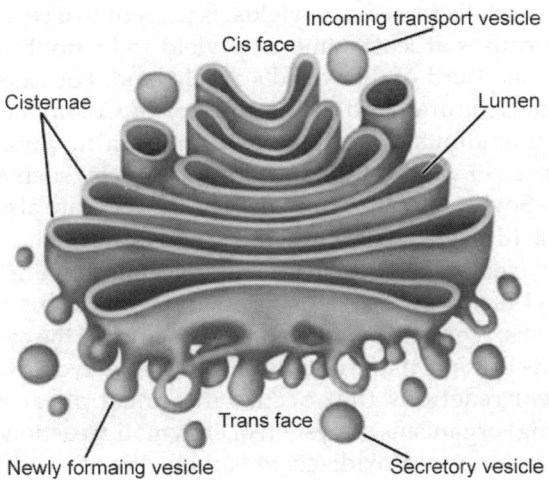

Fig. 22: Cisternae

- **Cisternal maturation:** A model for the mechanism of Cargo transport through the Golgi stack. It is also called cisternal migration or cisternal progression. In this model, a new Golgi cisterna forms at the *cis* face, then moves forward in the stack as the protein content of the cisterna changes from *cis* to medial to *trans*. Proteins that belong to earlier cisternae are retrived by retrograde in transport vesicles.

- **Cistron:** Segment of a DNA molecule within which two mutations cannot complement each other, coding for a single polypeptide chain, equated with a gene.

- **Citrate synthase gene:** A gene that codes for (i.e. causes to be produced by an organism possessing that gene) the enzyme known as citrate synthase.

- **Citrate synthase:** The enzyme utilized (by plants) to synthesize (create) citric acid.

- **Citric acid:** A tricarboxylic acid occurring naturally in plants, especially citrus fruits. It is used as a flavoring agent, as an antioxidant in foods, as an animal feed ingredient, and as a sequestering agent. The commercially produced form of citric acid melts at 153°C (307°F). Citric acid is found in all cells, its central role is in the metabolic process. Some plants naturally release citric acid from their roots into the surrounding soil, in order for that citric acid to chemically bind aluminum ions that are present in some soils. Such aluminum, which slows plant growth and decreases crop yields, is present to a certain degree (which causes at least some crop yield reduction) in approximately one-third of the world's arable land. For example, 70% of the agricultural land in the country of Colombia possesses harmful amounts/conditions of aluminum to damage crops. Corn (maize) yields are reduced up to 80% by such aluminum in soils. Soybeans, cotton, and field bean yields are also reduced.

- **Citric acid cycle:** Also known as the tricarboxylic acid cycle [TCA cycle because the citric acid molecule contains three (tri) carboxyl (acid) groups]. Also known as the Krebs cycle after H A Krebs, who first postulated the existence of the cycle in 1937 under its original name of citric acid cycle. A cyclic sequence of chemical reactions that occurs in almost all aerobic (air-requiring) organisms. A system of enzymatic reactions in which acetyl residues are oxidized to carbon dioxide and hydrogen atoms, and in which formation of citrate is the first step.

- **CLA:** Abbreviation for conjugated linoleic acid.
- **Clades:** The taxonomic subgroups within cladistics.
- **Cladistics:** Initially popularized by Willi Hennig's 1950 book, *Phylogenetic Systematics*, cladistics is a system of taxonomic classification of organisms (and/or their specimens) based upon (determined) similar lines of selected shared traits.
- **Claims:** The section of a patent that states in detail, the uses and possible applications of the invention described in the patent.
- **Class I, II molecules:** Proteins encoded by different clusters of genes within the major histocompatibility complex.
- **Class switching:** A change in Ig gene organization in which the C region of the heavy chain is changed but the V region remains the same.
- **Classical pathway (of complement activation):** Complement activation begins with soluble antigen-antibody complex (immune complex) formation or binding of antibody to an antigen present on a cell. IgM and certain subclasses of IgG activate the classical pathway.
- **Clathrin:** Proteins interact with adaptor proteins to form the coat on some of the vesicles that bud from the cytoplasmic face of the plasma membrane and the *trans*-Golgi network. Clathrin is composed of heavy and light chains that form triskelions, which then assemble into polyhedral curved lattices during the formation of clathrin-coated pits and vesicles.
- **Clathrin-coated vesicle:** A membrane-bound compartment that mediates endocytosis, formation of secretory granules at the *trans*-Golgi network, and transport from the *trans*-Golgi network to the endocytic pathway. In addition to clathrin, its major constitutes include cargo and adaptor proteins.
- **Clear plaque:** A plaque that contains only lyzed bacterial cells.
- **Cleavage and differentiation stage (of embryo development):** In morphogenetic terms, a zygote progresses through morphologically distinct stages of development, viz., globular, heart, torpedo and finally differentiated cotyledonary stages; this is termed as cleavage and differentiation stage of embryo development.
- **Cleavage furrow:** The constriction of the cell cortex that separates newly reformed nuclear after mitosis and results in the formation of two cells are the cleavage furrow (Fig. 23).

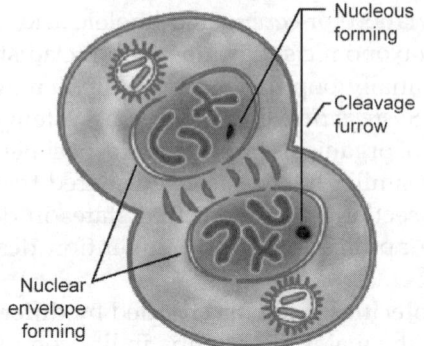

Fig. 23: Cleavage furrow

- **Cleavage stage:** The fertilized eggs of some species are very large and initially undergo several rounds of cell division without any growth of the cells between successive mitoses. As a result each embryo is progressively divided into smaller and smaller cells. This process is the cleavage stage of embryogenesis.
- **Cleave:** To break phosphodiester bonds of double stranded DNA, usually with a Type II restriction enzyme.
- **Cleaved amplified polymorphic sequence (CAPs):** Partial DNA sequence information for the locus of interest is used to create a set of PCR primers that are used to amplify the genome segment of interest. The amplification product is digested with the selected restriction enzyme, and digest is subjected to gel electrophoresis to detect polymorphism in the lengths of fragments, so generated.
- **Clinical trial:** One of the final stages in the collection of data (for drug approval prior to commercialization) in which the new drug is tested in human subjects. Used to collect data on effectiveness, safety, and required dosage.
- **Clonal anergy:** When extrathymic T-cells encounter antigens presented by such cells that lack the constimulatory molecules, they become nonresponsive; T-cell self-tolerance can also arise from clonal anergy.
- **Clonal deletion:** Describes the elimination of a clonal population of lymphocytes. At certain stages of lymphocyte development, clonal deletion can be induced when lymphocyte antigen receptors bind to their cognate antigen.
- **Clonal deletion:** B cells marked by negative selection, die by apoptosis.

- **Clonal propagation:** Vegetative propagation of plants considered to be physiologically and/or genetically uniform which originated from a single individual or explant is called clonal propagation.
- **Clonal selection:** Phenomenon of selective proliferation of lymphocytes, e.g. B-cells, in response to their interaction with an antigen.
- **Clone bank:** A population of organisms, each containing a DNA molecule inserted through cloning vector.
- **Clone:** A collection of genetically identical cells or organisms derived from a common ancestor where all members have similar genetic composition.
- **Clone-by-clone sequencing:** In this method, the fragments are first aligned into contigs, and each clone of the contig is then sequenced.
- **Cloning site:** A location on a cloning vector into which DNA can be inserted.
- **Cloned strain or line:** As train or line descended directly from a clone.
- **Cloning vector:** A carrier molecule, replicating autonomously, generally a plasmid or phage, into which any foreign DNA can be inserted, introduced into the host cell and many copies of the foreign DNA are produced (Fig. 24).

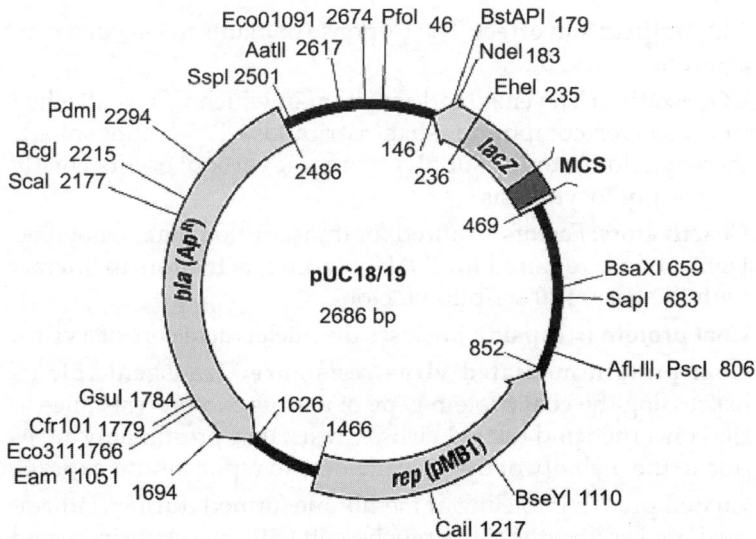

Fig. 24: Cloning vector

- **Cloning:** Incorporation of a DNA molecule into a chromosomal site or a cloning vector.
- **Clonotypic:** Characteristic of a clone, for example, T cells expressing the same T cell receptor are said to be clonotypic.
- **Closed continuous culture:** In this approach, a definite volume of culture is withdrawn regularly, cells are separated from the used medium and are added back to the culture so that cell biomass keeps on increasing.
- **Closed reading frame:** It contains termination codons that prevent its translation into protein.
- *Clostridium:* A genus of bacteria. Most are obligate anaerobes, and form endospores.
- **Cloverleaf:** Describes the structure of tRNA drawn in two dimensions, forming four distinct arm-loops.
- **CML:** Abbreviation for chronic myelogenous leukemia (also known as chronic myeloid leukemia, or chronic myelocytic leukemia).
- **CMV:** Acronym for cucumber mosaic virus.
- **Cocultivation:** Incubation of host cells or tissues with *Agrobacterium* or any other organism acting as a vehicle for a vector.
- **CO_2 fertilization effect:** The response of plants to elevated concentrations of CO_2.
- **CO_2 fixation:** The enzymatic reaction in which CO_2 is attached to a receiver compound, such as ribulose-1, 5-bisphosphate, thereby adding to the supply of organic carbon; occurs chiefly during photosynthesis.
- **Coactivators:** Factors required for transcription that do not bind DNA but are required for (DNA-binding) activators to interact with the basal transcription factors.
- **Coat protein (= capsid):** Encloses the nucleis acid core of a virus.
- **Coat protein-mediated virus resistance:** Transgenic plants expressing the coat protein gene of a virus exhibit resistance to the concerned and related viruses; resistance presumably arises due to the inability of the viral genome to replicate and express.
- **Coated pit:** An infolcling of membrane formed during clathrin-mediated endocytosis. It is pinched off to form a clathrin-coated vesicle.

- **Coated vesicles:** Vesicles whose membrane has on its surface a layer of a protein such as clathrin, COP-I, or COP-II.
- **Coatomer:** Another name for the complex of COPI coat proteins.
- **Coccus:** A spherical-shaped bacterium.
- **Cochaperonin:** A protein molecule inside living cells that works together with applicable chaperonin(s) to help ensure proper folding of the (new) protein molecules that are synthesized (manufactured) in the cell's ribosomes.
- **Cocloning (of molecules):** The additional (accidental) cloning (i.e. copying) of extra molecular fragments, other than the desired one, that sometimes occurs when a scientist is attempting to clone a molecule.
- **Coconut milk:** Liquid endosperm from immature nuts (before cellular endosperm formation has begun); boiled (to denature the proteins and enzymes), filtered and stored at –20°C.
- **Coconversion:** The simultaneous correction of two sites during gene conversion.
- **Cocoon:** A protective coverage for eggs and/or larvae produced by many invertebrates such as the silkworm moth.
- **Coculture:** Culture of plant cells/tissues of different species or even of different organisms (e.g. plant cell with bacteria) together in the same culture vessel.
- **Coculture with *Agrobacterium*:** Culture of plant cells/tissues with *Agrobacterium* cells, usually, to achieve genetic transformation.
- **Codex alimentarius commission:** An international regulatory body that is part of the United Nations Food and Agriculture Organization (UNFAO), it is one of the three international SPS (sanitary and phytosanitary) standard-setting organizations recognized by the World Trade Organization (WTO). Created in 1962 by the UN's FAO and the World Health Organization (WHO), the commission has 165 member nations. In Latin, *codex alimentarius* means food law or food code. Responsible for execution of the Joint FAO/WHO Food Standards Program, the Codex Alimentarius standards are a set of international food mandates adopted by the organization. With delegates from member country governmental agencies, the Codex Secretariat is headquartered in Rome, Italy. The commission periodically

determines, then publishes, a list of food ingredients and maximum allowable levels that it deems safe for human consumption (known as the *codex alimentarius*).

- **Coding:** The specification of a peptide sequence by the code contained in DNA molecules.
- **Coding end:** It is produced during recombination of immunoglobulin and T cell receptor genes. Coding ends are at the termini of the cleaved V and (D) J coding regions. The subsequent joining of the coding ends yields a coding joint.
- **Coding region:** A part of the gene that represents a protein sequence.
- **Coding sequence:** The region of a gene (DNA) that encodes the amino acid sequence of a protein.
- **Coding strand:** The strand of DNA in a gene that has the same sequence as the mRNA transcribed from the gene.
- **Codominance:** Both the alleles of a gene express themselves in heterozygotes.
- **Codominant alleles:** A pattern of inheritance in which both alleles of a gene are expressed in the heterozygote, three alleles A, B, and O determine human blood type. Three possible genotypes are AA, BB, OO that correspond to the phenotypes of blood type A, B, and O respectively; Two other genotypes are AO and BO that correspond to blood A and B, respectively because the O allele is recessive. The remaining genotype is AB, corresponding to blood type AB. Both the A and B alleles contribute to the phenotype of the heterozygote. Thus, the alleles A and B are said to be codominant, both the alleles produce effective product.
- **Codominant:** Two alleles are said to be codominant when they are each equally evident in the phenotype of the heterozygote.
- **Codon bias:** Preference for certain codons over the others from among the multiple codons specifying the same amino acid; each organism exhibits a different pattern of codon preference.
- **Codon:** A triplet of nucleotides that represents an amino acid or a termination signal.
- **Codon optimization:** An experimental strategy in which codons within a cloned gene—one not generally used by the host cell translation system, are changed by *in vitro* mutagenesis to the preferred codons without changing the amino acids of the synthesized protein.

- **Coefficient:** A number expressing the amount of some change or effect under certain conditions (e.g. the coefficient of inbreeding).
- **Coenzyme:** In case of enzymes; a specialized molecule that mediates electron transfer during redox catalysis.
- **Coevolution:** The evolution of complementary adaptations in two species caused by the selection pressure that each exerts on the other. It is common in symbiotic associations in insect-pollinated plants, etc.
- **Cofactor fermentation:** The simultaneous growth of two microorganisms in one bioreaction.
- **Cofactor recycle:** The regeneration of a spent cofactor by an auxiliary reaction such that it may be reused many times over by a cofactor- requiring enzyme during a reaction.
- **Cofactor:** In case of enzymes; a transition metal that mediates electron transfer during redox catalysis.
- **Cogeneration:** Production of both electricity and process heat (steam) in an industrial plant.
- **Cognate tRNAs:** Cognate tRNAs are those recognized by a particular aminoacyl – tRNA synthetase.
- **Cohesin** proteins form a complex that holds sister chromatids together. They include some SMC proteins.
- **Cohesive ends:** Single stranded complementary nucleotides on the ends of double stranded DNA molecule (Fig. 25).
- **Coincidence:** The ratio of the observed frequency of double

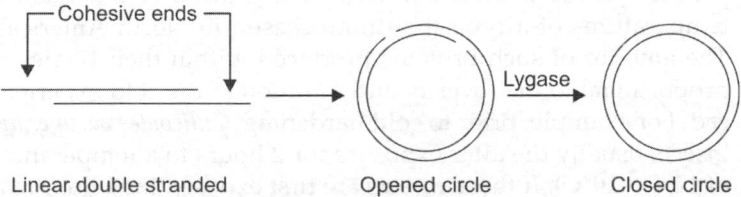

| Linear double stranded | Opened circle | Closed circle |

Fig. 25: Cohesive ends

crossing-over to the expected frequency where the expected frequency is calculated by assuming that the two crossing-over events occur independently of each other.
- **Coincidental evolution (coevolution):** It describes a situation in which two genes evolve together as a single unit.

- **Cointegrate:** A DNA molecule formed by the fusion of two different DNA molecules usually mediated by a transposable element.

C

- **Cointegrated structure:** Produced by fusion of two replicons, one originally possessing a transposon, the other lacking it; cointegrate have copies of the transposon present at both junctions of the replicons, oriented as direct repeats.
- **Cointegrated Ti vector:** A vector obtained by integration of an intermediate vector (IV) into the T-DNA region of a disarmed Ti plasmid; interaction by homologous recombination; IV contains the DNA fragment/gene to be transferred into plants.
- **Colplasmid:** These plasmids encode colicins, which are proteins that kill sensitive *E. coli* cells; they also carry genes that provide immunity to the particular colicins.
- **Colpretreatment of anthers:** Exposure of anthers to 5–9°C (rice) for 3–14 days before culturing them at 22–25°C; enhances the frequency of androgenesis.
- **Colchicines:** An alkaloid obtained from bulbs of autumn crocus (*Colchicum autumnale*); used for chromosome doubling as it prevents spindle formation.
- **Cold hardening:** A process of acclimatization in which certain organisms produce specific proteins that protect them from freezing to death during the winter. Among other organisms, the common housefly, the *Arabidopsis thaliana* plant, the fruit fly *Drosophila*, and no-see-ems (*Culicoides variipennis*) can produce these proteins (during the gradually decreasing temperatures of a typical autumn season in North America). The amount of such proteins produced within their bodies is proportional to the severity and duration of the cold experienced. For example, prior to cold hardening, *Culicoides variipennis* insects usually die after exposure for 2 hours to a temperature of 14°F (–10°C). If those insects are first exposed for 1 hour to a temperature of 41°F (5°C), approximately 98% of these insects can then survive exposure for 3 days to a temperature of 14°F (–10°C).
- **Cold-sensitive:** Cold-sensitive mutant is defective at low temperature but functional at normal temperature.
- **Coleoptile:** Protective sheath covering the shoot apex of the embryo in monocotyledons plants. It protects the plumule as it emerges through the soil.

- **Coleorhiza:** A protective sheath surrounding the radicle of monocotyledons plants.

- **Colicins:** Proteins produced by *Escherichia coli* (*E. coli*), that are toxic (primarily) to other closely-related strains of bacteria. The particular *E. coli* that produce a given colicin are generally unaffected by the colicin that they produce.

- **Colinear:** Relationship describes the 1:1 representation of a sequence of triplet nucleotides in a sequence of amino acids.

- **Collagen:** The major structural protein in connective tissue. It is instrumental in wound healing [stimulated by fibroblast growth factor (FGF), platelet-derived growth factor, and insulin-like growth factor-1].

- **Collagenase:** An enzyme that catalyzes the cleavage of collagen, such as when bacteria in the mouth cause production of collagenase that then cleaves (breaks down) the collagen that holds teeth in place. Some cancers use collagenase to break down connective tissues in the body they inhabit, enabling the cancers to form the (new) blood vessels that nourish those cancers and help those cancers spread through the body. Collagenase may also be responsible indirectly for certain autoimmune diseases such as arthritis, by breaking down the protective proteoglycan coat that covers cartilage in the body.

- **Collenchyma:** A tissue of living cells, the walls being unevenly thickened with cellulose and hemicellulose but never lignified. It functions in mechanical support in young, short-lived or non-woody organs and is thus found in midribs and leaf petioles.

- **Colony:** A growth of a group of microorganisms derived from one original organism. After a sufficient growth period, the growth is visible to the eye without magnification.

- **Colony blot:** The molecules (usually DNA) are from colonies of bacteria or yeast growing on a bacteriological plate.

- **Colony hybridization:** A technique for using *in situ* hybridization to identify bacteria carrying chimeric vectors whose inserted DNA is homologous with some particular sequence.

- **Colony stimulating factors:** Specific glycoprotein growth factors required for the proliferation and differentiation of hematopoietic progenitor cells. Different colony stimulating factors (CSFs) stimulate the growth of different cells.

- **Colorimetric biosensor:** It measures the heat released or absorbed during the reaction catalyzed by the biological component of the biosensor.
- **Color retention agents:** Agent that are used to preserve a food's existing color.
- **Combinatorial biology:** A term used to describe the set of DNA technologies used to generate a large number of samples of new chemicals (metabolites) via creation of non-natural metabolic pathways. The collection of samples, thus generated is called a library, and the samples are then tested for potential use (e.g. for therapeutic effect, in the case of a pharmaceutical). These technologies enable greater efficiency in a pharmaceutical researcher's screening process for drug discovery.
- **Combinatorial chemistry:** A term used to describe the set of technologies utilized to generate a large number of samples of (new) chemicals, which are then tested (screened) for potential use (e.g. for therapeutic effect, in the case of a pharmaceutical). These large numbers of chemical samples, thus generated, are called a library and are screened (e.g. for therapeutic effect) via a variety of laboratory, biosensor, computational, receptor, or animal tests. Combinatorial chemistry was made feasible by H Mario Geysen, who, during the 1980s, developed a methodology to synthesize arrays of peptides on pin-shaped solid supports. In addition, Richard Houghten developed a technique for creation of peptide libraries in small mesh bags by solid-phase parallel synthesis; thereby enabling automation of the process. For a library that is used for new drug (candidate) screening, high diversity in molecular structure among the chemicals in the library is desired to increase the efficiency of the screening process. One method used to measure diversity of the molecular structure among samples in a library is called molecular fingerprinting. If two samples are identical in molecular structure, the fingerprint coefficient is 1.0. If two samples are totally dissimilar in molecular structure, the coefficient is 0. The diversity of a library is measured by comparing each sample's molecular structure to that of all the others in the library.
- **Combinatorial library:** During the ligation, reaction with cDNAs of light and heavy antibody chains into a bacteriophage lambda (λ) vector, many novel combinations consisting of one

heavy and one light chain coding region are formed. The library comprises these combinations each in a separate vector.

- **Combining site:** The site on an antibody molecule that locks (binds) onto an epitope (hapten).
- **Combustion:** The practice of disposing of wastes by incineration in a special facility designed to handle large amounts of waste; modern combustion facilities also utilize some of the energy by generating electricity on the site.
- **Cometabolite:** The substrate, which induces the enzymes necessary for degradation of a xenobiotic, and serves as a source of energy, carbon and reducing power.
- **Commensal:** A term that literally means eating at the same table; it is used to refer to organisms such as the house mouse (*Mus musculus*), that tend to thrive alongside/among humans. For example, the numerous strains of *Salmonella* bacteria can live within the intestine of an adult cow without harming that cow, but would be pathogenic (disease causing) in a human's intestine. Similarly, the *E. coli* 0157:H7 strain of *Escherichia coli* form bacteria can live within the digestive system of an adult cow without harm, but is pathogenic in a human's digestive system. However, hundreds of other strains of *E. coli* bacteria live within the digestive system of humans, without causing harm to the human body.
- **Commensalism:** The interaction of two or more dissimilar organisms where the association is advantageous to one without affecting the other(s).
- **Commission E monographs:** Documents published by the Government of Germany, which detail the proven safety and efficacy of certain phytochemical-containing herbs (approved by the German Government). For example, consumption of St. John's Wort (a plant native to Europe) is approved in Germany for treatment of depressive mood disorders, anxiety, and nervous unrest.
- **Commission of biomolecular engineering:** An agency of the French Government, established to oversee and regulate all genetic engineering activities in France.
- **Committee for proprietary medicinal products:** The European Union's (EU's) scientific advisory organization dealing with new human pharmaceuticals approval. Its recommendations (e.g. to either approve or not approve a new product) are usually

adopted by the European Medicines Evaluation Agency (EEA), to which the Committee for proprietary medicinal products (CPMP) reports. Within 60 days of a CPMP "approval for recommendation" being adopted by the EMEA, each of the EU's member countries must advise the EMEA of its progress toward a regulatory decision on that pharmaceutical's submission for approvals.

* **Committee for veterinary medicinal products (CVMP):** The European Union's (EU's) scientific advisory organization dealing with approvals of new medicinal products intended for use in animals. Its recommendations (e.g. to either approve or not approve a new product) are usually adopted by the European Medicines Evaluation Agency (EMEA).

* **Committee on safety in medicines:** The British Government Agency that must approve new pharmaceutical products for sale within the United Kingdom. In concert with the Medicines Control Agency (MCA), it regulates all pharmaceutical products in the UK. It is the equivalent of the US Food and Drug Administration.

* **Community plant variety office:** An agency of the European Union established by council regulation 2100/94; and located in Angers, France. It applies UPOV rules across all countries of the European Union when a plant breeder registers a new plant variety at the community plant variety office. Thus, it confers and protects plant breeder's rights (PBR) across the entire European Union in a manner analogous to the way, the European patent office (EPO) confers patent rights (for patented inventions) across the entire European Union.

* **Companion cell:** Living cell associated with the sieve cell of phloem tissue in vascular plants.

* **Comparative genomics:** Study of differences and similarities in genome structure and organization of different organisms.

* **Compatibility group:** Group of plasmids contains members unable to coexist in the same bacterial cell.

* **Compatibility group:** Compatibility group of plasmids contains members unable to coexist in the same bacterial cell.

* **Compatible trait transgenics:** Those transgenics, which reduce the use of nonsustainable inputs without polluting the environment.

- **Competence for regeneration:** Ability of plant cells to regenerate plants via shoot or somatic embryo regeneration; same as totipotency.
- **Competence for transformation:** Ability of a cell to take up DNA and express the transgene.
- **Competence:** Ability of a bacterial cell to take up DNA molecules and become genetically transformed.
- **Competency:** An epidermal state, induced by treatment with cold cations during which bacterial cells are capable of taking-up foreign DNA.
- **Competent cell:** The cells those are capable of taking up DNA.
- **Complement cascade:** The precisely regulated, sequential interaction of proteins (in the blood) triggered by a complex of antibody and antigen to cause lysis of infected cells. The triggering of lysis by multivalent antibody-antigen complexes is mediated by the classical pathway, beginning with the activation of C1, the first component (protein) of the pathway. This activation step, in which C1 undergoes conversion from a zymogen to an active protease, results in sequential cleavage of the C4, C2, C3, and C5 components (proteins). C5b, a fragment of C5, then joins C6, C7, and C8 to penetrate the (cell) membrane bearing the antigen. Finally, the binding of some 16 molecules of C9 to this bridgehead produces large pores in the (cell) membrane, which cause the lysis and destruction of the target cell.
- **Complement:** Initially, it was defined as the activity of blood serum that completes the action of antibody; it consists of over 30 soluble and cell bound proteins and glycoproteins that interact in a highly regulated cascade, following the initial activation and carry out a number of basic functions.
- **Complement protein:** Proteins that bind to antibody-antigen complexes and help degrade the complexes by proteolysis.
- **Complementary (Molecular genetics):** Refers to strands of DNA that will hybridize (bind) to each other, due to one-for-one match-up of each strand's sequence of nucleotides. Any sequence (within the two strands) that does not match up one-for-one will not hybridize to the respective sequence (in the adjacent strand).
- **Complementary base pairing:** The formation of hydrogen bonds between adenine and thymine, and between guanine and cytosine is known as complementary base pairing.

C

- **Complementary-determining regions (CDRs):** The hyper variable regions of an antibody molecule consisting of three loops from the heavy chain and three from the light chain that together from the antigen-binding site.

- **Complementary DNA (cDNA):** Synthetic DNA transcribed from a specific RNA through the action of the enzyme reverse transcriptase.

- **Complementary entity:** One of a pair of nucleotide bases that from hydrogen bonds with each other.

- **Complementary gene:** Two or more interdependent genes such that (in the case of dominant complementaity) the dominant allele from either gene can only produce an effect on the phenotype of an organism if the dominant allele from the other gene is also present or (in the case of recessive complementary) only double homozygous recessive show the effect.

- **Complementary homopolymeric tailing:** The process of adding complementary nucleotide extensions to different DNA molecules, e.g. dG (deoxyguanosine) to the 3'-hydroxyl ends of another DNA molecule to facilitate after mixing the joining of the two DNA molecules by base pairing between the complementary extensions. Also called dG-dC tailing dA-dT tailing.

- **Complementary nucleotides:** Members of the pairs adenine-thymine, adenine-uracil and guanine-cytosine that have the ability to hydrogen bond to one another.

- **Complementary strand:** In case of nucleic acids; a polynucleotide strand that has complementary bases at every position of another polynucleotide strand.

- **Complementation assay:** See *in vitro* complementation assay.

- **Complementation group:** This is a series of mutations unable to complement when tested in pairwise combinations in *trans;* defines a genetic unit (the cistron).

- **Complementation test:** Determines whether two mutations are alleles of the same gene. It is accomplished by crossing two recessive mutations that have the same phenotype and determining whether the wild type phenotype can be produced. If so, the mutations are said to complement each other and are probably not mutations in the same gene.

- **Complementation:** It refers to the ability of independent (nonallelic) genes to provide diffusible products that produce wild phenotype when two mutants are tested in *trans*-configuration in a heterozygote.

- **Complete digestion (of DNA):** Complete digestion of DNA signifies that the restriction enzyme has cut the DNA at every recognition site for that enzyme present in the DNA.

- **Complete dominance:** The state in which the phenotype is the same, when the dominant allele is homozygous or heterozygous.

- **Complete linkage:** It describes the inheritance patterns for two genes on the same chromosome when the observed frequency for crossover between the loci is zero.

- **Complex locus:** Complex locus (of *D. melanogaster*) has genetic properties inconsistent with the function of a gene representing a single protein. Complex loci are usually very large (>100 kb) at the molecular level.

- **Complex medium:** In fermentation; it contain undefined constituents like soybean meal, molasses, cornsteep liquors, etc. and gives much higher yields of metabolites.

- **Complex oligosaccharide:** An N-linked oligosaccharide that is made during transit through the Golgi apparatus. Mannose residues are trimmed from the high mannose precursor in the rough endoplasmic reticulum and *cis* Golgi, and other sugars are added by enzymes in the medial and trans Golgi cisternae to form a complex oligosaccharide.

- **Complex organic additive:** A nutritive mixture of undefined composition, e.g. yeast extract, coconut milk, malt extract, tomato juice, etc.

- **Complex probes:** The labeled mRNA used as probe; represents the total mRNA produced by the cell.

- **Complexity:** The total length of different sequences of DNA present in a given preparation.

- **Composite transposons:** Composite transposons have a central region flanked on each side by insertion sequences, either, or both of which may enable the entire element to transpose.

- **Compositing:** The process of letting organic wastes decomposes in the presence of air; nutrient-rich compost is the resulting product.

- **Compost:** Fully decomposed organic material (Fig. 26).

C

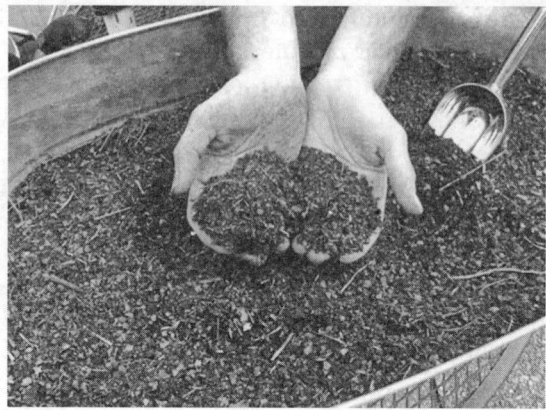

Fig. 26: Compost

- **Compound:** Any substance that is made up of two or more different kinds of atoms bonded together.
- **Compound chromosome:** A chromosome formed by the union of two separate chromosomes as in attached-X chromosomes or attached-X-Y chromosomes.
- **Computer:** It is device that can accept data, perform certain functions on that data and present the results of those operations with accuracy (Fig. 27).

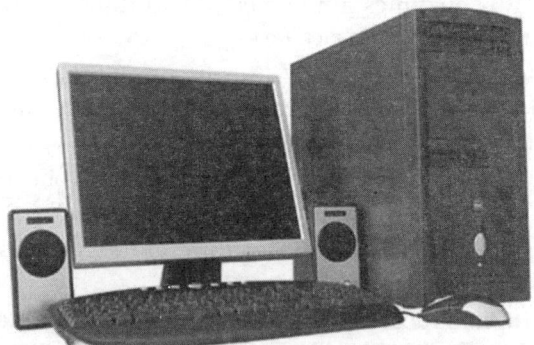

Fig. 27: Computer

- **Concatemer:** Concatemer of DNA consists of a series of unit genomes repeated in tandem.
- **Concentration gradient:** A change in the concentration of a molecule or ion from one point to another. The gradient might

be gradual (as in a solution that is not homogenous) or abrupt (created by a membrane).

- **Concerted evolution:** The ability of two related genes to evolve together as though constituting a single locus.
- **Concordance:** Identify of mathched pairs or groups for a given trait such as sibs expressing the same trait.
- **Condensation reaction:** One in which a covalent bond is formed with loss of a water molecule, as in the addition of an amino acid to a polypeptide chain.
- **Condensin:** Proteins are components of a complex that binds to chromosomes to cause condensation for meiosis or mitosis. They are members of the SMC family of proteins.
- **Conditional lethal mutations:** Kill a cell or virus under certain (non-permissive) conditions, but allow it to survive under other (permissive) conditions.
- **Conditioned medium:** In case of plant tissue culture; a cell-free medium in which cells/tissues had been grown for some time; permits culture of cells at a much lower density than in fresh medium. In case of animal tissue culture; a medium in which homologous cells were grown for a period of time.
- **Conditioning:** 1. The effects on phenotypic characters of external agents during critical developmental stages. 2. The undefined interaction between tissues and culture medium resulting in the growth of single cells or small aggregates. Conditioning may be accomplished by immerzing cell or callus contained within a porous material (such as dialysis tubing) into fresh medium for a period dependent on cell density and a volume related to the amount of fresh medium.
- **Configuration:** The three-dimensional arrangement in space of substituent groups in stereoisomers.
- **Conformation:** The three-dimensional arrangement of substituent groups in a protein or other molecular structure free to assume different positions. The geometric form or shape of a protein in three-dimensional space.
- **Conidium:** Asexual spore produced by a specialized hypha in certain fungi.
- **Conjugate:** A molecule created by fusing together (via recombination or chemically) two unlike (different) molecules. The purpose is to create a molecule in which one of the original

C

molecules has one function, i.e. a toxic, cell-killing function, while the other original molecule has another function, such as targeting the toxin to a specific site which might include cancerous cells. For example, molecules of interleukin-2 (IL-2) have been fused with molecules of diphtheria toxin to create a conjugate that does the following: It enters leukemia and lymphoma cells. Because these two types of cancer cells possess IL-2 receptors on their surfaces, the IL-2 (targeting function) binds to that receptor and is internalized. The diphtheria toxin (killing function) then shuts down protein synthesis within the cancer cells. It then kills the cancerous cells. This type of approach is widespread and there are many different types of conjugates. One consists of enzymes used in the treatment of certain molecular diseases attached covalently to polyethylene glycol (PEG). In this case, the PEG greatly diminishes both the immunogenicity (the ability to induce an immune reaction) and the antigenicity (the ability to react with preformed antibodies). Antibodies may be used as vectors to carry both relatively small molecules of destructive chemicals or proteins to specific sites (cells) within the body. Antibodies may be coupled to enzymes, toxins, and/or ribosome—inhibiting proteins, as well as to radioisotopes. These conjugates are known collectively as immunoconjugates.

- **Conjugated enzyme:** An enzyme made up of a protein part (apoenzyme) and a nonprotein part.
- **Conjugated linoleic acid:** A naturally occurring n-6 poly-unsaturated fatty acid (PUFA) discovered in 1979, whose consumption by humans has been linked to reduction in risk for atherosclerosis, reduction in blood triglyceride levels, reduction in body fat (adipose tissue) in obese humans, and reduction in risk for breast cancer, skin cancer, and some other types of cancer. Conjugated linoleic acid (CLA) exhibits powerful antioxidant properties (i.e. it "quenches" free radicals). Chemically, CLA consists of two linoleic acid molecules linked together by a chemical bond, so it is a dimer. Foods that are naturally highest in CLA content include beef, lamb, full-fat milk, butter, cheese, some creams, and full-fat yogurt. Feeding of soybean oil (in feed rations) to livestock has been proven to increase CLA content in the resultant meat. In 1998, TR Dhiman showed that feeding of soybean oil containing (i.e. whole) soybeans to dairy cattle also increased the content of CLA in

their milk. Research conducted during the 1990s indicated that consumption of CLA (by humans, swine, rats, etc.) causes the bodies of those animals to change the way they utilize and store energy. Thus, the body requires less food to perform at the same level. The body also tends to produce less body fat (adipose tissue) and more lean protein (muscle) tissue.

- **Conjugated protein:** A protein containing a metal or an organic prosthetic group, or both. For example, a glycoprotein is a conjugated protein bearing at least one oligosaccharide group.
- **Conjugation:** It describes mating between two bacterial cells, when (part of) the chromosome is transferred from one to the other.
- **Conjugative functions:** Plasmid-based gesen and their products that facilitates the transfer of a plasmid from one bacterium to another.
- **Conjugative plasmid:** Mediate DNA transfer through conjugation; as a result, they spread rapidly among the bacterial cells of a population, e.g. F-plasmids, many R-plasmids and some Col plasmids.
- **Consensus sequence:** A common, although not necessarily identical sequence of nucleotides in DNA or amino acids in proteins.
- **Consequence analysis (in recombinant DNA research):** Assessment of the consequences of GMOs producing adverse effects on the environment, including human health.
- **Conservation tillage:** Refers to crop production (farming) techniques/practices such as low-tillage crop production, no-tillage crop production, etc. that avoid or minimize the disturbance of topsoil.
- **Conservation:** Refers to the management of a resource in such a way as to assure that it will continue to provide maximum benefit to humans in the long run; it includes various degrees of use or protection, depending on what is necessary to maintain the resource over a long period.
- **Conservative recombination:** It involves breakage and reunion of pre-existing strands of DNA without any synthesis of new stretches of DNA.
- **Conservative replication:** DNA replication in which one new DNA molecule has parental strands and other contains both newly synthesized strands.

- **Conservative transposition:** The movement of large elements, originally classified as transposons, but now considered to be episomes. The mechanism of movement resembles that of phage lambda.

- **Conserved:** Positions are defined when many examples of a particular nucleic acid or protein are compared and the same individual bases or amino acids are always found at particular locations.

- **Conserved sequence:** A base sequence present without any change in all DNA sequence having the same function.

- **Consortia:** Microorganisms that interact with each other (or at least coexist peacefully when growing together. An example of such interaction/coexistence would be bioleaching.

- **Constant domains:** Regions of antibody chains that have the same amino acid sequence in different members of a particular class of antibody molecules.

- **Constant region:** Constant region of immunoglobulins are coded by C genes and are the parts of the chain that vary least. Those of heavy chains identify the type of immunoglobulin.

- **Constitutive enzymes:** Enzymes that are part of the basic, permanent enzymatic machinery of the cell. They are formed at a constant rate and in constant amounts regardless of the metabolic state of the organism. For example, enzymes that function in the production of cell-usable energy (such as ATP) might be good candidates. And this, in fact, is the case with the enzymes of the glycolytic sequence, which is the most ancient energy-yielding catabolic pathway.

- **Constitutive genes:** Expressed as a function of the interaction of RNA polymerase with the promoter, without additional regulation; sometimes also called housekeeping genes in the context of describing functions expressed in all cells at a low level.

- **Constitutive heterochromatin:** The inert state of permanently nonexpressed sequences, usually satellite DNA.

- **Constitutive mutations:** It causes genes that usually are regulated to be expressed without regulation.

- **Constitutive:** Process is one that occurs all the time, unchanged by any form of stimulus or external condition.

- **Constitutive enzyme:** Synthesized continually regardless of growth conditions.

- **Constitutive gene:** Continually expressed in all cells of an organism.
- **Constitutive promoter:** A promoter, which does not require any specific stimulus for activity; always active in all cell types.
- **Constitutive synthesis:** Continual production of RNA or protein by an organism.
- **Constitutively secreted:** Macromolecules are transported to the plasma membrane or secreted at a relatively co-nstant rate. They include lipids and soluble and membrane proteins. They are not secreted by regulated exocytosis and they exit to the plasma membrane from the trans-Golgi network.
- **Consultative Group on International Agricultural Research (CGIAR):** An organization that is co-sponsored by the Rome-based United Nations Food and Agriculture Organization (FAO), the United Nations Development Programme (UNDP), and the World Bank. The CGIAR is an association of 58 public and private donors that jointly support 16 International Agricultural Research Centers located primarily in developing countries. Twelve of the research centers have collectively assembled 500,000 different preserved samples (i.e. germplasm) of major food, forage, and forest plant species into a gene bank. This, the world's largest internationally held collection of genetic resources, was legally placed under the auspices of the FAO in 1994 in order to hold the collection in trust for the international community. Since 1970, CGIAR's collection has supported research efforts to develop better varieties of staple foods consumed primarily in developing countries of the world.
- **Contained use:** Any operation undertaken within a facility, installation or other physical structure, which effectively limit the contact with and the impact on the external environment.
- **Containment:** A combination of laboratory procedures, laboratory equipment and installations, and host-vector systems designed to minimize accidental release of organisms during laboratory operations, their dissemination and survival in the environment, and accident infection of laboratory workers and of persons outside the laboratory; includes two types: physical and biological.
- **Contaminant:** By definition, any unwanted or undesired organism, compound, or molecule present in a controlled environment. Unwanted presence of an entity in an otherwise clean or pure environment.

- **Contamination:** Presence of unwanted microorganisms in microbial, plant or animal cultures, food or any products in laboratory or industry.
- **Context:** Of a codon in mRNA refers to the fact that neighboring sequences may change the efficiency with which a codon is recognized by its aminoacyl-tRNA or is used to terminate protein synthesis.
- **Contig:** A set of overlapping clones that provides a physical map of a protein of chromosome. It refers to contiguous map.
- **Contiguous (contig) map:** The alignment of sequence data from large, adjacent regions of the genome to produce a continuous nucleotide sequence across a chromosomal region.
- **Con-Till:** An abbreviation that refers to conservation tillage farming practices.
- **Continuous bioreactor:** There is continuous inflow of fresh medium into the reactor, and outflow of used medium (with or without cells) during the entire incubation period; cell density can be maintained at a predetermined level; continuous source of biomass or inoculums.
- **Continuous cell line:** In animal cell culture; a cell line that can be maintained indefinitely.
- **Continuous culture:** A suspension culture held at constant volume and continuously supplied with nutrients by the inflow of fresh medium.
- **Continuous fermentation:** A process in which cells or micro-organisms are maintained in culture in the exponential growth phase, by the continuous addition of fresh medium that is exactly balanced by the removal of cell suspension from the bioreactor.
- **Continuous flow reactor:** Substrate solution is continuously pumped into reactor, while product is continuously withdrawn; based on immobilized enzymes.
- **Continuous flow stirred tank digesters:** These digesters are continuously fed as well as stirred to achieve a very high mixing; the spent substrate is also continuously removed; they are suited to treat medium to high strength (2–10% solids) wastes; these are the most common type of digesters used for sewage and animal excreta treatment.
- **Continuous flow stirred tank reactor:** Based on immobilized enzymes; substrate solution is continuously pumped in, and

product removed, and reaction mixture is continuously mixed by stirring.

- **Continuous free-flow zone electrophoresis:** In this electrophoresis, a continuous stream of buffer flows perpendicular to the electrical field between two cooled glass plates kept 0.5–1.0 mm apart; it separates even such particles that have minimal differences in the surface charge; it separates even cells.

- **Continuous perfusion:** A type of cell culture in which the cells (either mammalian or otherwise) are immobilized in part of the system, and nutrients/oxygen are allowed to flow through the stationary cells, thus, effecting nutrient-waste exchange. Ideally the system incorporates features that retard the activity of proteolytic enzymes, and reduce the need for anti-infective agents (e.g. antibiotics) and fetal bovine serum, which are required by most other cell culture systems. Continuous perfusion is used because, among other things, it eliminates the need to separate the cells from the culture medium when fresh medium is exchanged for old.

- **Continuous variation:** Variation not represented by distinct classes. Phenotypes grade into each other, and measurement data are required for analysis. Multiple genes are unusually responsible for this type of variation aka quantitative variation compare with discontinuous variation.

- **Contractile ring:** A ring of actin filaments that forms around the equator at the end of mitosis and is responsible for pinching the daughter cells apart (Fig. 28).

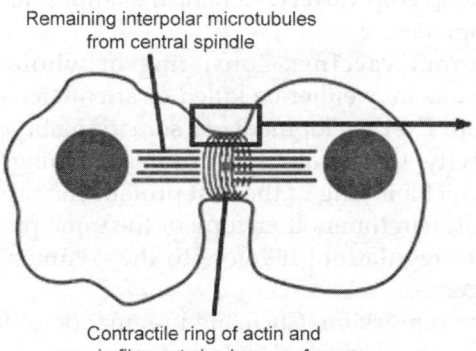

Remaining interpolar microtubules
from central spindle

Contractile ring of actin and
mysoin filaments in cleavage furrow

Fig. 28: Contractile ring

C

- **Control:** To direct or regulate cultures with addition of plant growth regulators. Unchanged protocol or treatment for comparison with the experimental treatment. The term is commonly used for untreated organisms.
- **Control of endophytic contamination:** In this case, surface sterilization is ineffective; a suitable systemic fungicide and/or an antibiotic is usually added to the culture medium; preferably, explants are taken from green-house grown plants.
- **Control sequences:** Those sequences of DNA adjacent to a gene (in genome) and turn on and/or turn off that gene.
- **Controlled environment:** The environment in which parameters, such as light, temperature, relative humidity and sometimes the partial gas pressure, are fully controlled.
- **Controlling elements:** Controlling elements of maize are transposable units originally identified solely by their genetic properties. They may be autonomous (able to transpose independently) or autonomous (able to transpose only in the presence of an autonomous element).
- **Convection:** Mass or bulk movement of one part of a solution relative to the rest, usually because of density differences.
- **Convention on biological diversity (CBD):** The international treaty governing the conservation and use of biological resources around the world that was signed by more than 150 countries at the 1992 United Nations Conference on Environment and Development. Article 19.4 of the CBD called for establishment of a protocol on biosafety to govern the transnational-boundary movement of nonindigenous living organisms.
- **Conventional crop variety:** Genetic makeup is not modified by genetic engineering.
- **Conventional vaccine:** Consisting of whole pathogenic organism, this may either be killed or attenuated.
- **Conversion:** The development of a somatic embryo into a plant.
- **Cooperativity:** Cooperativity in protein binding describes an effect in which binding of the first protein enhances binding of a second protein (or another copy of the same protein).
- **Coordinate regulation:** It refers to the common control of a group of genes.
- **Coordinate repression:** Correlated regulation of the structural genes in an operon by a molecule that interacts with the operator sequence.

- **Coordinated framework for regulation of biotechnology:** The regulatory framework through which the US evaluates and approves new products derived via biotechnology. The coordinated framework assigns specific regulatory tasks to each of the US Government's applicable agencies (see below). For example, the US Environmental Protection Agency (EPA) is assigned to evaluate and regulate all genetically modified pest protected (GMPP) new plants, in terms of their impact on pests. The US Food and Drug Administration (FDA) is assigned to evaluate and regulate all new food crops derived via biotechnology, in terms of their potential impact on food safety (allergenicity, toxicity, etc.). The US Department of Agriculture (USDA) is assigned to evaluate and regulate all new plants derived via biotechnology, in terms of field (outdoor) testing and of potential impact on the environment such as weediness.

- **COP-I:** Coated vesicle is a membrane-bounded compartment that buds from the cytoplasmic face of the Golgi complex and mediate retrograde transport from the Golgi complex to the rough endoplasmic reticulum. COP-I-coated vesicles may also mediate transport between Golgi cisternae.

- **COP-II:** Coat consists of a protein complex containing five major proteins. COP II-coated vesicles are membrane-bounded vesicles that bud from the cytoplasmic face of the rough endoplasmic reticulum and mediate anterograde transport from the rough endoplasmic reticulum (ER) to the Golgi.

- **Copolymers:** Mixtures consisting of more than one monomer. For example, polymers of two kinds or organic bases, such as uracil and cytosine (poly-UC) have been combined for studies of the genetic code.

- **Coppicing:** Production of young shoots, especially, after the main shoot has been cut off; the young shoots are juvenile.

- **Copy choice:** A type of recombination used by RNA viruses, in which the RNA polymerase switches from one template to another during synthesis.

- **Copy number:** The average number of molecules of a plasmid of a gene per genome present in a cell.

- **Cordycepin:** 3′ deoxyadenosine, an inhibitor of polyadenylation of RNA.

- **Core DNA:** The 146 bp of DNA contained on a core particle.

- **Core enzyme:** The complex of RNA polymerase subunits that undertakes elongation. It does not include additional subunits or factors that may needed for initiation or termination.
- **Core histone:** One of the four types (H2A, H2B, H3, H4) found in the core particle derived from the nucleosome (this excludes histone HI).
- **Core particle:** A digestion product of the nucleosome that retains the histone octamer and has 146 bp of DNA; its structure appears similar to that of the nucleosome itself.
- **Core promoter:** Of RNA polymerase I is the region immediately surrounding the startpoint. It is necessary and sufficient to initiate transcription, but only at a low level.
- **Core:** Sequence is the segment of DNA that is common to the attachment sites on both the phage lambda and bacterial genomes. It is the location of the recombination event that allows phage lambda to integrate.
- **Corepressor:** A small molecule that triggers repression of transcription by binding to a regulator protein.
- **Corn meal medium:** It is prepared by grinding degermed (de-embryonated) corn to fine powder, and 8–10% of this corn meal is heated to gelatinize the starch.
- **Corn rootworm:** A complex of several strains of beetles referring to the larva stage of the corn rootworm beetle (*Diabrotica virgifera virgifera*), which historically has laid its eggs on corn/maize (*Zea mays* L.) plants. When they hatch, the larva must feed on the roots of the corn/maize plant in order to live. Some strains of *Bacillus thuringiensis* (*B.t.*) have proven to be effective against the corn rootworm, when sprayed onto them or genetically engineered into the corn/maize plant. In 1992, a new genetic variant of corn rootworm known as the Western phenotype or Western corn rootworm (*Diabrotica virgifera virgifera* LeConte) was discovered in the US. It prefers to lay its eggs on soybean plants instead of corn plants.
- **Corn:** The domesticated plant *Zea mays* L. also known as maize. A green, leafy (grain) plant that is one of the world's largest providers of edible starch and fructose (sugar) for mankind's use. This summer annual varies in height from 2 feet (0.5 meter) to more than 20 feet (6 meters) tall. The seeds (kernels) are borne in cobs, ranging in size from 2 feet long to smaller than a man's thumb. Due to genetic variation (of different hybrids/varieties),

the fraction of kernel that consists of recoverable starch varies between 42 and 73% for different corn varieties. Due to genetic variation (of different hybrids/varieties), the fraction of kernel that consists of protein varies between 8 and 10%, but that protein content can be increased by 10% by inserting the glutamate dehydrogenase (GDH) gene into the corn plant. Due to genetic variation, the fraction of kernel that consists of oil varies between 3.5 and 8.5% for different varieties. Grown widely in the world's temperate zones, corn is grown as far north as latitude 58° in Canada and Russia and as far south as latitude 40° in the Southern Hemisphere. During the 1980s, scientists were able to insert genes from *Bacillus thuringiensis* (*B.t.*) bacteria into the corn plant to make that plant resistant to certain insects. During the 1990s, scientists were able to insert genes into the corn plant to make it tolerant to certain herbicides and to cause the corn plant to produce monoclonal antibodies (MAbs). Some of the major economic pests of corn include the European corn borer (*Ostrinia nubilalis*), corn earworm (*Helicoverpa zea*), corn rootworm (*Diabrotica virgifera virgifera*), and beet armyworm (*Pseudaletia unipuncta*) (Fig. 29).

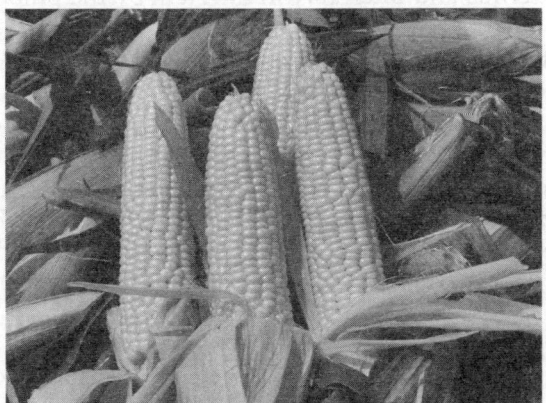

Fig. 29: Corn

- **Coronary heart disease (CHD):** A disease of the heart and arteries, in which (among other effects) cholesterol is deposited on the interior walls (lumen endothelium), where it can sometimes later break off and cause death (via heart attack). Risk factors (increased risk) for CHD include high blood levels of triglycerides, high levels of apolipoprotein B, high levels of LDLPs/VLDLs (the two lipoproteins that are most likely to deposit cholesterol on artery walls), and/or low levels of HDLPs (the lipoproteins that help to clear away cholesterol deposits from artery walls). A human diet containing a large amount of certain phytosterols (e.g. campesterol, beta-sitosterol, and stigmasterol) has been shown to lower total serum (blood) cholesterol and low-density lipoproteins (LDLP) levels by approximately 10%; and thereby lower the risk of CHD. A human diet containing a large amount of oleic acid causes lower blood cholesterol levels and thus lower risk of CHD and atherosclerosis.

- **Corpus:** The corpus is found below the tunica and is a part of the apical meristem. In the corpus, cell divide in all directions, giving them an increase in volume.
- **Correct PCR product:** At the second cycle of PCR, primers will anneal to the long product, i.e. amplification product of first cycle much before 3′-end where sequences complementary to them are located. Primer extension step in this cycle.
- **Correlation:** A statistical association between variables.
- **Cortex:** Primary tissue of a stem or root bounded externally by the epidermis and internally in the stem by the phloem and in the root by the pericycle.
- **Cos site (ends):** The 12-base, single strand, complementary extension of phage lambda (λ) DNA.
- **Cosegregation:** When two genetic conditions appear to be inherited together.
- **Cosmid:** Cosmid is a hybrid plasmid composed of the *cos* sites of lambda and antibiotic resistance genes of plasmids, enters into the host cell like a phage and replicate like a plasmid (Fig. 30).

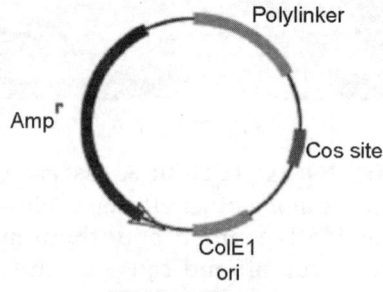

Fig. 30: Cosmid

- **Cosuppression:** A significant decrease (silencing) in the expression of a gene (within an organism's genome/DNA) that (often) results when man inserts and causes a homologous gene to be expressed. For example, high-oleic oil soybeans result when the GmFad2–1 gene (which codes for native $\Delta 12$ desaturase enzyme) is inserted and expressed in traditional varieties of soybeans. That is because the inserted gene silences itself and the endogenous GmFad2–1 gene (i.e. the one naturally/originally present in the soybean plant), prevents formation of the $\Delta 12$ desaturase enzyme (which normally causes most oleic acid within soybeans to be converted into polyunsaturated acid/linoleic acid).

- **Cosuppression:** Describes the ability of a transgene (usually in plants) to inhibit expression of the corresponding endogenous gene.

- **Cot curve:** A plot of the extent of renaturation of DNA against time.

- **Cot:** The product of DNA concentration and time of incubation in a reassociation reaction.

- **Cot$_{1/2}$:** The Cot required to proceed to half completion of the reaction; it is directly proportional to the unique length of reassociating DNA.

- **Cotransfection:** In baculovirus expression systems, the procedure by which the baculovirus and the transfer vector are simultaneously introduced into insect cells in culture.

- **Cotransformation:** In genetic engineering experiments, it is often necessary to transform with a plasmid for which there is no selectable phenotype and then screen for the presence of that plasmid within the host cell. Cotransformation is a technique of host cells that are incubated with two types of plasmid, one of which is selectable and the other not. Cells which have been transformed with the first plasmid are then selected. If transformation has been carried out at high DNA concentration, then it is probable that these cells will also have been transformed with the second (nonselectable) plasmid. The technique is frequently used in experiments with mammalian cells.

- **Cotranslational translocation:** Describes the movement of a protein across a membrane as the protein is being synthesized. The term is usually restricted to cases in which the ribosome binds to the channel. This form of translocation may be restricted to the endoplasmic reticulum.

- **CotV2:** The midpoint of a Cot curve. It is proportional to the complexity of the DNA sequences in the renaturation reaction.
- **Cotyledons:** Leaf like structures at the first node of the seedling stem. In some dicotyledons, they contain stored food for the young plant not yet able to photosynthesize its own food. Often referred to as seed leaves.
- **Counterion:** An ion of opposite charge to the one under consideration. Generally, a similar ion.
- **Countertranscript:** An RNA molecule that prevents an RNA primer from initiating transcription by base pairing with the primer.
- **Coupling:** The phase state in which either two dominant or two recessive alleles of two different genes occur on the same chromosome. Also called *cis* configuration, cf repulsion.
- **Covalent bond:** A bond in which an electron pair is equally shared by protons in two adjacent atoms (Fig. 31).

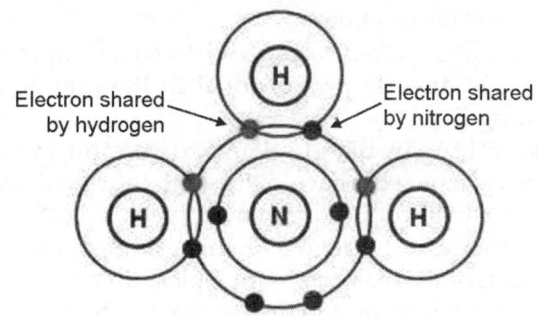

Fig. 31: Covalent bond

- **Covalent catalysis:** The chemical groups, e.g. amino groups, in the side chains of amino acids present in the active site of the enzyme become covalently bound to a group in the substrate molecule; another substrate may then react with the substrate bound to the enzyme to form the product.
- **Covalently closed circle (CCC):** A double-stranded DNA molecule with no free ends. The two strands are interlinked and will remain together even after denaturation. In its native form a CCC will adopt a super coiled configuration.
- **Covariance:** A measure of the statistical association between variables. The extent to which two variables vary together.

- **Cowpea mosaic virus (CpMV):** A virus that infects cowpea (*Vigna unguiculata*) plants (known as black-eyed peas in the US), but does not infect animals. Researchers have discovered how to cause CpMV to express certain animal virus proteins (i.e. antigens) on its surface, through genetic engineering. These virus antigens hold potential to replace the antigens currently used in vaccines, which are fraught with problems due to their production in animal cells, bacterial cells, or yeast cells. In addition, CpMV acts as an intrinsic, natural adjuvant to the (animal virus) antigens, since it provokes an immune response itself (Fig. 32).

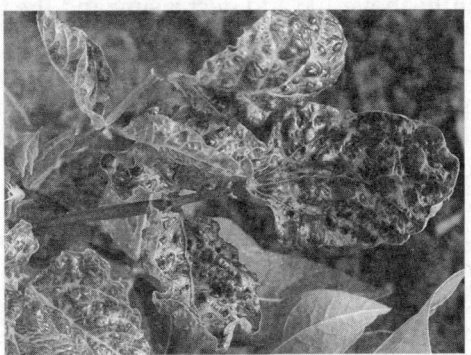

Fig. 32: Cowpea mosaic virus

- **Cowpea trypsin inhibitor (CpTI):** A chemical that is naturally coded by a certain cowpea (*Vigna unguiculata*) plant gene. It kills certain insect larvae by inhibiting digestion of ingested trypsin, thereby starving the larvae to death.
- **CP4 EPSPS:** The enzyme 5-enolpyruvyl-shikimate-3-phosphate synthase, which is naturally produced by an *Agrobacterium* species (strain CP4) of soil bacteria. CP4 EPSPS is essential for the functioning of that bacterium's metabolism biochemical pathway. CP4 EPSPS happens to be unaffected by glyphosate-containing or sulfosate-containing herbicides, so introduction of the CP4 EPSPS gene into crop plants (e.g. soybeans) makes those plants essentially impervious to glyphosate-containing or sulfosate-containing herbicides.
- **cpDNA:** The DNA of plant plastids including chloroplasts.
- **CpG island** is a stretch of 1–2 kb in a mammalian genome that is rich in unmethylated CpG doublets.

C

- **Crisis** is a state, reached when primary cells placed into culture are unable to replicate their DNA because their telomeres have become too short. Most cells die, but a few emerge by a process of immortalization that usually involves changes to bypass the limitations of telomeric length.

- **Crisscross inheritance:** Transmission of a gene from a male parent through female child to male grandchildren, e.g. X-linked inheritance.

- **Critical breed:** A breed where the total number of breeding females is less than 100 or the total number of breeding males is less than or equal to five or the overall population size is close to, but slightly above 100 and decreasing and the percentage of pure breed females is below 80%.

- **Critical maintained breed and endangered maintained breed:** Categories where critical or endangered breeds are being maintained by an active public conservation programme or within a commercial or research facility.

- **Critical micelle concentration:** Also known as the CMC of a surfactant, it is the lowest surfactant concentration at which micelles are formed. That is, the CMC represents that concentration of surfactant at which individual surfactant molecules aggregate into distinct, high molecular weight spherical entities called micelles. Or from another viewpoint, it represents the concentration of a surfactant, above which micelles or reverse micelles will spontaneously form through the process of self-aggregation (self-assembly).

- **Cross:** In genetic studies the mating of two individuals or populations. Also called mating.

- **Cross-breeding:** Mating between members of different populations (lines, breeds, races or species).

- **Cross-contamination:** Especially in animal cell cultures; presence of cells from other cell lines of the same species, or from some other species.

- **Cross-feeding:** Cells of one species (or genotype) provide the biochemicals needed by cells of another species (or genotype); in coculture or feeder layer technique.

- **Cross-hybridization:** The hydrogen bonding of a single-stranded DNA sequence that is partially but not entirely complementary to a single-stranded substrate. Often, this involves hybridizing a DNA probe for a specific DNA sequence to the homologous sequences of different species.

- **Cross over:** A recombinant chromosome.
- **Cross-pollination:** Fertilization of a plant from a plant with a different genetic makeup; hybrid.
- **Cross-pollination efficiency:** Efficiency of pollen from one plant reaching the stigma of another plant.
- **Cross-reaction:** In immunology; interaction of an antibody induced by one antigen with another antigen due to a similarity in their epitopes.
- **Crossing over:** The exchange of corresponding chromosome parts between homologous by breakage and reunion (Fig. 33).

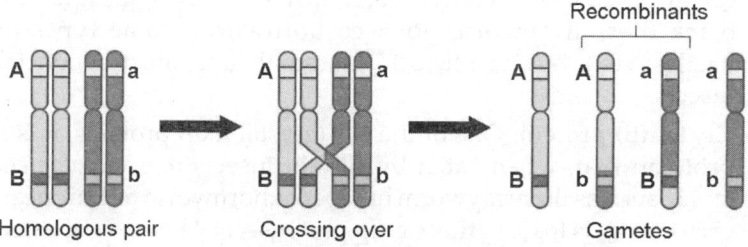

Fig. 33: Crossing over

- **Crossing over unit:** A measure of distance between two loci on genetic maps that is based on the average number.
- **Crossover control:** Limits the number of recombination events between meiotic chromosomes to 1–2 crossovers per pair of homologus.
- **Crossover fixation:** Refers to a possible consequence of unequal crossing-over that allows a mutation in one member of a tandem cluster to spread through the whole cluster (or to be eliminated).
- **Crown:** The region at the base of the stem of cereals and forage species from which tillers or branches arise. In woody plants, the root stem junction. In forestry, the top portions of the tree.
- **Crown gall:** A tumor occurring at the base of certain plants due to infection of the plant by *Agrobacterium tumifaciens*.
- **CRP activator (CAP activator):** A positive regulator protein activated by cyclic AMP. It is needed for RNA polymerase to initiate transcription of certain (catabolite-sensitive) operons of *E. coli*.

- **Cruciferae:** A taxonomic group (family) of plants that includes canola, mustard, oilseed rape, etc. (*See also* Brassica).

- **Cruciform:** The structure produced at inverted repeats of DNA if the repeated sequence pairs with its complement on the same strand (instead of with its regular partner in the other strand of the duplex).

- **CRW:** Refers to one type of corn (maize) that has been made resistant to the depradations of corn rootworm larvae (*Diabrotica virgifera virgifera*) via genetic engineering.

- **Cry proteins:** A class of proteins produced by *Bacillus thuringiensis* (*B.t.*) bacteria (or plants into which a *B.t.* gene has been inserted). Cry (crystal like) proteins are toxic to certain categories of insects (corn borers, corn rootworms, mosquitoes, black flies, armyworm, tobacco hornworm, some types of beetles, etc.), but harmless to mammals and most beneficial insects.

- **Cry1A (b) protein:** One of the cry (crystal like) proteins, it is a protoxin that, when eaten by certain insects (e.g. *Lepidoptera* larvae such as the armyworm or tobacco hornworm or European corn borer), is toxic to those crop pest insects. However, if eaten by a mammal, the Cry1A(b) protein is digested harmlessly within one minute.

- **Cry1A (c) protein:** One of the cry (crystal like) proteins.

- **Cry1F protein:** One of the cry (crystal like) proteins, it is a protoxin that, when eaten by the European corn borer, South Western corn borer, black cutworm, and fall armyworm, is toxic to those insects.

- **Cry3B(b) protein:** One of the cry (crystallike) proteins, it is a protoxin that, when eaten by certain insects (e.g. larvae of corn rootworm *Diabrotica virgifera virgifera*), is toxic to those insects.

- **Cry9C protein:** See Cry1F protein.

- **Cryobiological preservation (cryopreservation freeze preservation):** The preservation of germplasm resources in a dormant state by cryogenic techniques, as currently applied to storage of plant seeds and pollen, microorganisms, animal sperm and tissue culture cell lines.

- **Cryobiology:** The branch of science, which deals with preservation of cells, tissues, etc. in frozen state in liquid nitrogen.

* **Cryogenic injuries:** Injuries to cells due to the procedure of cryopreservation; chiefly during freezing and, also during thawing; may be physical (due to ice crystal formation, which may rupture cell organelles or even cells) or chemical (due to toxic solution effect and/or loss of vital solutes from cells through leakage during freezing/thawing).
* **Cryogenic:** At very low temperature.
* **Cryopreservation:** Culture preservation at ultra—low temperature of –196°C.
* **Cryoprotectant:** A chemical agent that inhibits freezing and thawing damage to cells.
* **Cryotherapy:** Prolonged exposure (4 months or more) of plants to a low temperature (e.g. 5°C), followed by shoot-tip culture for virus elimination; superior to thermotherapy.
* **Cryptic:** Structurally heterozygous individuals, not identifiable on the basis of abnormal meiotic-chromosome pairing configurations.
* **Cryptic satellite:** A satellite DNA sequence not identified as such by a separate peak on a density gradient; that is, it remains present in main-band DNA.
* **Crystal protein:** An insecticidal protein present as a crystalline inclusion in *Bacillus thuringiensis* spores; 17 distinct groups of 130 or 70 kDa proteins.
* **CryX protein:** One of the cry (crystal-like) proteins, it is a protein that, when eaten by corn rootworm larvae (*Diabrotica virgifera virgifera*), is toxic to those insects.
* **CT:** Refers to conservation Tillage practices of crop production.
* **CTAB method:** When CTAB (cetyltrimethyl-ammonium bromide) is added to the cell extracts, it forms an insoluble complex with nucleic acids, this precipitate is recovered through centrifugation and resuspended in 1M NaCl; carbohydrates, proteins, etc., are discarded with supernatant. The nucleic acid solution is treated with RNase, and DNA is concentrated by ethanol precipitation.
* **ctDNA:** Chloroplast DNA.
* **CTNBio:** Acronym for Brazil's National Technical Commission on Biosafety, the Brazilian government's regulatory body for granting formal approval to a new genetically engineered plant (e.g. a genetically engineered crop to be planted). CTNBio is analogous to Germany's ZKBS (Central Commission on

Biological Safety), Australia's GMAC (Genetic Manipulation Advisory Committee), Kenya's Biosafety Council, and India's Department of Biotechnology.

- **Cultivar:** Refers to the cultivated variety of a plant species. Genetically, all individuals of a cultivar are uniform.
- **Culture:** Any population of cells (bacteria, algae, protozoa, virus, yeasts, plant cells, mammalian cells, etc.) growing on, or in, a medium that supports their growth. Typically used to refer to a population of the cells of a single species or a single strain. A medium which contains only one specific organism (e.g. *E. coli* bacteria) is known as a pure culture. A culture may be preserved (stored alive) by freezing, drying (in which the cells go dormant), subculturing on an agar medium, or other methods.
- **Culture alteration:** A term used to indicate a persistent change in the properties of a culture's behavior (e.g. altered morphology, chromosome constitution, virus susceptibility, nutritional requirements, proliferate capacity, etc.). The term should always be qualified by a precise description of the change which has occurred in the culture.
- **Culture initiation:** Surface sterilization of explants and establishing them *in vitro*.
- **Culture medium:** The medium on which cells, tissues and organs are cultured; contains inorganic salts, vitamins, a carbon source and growth regulators as per need.
- **Culture room:** Room with controlled environment, e.g. regulated temperature, light, etc. and used for culture of cells/tissues/organs/organisms.
- **Curing:** The elimination of a plasmid from its host cell. Many agents which interfere with DNA replication, e.g. ethidium bromide, can cure plasmids from either bacterial or eukaryotic cells.
- **Curing agent:** A substance that increases the rate of loss of plasmids during bacterial growth.
- **Cut:** An enzyme-induced, highly specific break in both strands of a DNA molecule (opposite one another). The enzymes involved are called restriction enzymes.
- **Cuticle:** Layer of cutin or wax on the other surface of leaves and fruits and that reduces water loss.
- **Cutinization:** Impregnation of cell wall with cutin; cutinization of the outer-most cell wall is essential for somatic embryo development.

- **Cutting:** A detached plant part that under appropriate cultural conditions can regenerate the complete plant without a sexual process.
- **Cutting periodicity:** The spacing between cleavages on each strand when a duplex DNA immobilized on a flat surface is attacked by a DNAase that makes single-strand cuts.
- **C-value:** The total amount of DNA in the genome (per haploid set of chromosomes).
- **C-value paradox:** Describes the lack of relationship between the DNA content (C-value) of an organism and its coding potential.
- **Cybrid:** A cytoplasmically hybrid cell with organelles from both parental sources (obtained through fusion of cytoplast with a whole cell) and a nucleus of only one cell. Nucleus of the other cell denatured.
- **Cybridization:** The process of cybrid production; usually, to transfer cytoplasm from one species into other.
- **Cyclic AMP (cAMP):** A molecule of AMP in which the phosphate group is joined to both the 3′ and 5′ positions of the ribose; its binding activates the CAP, a positive regulator of prokaryotic transcription (Fig. 34).

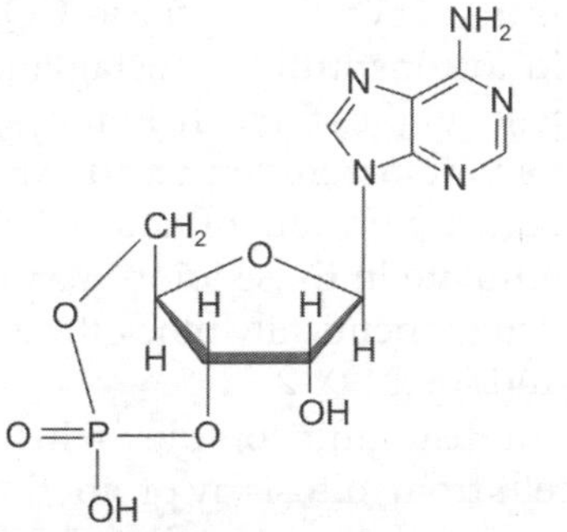

Fig. 34: Cyclic AMP

- **Cyclic phosphorylation:** Synthesis (manufacturing) of adenosine triphosphate (chemical reaction) that occurs during photosynthesis in plants. Also called photosynthetic phosphorylation (photophosphorylation).
- **Cyclin-dependent kinase (CDK):** One of a family of kinases which are inactive unless bound to a cyclin molecule. Most cyclin-dependent kinases participate in some aspect of cell cycle control.

- **Cyclin-dependent kinase inhibitors (CKI):** A class of proteins which inhibit cyclin-dependent kinases by binding to them. Inhibition lasts until the cki is inactivated, often in response to a signal for the cell cycle to progress.
- **Cyclins:** Proteins that accumulate continuously throughout the cell cycle and are then destroyed by proteolysis during mitosis.
- **Cyclodextrin:** A macrocyclic (doughnut-shaped) carbohydrate ring produced enzymatically from starch. The external surface is hydrophobic while the interior is hydrophilic in nature. The hole of the doughnut is large enough to accommodate guest molecules. Uses include solubilization, separation, and stabilization of molecules in the interior cavity of, or in association with, the cyclodextrin molecules.
- **Cycloheximide:** Also called actidione. A chemical that inhibits protein synthesis by the 80S eukaryotic ribosomes; it does not, however, inhibit the 70S ribosomes of prokaryotes. The chemical blocks peptide bond formation by binding to the large ribosomal subunits.
- **Cyclo-oxygenase:** Abbreviated COX, it is an enzyme that converts arachidonic acid to prostaglandins in the human body. There are two forms of cyclo-oxygenase: COX-1, which converts arachidonic acid to constitutive prostaglandins, which help to maintain the tissues of the stomach, kidneys, and intestines, and COX-2, which converts arachidonic acid to inducible prostaglandins, which can cause pain and inflammation in the body's joints when they accumulate in those joints. Aspirin and some other pain-relieving drugs chemically block the above described activity of COX-1 and/or COX-2.
- **Cyclosome:** A multisubunit complex which initiates anaphase and the exit of cells from mitosis by promoting the ubiquitination and proteolysis of a variety of proteins. These include the mitotic cyclins, several proteins required to hold sister chromatids together, and other proteins which control the dynamics of the mitotic spindle.
- **Cyclosporin:** An immune-system-suppressing drug isolated from a mold in the mid-1970s by the Swiss firm of F Hoffmann-LaRoche and Co. AG. The drug is used to prevent an (organ recipient's) immune system from rejecting a transplanted organ and typically must be taken by the organ recipient for the duration of his or her lifetime. Cyclosporin's

mechanism of action is to prevent the divalent calcium cation (Ca^{2+}) from entering T-lymphocytes to activate certain genes within those T-lymphocytes (that trigger the rejection process). In 1996, Thomas Eisner reported that the mold *Tolypocladium inflatum*, from which cyclosporin is harvested, prefers a natural (wild) substrate of a deceased dung beetle. During 2000, it was discovered that cyclosporin inhibits growth of the parasitic microorganism *Toxoplasma gondii* (which can cause loss of sight, and neurological disease in humans).

- **Cysteine (CYS):** An amino acid of molecular weight (mol. wt.) 121 Daltons. Incorporated in many proteins, it possesses a sulphydryl group (SH) that makes cysteine a mild reducing agent. Cysteine can cross-link with another cysteine located on the same or on a different polypeptide chain to form disulfide bridges. The free cysteine group is called a thiol group. High levels of cysteine content in certain genetically engineered corn (maize) kernels have been shown to inhibit in-field production of mycotoxins in corn (e.g. by several species of fungi that can be carried into corn plants by insects).

- **Cystic fibrosis transmembrane regulator protein (CFTR):** A protein that regulates proper chloride ion transport across the cell membranes of human lung airway epithelial cells. When the gene that codes for CFTR protein is damaged or mutated, the (mutant) CFTR protein fails to function properly, causing mucous (and bacteria) to accumulate in the lungs. This lung disease is known as cystic fibrosis.

- **CystX:** Refers to a naturally occurring gene present in the genome (DNA) in some varieties of soybean plant, that confers on those particular soybean varieties (some) resistance to the soybean cyst nematode. Discovered and developed during the 1990s by Jamal Faghihi, John Ferris, Virginia Ferris, and Rick Vierling.

- **Cytochrome:** Any of the complex protein respiratory pigments (enzymes) occurring within plant and animal cells. They usually occur in mitochondria and function as electron carriers in biological oxidation. Cytochromes are involved in the handing off of electrons to each other in a stepwise fashion. In the process of handing off, other events take place which result in the production of energy that the cell needs and is able to use.

- **Cytochrome P450:** An enzyme within the liver that contains an iron-heme cofactor. It catalyzes many different biological hydroxylation reactions. Essentially, the enzyme renders fat soluble (hydrophobic) molecules water soluble or more water soluble (by introduction of the hydrophilic hydroxyl group), so that the molecules may be removed (washed) from the body via the kidneys. This enzyme is being investigated for its potential as a catalyst in the hydroxylation of specific (valuable) industrial chemicals.

- **Cytochrome P4503A4:** An enzyme within the liver that, in humans, catalyzes reactions involved in the metabolism (breakdown) of certain pharmaceuticals. Those pharmaceuticals include some sedatives, antihypertensives, the antihistamine terfenadine, and the immunosuppressant cyclosporin.

- **Cytodifferentiation:** Development of various cell types from the relatively undifferentiated meristematic cells.

- **Cytogenetics:** Area of biology concerned with chromosomes and their implication in genetics. Cellular activity and variability.

- **Cytogenetic abnormalities:** Changes in chromosome number and/or structure.

- **Cytogenetic instability:** Origin of variation in chromosome number and/or structure; occurs in virtually all cell cultures.

- **Cytogenetic map:** It depicts the locations of various genes in a chromosome relative to specific microscopically visible landmarks in the chromosomes; commonly used in eukaryotes since they have relatively large microscopically observable chromosomes.

- **Cytokine:** A small polypeptide that affects the growth of particular types of cells.

- **Cytokines:** Hormone like proteins that act by binding to specific receptors on cell surface; needed to activate B cells and T cells.

- **Cytokinesis:** The final process involved in separation and movement apart of daughter cells at the end of mitosis (Fig. 35).

- **Cytokinins:** A class of plant growth regulators which causes cell division, cell differentiation, shoot differentiation and breaking of apical dominance, e.g. BAP, kinetin, zeatin.

- **Cytology:** The study of the structure and function of cells.

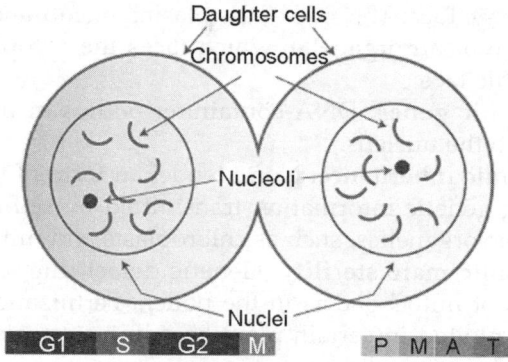

Fig. 35: Cytokinesis

- **Cytolysis:** The dissolution of cells, particularly by destruction of their surface membranes.
- **Cytomegalovirus (CMV):** A virus that infects different groups of people in varying amounts, depending on their behavior. For example, 40–90% of American heterosexuals, and about 95% of homosexuals are infected with CMV. CMV normally produces a latent (nonclinical, nonobvious) infection, but with AIDS or other events can cause immune system suppression. CMV produces a febrile (fever-causing) illness that is usually mild in nature but can become retinitis (eye infection). CMV can be treated (to half life-and sight-threatening infection) in immuno-compromised patients (i.e. transplant patients and AIDS victims) with Ganciclovir ™, an antiviral compound developed by Syntex or Foscarnet™, a compound developed by Astra Pharmaceuticals. In 1996, Stephen E Epstein found that latent CMV may cause changes in artery wall cells that aid clogging of arteries in adults (especially following balloon angioplasty).
- **Cytopathic:** Damaging to cells.
- **Cytoplasm:** The material between the plasma membrane and the nucleus.
- **Cytoplasmic DNA:** The DNA within an organism (e.g. plant) that is not inside the cell's nucleus. Cytoplasmic DNA (i.e. located in the cell's mitochondria and the chloroplasts) is not transferred from plant to plant via pollen, as nuclear DNA is.
- **Cytoplasmic domain:** The part of a transmembrane protein that is exposed to the cytosol.

- **Cytoplasmic face:** The side of the plasma membrane, or of the membrane of an organelle, which faces the cytoplasm is its cytoplasmic face.
- **Cytoplasmic genes:** DNA-containing bodies in the cell but external to the nucleus.
- **Cytoplasmic inheritance:** Non-Mendelian form of inheritance involving genetic information transmitted by self-replicating cytoplamic organelles, such as chloroplasts and mitochondria.
- **Cytoplasmic male sterility:** Genetic defect due to defective functions of mitochondria in the pollen. Fertilization will not occur. Exploited in certain plant breeding strategies, such as F1- hybrid maize cultivars.
- **Cytoplasmic organelles:** Discrete subcellular structures located in the cytoplasm of cells, these allow division of labor within the cell.
- **Cytoplasmic protein synthesis:** The translation of mRNAs representing nuclear genes; it occurs via ribosomes attached to the cytoskeleton.
- **Cytoplast:** A protoplast without an active nucleus.
- **Cytosine (c):** One of the pyrimidine (six-membered single ringed nitrogenous base) in DNA and RNA (Fig. 36).

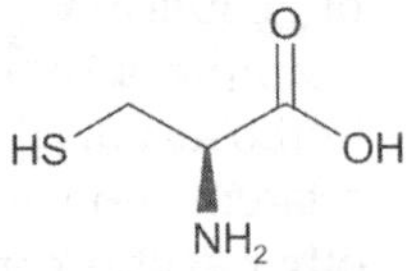

Fig. 36: Cytosine

- **Cytoskeleton:** Consists of networks of fibers in the cytoplasm of the eukaryotic cell.
- **Cytosol:** The general volume of cytoplasm in which organelles (such as the mitochondria) are located.
- **Cytotoxic:** Poisonous to cells.
- **Cytotoxic T cell:** A T lymphocyte (usually CD^{8+}) that can be stimulated to kill cells containing intracellular pathogens, such as viruses.
- **Cytotype:** A maternally inherited cellular condition in Drosophila that regulates the activity of transposable P elements.

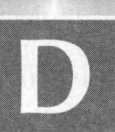

- **Desaturase:** One of the desaturases (enzymes).
- **D arm:** Of tRNA has a high content of the base dihydrouridine.
- **D Loop:** A region within mitochondrial DNA in which a short stretch of RNA is paired with one strand of DNA, displacing the original partner DNA strand in this region. The same term is used to describe the displacement of a region of one strand of duplex DNA by a single-stranded invader in the reaction catalyzed by RecA protein.
- **D segment:** It is an additional sequence that is found between the V and J regions of an immunoglobulin heavy chain.
- **Dabs (Single-domain antibodies):** Antibodies with only one (instead of two) protein chain derived from only one of the domains of the antibody structure. Dabs exploit the finding that, for some antibodies, half of the antibody molecule binds to its target antigen almost as well as the whole molecule. The potential advantages of dabs are that they can be made easily by bacteria or yeasts, and offer a way to clone antibody-like molecules into bacteria, and hence to be able to easily screen millions of antibodies. Related ideas are single-chain antigen (SCA), binding technology biosynthetic antibody binding sites (BABS), minimum recognition units (MRUs) and complementary determining regions (CDRs).
- **Daffodils:** Refers to the approximately 80 species of flowering plants within the genus *Narcissus*. Native to Southern Europe and Northern Africa, they are the source of golden rice and the Alzheimer's disease treatment compound galantamine hydrobromide.
- **Daidzin:** The β-glycoside form (isomer in which glucose is attached to the molecule at the seven position of the A ring) of the isoflavone known as daidzein (aglycone form).
- **Dalton (Da):** A unit of mass roughly equivalent to the mass of a hydrogen atom 1.67 × 10.24 g. Named after the famous

nineteenth century chemist John Dalton (1766–1844). Used in shorthand expression of molecular weight, especially as kilodaltons (kDa) or megadaltons (MDa), which are equal to respectively to 1×10^3 and 1×10^6 daltons.

- **Darwinian cloning:** Selection of a clone from a large number of essentially random starting points rather than isolating a natural gene or making a carefully designed artificial one. Molecules which are more similar to those needed are selected, mutated to generate new variants and reselected. The cycle proceeds until the required molecule is found. The advantage of the system is that the selection is from a vast number of possibilities.
- **Data cleaning:** A process whereby automated or semi-automated algorithms are used to process experimental data including noise, experimental errors and other artifacts, in order to generate and store high-quality data for use in subsequent analysis. Data cleaning is typically required in high-throughput sequencing where compression or other experimental artifacts limit the amount of sequence data generated from each sequencing run or read.
- **Data mining:** The ability to query very large databases in order to satisfy a hypothesis ('top-down' data mining) or to interrogate new hypothesis based on rigorous statistical correlations ('bottom-up' data mining).
- **Data processing:** Data processing is defined as the systematic performance of operations upon data such as handling, merging, sorting and computing. The semantic content of the processed data may be changed.
- **Data waterhouses:** Vast arrays of heterogeneous (biological) data stored within a single logical data respiratory that are accessible to different querying and manipulation methods.
- **Database mining tools:** Search engines and analysis tools needed for utilization of various databases.
- **Database mining:** Process of database utilization.
- **Database:** A repository of sequences (DNA or amino acids) which provide a centralized and homogenous view of its contents.
- **Daughter cells:** The two cells that result from a cell division are referred to as daughter cells. In budding yeast only the cell derived from the bud is called the daughter cell.
- **Daughter:** Strand or duplex of DNA refers to the newly synthesized DNA.

- **DBT:** An acronym used by some to designate the Indian Department of Biotechnology.
- **DDT (Dichlorodiphenyl trichloroethane):** The first and once most widely used synthetic organic pesticide; belongs to the chlorinated hydrocarbon class.
- *De Novo*: It means anew, afresh.
- *De Novo* **methylase:** Adds a methyl group to an unmethylated target sequence on DNA.
- *De Novo* **sequencing:** A procedure in which DNA sequence is ascertained by the hybridization of the test DNA to an array of all possible eightmer oligonucleotides (usually on a gene chip). All positive interactions are identified and then aligned using the overlapping sequences to delineate the complete DNA sequence.
- **Deacetylase:** It is an enzyme that removes acetyl groups from proteins.
- **Deacylated tRNA:** It has no amino acid or polypeptide chain attached because it has completed its role in protein synthesis and is ready to be released from the ribosome.
- **Deamination:** The removal of amino groups from molecules (e.g. in an animal's food) via the energy-consuming metabolism of excess amino acids eaten by that animal. For example, when livestock are fed more lysine (amino acid) than their body needs in a given day (animals' bodies can only utilize the essential amino acids in precise amounts/ratios of their daily diet), the excess lysine is metabolized to urea and then excreted.
- **Death domain:** It is a protein-protein interaction motif found in certain proteins of the apoptotic pathway.
- **Death phase:** The final growth phase during which nutrients have been depleted and cell number decreases.
- **Decamer (oligonucleotide):** An oligonucleotide 10 bases long; generally used in RAPD (Randomly amplified polymorphic DNA) analysis.
- **Decapitation:** Removal of the shoot tip/shoot apex, usually of the main shoot; relatives apical dominance.
- **Deceleration phase:** The phase of declining growth rate, following the linear phase and preceding the stationary-phase in most batch-suspension cultures.
- **Dedifferentiation:** Reversion of differentiated cell to the meristematic stage; induced by auxin and/or cytokinin.

- **Deep well injection:** Disposal of liquid chemical wastes by putting them into deep dry wells, where they permeate dry strata.
- **Defective viral genome mediated resistance:** In case of some viruses; a deleted version of their genomes, when integrated into host genome, leads to resistance to the concerned virus.
- **Defective virus:** A virus that, by itself, is unable to reproduce when infecting its host (cell), but that can grow in the presence of another virus. The other virus provides the necessary molecular machinery that the first virus lacks.
- **Defensins:** A class of peptides that inhibits certain fungal diseases. These are produced as a natural defense by some plants. For example, the alfalfa plant produces a defensin known as alfAFP (alfalfa antifungal peptide). In addition to protecting the plant from certain diseases, the alfAFP also inhibits a fungal disease known as potato early dying complex (also called *Verticillium* wilt), which is caused by the fungus *Verticillium dahliae*.
- **Deficiency:** Insufficiency or absence of one or more usable forms of enzymatic, nutritional or environmental requirements so that development, growth or physiological functions are affected.
- **Defined:** Fixed conditions of medium, environment and protocol for growth.
- **Defined molecular marker:** A DNA fragment whose function or specific features are known.
- **Degeneracy:** Degeneracy in the genetic code refers to the lack of an effect of many changes in the third base of the codon on the amino acid that is represented.
- **Degenerate codons:** Two or more codons that code for the same amino acid. For example, isoleucine is specified by the AUU, AUC, and AUA triplets. Since in this case more than one triplet codes for isoleucine, the codons are called degenerate.
- **Degenerate primer:** Set of primers having the same sequence, except for one or more positions where variation occurs.
- **Degeneration:** Changes in cells, tissues or organs due to disease.
- **Degradation:** A gradual wearing down or away. Also, with regard to soil, a lowering of the nutrient content and associated ability to support continuing crop growth.
- **Degradative plasmids:** These plasmids enable the host bacterium to metabolize unusual molecules like toluene and salicylic acid.

D

- **Degradosome:** It is a complex of bacterial enzymes, including RNAases, a helicase, and enolase (a glycolytic enzyme), which may be involved in degrading mRNA.
- **Dehalogenation:** The removal of halogen atoms (chlorine, iodine, bromine, fluorine) from molecules usually during biodegradation.
- **Dehiscence:** The spontaneous and often violent opening of a fruit, seed pod or anther to release and disperse the seeds or pollen.
- **Dehydrogenases:** Enzymes that catalyze the removal of pairs of hydrogen atoms from their substrates.
- **Dehydrogenation:** The removal of hydrogen atoms from molecules. When those molecules are the components of vegetable oils/fats, a lower content percentage of saturated fats results.
- *Deinococcus radiodurans*: A species of bacteria capable of surviving 1.5 million rads of gamma radiation (3,000 times the lethal radiation dose for humans), surviving long periods of dehydration, and surviving high doses of ultraviolet radiation. *Deinococcus radiodurans* was discovered in 1956 in some canned meat.
- **Deionized water:** Water which is free of most inorganic (not completely free, since Na is present in ample quantities) and most organic compounds.
- **Delaney clause:** Formerly part of American Federal Law (1959 Delaney amendment to the food, drug and cosmetic act), it was eliminated in 1996. The delaney clause had set a zero-risk tolerance level for carcinogenic pesticide residues in processed foods.
- **Delayed early:** Genes in phage lambda are equivalent to the middle genes of other phages. They cannot be transcribed until regulator protein(s) coded by the immediate early genes have been synthesized.
- **Deletion (deficiency):** It is a type of mutation in which an end of a chromosome breaks off or when two simultaneous breaks lead to the loss of a segment from the chromosome, even if only one member of pair of chromosomes is affected, a deletion can cause abnormalities. Cri du chat syndrome is deletion in which an individual has a small head, is mentally retarded, and has facial abnormalities, and abnormal glottis and larynx resulting in a cry resembling that of a cat.

- **Deletions:** Generated by removal of a sequence of DNA, the regions on either side being joined together.
- **Deliberate release:** Putting something into the outside world. In biotechnology it means putting a genetically modified organism (GMO) into field trials.

D

- **Delta 12 desaturase:** An enzyme present within the soybean plant and in other oilseed crops (canola, maize/corn, etc.). Delta 12 desaturase (Δ 12) is involved in the synthesis pathway utilized by oilseed crops to synthesize (manufacture) polyunsaturated fatty acids (e.g. linoleic acid) from monounsaturated fatty acids (e.g. oleic acid) in seeds (while those seeds are developing).
- **Deme:** A group of organisms in the same taxon.
- **Demethylase:** It is a casual name for an enzyme that removes a methyl group, typically from DNA, RNA, or protein.
- **Demethylation:** Removal of methyl ($-CH_3$) groups usually from methylated "C" residues.
- **Demineralize:** To remove the mineral content (salts, ions) from a substance especially water. Removal methods include distillation and electrolysis. The process is demineralization.
- **Denaturation (of DNA or RNA):** Conversion from the double-stranded to the single-stranded state; separation of the strands is most often accomplished by heating.
- **Denaturation (of protein):** Conversion from the physiological conformation to some other (inactive) conformation.
- **Denature:** To induce structural alterations that disrupt the biological activity of a molecule. Often refers to breaking hydrogen bonds between base pairs in double-stranded nucleic acid molecules to produce single-stranded polynucleotides or altering the secondary and tertiary structure of a protein destroying its activity.
- **Denatured DNA:** DNA converted from double-stranded to single-stranded form by a denaturation process such as heating the DNA solution. In the case of heat denaturation, the solution becomes very gelatinous and viscous (Fig. 1).
- **Denaturing polyacrylamide gel electrophoresis:** The use of polyacrylamide gel electrophoresis (PAGE) in order to separate and analyze DNA fragments (sequences) after that DNA is first denatured. This methodology can be employed to scan DNA in order to detect point mutations.

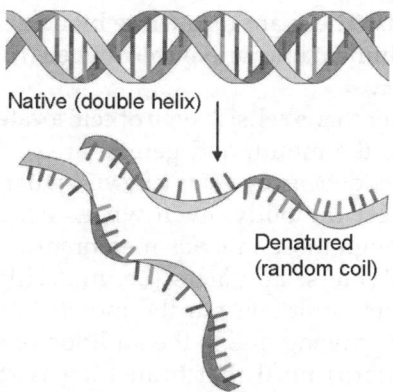

Native (double helix)

Denatured
(random coil)

Fig. 1: Denatured DNA

- **Dendrimers:** Polymers (i.e. molecules composed of repeating atomic units within the molecule) that repeatedly branch (while growing due to addition of more atoms in a repeating pattern) until that branching is stopped by the physical constraint of contacting itself (i.e. having formed a complete, hollow sphere). Discovered during the 1970s by Donald Tomalia, dendrimers possess sites on their exterior surface to which genetic material (e.g. genes or other portions of DNA) can be attached. Dendrimers bearing such genetic material have shown the capacity to successfully transfer that genetic material into more than thirty types of living animal cells.
- **Dendrites:** Highly branched structures that extend from the (nucleus of) neurons to (synapse junctions with) other neurons (e.g. in human brain tissue). The primary purpose of dendrites is to process signals that are generated/received at the synapses (e.g. from the dendrites of adjoining neurons). Neuron ribosomes are located in the dendritic spines, the dendrite projections that form synapses (the junctions between dendrites where signal transfer between neurons takes place). Thus, those ribosomes make the proteins that are crucial to learning and memory (e.g. accomplished via growth/changes of dendrites). Messenger RNAs are synthesized (manufactured) in the nucleus of the neuron, then transported on microtubules (filaments within the neuron cell) to the ribosomes in the dendrites, where they cause manufacture of proteins (e.g. enzymes) in response to synapse activity (i.e. signals).

- **Dendritic cells:** These are rare white blood cells, which act to stimulate the human immune system (T cells) to combat certain types of cancer.
- **Dendritic Langerhans cells:** A type of cell, located in the mucous membranes of the mouth and genital areas, that permits the human immunodeficiency virus (the virus that causes AIDS) to enter and infect the body, even when there are no cuts or abrasions through those mucous membranes.
- **Dendritic polymers:** Polymers (i.e. molecules composed of repeating atomic units within the molecule) that repeatedly branch (while growing due to the addition of more atoms in a repeating pattern) until that branching is stopped (e.g. by physical constraints, for those polymers within living tissues). In the absence of physical constraints, dendritic polymers can continue branching (and growing) until they form a complete (hollow) sphere. Such spheres are potentially useful for protecting and delivering a fragile pharmaceutical molecule to specific tissue(s) within the body.
- **Denitrification:** Reduction of nitrate to nitrites or into gaseous oxides of nitrogen, or even into free nitrogen by organisms.
- **Density gradient:** It is used to separate macromolecules on the basis of differences in their density. It is prepared from a heavy soluble compound such as CsCl.
- **Density-dependent inhibition:** Describes the limitation that eukaryotic cells in culture grow only to a limited density, because growth is inhibited, by processes involving cell-cell contacts.
- **Density gradient centrifugation:** High-speed centrifugation in which molecules float at a point where their density equals that in a gradient of cesium chloride or sucrose. The density gradient may either be formed before centrifugation by mixing two solutions of different density (as in sucrose density gradients) or it can be formed by the process of centrifugation itself (as in CsCl and Cs_2SO_4 density gradients).
- **Denticle:** It is a pigmented, hardened spike of cuticle protruding from the ventral epidermis of a *Drosophila* embryo.
- **Deoxynivalenol:** A mycotoxin (toxin that is naturally produced by a fungus under certain conditions) which, under specific temperature and moisture conditions, is sometimes produced by certain fungi (e.g. some *Fusarium*) growing in some grains

(e.g. corn/maize). Deoxynivalenol is also known as DON, and/ or vomitoxin, because certain animals (especially swine) will often vomit after they have consumed grain that contains deoxynivalenol due to its toxicity.

- **Deoxyribonuclease (DNAase):** It is an enzyme that specifically digests DNA. It may cut only one strand or may cut both strands.

- **Deoxyribonucleic acid (DNA):** It is a nucleic acid molecule consisting of long chains of polymerized (deoxyribo) nucleo- tides. In double-stranded DNA the two strands are held together by hydrogen bonds between complementary nucleotide base pairs.
- **Deoxyribonucleotide:** A deoxyribonucleotide having a phosphate residue at 3'- or 5'- position; *in vivo*, 5'- phosphate is the rule.
- **Deoxyribose:** A 5 carbon sugar with a hydrogen atom rather than a hydroxyl group attached to 2' carbon (Fig. 2).
- **Deoxyriboside:** Compound obtained by a linkage between deoxyribose sugar and an organic base.

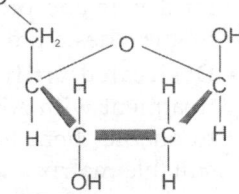

Fig. 2: Deoxyribose

- **Derepressed:** This state describes a gene that is turned on. It is synonymous with *induced* when describing the normal state of a gene; it has the same meaning as *constitutive* in describing the effect of mutation.
- **Derepression:** The process of "turning on" the expression of a gene or set of genes whose expression has been repressed (turned off). Displacement of a repressor protein from a promoter region of DNA. When attached to the DNA, the repressor protein prevents RNA polymerase from initiating transcription. The turning on of a gene.
- **Derivative:** 1. Resulting from or derived from. 2. Term used to identify a variant during meristematic cell division.
- **Desalinization:** Refers to the process, which purifies seawater into high-quality drinking water via distillation or micro- filtration.
- **Desaturase:** An enzyme (group) family that is present within the soybean plant and other oilseed crops (e.g. canola, corn/ maize). One or more desaturases is involved in the synthesis pathway through which oilseed crops produce unsaturated fatty

acids (e.g. linoleic acid). A desaturase is also involved in production of beta carotene (in some plants).

- **Descriptor:** Character used for evaluation and characterization of different accessions of germplasm.
- **Desferroxamine manganese:** An iron chelating agent (i.e. it chemically binds to iron atoms in the blood, thus trapping the iron atoms). The molecule also acts as an hSOD mimic by capturing harmful oxygen free radicals in the blood before they damage the walls of blood vessels. Recent research indicates that desferroxamine manganese may be useful in blocking the onset of cataracts.
- **Desicant:** Any compound used to remove moisture or water.
- **Desiccate:** To dry, exhaust or deprive of water or moisture. Any chemical used for this purpose is called a desicant. An apparatus for drying and preventing hygroscopic samples from rehydrating is a desiccator. The process is desiccation.
- **Desiccated artificial seeds:** Somatic embryos hardened by treatment with ABA and then coated with a suitable polymer to enable them to withstand desiccation; encapsulated in a suitable matrix and dried; afford easy handling and storage.
- **Desiccator:** Apparatus for drying or depriving of moisture.
- **Designer crops:** Crop varieties specially designed to meet certain specific consumer, industrial, etc. needs; they possess features that were specified before their development.
- **Desulfovibrio:** A genus of bacteria that reduces sulfate to H_2S (hydrogen sulfide). Energy is obtained by oxidation of H_2 or organic molecules. Not a strict autotroph because CO_2 cannot be used as a sole carbon source.
- **Desulfurization:** Technology for removing sulphur from oil and coal by use of bacteria. Sulphur residues in fuels end up as sulphur dioxide when the fuel is burned resulting in acid rain. Bacteria may oxidize sulphites (insoluble) into sulphates (soluble) which can be washed away with the bacteria.
- **Detergent:** Substance which lowers the surface tension of a solution improving its clearing properties (e.g. Tween-20 TM, a surfactant and wetting agent).
- **Determinate growth:** Growth determined and limited in time as in most floral meristems and leaves. The differentiation process is irreversibly established. Determinate growth contrasts with the usual culture growth which is infinite and indeterminate.

- **Determination:** Process by which undifferentiated cells in an embryo become committed to develop into specific cell types such as neurons fibroblasts or muscle cells.
- **Determined:** Describing embryonic tissue at a stage when it can develop only as a certain kind of tissue.
- **Development:** The sum total of events that contribute to the progressive elaboration of an organism. The two major aspects of development are growth and differentiation.
- **Development culture:** A research culture producing a compound of sufficient commercial interest and used for developing large-scale fermentation procedures.
- **Developmental determination:** During shoot regeneration; this phase follows morphogenic competence acquisition; during this phase, cells become irreversibly committed to a developmental path in response to the inductive condition.
- **Deviation:** 1. In statistics the difference between an actual observation and the mean of all observations. 2. An alteration from the typical from function or behavior. Mutation or stress are the common reasons behind deviation.
- **Dextran:** A polysaccharide produced by yeasts and bacteria as an energy storage reservoir (analogous to fat in humans). Consists of glucose residues, joined almost exclusively by alpha-1,6 linkages. Occasional branches (in the molecule) are formed by alpha-1, 2, alpha-1, 3, or alpha-1, 4 linkages. Which linkage is used depends on the species of yeast or bacteria producing the dextran.
- **Dextrin:** An intermediate polysaccharide compound resulting from the hydrolysis of starch to maltose by amylase enzymes.
- **Dextrorotary (D) isomer:** A stereoisomer that rotates the plane of plane-polarized light to the right. *Dextro* means right.
- **Diabetes:** A grouping of diseases in which the body either does not synthesize (manufacture) insulin, or else its tissues are insensitive to the insulin that it does synthesize. Approximately, 5–10% of all people with diabetes are unable to synthesize insulin (e.g. because their insulin-making tissue was destroyed by autoimmune disease). Approximately 90–95% of all people with diabetes are insensitive to the insulin their body synthesizes.
- **Diacylglycerols:** Molecules that consist of two fatty acids attached to a glycerol backbone. Research during the 1990s indicated

that consumption of vegetable oils (e.g. used in frying foods) containing primarily diacylglycerols (versus typical triacylglycerols), is less likely to result in it being deposited as body fat (adipose tissue).

- **Diagnostic procedure:** A test or assay used to determine the presence of an organism substance or nucleic acid sequence alteration.
- **Diagnostic:** A test or kit used to diagnose a disease or medical condition.
- **Diakinesis:** A stage of meiosis just before metaphase I in which the separation of homologous chromosomes is almost completed (Fig. 3).

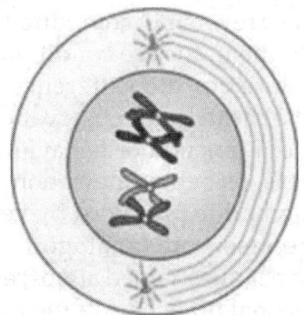

Fig. 3: Diakinesis

- **Dialysis:** The separation of low molecular weight compounds from high molecular weight components in solution by diffusion through a semipermeable membrane. Frequently utilized to remove salts and biological effectors (such as nicotinamide adenine dinucleotides, nucleotide phosphates, etc.) from polymeric molecules such as protein, DNA, or RNA. Commonly used membranes have a molecular weight cut-off (threshold) of around 10,000 daltons, but other membrane pore sizes are available.
- **Diastereoisomers:** Four variations of a given molecule, consisting of a pair of stereoisomers about a second asymmetric carbon atom for each of the two isomers of the first asymmetric carbon atom.
- **Diazotrophs:** The microorganisms that fix atmospheric nitrogen (N_2).

- **Dicentric chromosome:** The product of fusing two chromosome fragments, each of which has a centromere. It is unstable and may be broken when the two centromeres are pulled to opposite poles in mitosis.
- **Dichogamy:** The condition in which the male and the femal reproductive organs of a flower mature at different times thereby making self-fertilization improbable or impossible.
- **Dicotyledon:** A plant which has two cotyledons, or seed leaves. One of the two classes of plants in the angiosperms (the other class is the monocotyledons). Colloquially called a dicot. Examples include many crop plants (potato, pea, beans) ornamentals (rose, Ivy) and timber trees (oak, beech, lime).
- **Dideoxynucleotide (DDNTP):** Nucleotide in which oxygen is absent from the 2' and 3' positions of ribose; blocks further extension of a nucleotide chain beyond the point at which it incorporated into the chain.
- **Differential centrifugation:** A method of separating subcellular particles according to their sedimentation coefficients which are roughly proportional to their size. Cell extracts are subjected to a succession of centrifuge runs at progressively faster rotation speeds. Large particles, such as nuclei or mitochondria will be precipitated at relatively slow speeds and higher G forces will be required to sediment small particles such as ribosome.
- **Differentially permeable:** Referring to a membrane through which different substances diffuse at different rates. Some substances may be unable to diffuse through such a membrane.
- **Differentiation:** Formation of various cell types and organs like root, shoot, etc. either *in vivo* or in cell cultures.
- **Diffusion:** The movement of molecules from a region of lower concentration.
- **Digest:** To cut DNA molecules with one or more restriction endonucleases.
- **Digester:** A low technology reactor used for anaerobic bacterial digestion.
- **Digestion (within chemical production plants):** Breakdown of feed stocks by various processes (chemical, mechanical, and biological) to yield their desired building-block components for inclusion as raw materials in subsequent chemical or biological processes.

- **Digestion (within organisms):** The enzyme enhanced hydrolysis (breakdown) of major nutrients (food) in the gastrointestinal system to yield their building-block components (to the organism), such as amino acids, fatty acids, or other essential nutrients.
- **Dihaploid:** A haploid derived from tetraploid.
- **Dihybrid:** An individual that is heterozygous. For two pairs of alleles the progeny of a cross between homozygous parents differing at two loci.
- **Dihybrid cross:** A type of cross involving parents differing in only two traits or in which only two traits are considered.
- **Dimer:** Association of two molecules.
- **Dimethyl sulphoxide:** A highly hygroscopic liquid and powerful solvent with little odor or color. It is an organic co-solvent used in small quantities to dissolve neutral organic substances in tissue culture media preparation. DMSO also has uses as a cryoprotectant.
- **Dimorphism:** The existence of two distinctly different types of individuals within a species. An obvious example is the sexual dimorphism in certain animals.
- **Diplochromosome:** Chromosome having four chromatids; produced by endoreduplication.
- **Diploid:** Diploid set of chromosomes contains two copies of each autosome and two sex chromosomes.
- **Diploid cell:** A cell which contains two sets of chromosomes.
- **Diploidization:** Process of doubling the chromosome complement (genome) of a cell.
- **Diplonema:** Stage in prophase of meiosis I following the pachytene stage but preceding diakinesis in which one pair of sister chromatids begin to separate from the other pair, i.e. the centromeres begin to disjoin.
- **Diplophase:** A phase in the life cycle of an organism in which the cells of the organism have two copies of each gene. When this state exists the organism is said to be diploid.
- **Direct gene transfer:** Vector-independent gene transfer.
- **Direct organogenesis:** Embryoid formation of the surface of zygote or somatic embryos or a seedling plant tissue in culture, without an intervening callus phase.
- **Direct repeats:** Identical (or related) sequences present in two or more copies in the same orientation in the same molecule of DNA; they are not necessarily adjacent.

- **Direct selection:** Cells resistant to the selection pressure survive and divide to form colonies, while the wild type cells are killed by the selection agent.
- **Direct somatic embryogenesis:** Embryos develop directly from explants cells without any intervening callus phase; responding explants cells are themselves either embryogenic or quite close to this state.
- **Direct transfer:** Refers to methods of inserting a gene directly into a cell's DNA without the use of a vector. One example of direct transfer is electroporation.
- **Directed mutagenesis:** The process of generation of nucleotide changes in cloned genes by any one of several procedures including site-specific and random mutagenesis also called *in vitro* mutagenesis.
- **Directional cloning:** The technique by which DNA insert and vector molecules are digested with two different restriction enzymes to create noncomplementary sticky ends at either end of each restriction fragment so, allowing the insert to be ligated to the vector in a specific orientation and preventing the vector from recircularizing.
- **Disaccharides:** Carbohydrates consisting of two covalently linked monosaccharide units; hence *di* for two.
- **Disarm:** To delet from a plasmid or virus genes that are cytotoxic or tumor inducing.
- **Disarmed plasmid:** A plasmid from which some portion has been deleted.
- **Discontinuity:** The site in a DNA strand at which the phosphodiester bond between two adjacent nucleotides is broken.
- **Discontinuous replication:** The synthesis of DNA in short (Okazaki) fragments that are later joined into a continuous strand.
- **Discontinuous variation:** Phenotypic variation involving distinct classes such as red versus white, tall versus dwarf.
- **Discordant:** Members of a pair showing different rather than similar characteristics.
- **Discovery:** Isolation/identification of things which are already present in nature/universe; discovery only indicates their presence.
- **Disease:** The opposite of ease. Any alteration from the state of metabolism necessary for the normal development and

functioning of an organism usually associated with infection by a pathogen or the malfunction or absence of one or more genes.

- **Disease free:** A plant or animal certified through specific tests as being free of specified pathogens. Disease-free should be interpreted to mean 'free from any known diseases' as 'new' diseases may yet be discovered to be present.
- **Disease indexing:** Disease indexed organisms have been assayed for the presence of known diseases according to standard testing procedures.
- **Disease resistance:** The ability to remain healthy by resisting disease or the disease agent. Disease resistance or tolerance is a subject of intense interest in biotechnology.
- **Disinfection:** Killing of microorganisms in water or other media where they might otherwise pose a health threat, e.g. chlorine is commonly used o disinfect water supplies. Inactivation of microorganisms present on the surface of explants, etc. *see also Surface sterilization.*
- **Disjunction:** The movement of members of a chromosome pair to opposite poles during cell division. At mitosis and the second meiotic division, disjunction applies to sister chromatids; at first meiotic division it applies to sister chromatid pairs.
- **Disomic:** A cell/an individual having normal somatic chromosome complement of a species; each chromosome of the genome(s) is present in two copies.
- **Disomy:** The presence of a pair of specific chromosome. This is the normal condition and abnormal occurrences are monosomy, trisomy and nullisomy (with respectively one chromosome of a pair, three or none). There are also abnormal disomic conditions such as when both chromosomes of the pair were inherited from the same parent.
- **Dispense:** To portion out a nutrient medium into containers such as test tubes, jars, Erlenmeyer flasks, petri dishes, etc.
- **Dispersed growth digesters:** In such digesters, the microbial population is dispersed throughout the sewage being treated.
- **Dissecting microscope:** A microscope with a low magnifying power of about 50x used to examine or excise small plant or animal parts.
- **Dissection:** Separation of a tissue by cutting for analysis or observation.

- **Dissimilation:** The breakdown of food material to yield energy and building blocks for cellular synthesis.
- **Dissolve:** Pass chemicals into solution.
- **Dissolved oxygen (DO):** Oxygen gas dissolved in water; concentration of DO is a measure of water quality.
- **Distant hybridization:** Hybridization between distantly related taxa, e.g. two different species, genera, etc.
- **Distillation:** The process of heating a mixture to separate the more volatile from the less volatile parts and then cooling and condensing the resulting vapor so as to produce a more nearly pure or refined substance.
- **Distinctiveness:** In case of PBR, the new variety must be distinguishable from other varieties by one or more identifiable morphological, physiological or other characteristics.
- **Distribution coefficient (K_d):** The ratio of the concentration of a sample component in one phase to its concentration in a second phase equilibrium. The two phases may be immiscible liquids or the mobile phase and the stationary phase.
- **Disulfide bond:** An important type of covalent bond formed between two sulfur atoms of different cysteines in a protein. Disulfide bonds (linkages, bridges) contribute to holding proteins together and also help provide the internal structure (conformation) of the protein.
- **Ditype:** In fungi a tetrad that contains two kinds of meiotic products (spores), e.g. 2AB and 2ab.
- **Diurnal:** Term describing the occurrence of an event at least once every 24 hours.
- **Divergence:** The percent difference in nucleotide sequence between two related DNA sequences or in amino acid sequences between two proteins.
- **Divergent transcription:** The initiation of transcription at two promoters facing in the opposite direction, so that transcription proceeds away in both directions from a central region.
- **Diversity (within a species):** Refers to the genetic variation that exists within a population (of organisms) in a species. For example, black cattle and white cattle; or both toxic and nontoxic strains/serotypes of *Escherichia coliform* (*E. coli*) bacteria. This diversity is due to one or more single-nucleotide polymorphisms (SNPs) in each individual's genome (DNA) within the population of organisms.

D

- **Diversity biotechnology consortium:** A nonprofit US organization formed in August of 1994 by a group of research institutions and companies. The consortium's first president was Stuart A Kauffman of the Santa Fe Institute. The consortium's purpose is to further use of molecular diversity as a tool in drug design, and in the study of mutating viruses.
- **Dizygotic twins:** Two-egg twins, i.e. a pair of individuals that shared the same uterus at the same time but which arose from separate and independent fertilization of two ova.
- **DNA amplification:** Multiplication of a piece of a DNA in a test tube into many thousand or million of copies by using PCR.
- **DNA array:** A series DNA sequences fixed as distinct spots on a suitable solid support, like a glass chip; basically two types; spotted DNA array and printed oligonucleotide chips.
- **DNA bank:** Storage of DNA which may or may not be the complete genome but should always be accompanied by inventory information. (*Note:* Present time, animals cannot be re-established from DNA alone).
- **DNA bridges:** Large segments of DNA whose sequence (i.e. composition) is known and mapped in total. Those sequences are then utilized by scientists to piece together (bridging the DNA segments) and assemble a (more) complete map (e.g. of an organism's chromosome or genome).
- **DNA carrier:** Substance or particle that can transfer genes into a cell. These include viruses, liposomes (fat globules) and artificial chromosomes (sequences of DNA created in a laboratory) that can transport large amounts of DNA.
- **DNA chimera:** One DNA molecule composed of DNA from two different species.
- **DNA chip:** The solid supports of glass or silicon about the size of a microscope slide consisting of DNA attached in highly organized arrays. It is available commercially also, e.g. GeneChip® Probe Array.
- **DNA construct:** A suitable DNA which has been prepared for cloning purpose.
- **DNA delivery system:** A genetic term for any procedure that transports DNA into a recipient cell.
- **DNA diagnosis:** The use of DNA polymorphisms to detect the presence of a specific allele (often associated with a disease or syndrome) or DNA sequence.

- **DNA fingerprint:** Molecular marker pattern of an individual obtained by using highly polymorphic markers; used for unequivocal identification of strains, individuals, criminals, etc.
- **DNA fingerprinting:** It analyzes the differences between individuals of the fragments generated by using restriction enzymes to cleave regions that contain short repeated sequences. Because these are unique to every individual, the presence of a particular subset in any two individuals can be used to define their common inheritance (e.g. a parent-child relationship).
- **DNA footprinting:** It enables identification of the site on a DNA molecule to which a protein, such as RNA polymerase, binds.
- **DNA helicase (gyrase):** An enzyme that catalyzes the unwinding of the complementary strands of a DNA double helix.
- **DNA hybridization:** The pairing of two DNA molecules often from different sources by hydrogen bonding between complementary nucleotides. This technique is frequently used to detect the presence of a specific nucleotide sequence in a DNA sample.
- **DNA insert:** The DNA segment to be cloned.
- **DNA kinase:** An enzyme that catalyzes the addition of phosphate groups at the 5′ terminus of DNA.
- **DNA ladder:** A set of precisely sized DNA fragments that can be run on a gel in parallel with test samples to estimate the size of an unknown DNA fragment.
- **DNA ligase:** An enzyme that seals nicks in DNA strands by catalizing the formation of phosphodiester bond between the contiguous nucleotides.
- **DNA methylation:** Addition of methyl ($-CH_3$) residues, chiefly to cytosine residues, usually, located in CG or CNG (N means any one of the four DNA bases) sequences, after they are incorporates in DNA.
- **DNA microarray:** An assembly of a very large number of small dots onto a solid support, each dot containing a short sequence of a different gene of the organism concerned.
- **DNA mutant:** Of bacteria is temperature-sensitive; it cannot synthesize DNA at 42°C, but can do so at 37°C.
- **DNA polymerase:** An enzyme that synthesizes a daughter strand(s) of DNA (under direction from a DNA template). May be involved in repair or replication.
- **DNA polymorphism:** The existence of two or more alternative forms (alleles) of a chromosomal locus that differ in nucleotide

sequence or have variable numbers of repeated nucleotide sequence or have variable numbers of repeated nucleotide units.

- **DNA primase:** An enzyme that catalyzes the synthesis of short strands of RNA that initiate the synthesis of DNA strands.

- **DNA probe:** Isolated single radiolabelled ^{32}P-DNA strands (oligonucleotides) used to detect the presence of the complementary (opposite) strands, and as a very sensitive biological detectors.

- **DNA profiling:** Invented in 1985 by Alec Jeffreys, this technique is used by forensic (i.e. crime-solving) chemists to match biological evidence (e.g. a blood stain) from a crime scene to the person (e.g. the assailant) involved in that particular crime. DNA profiling involves the use of restriction fragment length polymorphism (RFLP) analysis or allele-specific oligonucleotide/polymerase chain reaction (ASO/PCR) analysis to identify the specific sequence of bases (i.e. nucleotides) in a piece of DNA taken from the biological evidence. Since the specific sequence of bases in DNA molecules is different for each individual (due to DNA polymorphism), a criminal's DNA can be matched to that of the evidence to prove guilt or innocence. Biological evidence may include, among other things, blood, hair, nail fragments, skin, and sperm.

- **DNA repair:** A variety of mechanisms that repair errors which occur during DNA replication.

- **DNA repair enzymes:** Enzymes that catalyzes the repair of DNA.

- **DNA replicase:** A DNA-synthesizing enzyme required specifically for replication.

- **DNA replication:** The use of existing DNA as a template fo the synthesis of new DNA strand. In humans and other eukaryotes, replication occurs in the cell nucleus (Fig. 4).

- **DNA sequence:** The relative order of base pairs, whether in a fragment of DNA, a gene, a chromosome or an entire genome.

- **DNA sequencing:** Determination of the base sequence of a DNA fragment.

- **DNA topoisomerase:** It is an enzyme that changes the number of times the two strands in a closed DNA molecule cross each other. It does this by cutting the DNA, passing DNA through the break, and resealing the DNA.

- **DNA vaccine:** It contains a gene encoding an immunogenic protein from the concerned pathogen.

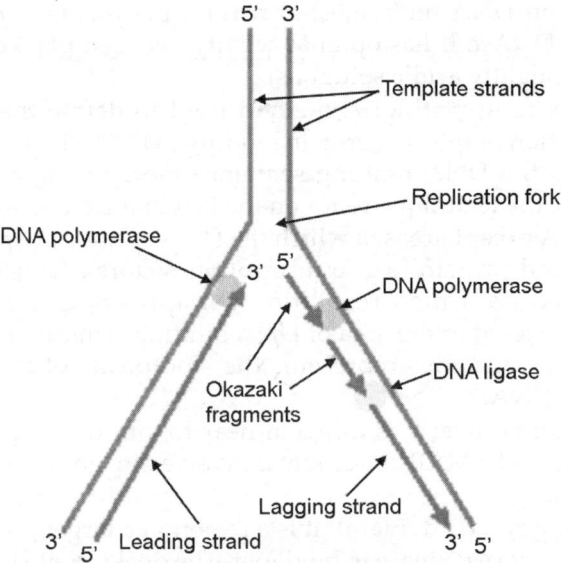

Fig. 4: DNA replication

- **DNA vector:** A vehicle (such as a virus) for transferring genetic information (DNA) from one cell to another.
- **DNA:** A macromolecule in which deoxyribonucleotides are joined together by phosphodiester linkage; usually, double-stranded.
- **DNAase I hypersensitive site:** A short region of chromatin detected by its extreme sensitivity to cleavage by DNAase I and other nucleases; probably comprises an area from which nucleosomes are excluded.
- **DNA-delivery system:** Any procedure that introduce DNA into a recipient cell.
- **DNA-driven hybridization:** The reaction of an excess of DNA with RNA.
- **DNA-RNA hybrid:** A double-helix that consists of one chain of DNA hydrogen bonded to a chain of RNA by means of complementary base pairs.
- **DNAse:** Deoxyribonuclease, an endonuclease enzyme family that degrades (cuts up) DNA molecules. DNAse I is produced and secreted by the salivary glands, intestines, liver, and pancreas of animals. It has optimal activity (i.e. greatest ability

D

to cut up DNA molecules) at neutral pH (neither acidic nor basic). DNAse II has optimal activity between pH 4.6 and 5.5 (i.e. in slightly acidic solutions).

- **DNAse footprinting:** A method used to define the specific interaction points of a protein binding to DNA. Typically used to map the DNA binding sequence motifs of transcription factors, the technique relies on the fact that DNase will digest all DNA except areas in which the DNA strands are protected by bound protein (e.g. transcription factors). Labeled DNA resolved on a high-resolution gel appears as a sequence ladder except in the area of DNA binding. This area contains no bands and thus represents the "footprint" of the protein on the DNA.

- **Docking groove:** It is a region near to, but distinct from the active site of a MAP kinase that is involved in binding to a target protein.

- **Docking site (D domain):** It is a region in a target protein that used by a MAP kinase to bind to it. The docking site has a high concentration of hydrophobic residues separated from two basic residues.

- **Docking:** The initial association of a translating ribosome with the translocation channel in the membrane of the ER.

- **Docosahexaenoic acid (DHA):** One of the omega-3 (n-3) highly unsaturated fatty acids (HUFA), DHA is an important in the development of the human infant's brain, spinal cord, and retina tissues. DHA aids optimal brain and nervous system development in human infants, and is required for optimal brain function throughout life. Naturally present in human breast milk and fish oil. The human body converts linolenic acid (e.g. from consumption of soybean oil) to the two highly HUFA, DHA and eicosapentaenoic acid (EPA). Research indicates that consumption of DHA also helps to reduce the risk of heart disease (by lowering blood pressure) and depression (via its effect in the brain).

- **Dolichol:** It is a lipid that consists of a long chain of isoprenoid units and is present in the membrane of the rough endoplasmic reticulum. It is part of the precursor in the synthesis of N-linked oligosaccharides. An oligosaccharide is assembled onto dolichol via a pyrophosphoryl linkage, then transferred to particular asparagine residues of a nascent polypeptide.

- **Dolly:** The (name of the) first mammal to be created by cloning a cell from an adult animal. In this particular case the cell came from the mammary tissue of an adult ewe. The creation of Dolly showed that the process of differentiation into adult tissue is not as previously thought irreversible. The result was achieved by nuclear transfer. Dolly's birth was announced in 1997. Since then cattle and mice have also been cloned from adult cells.

- **Domain (of a chromosome):** May refer either to a discrete structural entity defined as a region within which supercoiling is independent of other domains, or to an extensive region, including an expressed gene that has heightened sensitivity to degradation by the enzyme DNase I.

- **Domain (of a protein):** A discrete continuous part of the amino acid sequence that can be equated with a particular function.

- **Domestic animal diversity (DAD):** The spectrum of genetic differences within each breed and across all breeds within each domestic animal species together with the species differences all of which are available for the sustainable intensification of food and agriculture production.

- **Dominance:** It is the over-riding effect of a gene over its allele in such a way that the heterozygote is phenotypically indistinguishable from the dominant homozygote.

- **Dominant** allele determines the phenotype displayed in a heterozygote with another (recessive) allele. An allele is one of several alternative forms of a gene occupying a given locus on a chromosome.

- **Dominant allele:** The allele expresses itself in the heterozygous state.

- **Dominant marker selection:** Selection of cells via a gene encoding a product that enables only the cells that carry the gene to grow under particular conditions. For example, plant and animal cells, that, express the introduced NeoR gene are resistant to the compound G_{418}.

- **Dominant negative:** Mutations are frans-acting and are a hallmark of negative complementation occurring in multimeric proteins where one mutant subunit may poison the whole multimer even though the other subunits are wild-type.

- **Dominant selection marker gene:** A gene that allows the host cell to survive under conditions where it would otherwise die.

D

- **Dominant oncogene:** A gene that stimulates cell proliferation and contributes to oncogenesis when present in a single copy.
- **Dominant trait:** A trait expressed preferentially over another trait.
- **Dominant:** Dominant allele determines the phenotype displayed in a heterozygote with another (recessive) allele.
- **DON:** Abbreviation for the mycotoxin deoxynivalenol produced by *Fusarium* fungi DON. Also known as "vomitoxin", because it can cause some animals to vomit if they consume it.
- **Donor junction:** The junction between the left 52'end of an exon and the right 32'end of an intron.
- **Donor plant:** Plant from which explants are obtained for *in vitro* culture. syn. *Mother plant*.
- **Dormancy:** An inactive period in the life of an animal or plant during which growth slows or completely ceases. Physiological changes associated with dormancy help the organism survive adverse environmental conditions. Annual plants survive the winter as dormant seeds while many perennial plants survive as dominant tubers, rhizomes or bulbs. Hibernation and estivation in animals help them survive extremes of cold and heat, respectively.
- **Dorsalventral axis:** It is the line running from the back to the belly of an animal.
- **Dosage compensation:** Mechanisms employed to compensate for the discrepancy between the presence of two X chromosomes in one sex but only one X chromosome in the other sex.
- **Dose:** It is the mathematical product of the concentration of hazardous material and the length of exposure to it. The effects of any given material or radiation corresponds to the dose received.
- **Dot blot technique:** In this technique, total DNA (or RNA) isolated from each of several test individuals/tissues are placed onto nitrocellulose filter as dots; DNA is denatured, fixed to the filter and hybridization is detected by autoradiography or fluorescence.
- **Double crossing over:** Two simultaneous reciprocal breakage and reunion events between the same two chromatids.
- **Double fertilization:** In plants; fusion of one sperm with the egg cell and of the other sperm with the secondary nucleus (produces endosperm); both fusion must occur in the same embryo sac to ensure normal seed development.

- **Double haploid (DH):** A disomic obtained by doubling the chromosome number (usually, by colchicine treatment) of a haploid; as a rule homozygous.
- **Double helix:** The natural coiled conformation of two complementary, antiparallel DNA chains. This structure was first put forward by Watson and Crick in 1953.
- **Double-minute chromosomes:** They are extrachromosomal elements formed by amplification of DHFR genes in response to methotrexate treatment. They are large enough to be visible in the light microscope.
- **Double recessive:** An organism homozygous for a recessive allele at each of two loci.
- **Double-strand break (DSB):** Occurs when both strands of a DNA duplex are cleaved at the same site. Genetic recombination is initiated by double-strand breaks. The cell also has repair systems that act on double-strand breaks created at other times.
- **Double-stranded complementary DNA (dscDNA):** A double strand DNA molecule created from a cDNA template.
- **Doubling time:** The time required to double the number of cells.
- **Down mutation** in a promoter decreases the rate of transcription.
- **Down promoter mutations:** Those mutations that decrease the frequency of initiation of transcription. Down promoter mutations lead to the production of less mRNA than is the case in the nonmutated state.
- **Down regulating:** Phrase referring to regulatory sequences, chemical compounds (e.g. transcription factors), mutations (e.g. down promoter mutations), etc. that cause a given gene to express less of the protein that it normally codes for.
- **Down:** Down promoter mutations decrease the frequency of initiation of transcription.
- **Downstream processing:** Separation and purification of product(s) from a fermentation process.
- **Downstream:** It identifies sequences proceeding farther in the direction of expression; for example, the coding region is downstream of the initiation codon.
- **Down syndrome:** An inherited condition due to an extra chromosome 21, either as a third chromosome 21 or attached to chromosome 13, 14 or 15. Also called trisomy 21.
- **DP thymocyte:** It is a double positive thymocyte. It is an immature T cell that expresses cell surface CD4 and CD8.

Selection of DP thymocytes in the thymus yields mature T cells expressing either CD4 or CD8.

- **Driver mRNA:** The biotin-labeled mRNA from nonstressed cell.
- *Drosophila:* The name of a type of fly (*Drosophila melanogaster*) that reproduces rapidly, and that is commonly utilized in genetics experiments due to its short life cycle (14 days) and simple genome (four chromosome pairs). Because of these factors, a large base of knowledge about *Drosophila* genetics has been accumulated by the world's scientific community. For example, of the nearly 300 disease-causing genes in the human genome, more than half have an analogous gene in the *Drosophila* genome. *Drosophila* was one of the first organisms to have its entire genome sequenced by man.
- **Drug:** Any molecule that affects a biological process. More strictly a molecule whose pharmacological activity can be correlated with its chemical structure.
- **Drug delivery:** Method by which a therapeutic agent is delivered to its site of action.
- **Dry heat sterilization:** Sterilization by heating in an oven at 160–180°C for 3 hours.
- **Dry weight:** Weight of cells/tissues after drying them at 60°C for 12 hours.
- **dsDNA:** Double-stranded DNA.
- **Dual culture:** A culture made of a plant tissue and one organism (such as a nematode) or an obligate parasite/microorganism (such as a fungus). Dual culture techniques are used for a variety of purposes including assessing host-parasite interactions and the production of axenic cultures.
- **Dual specificity kinase:** It is a protein kinase that can phosphorylate tyrosine or threonine or serine amino acids.
- **Duplex:** The double-helical structure of deoxyribonucleic acid (DNA).
- **Duplications:** The are a doubling of a chromosomal segment. A broken segment from one chromosome can simply attach to its homologue.
- **Dynamin:** It is a cytosolic protein that is a GTPase and is required for clathrin-mediated vesicle formation. Although the exact role of dynamin is debated, dynamin polymers are involved in the scission of clathrin-coated pits from membranes. A variant of dynamin functions in mitochondrial septation.

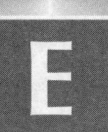

- **Early development:** The period of a phage infection before the start of DNA replication.
- **Early endosome:** It is the part of the endosomal compartment in which endocytosed molecules appear after a minute or so. Early endosomes are located near the plasma membrane, function in sorting of endocytosed molecules, and have a pH of about 6.
- **Early gene:** Genes are transcribed before the replication of phage DNA. They code for regulators and other proteins needed for later stages of infection.
- **Early infection:** The part of the phage lytic cycle between entry and replication of the phage DNA. During this time, the phage synthesizes the enzymes needed to replicate its DNA.
- **Early region replacement vector:** SV 40 (mammalian) transducing vector; early region of virus is replaced by DNA insert.
- **Early vs late genes:** Those genes transcribed early in a bacteriophage-mediated infection process as compared to those genes transcribed some time later. May require different "p factors" (sigma) for recognition of promotors.
- **Early vs late proteins:** During viral infection, viral-specific proteins are synthesized at characteristic times after infection. They are called "early" and "late." Often under positive control of bacterial and viral sigma factors.
- **Earthworms (*Eisenia foetida*):** These worms live in the soil and consume up to ten tons of organic matter (old crop plant stalks, husks, etc.) per acre (approximately 0.4 hectare) per year. In so doing, earthworms make the soil more fertile, since the process breaks down that organic matter into soil (when excreted by those earthworms). Earthworm tunnels also help aerate soil, which encourages healthy plant root systems (Fig. 1).
- **Ecdysone:** A steroid hormone in insects that stimulates moulting and metamorphosis. It acts on specific genes stimulating the synthesis of proteins involved in these bodily changes.

E

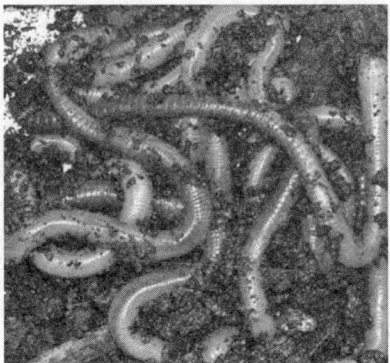

Fig. 1: Earthworms

- **Eciosion:** Emergence of an adult insect from the pupil stage.
- **Ecocentrism:** The view that consider the whole environment or ecosphere as important and deserving of consideration, without giving preference to organisms such as animals and humans. It states that all elements of the environment have worth and should be valued and cared for.
- **Ecology:** The study of the inter-relationships between organisms and their environments.
- **Economic threshold:** The level of pest damage below which an application of pesticides to control the pest is more costly than the economic loss caused by the pest.
- **Economic trait locus (ETL):** A locus influencing a trait that contributes to income. The plural form is also abbreviated as economic trait loci (ETL).
- **Ecosystem:** The complex of a living community and its environment functioning as an ecological unit in nature of abiotic factors and biotic factors.
- **Ecosystem diversity:** The differences among ecosystems including habitat diversity and ecological processes in an ecosystem.
- **Ecotype:** A population or a strain of an organism that is adapted to a particular habitat.
- **Ectodermal adult stem cells:** Certain stem cells present within (adult) bodies of organisms, that can be differentiated (via chemical signals) to give rise to cells of skin, hair, tooth enamel, mucous membranes, and some glandular tissues.

- **Ectopic expression:** The expression of a gene in a tissue in which it is not usually expressed; for example, in a transgenic animal or as the result of injection into an unusual location in an embryo.
- **Ectopic:** Refers to something being out of place. EF-G is an elongation factor needed for the translocation stage of bacterial protein synthesis.
- **Edible vaccine:** An edible plant part in which an antigenic protein of a pathogen is produced and accumulated; feeding of this part generates immunity against the concerned pathogen.
- **Ethylenediamine tetra-acetate (EDTA):** An organic molecule which, due to the chemical groups it contains and their juxtaposition within that molecule, is able to chelate (bind) certain other molecules such as divalent metal cations. EDTA thus inhibits some enzymes requiring such ions for activity.
- **Effector:** It is the target protein for the activated G protein.
- **Effector cells:** Cells of the immune system that are responsible for cell-mediated cytotoxicity.
- **Effector molecule:** A molecule that influences the behavior of a regulatory molecule such as a repressor protein thereby influencing gene expression.
- **Effector site:** It is the site that is bound by a small molecule on an allosteric protein. The result of binding is to change the activity of the active site, which is located elsewhere on the protein.
- **Effluent:** Mobile phase that has exited from the column.
- **EGF receptor:** A protein embedded in the surface of the membranes of skin cells. The receptor consists of: 1. an outside (of the cell membrane) enzyme that recognizes epidermal growth factor (EGF) and binds to it, and; 2. an enzyme on the inside of the cell membrane, which is of the tyrosine kinase class. When free EGF comes in contact with an EGF receptor, they bind (in a lock-and-key fashion) and then enter the cell together (through the cell membrane. There EGF stimulates growth or division of the cell via ras protein and ras gene). The EGF receptor (and receptors in general) is like a butler who allows the EGF (a guest) to enter the cell (home).
- **EGS:** External guide sequence.
- **Eicosanoids:** A group of chemical compounds which the human body synthesizes (manufactures) from arachidonic acid, docosahexanoic acid, and other starting materials. One subgroup of eicosanoids is that of the prostaglandins (cyclic fatty

acids that act as hormones in the body). For example, the COX-1 enzyme converts arachidonic acid to constitutive prostaglandins, and the COX-2 enzyme converts arachidonic acid to inducible prostaglandins.

- **Eicosapentanoic acid (EPA):** One of the omega-3 (n-3) polyunsaturated fatty acids (PUFA), EPA is important for the development of the human brain, retina tissue, prevention of high blood pressure, coronary heart disease (CHD), and some cancers. The human body converts linolenic acid (e.g. from consumption of soybean oil) to the two highly unsaturated fatty acids (HUFA), eicosapentanoic acid (EPA) and docosahexanoic acid (DHA).

- **ELAM-1:** Also known as E-selectin, it is a selectin molecule that is synthesized by endothelial cells after (adjacent) tissue is infected. ELAM-1 molecules then help leukocytes, leave the bloodstream to fight the infection.

- **Elastase:** An enzyme secreted by neutrophils (white blood cells that engulf pathogens) which catalyzes the cleavage (breakdown) of specific proteins that function to provide elasticity to certain tissues. May be indirectly responsible for some autoimmune diseases, such as arthritis (which results from breakdown of cartilage tissue). Elastase may also be indirectly responsible for the emphysema (caused by loss of lung elasticity) that results from prolonged smoke inhalation. When a-1 antitrypsin (anti-elastase) efficacy is reduced (via smoke), the now-unrestrained excess elastase destroys alveolar walls in the lungs by digesting elastic fibers and other connective tissue proteins.

- **Elastin:** A fibrous protein that is the major constituent of the yellow elastic fibers of connective tissue.

- **Electrical gradient:** A change in the amount of charge from one point to another.

- **Electrical polarity in embryogenesis:** K^+ ions enter from the end that would later develop into plumule, while H^+ ions pass out of the redicular end; redicular end exhibits a high concentration of calmodulin.

- **Electroblotting:** A couple of sheets of filter paper soaked in anode buffer are placed on the anode plate, and blotting membrane is placed on top of these sheets. The gel is then laid on the top of the membrane and is covered with a couple of sheets of filter paper soaked in cathode buffer; the cathode plate is then placed on the top of these filter papers. The anions migrate from the gel onto the blotting membrane surface at the same speed; as a result, a regular transfer of molecule takes place.

- **Electrochemical gradient:** A change in the concentration of ions from one point to another produces an electrochemical gradient. The term indicates that there is a change in the concentration of both electrical charge and of a chemical species.
- **Electrochemical sensor:** Type of biosensor in which a biological process is harnessed to an electrical sensor system such as an enzyme electrode. Other types couple a biological event to an electrical one via a range of mechanisms such as those based on oxygen and pH.
- **Electrode:** Substances in contact with a conductor. The substances are connected to a source of an electric field.
- **Electrofusion:** Fusion of, usually two, protoplasts induced by an exposure to a very short (few milliseconds) duration of a high voltage current.
- **Electrolysis:** Refers to the use of electrical energy to split water molecules into hydrogen and oxygen atoms.
- **Electrolyte:** Any compound (salt, acid, base, etc.) which in aqueous solution dissociates into ions (charged atom-sized particles). Electrolytes may either be strong (completely or nearly completely dissociated) or weak (only partially dissociated).
- **Electromagnetic radiation:** Electromagnetic waves including ultraviolet (UV), X-rays and gamma radiation (γ-rays). Electromagnetic radiation is used to produce mutant cells or organism or in the case of UV disinfestations and sterilization in tissue culture.
- **Electromagnetic spectrum:** The range of wavelengths or frequencies over which electromagnetic radiation extends.
- **Electron carrier:** A protein, such as flavoprotein or a cytochrome, that can gain and lose electrons reversibly and function in the transfer of electrons from one carrier to another until the electron is taken up by a final molecule or atom such as oxygen.
- **Electron microscope:** A microscope that uses an electron beam focused by magnetic 'lenses'.
- **Electron microscopy (EM):** A technique for greatly magnifying and visualizing very small entities such as viruses and even large molecules. The technique uses beams of electrons instead of light rays. Because of the physics involved, beams of electrons permit much greater magnification than is possible with a light

microscope. Electron microscopes have been used to examine the structures of viruses, bacteria, pollen grains, molecules, etc.

- **Electro-osmosis:** Migration of water toward an electrode as a result of the supporting medium and/or the surface of the separation equipment, e.g. of capillaries, also carrying charge.
- **Electrophoresis:** The method of separation of molecules such as DNA, RNA or protein based on their relative migration applying a strong electric field (Fig. 2).

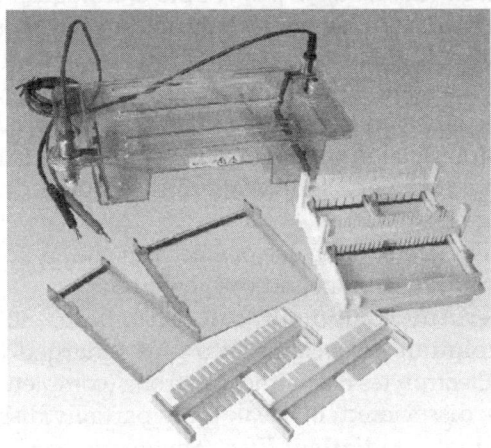

Fig. 2: Electrophoresis

- **Electrophoretic mobility:** The speed of migration of a charged molecule under the influenced of an electric field; depends on the charge to mass ratio of the molecule.
- **Electroporation:** A technique where electric field is applied to facilitate protoplast fusion derived from two different plants.
- **Electroporator:** A specially designed equipment used for protoplast fusion.
- **Element:** *In genetics*; a sequence of DNA that serves as a protein binding site, e.g. promoter, operator, etc.; it functions only in *cis* position. *In chemistry*; a substance made up of one and only one distinct kind of atom.
- **Elicitation:** Use of an elicitor to enhance secondary metabolite production.
- **Elicitor:** Compounds, which dramatically enhance the production of secondary metabolites; may be biotic or abiotic; the term was

originally used for molecules of pathogen origin, which induced the expression of pathogenesis related proteins in resistant varieties of the host.

- **ELISA:** Enzyme linked immunosorbant assay; uses an enzyme conjugated to an antibody for detection of a specific antigen/ antibody based on antigen-antibody interaction; the enzyme linked to the antibody produces detectable color, which enables an easy and highly sensitive detection.

E

- **Elite germplasm:** Refers to germplasm that is adapted (selectively breed) and optimized to new surroundings (i.e. environment). For example, corn/maize (*Zea mays* L.), which is native to Mexico, has been adapted and optimized to grow in field conditions in many of the world's countries.
- **Ellagic acid:** A naturally occurring plant phenol (phytochemical) that, when consumed by humans, has been shown to help inhibit some cancers. Ellagic acid is naturally present in strawberries, the pomegranate (*Punica granatum*), etc.
- **Elongation factors (EF in prokaryotes, eEF in eukaryotes):** Proteins that associate with ribosomes cyclically, during addition of each amino acid to the polypeptide chain.
- **Elongation:** It is the stage in a macromolecular synthesis reaction (replication, transcription, or translation) when the nucleotide or polypeptide chain is being extended by the addition of individual subunits.
- **Eluate:** A compound or mixture that has been separated in the exit from the column.
- **Eluent:** Mobile phase.
- **Elution volume:** The volume of mobile phase required to eluate a solute from a chromatographic column.
- **Elution:** Removal of a solute from a stationary phase by passage of suitable mobile phase.
- **EMAS:** Eco-management and audit scheme.
- **Emasculation:** Removal of anthers in the bud condition before the shed of the pollen.
- **Embryo cloning:** The creation of identical copies of an embryo by embryo splitting or by nuclear transfer from undifferentiated embryonic cells.
- **Embryo culture:** Culture of young embryos aseptically excised from developing seeds on suitable media to raise young seedlings.

E

- **Embryo rescue:** Recovery, by embryo culture, of seedlings by culturing such young embryos that would die due to endosperm abortion; usually, in cases of distant hybridization.
- **Embryo sac:** Female gametophyte; derived from megaspore by, usually, three successive mitotic divisions yielding eight haploid nuclei; three nuclei migrate to one pole and form three antipodal cells, three nuclei move to the opposite pole and form a central egg cell and two synergids, and two nuclei remain in the center and fuse to produce the secondary nucleus.
- **Embryo sexing:** The determination of the sex of an embryo typically by means of PCR involving amplification from a small sample of embryonic tissue using primers specific for a locus on the Y chromosome.
- **Embryo splitting:** Young animal embryos (4–8 cells) treated with trypsin to separate the individual cells; each such cell can develop into a separate embryo.
- **Embryo technology:** Generic name of any modification of mammalian embryos. It encompasses embryo cloning, embryo splitting, *in vitro* fertilization and embryo storage.
- **Embryo transfer:** Implantation of embryos from donor animals or generated by *in vitro* fertilization into the uterus of the recipient animals.
- **Embryo transplantation:** Implantation of young embryos developed *in vitro* or obtained from the uterus of donor females into the womb of surrogate females.
- **Embryo:** A very young individual (animal/plant) developing usually, from zygote.
- **Embryogenesis:** Process of development of embryo from a fertilized egg cell.
- **Embryogenic culture:** A culture containing cells capable of producing SEs; usually, has embryogenic clumps and even globular stage SEs.
- **Embryoids:** Embryo-like structure produced as a result of differentiation process such as embryogenesis and androgenesis.
- **Embryology:** The study of the early stages in the development of an organism. In these stages a single highly specialized cell, the egg, is transformed into a complex many celled organism resembling its parents.
- **Embryonic clump:** A localized group of meristematic and embryogenic cells, which are produced on somatic embryo induction

medium; they give rise to somatic embryos when cultured on a suitable medium or proliferate and remain in embryogenic state on the induction medium.

- **Embryonic stem (ES) cell:** Cells of early embryo that give rise to all differentiated cells including germ line cells.
- **Empirical:** Relating to or based upon practical experience, trial and error, direct observation or observation alone, without benefit of scientific method, knowledge or theory.
- **Emulsifiers:** Substances which allow water and oils to remain mixed together in form of an emulsion, e.g. in icecream, homogenized milk and mayonnaise.
- **Emulsion:** A stable dispersion of one liquid in a second, immiscible (i.e. nonmixable) liquid. For example, milk is an emulsion of oil (fat) in water, and latex paint is an emulsion of paint resin in water. Certain ingredients (e.g. β-conglycinin protein) help enable a greater content of the first liquid to be dispersed in the second liquid. Certain ingredients (e.g. β-conglycinin protein) make a given emulsion more stable (i.e. prevent the two liquids from separating over an extended period of time).
- **Enabling technologies:** The term "enabling technology" is used to describe technical processes that allow genetic modifications in organisms. This includes the ability to activate genes specifically or to influence them in their activity. The use of marker genes is also an enabling technology.
- **Enantiomers:** From the Greek word *enantios*, which means opposite. Enantiomers are a pair of nonidentical, mirror-image molecules. This means that both molecules are made up of the same atoms, i.e. they have the same molecular formula, but the constituent groups that are attached to a carbon atom can be arranged in two different ways (forms) around the carbon atom. This gives rise to an asymmetric molecule that can exist in either of two mirror-image forms whose mirror images are not superimposable. A pair of these molecules is known as enantiomers. The four-attached groups are all different from each other.
- **Enantiopure:** Refers to a compound (e.g. a pharmaceutical) that consists of only one of that compound's two possible enantiomers. Sometimes expressed in relative terms. For example, 98% enantiopure would refer to a compound that consists of 98% (of) desired enantiomer.

E

- **Encapsidation:** Process by which a virus nucleic acid is enclosed in a capsid.
- **Encapsulating agents:** Anything which forms a chell around an enzyme or bacterium although the agents used are usually polysaccharides such as alginate or agar. The agents are inert and allow nutrients and oxygen to diffuse into and out of the sphere readily and are easy to convert from gel (solid) to sol (liquid) or solution formed by altering the temperature or the concentration of ions.
- **Encapsulation:** Any method of getting something usually an enzyme or bacterium into a small package or capsule while it is still working or alive. It is a method for immobilizing cells for use in a bioreactor.
- **Encode:** To specify the sequence of amino acids in a protein.
- **End filling:** This method is used with those DNA molecules that have 5'-protruding ends; Klenow fragment is used to extent the recessed 3'-ends, thereby filling up the single-stranded ends.
- **End labeling:** The addition of a radioactively labeled group to one end (5' or 3') of a DNA strand.
- **Endangered breed:** A breed where the total number of breeding females is between 100 and 1000 or the total number of breeding males is less than or equal to 20 and greater than five or the overall population size is close to but slightly above 100 and increasing and the percentage of pure-breed females is above 80% or the overall population size is close to but slightly above and the percentage of pure-breed females is below 80%.
- **Endangered species:** A species whose total population is declining to relatively low levels such that if the trend continues, the species will most likely become extinct.
- **Endemic:** Describing a plant or animal species whose distribution is restricted to one or a few localities.
- **Endergonic reaction:** A chemical reaction with a positive standard free energy change (i.e. an "uphill" reaction). An (heat) energy-requiring reaction. A nonspontaneous reaction at ambient temperature.
- **End-labeling:** The introduction of a radioactive atom at the end of a DNA or RNA molecule. A commonly used method is to use T4 polynucleotide kinase to introduce a 32P atom onto the end of a DNA molecule.

- **Endocrine glands:** Glands that secrete their products (hormones) into the blood, which then carries them to their specific target organs. For example, adrenalin, produced in the adrenal glands, is carried to the heart (and other muscles) when needed during periods of stress. The endocrine glands are: the pituitary, thyroid, adrenals, pancreas, ovaries (in females) and testes (in males). Endocrine glands are found in some invertebrates as well as in vertebrates.

- **Endocrine hormones:** The products secreted by the endocrine glands. These help control long-term bodily processes, such as growth, lactation, sex cycles, and metabolic adjustment. The endocrine system and the nervous system are interdependent and often referred to collectively as the neuroendocrine system. For example, the juvenile hormone, found in insects and annelids, affects sexual maturation. There is currently great interest among scientists in the potential use of such hormones in the control of destructive insects.

- **Endocrine interference:** Interference with the normal balance hormones.

- **Endocrinology:** The branch of science that studies the endocrine glands, hormones, and hormone-like substances.

- **Endocytic vesicles:** These are membranous particles that transport proteins through endocytosis; also known as clathrin-coated vesicles.

- **Endocytosis:** A process by which proteins at the surface of the cell are internalized, being transported into the cell within membranous vesicles (Fig. 3).

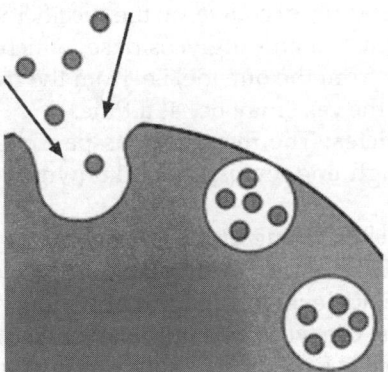

Fig. 3: Endocytosis

- **Endoderm:** The internal layer of cells of the gastrula which will develop into the alimentary canal (gut) and digestive glands of the adult.
- **Endodermal adult stem cells:** Certain stem cells present within (adult) bodies of organisms, that can be differentiated (via chemical signals) to give rise to cells of tongue, tonsils, the bladder/urethra, digestive tract, liver, pancreas, lung tissues, etc.
- **Endodermis:** The layer of living cells with various characteristically thickened walls and no intercellular spaces which surrounds the vascular tissue of certain stems and leaves. The endodermis separates the cortical cells from cells of the pericycle.
- **Endogamy:** The fusion of reproductive cells from closely related parents, i.e. inbreeding.
- **Endogenote:** The part of the bacterial chromosome that is homologous to a genome fragment (exogenote) transferred from the donor to the recipient cell in the formation of a merozygote.
- **Endogenous:** Developed or added from within the cell or organism.
- **Endogenous retrovirus:** Integrated retrovirus DNA (provirus) derived from infection of the germline of an ancestral animal. All animal are thought to carry numerous endogenous (but nonfunctional) retroviruses, some of which were inserted many millions of years ago.
- **Endoglycosidase:** An enzyme capable of hydrolyzing (breaking) interior bonds in the oligosaccharide molecular branches of a glycoprotein molecule. That is, the enzyme is capable of cutting a sugar-to-sugar bond anywhere within the sugar polymer molecule (depending, of course, on the specificity of the enzyme). This is in contrast to an exoglycosidase, which must cut away at the polymer from the outside, i.e. from the free-end, one unit (or section, as the case may be) at a time.
- **Endolytic vesicles:** The membranous particles that transport proteins through endocytosis; also known as clathrin-coated vesicles.
- **Endometrium:** The lining of the uterus.
- **Endomitosis:** Doubling of the number of chromosomes without division of the nucleus, resulting in polyploidy.
- **Endonucleases:** Cleave bonds within a nucleic acid chain; they may be specific for RNA or for single-stranded or double-stranded DNA.

- **Endophyte:** A microorganism (fungus or bacterium) that lives inside vascular tissues of plants (in spaces between plant cells). At least one company has incorporated the gene for a protein toxic to insects (taken from *Bacillus thuringiensis*) into an endophyte to confer insect resistance to a crop plant. When endophyte-infested fescue grass is fed to cattle, sheep, horses, or rabbits, it is generally toxic to those animals, due to mycotoxin(s) or alkaloids produced by that endophyte.

- **Endoplasmic reticulum (ER):** A highly convoluted sheet of membranes, extending from the outer layer of the nuclear envelope into the cytoplasm (Fig. 4).

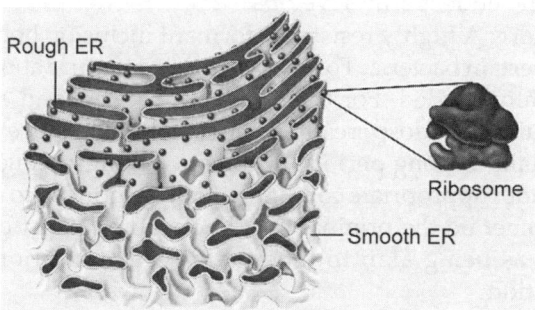

Fig. 4: Endoplasmic reticulum

- **Endopolyploidy:** The result of nuclear divisions without subsequent cytoplasmic division (cytokinesis), the polyploids so obtained are called endopolyploids.

- **Endoprotease:** An enzyme that cleaves the peptide bonds between amino acids within a protein cleavage is usually at one or more specific sites.

- **Endoreduplication:** Two or more successive rounds of DNA replication take place in nuclei without attendant cell division.

- **Endorphins:** Discovered during the 1970s by US and Scottish scientists, these hormones are produced in the brain, and act as natural painkillers. For example, runners and long-distance walkers achieve something of a "high" due to endorphins released during long runs or walks.

- **Endosome:** An organelle that functions to sort endocytosed molecules and molecules delivered from the trans-Golgi network and deliver them to other compartments, such as lysosomes. It consists of membrane-bounded tubules and vesicles.

- **Endosperm culture:** Culture of endosperm cells, usually, for obtaining triploid plants.
- **Endosperm:** The interior portion of a plant seed, beneath the outer hull (the portion that people tend to eat, in food crops). In grains (e.g. rice or corn/maize), the endosperm consists primarily of starch (carbohydrate). In legumes (e.g. beans), the endosperm contains mainly protein, a small amount of carbohydrates, and sometimes vegetable oil.
- **Endosperm mother cell:** One of the seven cells of the mature embryo sac containing the two polar nuclei and after reception of a sperm cell gives rise to the primary endosperm cell from which the endosperm develops.
- **Endospore:** A highly resistant, dormant inclusion body formed within certain bacteria. To kill spores, temperature above boiling are usually needed. For this, pressure cookers and autoclaves are required. Endospores have survival value since the spore can remain for long periods of time in a nongrowing state and then, under appropriate conditions, can be induced to germinate and regenerate the original cell. Endospore formation may be viewed as being akin to hibernation, i.e. a kind of bacterial hibernation.
- **Endostatin:** An antiangiogenesis human protein discovered by Judah Folkman. In concern with angiostatin, it causes certain cancer tumors in mice to shrink.
- **Endothelial cells:** These are the flat, sort of plate-shaped cells that line the surface of all blood vessels, heart, and lymphatics within the body. Endothelial cells possess transmembrane (through the cell membrane) molecules known as adhesion molecules, which selectively allow the passage (from blood-stream to tissues) of some molecules (leukocytes, monocytes, hormones, etc.). Endothelial cells are packed much tighter together in the capillaries that provide blood to the brain. This tighter packing limits, the size and kind of molecules that can pass into the brain. This blood-brain barrier serves to protect the sensitive brain tissue from pathogens or harmful molecules (e.g. toxins).
- **Endothelin:** A peptide that causes arteries to contract (which consequently causes blood pressure to increase).
- **Endothelium:** The layer of epithelial cells that line blood vessels throughout the body. The layer selectively allows the passage

(from bloodstream to tissues) of nutrients, hormones, and other molecules essential for tissue growth and function. The endothelium is involved in the recovery and recycling of old red blood cells. It also produces nitric oxide, which causes neighboring smooth muscle (blood vessel) cells to relax so that those (neighboring) blood vessels dilate and the body's blood pressure is lowered, and two compounds, prostacyclin and Von Willebrand factor, that prevent blood clotting.

- **Endotoxin:** Cell wall portion (lypopolysaccharide) of gram-negative bacteria that shows antigenic properties and trigger immune system.
- **End-product inhibition:** The ability of a product of a metabolic pathway to inhibit the activity of an enzyme that catalyzes an early step in the pathway.
- **Energy crops:** Crops that use solar energy efficiently to convert CO_2 into biomass.
- **Engineered antibodies:** Chimeric monoclonal antibodies, produced via genetic engineering of human antibody-producing cells (clones). For example, the genes coding for antilymphoma binding sites from a rat have been inserted into human antibody-producing cells to yield rat (antigen) binding sites mounted on human antibody stems.
- **Enhanceosome:** It is a complex of transcription factors that assembles cooperatively at an enhancer.
- **Enhancer:** A *cis*-acting sequence that increases the utilization of (some) eukaryotic promoters, and can function in either orientation and in any location (upstream or downstream) relative to the promoter.
- **Enkephalins:** A class of hormones produced in the brain that act as natural painkillers. Discovered by John Hughes and Hans Kosterlitz in 1975, they are some of the endorphins.
- **Enoyl-acyl protein reductase:** An enzyme that is utilized by bacteria in their synthesis (manufacture) of fatty acids.
- **Ensiling:** The fermentation of (usually chopped up) agricultural vegetation in order to preserve it. It is carried out for 1–2 weeks, using either indigenous microorganisms (e.g. *Lactobacillus* spp.) or introduced microorganisms (to speed up the process, yield product containing more nutrients for livestock, etc.), in the absence of oxygen (to prevent the growth of aerobic mold fungi). When indigenous microorganisms are used, *Lactobacillus* spp.

become the dominant microorganisms present, and heat is generated by the microorganisms within the vegetative mass (optimum temperature is 25–30°C, which is 77–86°F). Lactic acid produced by the microorganisms inhibits the growth of bacteria that would normally putrefy the vegetation.

- **Enterohemorrhagic *E. coli*:** The several dozen (approximately 60 known) serotypes (strains) of *E. coli* bacteria that cause internal hemorrhaging in humans that ingest those bacteria. The toxin produced by these particular *E. coli* bacteria attacks the human kidney, which often leads to kidney failure and/or death.

- **Enterotoxin:** The category (i.e. intestinally active) of toxins, produced by certain bacterial strains and/or serotypes, which attack the body's internal organs. For example, the serotype of *Escherichia coliform* bacteria known as *E. coli* 0157:H7 attacks the kidneys and other internal organs of humans, also causing internal bleeding and sometimes death.

- **Entrapment culture:** Cells are entrapped in an open matrix through which medium flows freely.

- **ENTREZ:** It is the integrated information database similarity search.

- **Enucleate:** A cell or protoplast without nucleus.

- **Enucleated ovum:** Egg cell from which the nucleus has been removed.

- **Envelopes:** Surround some organelles (for example nucleus or mitochondrion) and consist of concentric membranes, each membrane consisting of the usual lipid bilayer.

- **Environment:** The sum total of all surroundings of a living organism, including natural forces and other living things, which provide conditions for development and growth as well as of danger and damage.

- **Environmental impact:** The effect on the natural environment caused by human actions; it includes indirect effects, for example, through pollution, as well as direct effects such as cutting down of trees.

- **Environmental stewardship:** The view that humans have a duty to manage and care for the whole natural environment; that we are responsible for the continued health of the whole ecosystem, not just the parts that benefit the human race. It involves integrating and applying environmental values into a process.

- **Enzyme bioreactor:** A reactor in which a chemical conversion reaction is catalyzed by an enzyme.
- **Enzyme commission (EC) number:** Systematic name and number which identify an enzyme in technical literature. Assigned by the enzyme commission the EC number consists of four numbers separated by dots (:).
- **Enzyme denaturation:** The loss of enzyme (catalytic) activity due to loss of the correct functional structure of the protein. Denaturation may be caused by factors such as exposure to heat and organic solvents, degradation of the enzyme molecule by proteases, oxygen and acid or alkaline pH.
- **Enzyme derepression:** Commonly known as induction (of an enzyme). Initially, a repressor protein is bound to a specific region of DNA. This binding inhibits transcription to mRNA, thus blocking the synthesis of the protein (enzyme) specified by the mRNA. When present, the inducer molecule binds to the repressor protein and inactivates it. Thus, the inhibition caused by the repressor protein is overcome and mRNA can be synthesized, which consequently leads to synthesis of the mRNA-specified protein (enzyme). The word derepression is sometimes used because the repressor protein is, by itself, active in repressing protein (enzyme) synthesis. Its repressive action is mitigated (derepressed) by the inducer molecule. Hence, derepression (or unrepression) of repression equals induction.
- **Enzyme electrode:** A type of biosensor in which an enzyme is immoblized onto the surface of an electrode. When the enzyme catalyzes its reaction, electrons are transferred from the reactant to the electrode and so a current is generated.
- **Enzyme engineering:** Improvement in the activity and usefulness of an existing enzyme or creation of a new enzyme activity by making suitable changes in the amino acid sequence of concerned enzyme by recombinant DNA technology.
- **Enzyme immobilization:** Confining the enzyme molecule to a distinct phase from the one in which the substrate and the products are present.
- **Enzyme repression:** Inhibition of enzyme synthesis caused by the availability of the product of that enzyme. On a molecular level a repressor molecule (which could be, e.g. the amino acid arginine) combines with a specific repressor protein that is present in the cell. This repressor molecule/repressor protein

complex is then able to bind to a specific region of DNA at the initial end of the gene which is called the operator region. It is in this region where the synthesis of mRNA is initiated. The repressor "roadblock" thus stops the synthesis of mRNA, and therefore the synthesis of the protein is also blocked.

- **Enzyme stabilization using antibodies:** A method of stabilizing enzymes by binding antibodies to them. The antibodies should not block the active site of the enzyme as otherwise the protein is established but is inactive as a catalyst. Monoclonal antibodies are usually used as they bind to specific bits of the protein surface. If the enzyme tries to unfold into an inactivate structure, must not only overcome its own binding energy but also throw-off all the bound antibodies, this requires more energy and so is a correspondingly slower process.

- **Enzyme technology:** Use of purified enzymes for generating useful products or services.

- **Enzyme turnover:** The process through which the enzyme returns to its original shape, enabling the enzyme to catalyze another reaction.

- **Enzyme:** Generally, a protein that catalyzes or speeds up a specific chemical reaction; biosynthetic or degradative function; usually, occur in living cells/living systems.

- **Enzyme-product complex:** Enzyme molecule having the product molecule bound to its binding site.

- **Enzyme-reactor:** A vessel employed to carry out the desired conversion using an enzyme.

- **Enzyme-substrate complex:** Enzyme molecule having the substrate molecules bound to its active/binding site; this state precedes catalysis.

- **Eosinophils:** Polymorphonuclear leukocytes made in the bone marrow. They circulate in the blood for a number of hours (three to eight) and then migrate into the tissue where they reside. They kill parasites too large to be phagocytized by secreting substances that kill the parasites (hookworms, trichinosis, etc.), inhibit histamine release from mast cells, and secrete chemicals that neutralize histamine. Allergy causes an increase in eosinophils. GM-CSF stimulates eosinophil production.

- **EPG fragments:** Oligonucleotides produced from cell wall by endopolygalacturonase hydrolysis; affect morphogenic response of cell cultures; included under the general term *oligosaccharins*.

- **Epicotyl:** The upper portion of the axis of a plant embryo or seedling above the cotyledons.
- **Epidermal growth factor (EGF):** A protein of 53 amino acids that greatly increases growth/reproduction of epidermal (skin) cells. This protein also increases growth of wool in sheep and growth in more than 50% of human tumors. High concentrations of epidermal growth factor are found in human tears. EGF was discovered by Stanley Cohen.
- **Epidermis:** The outermost single (usually) layer of cells covering the entire plant body (primary body); forms a protective layer.
- **Epidermology:** The science of disease epidermics.
- **Epigenesis:** Describes the developmental process whereby each successive stage of normal development is built up on the preceding stages of development. An embryo is built up from a zygote, a seedling from an embryo and so on.
- **Epigenetic variation:** When a variant trait shows stability during miotic division in cell cultures, but disappears either during plantlet regeneration from them or during meiosis in the regenerated plants; may relate to up or down regulation of the promoter of the concerned gene.
- **Epigenetic:** Epigenetic changes influence the phenotype without alerting the genotype. They consist of changes in the properties of a cell that are inherited but that do not represent a change in genetic information.
- **Epimerase:** An enzyme capable of the reversible interconversion of two epimers.
- **Epimers:** Two stereoisomers differing in configuration.
- **Epinasty:** A process by which the growth of branches or petrioles is abnormally pointing downward. This phenomenon is caused by the more rapid growth of the upper side. Epinasty may result from either nutritional deficiencies or irregularities at the plant growth regulator level. Not to be confused with wilting as epinastic tissues are turgid.
- **Epiphyte:** A plant that grows upon another plant but is neither parasitic on it nor rooted in the ground.
- **Episome:** A genetic element in bacteria that can replicate freely in the cytoplasm or can be inserted into the main bacterial chromosome and replicate with the chromosome.
- **Epistasis:** One gene masks the expression of another nonallelic gene, absence of expected phenotype as a result of masking

E

expression of another gene pair. The crossing between two white sweet pea plants (CCpp × ccPP) produces purple flowered (CcPp) plants, F_2 generation results a 9 colored (9C-P-) : 7 white (3C-pp + 3ccP- + 1 ccpp) rather than 9:3:3:1 dihybrid ratio.

- **Epithelial projections:** Projections that anchor the epidermis (surface skin) to the dermis (subsurface tissue). Growth of these projections is increased by epidermal growth factor during the wound healing process.

- **Epithelium:** The prefix *epi-* means on, above, or upon. The membranous cellular tissue that covers a free surface or lines a tube or cavity of an animal body. It serves to enclose and protect the other tissues, to produce secretions and excretions, and to function in assimilation.

- **Epitope:** A specific chemical domain present on an antigen recognized by an antibody. Each epitope elicits synthesis of different antibodies.

- **Epizootic:** A disease affecting a large number of animals simultaneously.

- **Enolpyruvyl-shikimate phosphate synthase (EPSP):** An enzyme produced by virtually all plants and internally transported into their cells' chloroplasts, it is essential in a plant's metabolism biochemical pathway and for the biosynthesis (creation) of the aromatic (ring-shaped molecule) amino acids tyrosine, phenylalanine, and tryptophan, which are needed for plants to live. Some (glyphosate-containing and sulfosatecontaining) herbicides kill unwanted plants (e.g. weeds) by inhibiting EPSP synthase. By incorporating a gene that causes (over-) production of CP4 EPSP synthase into several crops (soybeans, cotton, etc.), scientists have been able to help those crops survive post-emergence application(s) of glyphosate-containing herbicide. Additional resistance to glyphosate-containing and sulfosate-containing herbicides can be conferred to plants by incorporating into plants a gene (GO) which causes those plants to produce glyphosate oxidase.

- **Equational division:** Mitotic type division that is usually the second division in the meiotic sequence somatic mitosis and the nonreductional division of meiosis. A chromosome division in which the two chromatids of each duplicated chromosome separate longitudinally prior to being incorporated into two daughter nuclei.

- **Equatorial plate:** The figure formed by the chromosomes in the center (equatorial plane) of the spindle in mitosis (Fig. 5).

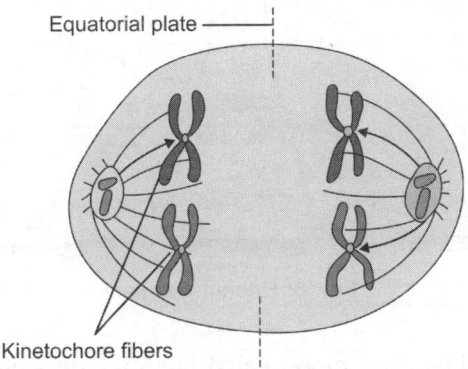

Equatorial plate ⎯⎯⎯⎯

Kinetochore fibers

Fig. 5: Equatorial plate

- **Equilibrium:** A state, in which the forward and the reverse reactions proceed at identical rates and there is no net product formation.
- **Equilibrium density gradient centrifugation:** A procedure used to separate macromolecules based on their density (mass per unit volume).
- **Equimolar:** Identical molar concentrations.
- **Ergotamine:** A mycotoxin (i.e. metabolite produced by a fungus, that is toxic to animals and humans) produced by the fungus (*Claviceps* spp.) known as ergot. Ergotamine is an alkaloid vasoconstrictor, whose consumption can lead to severe constriction of blood vessels in the brain and extremities, causing hallucinations and dry gangrene. Humans whose bodies are deficient in vitamin A are especially vulnerable to ergotism (ergot poisoning).
- **Erlenmeyer flask:** A conical flat-bottomed laboratory flask with a narrow neck designed by E Erlenmeyer. Widely used for culturing microorganisms (Fig. 6).
- **Error-prone:** Synthesis occurs when DNA incorporates noncomplementary bases into the daughter strand.
- **Erwinia caratovora:** A species of bacteria that can cause significant postharvest losses to potato farmers, when it infects potatoes and causes "soft rot" (spoilage).

E

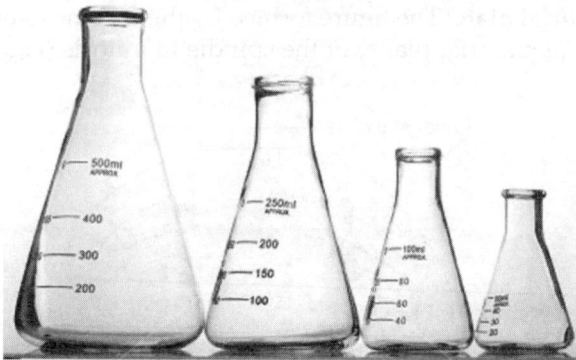

Fig. 6: Erlenmeyer flast

- **Erythrocytes:** (Red blood cells) Hemoglobin-containing cells (manufactured in the bone marrow) that transport the oxygen from the lungs to the body tissues where it is needed.
- **Erythropoiesis:** The formation of red blood cells from certain stem cells. Stimulated by the protein erythropoietin.
- **Erythropoietin (EPO):** A glycoprotein hormone produced in the kidneys that stimulates stem cells in the bone marrow to increase the number of red blood cells. Erythropoietin can be used to help correct a variety of anemias.
- **Escape:** A susceptible cell/individual being classified as resistant due to errors in evaluation/classification.
- *Escherichia coliform (E. coli):* A bacterium that commonly inhabits the human intestine as well as the intestine of other vertebrates (animals possessing a skeleton). The most thoroughly studied of all bacteria, *Escherichia coli* is used in many micro-biological experiments. It has historically been considered the workhorse of genetic engineering research, and genetically engineered versions have been used to produce human proteins (e.g. insulin). One of the more exotic uses of genetically engineered *E. coli* was to make indigo dye (originally discovered in 1983, using indole or tryptophan as starting materials). In 1993, Burt D Ensley and coworkers at Amgen discovered a way to genetically engineer *E. coli* to produce indigo from glucose starting material. *E. coli* has 4,288 genes (Fig. 7).
- *Escherichia coliform 0157:H7:* The particular strain (serotype) of *Escherichia coliform (E. coli)* bacteria that causes often-fatal

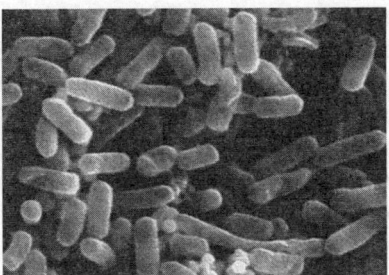

Fig. 7: Escherichia coliform (*E. coli*)

diarrhea, internal bleeding, and kidney damage in humans. Children are more susceptible to *E. coli* 0157:H7 than adults, because children possess more of the receptors (on cells inside the digestive tract) that are utilized by *E. coli* 0157:H7 to enter the body from the digestive tract. Although cattle were susceptible to *E. coli* 0157:H7's toxins prior to the 1980s, they eventually developed resistance. That meant that the cattle could carry these bacteria without getting sick, and transmit *E. coli* 0157:H7 to humans whenever conditions allow (e.g. when *E. coli* 0157:H7- infected cattle are slaughtered and people consume the meat without first heating it to a high enough temperature to kill the *E. coli* 0157:H7). Some varieties of *E. coli* 0157:H7 are resistant to the antibiotics tetracycline and streptomycin. In 1996, researchers at Cornell University in New York state, USA, discovered that nonambulatory cows (that could not walk) were approximately four times as likely as other cows to test positive for *E. coli* 0157:H7. Other research in Canada indicates that fasting of cattle (common occurrence for nonambulatory cows) tends to alter the pH inside the cow's rumen (stomach) in a way that encourages the proliferation of *E. coli* 0157:H7 instead of the bacteria that normally populate the rumen.

- **Essential amino acids:** Those amino acids that cannot be synthesized by humans and most other vertebrates, and therefore must be obtained from the diet. They are phenylalanine, valine, threonine, tryptophan, isoleucine, methionine, histidine, arginine, leucine and lysine (glycine and proline for poultry).
- **Essential element:** Any of a number of elements required by living organisms to ensure normal growth, development and maintenance.

E

- **Essential fatty acids:** Mammals (including humans) cannot synthesize linoleic (18:2) and linolenic (18:3) fatty acids; therefore, they must be supplied in their diet, and are called essential fatty acids.
- **Essential gene:** One whose deletion is lethal to the organism.
- **Essential nutrients:** Chemical compounds in foods required for (consuming organism's) life, growth, or tissue repair, and cannot be synthesized by that organism.
- **Essential requirement:** A nutrient is essential when it is manadatory for growth, development and reproduction. In tissue culture, it comprises inorganic salts including all of the element necessary for plant metabolism organic factors (amino acids, vitamins) usually also endogenous plant growth regulators (auxins, cytokines and often gibberellins) as well as a carbon source (sucrose or glucose).
- **Established cell lines:** Consist of eukaryotic cells that have been adapted to indefinite growth in culture (they are said to be immortalized).
- **Established culture:** An aseptic viable explant. Or A suspension culture subjected to several passages with a constant cell number per unit time.
- **Estimated breeding value (EBV):** Twice the expected progeny difference. The difference is doubled because breeding value is a reflection of all the genes of an animal, in contrast to progeny difference which is a reflection of a sample half of an animal genes. The predicted performance of the offspring of the mating between any two animals is the average of their EBVs (averaged because each parent makes an equal contribution to each offspring).
- **Estrogen:** A female sex hormone, secreted by the ovaries, that promotes estrus and helps to regulate the pituitary gland's production of luteinizing hormone (LH) and follicle stimulating hormone (FSH). Estrogen causes proliferation of breast tissue (cells) and is also responsible for the development of female secondary sex characteristics (e.g. smaller body size, lack of facial hair, higher pitch voice in humans). Research indicates that lack of estrogen (e.g. in postmenopausal women) makes humans more prone to colon cancer and heart disease, but less prone to the "hormone dependent" cancers (ovarian cancer, uterine cancer, etc.).

- **Ethanol (ethyl alcohol):** Commonly used to disinfest plant tissues, glassware utensils and working surfaces in tissue culture manipulations.
- **Ethephon (2-chloroethyl phosphonic acid ($ClC_2PO_3H_6$):** Through a spontaneous degradation of ethephon, ethylene is produced. Ethephon is a synthetic compound commonly used to treat cultured cells or unripe fruit with ethylene.
- **Ethics:** A branch of philosophy that deals with morality. It is concerned with distinguishing between right and wrong human actions, both at an individual and societal level. Ethics may also apply to the rules or standards that specify how particular members of an organization should conduct themselves.
- **Ethidium bromide:** A fluorescent dye used to stain DNA and RNA. The dye fluoresces when exposed to UV light.
- **Ethylene ($CH_2 = CH_2$):** A plant hormone, which is involved in fruit ripening, leaf abscission, flower senescence, etc.
- **Ethylenediamine tetra-acetic acid (EDTA):** A chelating compound. In tissue culture, it is used to keep nutrients such as iron, bound in a form that leaves them still available to the plant but which prevents them from precipitaining out.
- **Etiolation:** An abnormal increase in stem elongation accompanied by poor or absent leaf development. Physiological etiolation is caused by a lack of chlorophyll and is typical for plants growing under low light intensity or in complete darkness. It can also be caused by disease.
- **Etiological agent (of a disease):** The microorganism (or other agent) that causes the disease.
- **Etiology:** The science (study) of the cause (source) of a disease.
- **Eubacteria:** Comprises the major line of prokaryotes.
- **Eucaryote:** Also spelled eukaryote. A cell characterized by compartmentalization (by membranes) of its extensive internal structures; or an organism made up of such cells. For example, eukaryotes possess a distinct membrane-surrounded nucleus containing the DNA. Eukaryotic cells (e.g. human cells) are much larger and more complex than prokaryotic cells (e.g. bacteria). The cells of all higher organisms, both plant and animal, are eukaryotic, so those higher (complex) organisms are often referred to as eukaryotes. Most eukaryotic organisms cannot survive temperatures greater than 131°F (55°C). However, one called the Pompeii worm (*Alvinella pompejana*)

can withstand long-term exposure in water up to a temperature of 176°F (80°C).

- **Euchromatin:** Comprises all of the genome in the interphase nucleus except for the heterochromatin.

- **Eugenics:** First formulated by Francis Galton, who was a contemporary of Gregor Mendel in the 19th century, eugenics is the concept that a species can be "improved" by encouraging reproduction of only those organisms in that species that possess "desired" traits. This belief became popular in a number of countries during the early 20th century. Margaret Sanger, founder of America's Planned Parenthood organization, referred to African-Americans as "human weeds" and called for "more children from the fit, less from the unfit." Based upon Charles Darwin's written assertion that "the civilized races of man will almost certainly exterminate and replace the savage races," a number of large genocides were committed by national governments.

- **Euploid:** A cell carrying an exact multiple of the haploid chromosome number. For example, a diploid possesses twice the haploid number of chromosomes.

- **European corn borer (ECB):** Also known as pyralis. Latin name *Ostrinia nubilalis*, it is an insect whose larvae (caterpillars) eat and bore into the corn/maize plant (*Zea mays* L.). In doing so, they can act as vectors (i.e. carriers) of the fungi known as *Aspergillus flavus* (source of aflatoxin) or *Fusarium moniliforme* (source of fumonisin) or *Aspergillus parasiticus* (source of aflatoxin). Full-grown ECB larvae winter by sheltering inside a variety of vegetative materials (e.g. plant stalks lying on top of soil in some fields). ECB control can be effected by some of the following methods: 1. Spraying of conventional synthetic chemical pesticides 2. Spraying of pesticides produced via promulgation of *Bacillus thuringiensis* (*B.t.*) bacteria 3. Incorporating a (protoxin) gene from *B.t.* into the DNA of the corn plant, so that the plant itself produces *B.t.* protoxin. As part of Integrated Pest Management (IPM), farmers can utilize: 1. Corn possessing *B.t.* gene(s) to control populations of ECB without applying insecticides 2. The parasitic *Euplectrus comstockki* wasp to help control the ECB. (When that wasp's venom is injected into ECB larva, it stops the larva from molting and thus maturing) 3. Additional methods, alone or in concert with above.

- **European Medicines Evaluation Agency (EMEA):** A London-based agency of the European Union (EU) that began operation in 1995. It coordinates drug licensing and safety matters throughout the nations of the EU. Its licensing/approval process is compulsory throughout the EU.
- **European patent convention:** An international patent treaty signed in 1973, by which the countries of Europe agreed to recognize and honor the patents granted by each country, and those patents granted by the European Patent Office (EPO). Plant varieties or animal breeds were initially excluded from patentability by the European Patent Convention. In 1998, the European Parliament removed that exclusion.
- **European Patent Office (EPO):** The Munich, Germany-based agency of the European Union (EU)—established in 1977—that is responsible for common patent protection matters for all of the EU member countries, and the non-EU countries of Switzerland and Liechtenstein. The European Patent Office originally did not allow a "plant or animal breed" to be patented, whereas its US counterpart—the US Patent and Trademark Office (USPTO)—does allow patenting of microbes, plants, and animals (e.g. those which have been genetically engineered by man). In 1998, the European Parliament removed that exclusion, and in 1999, the European Patent Court issued a ruling which caused the European Patent Convention to allow patents on novel plants, thus making the two patent systems compatible.
- **European Plant Protection Organization (EPPO):** One of the international SPS standard- setting organizations that develops plant health standards, guidelines, and recommendations (e.g. to prevent transfer of a plant disease or plant pest from one country to another). Its secretariat is in Paris, France. EPPO, one of the organizations within the International Plant Protection Convention (IPPC), covers the countries of Europe.
- **Eutrophication:** Presence of organic materials and inorganic nutrients in river waters; contributed by waste water.
- **Evaluation:** Measurement of the characteristic those are important for production and adaptation either of individual animals or of populations most commonly in the context of comparative evaluation of the traits of animals or of populations.

E

- **Evapotranspiration:** The process of water loss in vapor form from a unit surface of land both directly and through leaf surfaces during a specific period of time.
- **Event:** Refers to each instance of a genetically engineered organism. For example, the same gene inserted by man into a given plant genome at two different locations (*loci*) along that plant's DNA would be considered two different events. Alternatively, two different genes inserted into the same *locus* of two same-species plants would also be considered two different events. Generally speaking, the world's regulatory agencies confer new biotech-derived product approvals in terms of events.
- **Evolution:** The process by which the present diversity of plant and animal life arose from the earliest organisms, a process believed to have been continuing for at least 3,000 million years.
- **Evolutionary clock:** It defined by the rate at which mutations accumulate in a given gene.
- ***Ex situ* germplasm conservation:** Collection and conservation of germplasm away from the area of their origin as seed banks, field banks, shoot-tip banks, cells and tissue culture banks and DNA banks.
- ***Ex vitro* hardening:** Hardening of plantlets outside culture vessels.
- ***Ex vivo* (testing):** The testing of a substance by exposing it to (excised) living cells (but not to the whole, multicelled organism) in order to ascertain the effect of the substance (e.g. pharmaceutical) on the biochemistry of the cell.
- ***Ex vivo* (therapy):** Removal of cells (e.g. certain blood cells) from a patient's body, alteration of those cells in one or more therapeutic ways, followed by reinsertion of the altered cells into the patient's body.
- **Excise:** To remove a tissue or an organ, usually, by cutting with a scalpel, to obtain explants or during subculture, etc.
- **Excision:** Phage or episome or other sequence describes its release from the host chromosome as an autonomous DNA molecule.
- **Excision-repair:** Systems remove a single-stranded sequence of DNA containing damaged or mispaired bases and replace it in the duplex by synthesizing a sequence complementary to the remaining strand.

- **Excitatory amino acids (EAAs):** Amino acids present in the brain (when released by certain immune system cells) that can kill brain cells when in excess (e.g. results from strokes, which cause the release of too many EAAs in the brain). Another source of harmful EAAs (e.g. glutamate) is the disease known as multiple sclerosis. Some spiders paralyze their prey with venom that contains a substance that blocks the action of EAAs; thus, pharmaceuticals based on an active ingredient in that venom may someday be used to prevent brain damage in stroke and in multiple sclerosis victims.
- **Excrete:** To transport a compound out of a cell aka to secrete to export.
- **Exergonic reaction:** A chemical reaction with a negative standard free energy change (i.e. a "downhill" reaction). A reaction which releases energy (exothermic; in the form of heat).
- **Exobiology:** Extraterrestrial biology.
- **Exocyst:** It is a complex of 8 proteins that is found at sites on the plasma membrane where secretion occurs. It tethers secretory vesicles to the membrane as the first step in the process of membrane fusion.
- **Exocytosis:** The process of secreting proteins from a cell into the medium, by transport in membranous vesicles from the endoplasmic reticulum, through the Golgi, to storage vesicles, and finally (upon a regulatory signal) through the plasma membrane (Fig. 8).

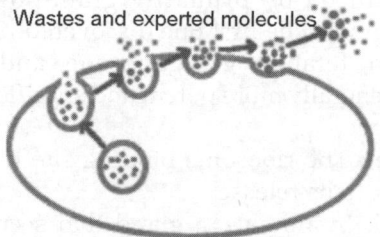

Fig. 8: Exocytosis

- **Exogenous elicitor:** Elicitor produced by an organism, e.g. a microorganism, other than the organism in question.
- **Exoglycosidase:** An enzyme that hydrolyzes (cuts) only a terminal (end) bond in the oligosaccharide (molecular) branch(es) of a glycoprotein.

E

- **Exon definition:** Describes the process when a pair of splicing sites are recognized by interactions involving the 5′ site of the intron and also the 5′ of the next intron downstream.
- **Exon shuffling:** New combinations of exons produced by recombination within the intervening sequences; produces new genes that encode proteins with altered functions.
- **Exon trapping:** Inserts a genomic fragment into a vector whose function depends on the provision of splicing junctions by the fragment.
- **Exon:** Any segment of interrupted gene that is represented in the mature RNA product.
- **Exonuclease III (ExoIII):** An enzyme from *E.coli* that removes nucleotides from 3′OH ends of double-stranded DNA.
- **Exonuclease:** Cleaves nucleotides one at a time from the end of a polynucleotide chain; they may be specific for either the 5′ or 3′ end of DNA or RNA.
- **Exosome:** It is a complex of several exonucleases involved in degrading RNA.
- **Exotic germplasm:** Germ plasm that has not been adapted (selectively breed) to the environment intended (for its offspring, via selective breeding by man).
- **Exotic species:** A species introduced into a geographical area to which it is not native.
- **Exotoxin:** Proteins (toxins) produced by certain bacteria that are released by the bacteria into their surroundings (growth medium). Produced by primarily gram-positive bacteria. Diphtheria toxin was the first one discovered. Other exotoxins cause botulism, tetanus, gas gangrene, and scarlet fever. Exotoxins are generally more potent and specific in their actions than endotoxins.
- **Exit site (e site):** The ribosome binding site that contains the free tRNA prior to its release.
- **Exocrine gland:** In animals, a gland that secretes through a duct.
- **Exogamy:** The fusion of reproductive cells from distantly related or unrelated organisms, i.e. outbreeding.
- **Exogenote:** Chromosomal fragment hormologous to an endo-genote and donated a merozygote.
- **Exogenous:** Produced outside of originating from or due to external causes. Opposite of endogenous.

- **Exogenous DNA:** DNA that has been derived from a source organism and has been cloned into a vector and introduced into a host cell. Also referred to as foreign DNA or heterogenous DNA.
- **Exon amplification:** A procedure that is used to amplify exons.
- **Expolysaccharide:** A high-molecular-weight polymer that is composed of sugar residues and is secreted by a micro-organism into the surrounding environment.
- **Expected progeny differences (EPD):** Numerical rankings of (livestock) parental genetics, in terms of an animal's genetic impact on progeny's has four following commercial traits: 1. Number of progeny born alive; 2. Weight of progeny at weaning age; 3. Number of days required to reach slaughter weight, when fed adequately; 4. Carcass lean meat vs fat percentages EPDs allow a farmer to estimate differences in performance of future offspring (of a given parent) vs offspring produced by parents of average genetic value. For example, a boar (male pig) possessing an EPD of –4 for "number of days required to reach slaughter weight" produces offspring that reach slaughter weight in four fewer days (of feeding time) than offspring that are sired by a boar possessing an EPD of 0.
- **Explant:** The tissue taken from a plant or seed and transferred to a culture medium to establish a tissue culture system or regenerated a plant.
- **Explant donor:** The source plant or mother plant from which is taken the explant used to initiate a culture.
- **Explantation:** The removal of cells, tissues or organs of animals and plants for observation of their growth and development in appropriate culture media.
- **Exponential phase:** A phase of cell growth where they undergo maximum rate of cell division.
- **Exportins:** Transport receptors that bind their cargo and associate with RanGTP in the nucleus. The trimeric complex translocates across the nuclear envelope into the cytoplasm, where hydrolysis of GTP bound to Ran results in release of cargo.
- **Express:** To translate the cell's genetic information stored in the DNA (gene) into a specific protein (synthesized by the cell's ribosome system). Certain proteins (i.e. when present in relevant cells) regulate the expression (e.g. increase/decrease/timing) of some genes.

E

- **Explosion method [to introduce foreign (new) genes into plant cells]:** A technique for gene-into-cell introduction in which the gene (genetic material) is driven into plant cells by the force of an explosion (vaporization) of a drop of water (to which the gene and gold particles have been added). The explosion is caused by application of high-voltage electricity to the drop of gene-laden water; the water is then vaporized explosively, driving the "shot" (gold particles) and genetic material through the cell membrane. The plant cell then heals itself (reseals the hole where the gene entered), incorporates the new gene into its genetic complement, and produces whatever product (e.g. a protein) for which the newly introduced gene codes.
- **Expressed sequence tags (ESTs):** These are 200–300 bp long cDNA sequences generated by picking thousands of random clones from cDNA libraries and using them for single-pass sequencing; represents a partial gene sequence; used in microarrays.
- **Expression cassette:** When an expression vector contains the promoter, ribosome binding site and transcription termination sequences in a cluster, it is termed as an expression cassette.
- **Expression library:** A collection of recombinant clones that together contains all the available cDNAs from a cell type/tissue/organism; cDNAs are integrated in an expression vector so that they are able to generate their protein product.
- **Expression profiling:** Determination of the cell types/tissues in which a gene is expressed as well as when, the given gene is expressed.
- **Expression site (in a trypanosome genome):** A locus near a telomere that can express the VSG gene that is located there.
- **Expression system:** Combination of host and vector which provides a genetic context for making a cloned gene function, i.e. produce peptide in the host cell.
- **Expression vector:** A vector, such as a plasmid, yeast, or animal virus genome, used to introduce foreign genetic material into a host cell in order to replicate and amplify the foreign DNA sequences as a recombinant molecule.
- **Expression-linked copy (ELC) (in a trypanosome genome):** The one copy of a VSG gene that is expressed.
- **Expressivity:** The intensity with which the effect of a gene is realized in the phenotype. The degree to which a particular effect is expressed by individuals.

- **Extant variety:** A notified variety or a farmer variety that is in public domain.
- **Extein:** Sequences remain in the mature protein that is produced by processing a precursor via protein splicing.
- **Extension (in nucleic acids):** The nucleic acid strand elongation (lengthening) that occurs in a polymerization reaction.
- **External domain:** The part of a plasma membrane protein that extends outside of the cell. Upon internalization, the protein's external domain extends into the lumen (the topological equivalent of the outside of the cell) of an organelle.
- **Extinction:** Refers to the death of all the individuals of a species; it leads to loss of all the genes of that species.
- **Extra arm (of tRNA):** It lies between the TyC and anticodon arms. It is the most variable in length in tRNA, from 3–21 bases. tRNAs are called class 1 if they lack it, and class 2 if they have it.
- **Extracellular matrix (ECM):** A relatively rigid layer of insoluble glycoproteins that fill the spaces between cells in multicellular organisms. These glycoproteins connect to plasma membrane proteins.
- **Extrachromosomal genome (in a bacterium):** A self-replicating set of genes that is not part of the bacterial chromosome. In many cases, the genes are necessary for bacterial growth under certain environmental conditions.
- **Extraction:** The process of recovering a compound or a group of compounds from a mixture or from cells into a solvent phase.
- **Extranuclear genes:** Reside outside the nucleus in organelles such as mitochondria and chloroplasts.
- **Extremophilic bacteria:** Bacteria that live and reproduce outside (either colder or hotter) the typical temperature range of 40°F (4°C) to 140°F (60°C) that bacteria tend to be found in, on earth. Other extremes are high pressure (e.g. at the ocean bottom), salt saturation, (e.g. the Dead Sea), pH lower than 2 (e.g. coal deposits), pH higher than 11 (e.g. sewage sludge), high levels of radiation, etc.
- **Extremozymes:** Enzymes that function optimally under extreme conditions of temperature, pH, etc.
- **Exude:** Slowly discharge or leak liquid material (exudate such as tannins or oxidized polyphenols) through pores or cuts or by diffusion into the medium. In some woody plant species exudation is associated with a lethal browning of explants.

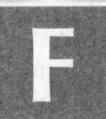

- **10 nm fiber:** It is a linear array of nucleosomes, generated by unfolding from the natural condition of chromatin.
- **30 nm fiber:** It is a coiled coil of nucleosomes. It is the basic level of organization of nucleosomes in chromatin.
- **F factor:** A bacterial episome that confers the ability to function as a genetic donor in conjugation the fertility factor in bacteria.
- **F plasmid:** It is an episome that can be free or integrated in *E. coli,* and which in either form can sponsor conjugation.
- **F:** Symbolizes filial from the latin meaning progeny.
- **F⁺ cell:** A bacterial cell that contains a fertility (F) factor, acts as a donor in bacterial conjugation.
- **F_1 generation:** First filial generation, offspring of a cross involving the F_1 generation.
- **F_1 hybrids:** The first-generation offspring of cross breeding; also known as first filial hybrids. They tend to be more healthy, productive, and uniform than their parents.
- **F_2 generation:** Second filial generation, offspring of a cross involving the F_1 generation.
- **Factor IX:** A protein factor in the blood serum that is instrumental in the cascade of chemical reactions (involving 17 blood components) that leads to clot formation, following a cut or other wound to body tissue. A deficiency of factor IX is the cause of the disease known as hemophilia B (approximately 15% of all hemophilia patients).
- **Factor VIII:** Also known as antihemophilic globulin (AHG) or antihemophilic factor VIII. A protein factor in the blood serum that is instrumental in the "cascade" of chemical reactions (involving 17 blood components in the intrinsic pathway) that leads to clot formation following a cut or other wound to body tissue. Also, a deficiency of AHG is the cause of the classical type of hemophilia sometimes known as hemophilia AM (approximately 85% of all hemophilia patients).

- **Factor:** A bacterial sex or fertility plasmid.
- **Facultative anaerobe:** An organism that will grow under either aerobic or anaerobic conditions.
- **Facultative cells:** Cells that can live either in the presence or absence of oxygen.
- **Facultative heterochromatin:** The inert state of sequences that also exist in active copies—for example, one mammalian X-chromosome in females.
- **Facultative parasites:** Refer to those saprophytes which mostly feed on dead organic matter, but if they reach the living plants they also attack the same.
- **Facultative saprophytes:** Refer to those parasites, which mostly feed on their living host plants but when living plants are not available, they feed on the dead residues of their hosts.
- **FAO:** Food and Agriculture Organization of the United Nations.
- **False negative:** A negative assay result that should have been positive.
- **Farnesyl transferase:** An enzyme utilized by the ras gene (to help "signal" certain cells to divide/grow).
- **Fast component (Of a reassociation reaction):** The first to renature and contains highly repetitive DNA.
- **Fate map:** A map of an embryo showing the adult tissues that will develop from the descendants of cells that occupy particular regions of the embryo.
- **Fats:** Energy storage substances produced by animals and some plants (e.g. soybeans), which consist of a combination of fatty acids and glycerol that form predominantly triglyceride molecules (although some diglyceride molecules are also often present in fats).
- **Fatty acid:** A long-chain aliphatic acid found in natural fats and oils. Fatty acids are abundant in cell membranes and (after extraction/purification) are widely used as industrial emulsifiers, e.g. phosphatidylcholine (lecithin). In general, fats possessing the highest levels of saturated fatty acids tend to be solid at room temperature, and those fats possessing the highest levels of unsaturated fatty acids tend to be liquid at room temperature. That rule of thumb was the original "dividing line" between compounds called fats and oils, respectively. In general, saturated fatty acids tend to be more stable (resistant to oxidation and thermal breakdown) than unsaturated fatty acids. Fatty

acids in biological systems (e.g. produced by plants in oilseeds) tend to contain an even number of carbon atoms in their molecular "backbone," typically between 14 and 24 carbon atoms. The molecular backbone (alkyl chain) may be saturated (no double bonds) or it may contain one or more double bonds. The configuration of the double bonds in most unsaturated fatty acids is CIS.

- **Fatty acid synthetase:** A group of seven related enzymes that catalyze synthesis (manufacturing) of fatty acids within the soybean plant (*Glycine max* (L.) Merrill).

F

- **F-Box proteins:** Proteins produced (manufactured) within some eukaryotic cells, that play an essential role in the degradation (i.e. breakdown) of cellular regulatory proteins, after those regulatory proteins have "completed there job" in the cell.

- **Fed-batch culture:** Microbial growth where nutrients are added into the fermenter without removing the product.

- **Federal coordinated framework for regulation of biotechnology:** The legal framework created by the US government in 1986, which divided regulation of biotechnology among the US Department of Agriculture, the US Environmental Protection Agency, and the US Food and Drug Administration.

- **Federal Insecticide Fungicide and Rodenticide Act (FIFRA):** A law enacted by the US congress in 1972. During 1994, the US environmental protection agency (EPA) proposed that the substances produced by plants (e.g. genetically engineered crops) for their defense against pests and diseases would be regulated by EPA under FIFRA.

- **Feedback inhibition:** Activity of an enzyme is inhibited by the end product of the biosynthetic pathway in which the enzyme participates.

- **Feedstock:** Raw material(s) used for the production of chemicals; or growth substrates of microbes (e.g. yeasts or bacteria that require a solid phase on which to attach themselves).

- **Female sterile:** In *Drosophila*, a female sterile mutation is one in that causes sterility in the female, often because of abnormalities in oogenesis.

- **Feminization:** The staminodes present in female flowers develop into fleshy carpels around the fruit leading to abnormal fruit development and partial to complete sterility.

- **Feral:** Refers to an individual or population that has returned to the wild after a history of domestication.

- **Fermentation:** The process by which microorganisms turn raw materials such as glucose into products such as alcohol.
- **Fermentation substrates:** Materials used as food for growing microorganism. The fermentation substrates and the trace materials needed together with chemicals added to make the fermentation easier form the culture medium.
- **Fermentor:** A large sized bioreactor/culture vessel used to produce products under controlled conditions.
- **Ferritin:** An iron-protein complex (a metalloprotein) that occurs in living tissues. Functions in iron storage in the spleen.
- **Ferrobacteria:** Also called iron bacteria. Any of a group of bacteria that oxidize iron as a source of energy. The oxidized iron in the form $Fe(OH)_3$ is then deposited in the environment by secretion from the bacterium. The energy obtained from these reactions is used to carry on processes in which the basic substances needed by the bacterium are manufactured. These bacteria are commonly found in seepage waters of coal and iron mining areas where iron compounds abound. Ferrobacteria are not disease producers (i.e. pathogenic), but they are important as scavengers. Sometimes they create a nuisance by multiplying so profusely in iron water pipes that they stop the flow of water. Ferrobacteria have been active through long periods of geologic time. For example, the great Mesabi iron (ore) seam of America's lake superior region is thought to be a product of ferrobacteria activity.
- **Ferrochelatase:** A mitochondrial enzyme that catalyzes the incorporation of iron into the protoporphyria molecule.
- **Ferrodoxin:** An iron-and sulfur-containing protein important in the electrontransfer processes of photosynthesis in plants. It also plays a role in the metabolism of some bacteria and was first found in an anaerobic bacterium.
- **Fertile (Of an organism):** Which are capable of breeding and reproduction.
- **Fertility factor (F):** A type of transmissible (i.e. can enter other cells) plasmid that is often found in *Escherichia coli* (*E. coli*).
- **Fertilization:** Fusion of egg cell with a sperm leading to zygote production, which gives rise to embryo (2n).
- **Fertilizer:** Any substance that is added to soil in order to increase its productivity. Fertilizers can be of natural origin such as composts or they can be inorganic (artificial fertilizer) chemical particularly nitrates and phosphates (Fig. 1).

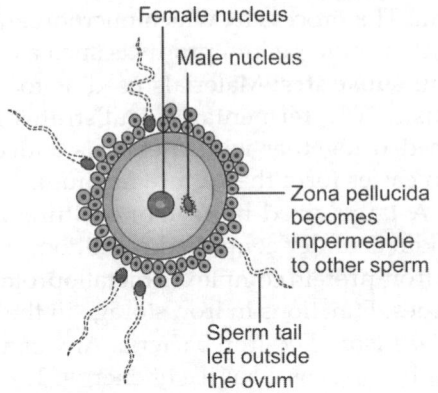

Female nucleus
Male nucleus
Zona pellucida becomes impermeable to other sperm
Sperm tail left outside the ovum

Fig. 1: Fertilization

- **Feulgen's test:** A histochemical test in which the distribution of DNA in the chromosomes of dividing cell nuclei can be observed.
- **FIA:** Refers to immunodiagnostic tests that are based on fluorescence tracers (labels).
- **Fibers:** Elongated cells with tapering pointed ends the cells interlock to form a strong, rigid tissue, pits in the walls are usually very marrow and not very numerous.
- **Fibrin:** The ordered fibrous array of fibrin monomers, called a fibrin-platelet clot (blood clot), which spontaneously assembles from fibrin monomers (which themselves are formed by the thrombin-catalyzed conversion of fibrinogen into fibrin). Fibrinogen itself is the product of a controlled series of zymogen activation steps (enzymatic cascade) triggered initially by substances released from body tissues as a consequence of trauma (harm).
- **Fibrinolytic agents:** Bloodborne compounds that activate fibrin in order to dissolve blood clots.
- **Fibroblast growth factor (FGF):** First described in the mid-1970s by Dr Gospodarowicz and fellow researchers at the University of California, San Francisco. It is a protein that stimulates the formation/development of blood vessels and fibroblasts (precursors to collagen, the connective tissue "glue" that holds cells together). FGF also is mitogenic (causes cells to divide and multiply) for both fibroblasts and endothelial cells, and attracts those two cell types (i.e. is chemotactic). Dr Gospodarowicz

named the FGF originally derived from bovine (cow) brain tissue to be acidic FGF. Dr Gospodarowicz named the FGF originally derived from bovine pituitary tissue to be basic FGF. This was due to their identical biological activity, but differing isoelectric points (the former being acidic, and the latter being basic). Basic FGF is, however, ten times more "potent" than acidic FGF in most bioassays.

- **Fibroblast:** Flattened cells of connective tissue.
- **Fibronectin:** An adhesive glycoprotein that forms a link between the epithelial cells and the connective tissue matrix (essential for blood clotting). Research has indicated that fibronectin may solve the problem of getting new cells to stick to existing tissue, once a growth factor has caused them to grow (e.g. when growth factor is administered after a serious wound to tissue).
- **Fibrous root:** Root system in which both primary and lateral roots have approximately equal diameters. Opposite is tap root.
- **Field collection:** Maintenance of germplasm by growing different accessions in the field; ordinarily, in case of fruit and forest trees, tuber crops, etc.
- **Field inversion gel electrophoresis (FIGE):** A chromatographic procedure for the separation of a mixture of molecules by means of a two-dimensional electrical field, applied across a gel matrix containing those molecules. For example, FIGE is commonly used to separate mixtures of large DNA molecules by their size and (electrical) charge. FIGE can be used to separate (resolve) DNA molecules up to 2,000 Kbp in length.
- **Field strategies for transgene containment:** These strategies are based on spatial isolation of the transgenic crops coupled with planting of continuous borders of a nontransgenic variety to serve as a pollen trap.
- **Figure eight:** Two circles of DNA linked together by a recombination event that has not yet been completed.
- **Filler epithelial cells:** Skin cells that initially form under a scab in the wound healing process, in response to stimulation by epidermal growth factor (EGF).
- **Film reactors:** These reactors contain a support for attachment of the bacterial cells to avoid their washout due to higher waste flow rates; support forms anaerobic filter through which the waste passes and is degraded; used to treat vegetable processing wastes of medium to high strength (1–10% solids), and animal wastes.

- **Filter hybridization:** Performed by incubating denatured DNA preparation immobilized on a nitrocellulose filter with a solution of radioactively labeled RNA or DNA.
- **Filter paper bridge:** A platform formed in a culture tube above the surface of liquid medium by inserting the two arms of a filter paper strip into the medium; explants are placed on the platform.
- **Filter sterilization:** Thermolabile compounds are sterilized by passing their solutions through a membrane of 0.45 µ or lower pore size.
- **Filtration:** Separation of solids from liquids by using a porous material that only allows passage of the liquid or solids smaller than the pore size of the filter. The material passing the filter forms the filtrate.
- **Fingerprint (of DNA):** A pattern of polymorphic restriction fragments that differ between individual genomes.
- **Fingerprint (of protein):** The pattern of fragments (usually resolved on a two-dimensional electrophoretic gel) generated by cleavage with an enzyme such as trypsin.
- **Finite cell lines:** In animal cell culture; cell lines that die after several subculture.
- **Fission:** Asexual reproduction involving the division of a single celled individual into two new single celled individuals of equal size.
- **Fitness:** The ability to survive to reproductive age and produce viable offspring. Fitness also describes the frequency distribution of reproductive success for a population of sexually mature adults.
- **Fixation:** Fixation is the process by which a new allele replaces the allele that was previously predominant in a population.
- **Fixed film digestors:** The biological components or micro-organisms are present in the form of a film on filter particles or large discs.
- **Flagella:** A protein-based, flexible, whip-like organ of loco-motion found on some microorganisms. With these, micro-organisms are able to swim. Flagella are usually very long and there are usually only one or two per cell. The tails of sperm cells are examples of flagella. Flagella are used in the swimming motion of bacteria toward sources of nutrients in a process called chemotaxis (Singular: Flagellum).

- **Flame sterilization:** Instruments like forceps, scalpels, etc. are ordinarily sterilized by dipping them in 95% ethyl alcohol followed by flaming.
- **Flamining:** A technique used to sort cells, nuclei or other biological materials by means of flow through apertures of defined size.
- **Flanking region:** The DNA sequences extending either side of a specific sequence.
- **Flanking sequences:** The sequences lying upstream and downstream of a given DNA sequence, i.e. usually, on either side of the coding region of a gene.
- **Flash point:** It is the temperature at which a substance catches fire.
- **Flavin adenine dinucleotide (FAD):** The coenzyme of some FAD oxidation-reduction enzymes; it contains riboflavin.
- **Flavin:** Also known as lyochrome. One of a group of pale yellow, greenly fluorescing biological pigments widely distributed in small quantities in plant and animal tissues. Flavins are synthesized only by bacteria, yeast, and green plants; for this reason, animals are dependent on plant sources for riboflavin (vitamin B2), the most prevalent member of the group.
- **Flavin mononucleotide (FMN):** Riboflavin phosphate, a coenzyme of certain oxidoreduction enzymes.
- **Flavin nucleotides:** Nucelotide coenzymes (FMN and FAD) containing riboflavin.
- **Flavin-linked dehydrogenases:** Dehydrogenases are enzymes (involved in removing hydrogen atoms from their substrate) which require one of the riboflavin coenzymes, FMN or FAD, in order to function.
- **Flavonoids:** A category of phytochemicals, that are typically beneficial to the health of humans that consume them. Hundreds of flavonoids are naturally produced (by plants) in common human foods. For example, the three isoflavones (genistein, daidzein, and glycitein) produced in seeds of the soybean plant (*Glycine max* (L.) Merrill) are flavonoids, and they confer several health benefits to humans that consume them. Coffee, tea, and chocolate products contain a number of antioxidant flavonoids (i.e. polyphenols). Because oxidation of lipids (lowdensity lipoproteins) in the bloodstream is the initial step in atherosclerosis

disease, consumption of large amounts of coffee may help to prevent atherosclerosis. Research conducted by Joe Vinson in 1999 indicated that high coffee consumption by humans reduced oxidation of lipids in the bloodstream by 30%. Cranberries (*Vaccinium macrocarpon*) contain a number of antioxidant flavonoids, and research indicates that consumption of large amounts on a regular basis may inhibit development of breast cancer. Blueberries (genus *vaccinium*) contain a number of flavonoids, and research indicates that consumption of large amounts on a regular basis helps to strengthen eyesight, improve memory, and inhibit some physical aspects of the aging process. Other subcategories of flavonoids are flavones, flavonols, flavonols, aurones, chalcones, etc. One example of a not-very-beneficial flavonoid is quercetin, a non-nutritive antioxidant produced in almonds.

- **Flavonols:** A group of phytochemicals, consisting of a subcategory of the flavonoid "family" of phytochemicals. Flavonols are typically beneficial to the health of humans that consume them, and are found in citrus fruits such as grapefruit, oranges, etc. However, at least one flavonol (quercitin glycoside) is found in tomato peels.
- **Flavoprotein:** An enzyme containing a flavin nucleotide as a prosthetic group.
- **Floatation:** Raising of microbial cells to the surface of medium by fine gas bubbles adsorbed to their surface.
- **Flocculant:** Agent that causes small particles to aggregate (flocculate).
- **Flocculation:** Sticking together of bacterial and other cells induced by inorganic salts, mineral hydrocolloids, etc.
- **Floccule:** Microorganism aggregate or colloidal particle floating in or on a liquid. Contaminated liquid media are usually cloudy illustrating this flocculation phenomenon.
- **Flora:** The microorganisms found in a given situation, e.g. reservoir flora (the microorganisms present in a given municipal water reservoir) or intestinal flora (the microorganisms found in the intestines).
- **Floury-2:** A gene in corn/maize (*Zea mays* L.) that (when present in the DNA of a given plant) causes that plant to produce seed that contains higher-than-traditional levels of the amino acids methionine and tryptophan.

- **Flow cytometry:** A technique used to sort cells or other biological materials by means of flow through apertures of defined size or by laser sorting.
- **Flower:** The structure in angiosperms (flowering plants) that bears the organs for sexual reproduction.
- **Fluidity:** A property of membranes; it indicates the ability of lipids to move literally within their particular monolayer.
- **Fluorescence activated cell sorter (FACS):** A machine used to sort cells from a mixed group of cells (e.g. to remove only the cells into which a new gene has been inserted via genetic engineering techniques). The desired cells are first labeled with a specific fluorescent dye, then passed through a flow chamber that is illuminated by a laser beam, which causes the labeled cells to fluoresce (glow). The molecules of the fluorescent dye, which "stick" to only one type of cell in the mixture, contain chromophores that can be elevated to an excited, unstable state via irradiation with specific wavelength(s) of light. Those chromophores remain in that excited state for a maximum of 10–9 seconds before releasing their energy by emitting light, and returning to their unexcited "ground" state. This fluorescence (glow) is a measurable property and the FACS machine utilizes it to separate the desired cells from the rest of the mixture.
- **Fluorescence:** The reaction of certain molecules upon absorption of specific amount/wavelength of light; in which those molecules emit (reradiate) light energy possessing a longer wavelength than the original light absorbed. All cells will naturally fluoresce, at least a bit. Human colon cancer cells, and precursor cells, fluoresce much more (and emit much more red light when they fluoresce) than noncancerous cells; which may lead to a new and better means of early detection.
- **Fluorescent probe:** Probe whose response is based on the fluorescence intensity of individual cells or cell components.
- **Fluorescent *in situ* hybridization (FISH):** *In situ* hybridization using a probe coupled to a fluorescent molecule.
- **Focus formation:** The ability of transformed eukaryotic cells to grow in dense cluster, piled up on one another.
- **Focus formatting unit (FFU):** A quantitative measure of focus formation.
- **Focus:** Transformed cells grow as a compact mass of rounded-up cells that grows in dense clusters, piled up on one another.

F

They appear as a distinct **focus** on a culture plate, contrasted with normal cells that grow as a spread-out monolayer attached to the substratum.

- **Fetus:** Prenatal stage of a viviparous animal between the embryonic stage and prinutrition.
- **Fog:** Fine particles of liquid suspended in the air such as of water in a fog chamber used for acclimatizing recent *ex vitro* transplants.
- **Foldback DNA:** DNA consists of inverted repeats that have renatured by intrastrand reassociation of denatured DNA.
- **Follicle:** Any enclosing cluster of cells that protects and nourishes a cell or structure within. Thus, a follicle in the ovary contains a developing egg cell while a hair follicle envelops the root of hair.
- **Follicle stimulating hormone (FSH):** A protein hormone used in conventional medical therapy in an attempt to increase production of sperm in men (inside the follicles of the testes).
- **Food and Drug Administration (FDA):** The federal agency charged with approving all pharmaceutical and food ingredient products sold within the US. In 1992, prior to approval of any of the biotechnology derived food crop plants, the FDA decided that food crops produced via "biotechnological (i.e. recombinant) technologies" must meet the same rigorous safety standards as those created via "traditional breeding methods," both categories of which are regulated by the FDA. Historically, new food crops created via "traditional breeding technologies" (e.g. crossing with wild type in order to confer disease resistance, increased yield, etc. on the resultant domesticated plant varieties/strains) have sometimes contained unexpectedly high levels of known (and naturally occurring) toxins (e.g. solanine, a naturally occurring toxin in potatoes and some other plants, psoralene, a naturally occurring toxin in celery, etc.).
- **Food good manufacturing practice (FGMP):** The Food and Drug Administration's (FDA's) approval mechanism for a process to manufacture a given food or food additive. It is implemented instead of specific regulations (such as those used to dictate processes in simple food manufacture, as in beef packing), due to the newness of the technology, and may later be superceded due to further advances in the technology.
- **Food processing enzyme:** Enzyme used to control food texture, flavor, appearance and to a certain extent, nutritional value.

Amylases break down complex polysaccharide to simplex sugars proteases tenderize meat proteins.

- **Foot candle:** An obsolete photometric measure of light intensity. Now superseded by the lux (symbol- lx; 1 fc = 10.7 lx).
- **Footprinting:** It is a technique to identify the site on DNA which is protected from the attack by nucleases by some protein.
- **Foreground selection:** In a backcross programme; selection for the gene/allele being transferred.
- **Foreign DNA:** A DNA molecule which is incorporated into a cloning vector or chromosome.
- **Forced cloning:** The insertion of foreign DNA into a cloning vector in a predetermined orientation.
- **Formaldehyde dehydrogenase:** An enzyme which catalyzes the oxidation of formaldehyde to formic acid (formate at intracellular pH). It requires nicotinamide-adenine dinucleotide (NAD) as an electron acceptor. It is important in the metabolism of methanol.
- **Formulation:** For traditional therapeutic agents this refers to the method by which a therapeutic agent is delivered to its site of action.
- **Fortification:** Addition of vitamins or minerals to a food at levels higher than those it originally present in the food.
- **Fortify:** To add strengthening components or beneficial ingredients to a nutrient medium.
- **Forward mutation:** Inactivate a wild-type gene.
- **FOSHU:** A Japanese government designation meaning "Foods of Specified Health Use." Introduced in the early 1980s, these are foods or food ingredients that meet the following specific criteria: 1. Must improve human nutrition and health. A benefit to human health and nutrition must be proven for that food/ingredient; 2. An appropriate daily dose (amount to be consumed) must be confirmed by doctors or dieticians; 3. The food/ingredient must guarantee balanced nourishment; 4. The active component (e.g. phytochemical) must be scientifically confirmed regarding its quantitative and qualitative definition, and its chemical and/or physical features; 5. The active component must not lower nutritional value (e.g. of the food it is added to); 6. The food/ingredient must be consumed in a normal fashion (i.e. eaten or drank, not as pill or powder form); 7. The active component must be of natural origin. Some of the

foods/ingredients designated "FOSHU" have been those containing polyphenols, anthocyanins, and diacylgycerols.

- **Fosmid:** A useful derivative of BAC vector that contains ë phage cos sites to facilitate its packaging in heads of phage ë.
- **Fossil fuel:** Fuel derived from coal or petroleum.
- **Fouling:** The coating or plugging (by materials or microorganisms) of equipment thus preventing it from functioning property.
- **Foundation on economic trends:** A small organization that lobbies against agricultural biotechnology.
- **Founder effect:** The presence in a population of many individuals all with the same chromosome (or region of a chromosome) derived from a single ancestor.
- **Frameshift mutation:** The insertion or deletion of a nucleotide pair or pairs, causing a disruption of the translational reading frame.
- **Frameshift:** Mutations arise by deletions or insertions that are not a multiple of 3 bp; they change the frame in which triplets are translated into protein.
- **Free energy:** The component of the total energy of a system that can do work at a constant temperature and pressure. Also known as Gibbs free energy. Free energy is a key variable calculated and monitored for different (proposed) drug molecules or drug/target interactions during rational drug design activities (e.g. molecular modeling).
- **Free fatty acids (FFA):** Individual fatty acid molecules within a vegetable oil, which exist in an uncombined-with-glycerine molecular state. The presence of FFA can be caused by naturally occurring noncombination (e.g. in some varieties of oilseeds), sprouting of the oilseeds prior to processing into vegetable oil, or breakdown of the fat (oil) during processing or usage.
- **Free probe:** Probe molecules that are not paired with the test nucleic acid sequence.
- **Free radical:** Sometimes called reactive oxygen species, singlet oxygen, or oxygen free radical. Term utilized to refer to an oxygen (atom) bearing an "extra" electron. Because of that, it possesses a large amount of energy, and in a biological system (i.e. inside the body of an organism), it can damage body tissues when it "discharges" that energy.
- **Freezing:** In case of cryopreservation; lowering of the temperature of cells from 0°C–196°C.

- **Frequency distribution:** A graph showing either the relative or absolute invidence of classes in a population.
- **Fresh weight:** Weight of cells/tissues, cultures in their native state after removal of medium (by washing) and extracellular water (by partial vacuum).
- **Friable:** Crubling or fragmenting callus. A friable callus easily dissected and readily digested into single cell or clump of cells in solution.
- **Frictional coefficient:** A measure of the resistance a particle offers to movement through a solvent.
- **Fructan:** A general term utilized to refer to any carbohydrate in which fructosyl-fructose (molecule) linkages constitute the majority of the molecule's glycosidic bonds (i.e. between atoms in the molecule).
- **Fructose oligosaccharides:** A "family" of oligosaccharides, some of which help foster the growth of bifidobacteria in the lower colon of monogastric animals (humans, swine, etc.). Those bifidobacteria generate certain short-chain fatty acids, which are absorbed by the colon and result in a reduction of triglyceride (fat) and cholesterol levels in the bloodstream, thereby lowering risk of coronary heart disease and thrombosis. Research indicates they also promote absorption of calcium from foods (in the large intestine). Fructose oligosaccharides are classifed as a "water soluble fiber" (by the European Union's Government Food Regulatory Agencies), because humans cannot digest them.
- **Fuel biotechnology:** Use of biological agents or their components to generate various energy rich compounds from different substrate/resources, which can be used as fuel.
- **Fully methylated:** Site is a palindromic sequence that is methylated on both strands of DNA.
- **Fumarase (fum):** An enzyme that catalyzes the hydration (addition of hydrogen atoms) of fumaric acid to maleic acid, as well as the reverse dehydration reaction (removal of hydrogen atoms).
- **Fumaric acid $(C_4H_4O_4)$:** A dicarboxylic organic acid produced commercially by chemical synthesis and fermentation; the trans-isomer of maleic acid; colorless crystals, melting point 87°C (191°F); used to make resins, paints, varnishes and inks, in food as a mordant (dye fixer/stabilizer), and as a chemical intermediate. Also known as boletic acid.

- **Fumonisins:** Mycotoxins that are primarily produced by the fungus *Fusarium moniliforme* (e.g. in insect-damaged corn/maize). Consumption of fumonisins by horses and swine can be fatal to those animals. Consumption of fumonisins by other animals (including humans) can result in tumors (e.g. cancer of the esophagus, in humans).
- **Functional foods:** Refers to foods that provide health benefits beyond basic nutrition.
- **Functional genomics:** The study of the pattern of expression of the genes present in the genome of organisms that leads to the growth and development of the organisms.
- **Functional group:** A molecule, or portion of a molecule, that will react with other molecule(s). For example, "hedgehog proteins" must first add a cholesterol molecule (to themselves) before they can carry out their task of directing/controlling tissue differentiation during mammal embryo development (into various organs, limbs, etc.). An "acetyl (functional) group" must be added to a choline molecule for the body in order to have the critical neurotransmitter acetylcholine.
- **Functional proteomics:** Use of proteomics techniques to analyze the characteristics of molecular protein networks involved in a living cell.
- **Functionally redundant:** Genes fulfill the same function in the same time and place, so that mutation of every member of the set is necessary to show a deficient phenotype.
- **Fungi:** They are numerous species of molds, mushrooms, brackens and other forms of nonphotosynthetic plants; derive energy and nutrients by consuming organic material.
- **Fungicide:** Any chemical compound toxic to fungi.
- **Fungus (plural: fungi):** Any of a major group of saprophytic and parasitic plants that lack chlorophyll and flowers, including molds, toadstools, rusts, mildews, smuts, ergot, mushrooms *Aqaricus bisporus*, and yeasts. Under certain conditions (temperature, humidity, etc.), some fungi can produce mycotoxins via their metabolism.
- **Furanose:** A sugar molecule containing the five-membered furan ring.
- *Fusarium*: A genus of fungus, also known as "scab," that infests certain grains (e.g. wheat *Triticum aestivum*, corn or maize *Zea mays* L., etc.) during growing seasons in which climate (e.g. high

humidity, cool weather) and other conditions combine to enable rapid growth/proliferation of the fungus. In wheat, fungus infestation (*Fusarium* head blight) causes the wheat plant to weaken and to produce empty seed heads, which reduces yield. As a by-product of their metabolism, some of the *Fusarium* types (species) produce deoxynivalenol (also known as DON or "vomitoxin"), zearalenone, and fumonisins (a group of very potent mycotoxins that are produced by *Fusarium moniliforme* and *Fusarium proliferatum* fungi). Fumonisin B1 is the most prevalent *Fusarium*-produced mycotoxin in corn (maize).

- *Fusarium moniliforme*: One of the Fusarium fungi; therefore, it can produce one or more fumonisins (a group of mycotoxins) under certain environmental conditions, when it grows in some grains. When *Fusarium moniliforme* grows within growing plants of domesticated rice (*Oryza sativa*), it can cause the plant disease known as Bakanae (also known as "foolish seedling" disease). Symptoms of Bakanae include rice plants that are much taller than normal rice plants, and leaves that are much longer than normal. That abnormal growth (of rice plant/leaves) is caused by a gibberellin compound excreted by the *Fusarium moniliforme* fungus. The fungus also excretes fusaric acids, which can stunt or kill rice plants.

- **Fusion gene:** A hybrid gene created by joining portions of two different genes (to produce a new protein) or by joining a gene to a different promoter (to alter or regulate gene transcription).

- **Fusion protein:** A single protein molecule encoded by parts of two or more genes combined together as one unit.

- **Fusion toxin:** A fusion protein that consists of a toxic protein (domain) plus a cell receptor binding region (protein domain). The cell receptor portion (of the total fusion toxin molecule) delivers the toxin directly to the (diseased) cell, thus sparing other healthy tissues from the effect of the toxin.

- **Fusion:** The process of joining the membranes of two cells to create another cell that contains the nuclear material from both parent cells.

- **Fusogen:** A fusion including agent used for agglutination of protoplast in somatic hybridization.

- **Fusogenic agent:** Any compound, virus, etc. that causes cells to fuse together. For example, one of the effects of the HIV (i.e. AIDS causing) viruses is to cause the T cells of the human immune system to fuse (causing collapse of the immune system).

- **Futile cycle:** An enzyme-catalyzed set of cyclic reactions that results in release of thermal energy (heat) through the hydrolysis of adenosine triphosphate (ATP). The hydrolysis of ATP is normally coupled to other cycles and reactions in which the energy released is metabolically used. However, futile cycles would appear to waste the energy of ATP as heat, except when one is shivering to keep warm. The production of heat by shivering is an example of the futile cycle.

F

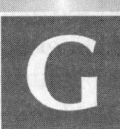

G

- **G banding:** A technique that generates a striated pattern in metaphase chromosomes that distinguishes the members of a haploid set.
- **G cap:** The 5′-terminal methylated guanine nucleoside that is present on many eukaryotic mRNAs. It is joined after transcription to the mRNA.
- **G proteins:** Guanine nucleotide-binding trimeric proteins that reside in the plasma membrane. When bound by GDP the trimer remains intact and is inert. When the GDP bound to α-subunit is replaced by GTP, α-subunit is released from the β-γ-dimer. One of the separated units (either α-monomer or the β-γ-dimer) then activates or represses a target protein.
- **G_1:** The period of the eukaryotic cell cycle between the last mitosis and the start of DNA replication.
- **G_2:** The period of the eukaryotic cell cycle between the end of DNA replication and the start of the next mitosis.
- **GA_{21}:** A naturally occurring gene (i.e. expressed at low levels in some plants) which confers resistance to glyphosate-containing herbicides. When the GA_{21} gene is inserted by man into crop plants (e.g. maize/corn) in a way that causes high expression, those crop plants are subsequently unaffected when glyphosate-containing herbicides are applied to fields to control weeds in those crops.
- **Gain-of-function:** Mutation represents acquisition of a new activity. It is dominant.
- **Galactose (gal):** A monosaccharide occurring in both levo (L) and dextro (D) forms as a constituent of plant and animal oligosaccharides (lactose and raffinose) and polysaccharides (agar and pectin). Galactose is also known as cerebrose.
- **GalNAc:** *N*-acetyl-D-galactosamine.
- **Gall:** A tumorous growth in plants.
- **Gamete:** A germ or reproductive cell. In animals (and humans) the functional, mature, male gamete is called a spermatozoan;

in plants it is called a spermatozoid. In both animals and plants the female gamete is called the ovum, or egg.

- **Gametoclonal variation:** Phenotypic variation apart from normal segregation occurring during gamete formation arising from the culture of gametophytic cells or tissues such as in anther culture or unfertilized ovule culture.
- **Gametogenesis:** The process of the formation of gametes.
- **Gametophyte:** That phase of the plant life cycle that bears the gamete producing organs in which the cells have n chromosomes. In angiosperms the pollen grain is the male gametophyte and the embryo sac is the female gametophyte.
- **Gamma globulin:** A type of blood protein that plays a major role in the process of immunity (immune system response). Sometimes the term "γ-globulin" refers to a whole group of blood proteins that are known as antibodies or immunoglobulins (Ig). Most often, however, it applies to a particular immunoglobulin, designated as IgG, believed to be the most abundant type of antibody in the body.
- **Gamma interferon:** Produced by T lymphocytes.
- **GAP:** A double-stranded DNA is said to be "gapped" when one strand is missing over a short region of the molecule.
- **Gapped DNA:** A duplex DNA molecule with one or more internal single stranded regions.
- **Gap genes:** In *Drosophila* the gap genes are a set of genes that helps setup in the segmentation of the embryo. Gap genes encode transcription factors that are expressed in broad regions of the embryo. Gap genes activate transcription of the pair-rule genes. A channel which only allows passage of its substrate under certain conditions is referred to as "gated". Gated channels can exist in at least two conformations, one of which is open and the other closed.
- **Gas transfer:** The rate at which gases are transferred from gas into solution. It is an important parameter in fermentation systems because it controls the rate at which the organism can metabolize.
- **Gastrula:** An early animal embryo consisting of two layers of cells. An embryological stage following the blastula.
- **Gated transport (of a protein):** One of three means for a protein molecule to pass between compartments within eukaryotic cells. The compartment "wall" (membrane) possesses a "sensor"

G

(receptor) that detects the presence of a correct protein (e.g. after that protein has been synthesized in the cell's ribosomes), then opens a "gate" (pore) in the membrane to allow that protein to pass from the first compartment to the second compartment.

- **G-bands:** Bands generated on eukaryotic chromosomes by staining techniques and appear as a series of lateral striations. They are used for karyotyping (identifying chromosomal regions by the banding pattern). GO is a noncycling state in which a cell has ceased to divide.

- **GC box:** It is a common pol II promoter element consisting of the sequence GGGCGG.

- **GEAC:** The country of India's Genetic Engineering Approval Committee. The GEAC must approve a rDNA product (e.g. a genetically engineered crop plant that earlier received its "bio safety clearance" from the Indian Department of Biotechnology) before that rDNA product is allowed to be commercially planted.

- **Gel electrophoresis:** Electrophoresis, in which a variety of chemically inert gel matrices having adjustable and regular pore size and used as matrix.

- **Gel filtration:** Also known as exclusion chromatography. An effective technique for separating molecules (such as peptide mixtures) on the basis of size. This is accomplished by passing a solution of the molecules to be separated over a column of Sephadex®, for example, which is a polymerized carbohydrate derivative that contains tiny holes. The holes are of such a size that some of the smaller molecules diffuse into them and are in this way retained (held back) while the larger molecules are not able to get into the holes and pass on by the solid phase (Sephadex®, in this example). This, simplistically, is how separation is effected.

- **Gel matrix:** Agarose or polyacrylamide or starch chemicals can be included in the gel to help separation such as the detergent sodium dodecyl sulphate (SDS) in protein gels to unfold proteins or urea in DNA sequencing gels which unfolds DNA.

- **Gel retardation analysis:** A technique used to identify those DNA fragments to which a specific protein, such as DNA polymerase, binds.

- **Gel:** A network of interacting fibers, or a polymer that is solid but traps large amounts of solvent in pore channel inside.

- **Gelatinization:** Starch becomes dissolved to form a viscous suspension.
- **GEM (Germ plasm enhancement for maize):** A project conducted under the auspices of the US Department of Agriculture, in concern with 16 American Universities and 20 corn (maize) seed companies. GEM's intent is to cross exotic (not in current use) germ plasm with commercial maize lines in order to increase corn yield.
- **Gene action:** Mode of expression of gene in a genetic population.
- **Gene addition:** The addition of a functional copy of a gene to the genome of an organism.
- **Gene amplification:** The copying of segments (e.g. genes) within the DNA or RNA molecule. This can be done by man (e.g. polymerase chain reaction), can be caused by certain chemical carcinogens (e.g. phorbol ester), or occur naturally (e.g. in prokaryotes and certain lower eucaryotes). The five primary techniques used by man to perform gene amplification are: 1. Polymerase chain reaction (PCR); 2. Ligase chain reaction (LCR); 3. Self-sustained sequence replication (SSR); 4. Q-beta Replicase Technique; 5. Strand displacement amplification (SDA).
- **Gene bank:** A collection of cells or artificial chromosomes containing known genetic information.
- **Gene cloning (Molecular cloning):** Insertion of a gene into a vector from a new DNA molecule that can be perpetuated into host cell.
- **Gene cluster:** A group of adjacent genes that are identical and related.
- **Gene conversion:** The process of nonreciprocal recombinant by which one allele in a heterozygote is converted into the corresponding allele.
- **Gene delivery (gene therapy):** The insertion of genes (e.g. via retroviral vectors) into selected cells in the body in order to: 1. Cause those cells to produce specific therapeutic agents (growth hormone in livestock, factor VIII in hemophiliacs, insulin in diabetics, etc.). A potential way of curing some genetic diseases, in that the inserted gene will produce the protein and/or enzyme that is missing in the body due to a defective gene (thus causing the genetic disease). Approximately, 3,000 genetic diseases are known to man. Examples of genetic diseases

G

include—cystic fibrosis, sickle cell anemia, Huntington's disease, phenylketonuria (PKU), Tay-Sach's disease, ADA deficiency (adenosine deaminase enzyme deficiency), and thalassemia; 2. Cause those cells to become (more) susceptible to a conventional therapeutic agent that previously was ineffective against that particular condition/disease (e.g. insertion of Hstk gene into brain tumor cells to make those tumor cells susceptible to the Syntex drug Ganciclovir); 3. Cause those cells to become less susceptible to a conventional therapeutic agent (e.g. insert genes into healthy tissue in order to enable that healthy tissue to resist the harmful effects of such conventional chemotherapy agents as vincristine); 4. Counter the effects of abnormal (damaged) tumor suppressor genes via insertion of normal tumor suppressor genes; 5. Cause expression of ribozymes that cleave oncogenes (cancer-causing genes); 6. Be used for other therapeutic uses of genes in cells.

- **Gene desert:** In human genome; gene-poor regions separating gene-rich regions.
- **Gene disruption:** Integration of a DNA sequence within another gene so that the latter is inactivated; used to produce "knockout" mice.
- **Gene dosage:** Gives the number of copies of a particular gene in the genome.
- **Gene expression analysis:** Generally done via use of "biochips" (which have numerous detection/analysis devices fabricated onto their silicon surface) or "microarrays," gene expression analysis involves evaluation of the expression (and expression levels) of numerous genes in a biological sample, to analyze/compare any differences between gene expression/products in: 1. Normal cells vs diseased cells; 2. Normal cells vs those responding to a stimulus; 3. Cells from the same organism, at different stages of development (e.g. embryo versus adult); 4. Normal (historic wild type) cells vs genetically engineered cells (those that have been engineered to cure a disease, resist a herbicide, etc.); 5. Normal cells vs. those same cells treated with a given pharmaceutical (candidate). Analysis generally involves measurement of gene expression markers (i.e. molecules synthesized, or cellular consequences such as apoptosis) to determine which genes are expressed (and when/how much, etc.).

- **Gene expression cascade:** A sequential series of individual gene expressions (i.e. each gene causing a separate/different protein to be "manufactured"), that is initiated ("set off") by the first gene expression. For example, a gene expression cascade is often initiated by the first gene causing expression of a transcription factor (i.e. protein that itself interacts with cell's DNA to either cause or speed up yet another gene expression). The protein resulting from that second gene expression could be yet another transcription factor that triggers another (i.e. third) gene expression, and so on.

G

- **Gene expression markers:** Refers to molecules (e.g. synthesized due to a specific gene's expression) or consequences (e.g. cell apoptosis due to a specific gene's expression) that can be measured as proof of gene's expression in gene expression analysis.
- **Gene expression profiling:** Determination of specifically which genes are "switched on" (e.g. in a cell), thereby enabling precise definition of the phenotypic condition of that cell (i.e. the phenotype of that cell at that moment). Typical uses (i.e. comparison of such tissue phenotypes) include: 1. Comparing diseased cell with normal cell; 2. Defining quantitatively the "normal" state; 3. Comparing a given drug's impact (i.e. treated cell with normal cell); 4. Comparing old cell with young cell. In subsequent gene expression analysis, the quantitative amounts of each protein being expressed can be determined via use of such technologies as two-dimensional (2D) gel electrophoresis, Southern blot analysis, fluorescence tagging, radiolabeling, RT-PCR, QPCR, plane polarimetry, etc.
- **Gene expression:** When a gene performs the specific function, which it is capable of, it is called gene expression; it begins with transcription of the gene and ends with the development of the specific phenotype; ordinarily, it refers to transcription of the concerned gene.
- **Gene family:** A set of genes whose exons are related; the members were derived by duplication and variation from some ancestral gene.
- **Gene farming:** Production of proteins encoded by transgene in animals/plants; the protein is recovered from milk, urine, blood (in animals), seeds, etc. (in plants).
- **Gene flow:** Introgression of genes from improved varieties of crop plants into their wild relatives.

- **Gene frequency:** The proportion in which alternative alleles of a gene occur in a population.
- **Gene function analysis:** The determination of which protein is expressed (i.e. caused to be "manufactured") by each gene in an organism's genome/DNA. Typically, gene function analysis follows after discovery of gene sequences found via structural genomics study. Some methods utilized to determine which proteins result from which gene(s) are: 1. Site-directed mutagenesis (SDM) to compare two same species organisms possessing two different genes at the same site (SNP) on the genome (i.e. on organism's DNA); 2. Antisense DNA sequences to compare two same-species organisms, one of which has a gene at the same site "turned off" (silenced) via antisense DNA; 3. Reporter gene, to compare two samespecies organisms (possessing two different genes at the same site on genome/DNA) via a reporter gene adjacent to the gene/site, to detect presence or absence of the desired trait/function; 4. Comparison of same organism (e.g. crop plant) when one of the two is "challenged" by a specific plant disease; 5. Chemical genetics, to compare two same-species organisms (one of which has gene at the specific site at least partially inactivated by a specific chemical); 6. "Silencing" or "knocking out" a particular gene via other methods than antisense or chemical genetics, to compare; 7. Use of already-known "model organisms" (e.g. *Drosophila* for comparing insect genes, *Arabidopsis thaliana* for plant genes, *Caenorhabditis elegans* for animal genes).
- **Gene fusion:** Refers to the technology/methods utilized to fuse together two or more genes. When such a "fused gene" is then inserted into a genome (e.g. the DNA of a plant), it causes production (in plant's ribosomes) of protein(s) consisting of all or part of the amino acid sequences (known as the "domain") of the two proteins typically coded for by those two genes. This fusion is often done in order to put expression of the second (fused) gene under the control of the (strong) promoter of the first gene. During 2001, Rajbir Sangwan and colleagues inserted a fused gene into a potato plant (*Solanum tuberosum*), a major source of plant starch. That fused gene coded for production of the two proteins α-amylase and glucose isomerase; both are enzymes. α-amylase catalyzes the conversion of potato starch into glucose (a sugar), and glucose

isomerase catalyzes conversion of glucose to fructose (a more valuable sugar).

- **Gene gun (biolistic):** A device to accelerate particles for physically delivering the recombinant DNA, typically precipitated onto microprojectile, into a cell using an explosive propellant (Fig. 1).

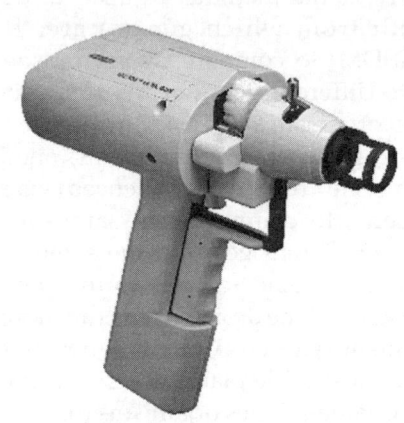

Fig. 1: Gene gun

- **Gene imprinting:** The differential expression of a single according to its parental origin.
- **Gene insertion:** The incorporation of one or more copies of a gene into a chromosome.
- **Gene interaction:** Modification of gene action by a nonallelic gene.
- **Gene library:** Random collection of cloned fragments in a vector that ideally includes all the genetic information of that species, e.g. wheat, rice, etc.
- **Gene linkage:** The hereditary association of genes located on the same chromosome.
- **Gene machine:** An instrument which, when fed information on the amino acid sequence of a protein (usually via a protein sequencer), will automatically produce polynucleotide gene segments to code for that protein.
- **Gene mapping:** The process of determining where genes are located on individual chromosomes, their position in relation to other genes and the distance between them.

- **Gene modification:** Chemical change to a gene's DNA sequence.
- **Gene pool:** All of the geetic information, including all variations, contained within a population of a particular species at a particular time.
- **Gene probe:** A single-stranded DNA or RNA fragment used in genetic engineering to search for a particular gene or other DNA sequence.
- **Gene product:** The biochemical material, either RNA or protein, resulting from expression of a gene. The amount of gene product is used to measure how active a gene is and abnormal amounts can be correlated with disease causing alleles.
- **Gene pyramiding:** Bringing two or more different genes conferring resistance to the same pathogen in the same line/variety.
- **Gene recombination:** The appearance of gene combinations in the progeny that differ from the combinations present in the parents.
- **Gene regulation:** The study of on-off mechanism of protein synthesis regulated by the gene in an organism.
- **Gene repair (done by man):** The "repair" of a damaged gene (e.g. mutation) or replacement of a given gene, via a process invented by Eric Kmiec in 1993. The desired DNA (gene) is added to a cell, along with RNA, in a paired-group known as a chimeraplast. The chimeraplast attaches itself to the cell; DNA at the site of the specific gene (i.e. the one that is to be changed), and "repairs" it using its (new) chimeraplast-DNA as a "template."
- **Gene repair (natural):** Refers to the natural processes via which all cells in an organism are continually repairing their DNA (which can be damaged by ultraviolet light, various chemicals, etc.). In these natural cell (gene repair) processes, first, an enzyme complex detects the damaged DNA (e.g. on one of the two strands of the DNA molecule). Next, an enzyme cuts out the damaged portion of the DNA (on that one strand, leaving the other—good—strand intact). Then a DNA polymerase enzyme enters the gap and synthesizes (manufactures) the new DNA (to replace the portion that was cut out), using the intact—good—DNA strand as a template. Finally, the new DNA is joined to the old DNA via the help of DNA ligase enzyme.
- **Gene replacement:** The incorporation of a transgene into a chromosome at its normal location by homologous recombination thus replacing the copy of the gene originally present at the locus.

- **Gene sequencing:** The technique of determining the order of bases of DNA molecule, which constitute a gene.
- **Gene silencing:** Suppression of transgene expression in later generations of transgenic plants; usually, due to transgene (including promoter) methylation; more common when the transgene is integrated in higher copy number.
- **Gene splicing:** The enzymatic attachment (joining) of one gene (or part of a gene) to another; also removal of introns and splicing of exons during mRNA synthesis.
- **Gene stacking:** Many transgenes are transferred into a single variety through a single transformation event.
- **Gene tagging:** Use of *Agrobacterium* T-DNA, transposons, etc. for identification and/or isolation of a gene by first integrating it into the concerned gene and isolating mutants so produced.
- **Gene technology office:** An agency of the Australian government, established in 1997, to oversee and regulate all genetic engineering activities conducted in the country of Australia. Replaced/superceded by Australia's newly formed Interim Office of the Gene Technology Regulator (IOGTR) in 1999.
- **Gene technology regulator:** The regulatory body of the Australia's government that is responsible for approvals of new rDNA products (e.g. new genetically engineered crops) before they can be introduced into Australia. Gene technology regulator (GTR) replaced Australia's Interim Office of the Gene Technology Regulator (IOGTR) in this role on June 21, 2001.
- **Gene testing:** Methods that identify the presence, absence or mutation of a particular gene in an individual.
- **Gene therapy:** The correction of a gene deficiency in a cell by the addition of new DNA and its insertion into the genome.
- **Gene tracking:** Following the inheritance of a particular gene from generation to generation.
- **Gene transfer:** The use of genetic or physical manipulations to introduce foreign genes into host cell to achieve desired characteristics in progeny.
- **Gene translocation:** The movement of a gene fragment from one chromosomal location to another, which often alters or abolishes expression.
- **Gene:** A particulate hereditary determiner, a unit of inheritance, a unit of DNA, located at a fixed point along a chromosome. Conceptually, a gene is an informational storage unit capable of

undergoing replication, expression, and mutation. Biochemically, a gene is a length of DNA that specifics a product or action. A region on DNA encoding a particular polypeptide chain or functional RNA such as rRNA or a tRNA.

- **Generalized transduction:** The transduction of any gene in the bacterial genome by a phage.
- **Generate:** To propagate or (mass) proliferate. The process is generation or regeneration.
- **Generation time:** The time required for a population of cells to double. The average time required for a round of cell division.
- **Generative nucleous:** One of the two male gametes in the pollen tube of angiosperms.
- **Genetic assimilation:** Eventual extinction of a natural species as massive pollen flow occurs from another related species and the natural species becomes more like the related species.
- **Genetic code:** The correspondence between triplets in DNA (or RNA) and amino acids in protein.
- **Genetic complementation:** When two DNA molecules that are in the same cell together, produce a function that neither DNA molecule can supply on its own aka complementation.
- **Genetic counseling:** Analysis of risk for genetic defects in a family and the presentation of options available to avoid or ameliorate possible risks.
- **Genetic disease:** A disease caused by a mutant gene; generally, due to the recessive allele.
- **Genetic distance:** A measure of the genetic similarity between any pair of populations. Such distance may be based on phenotypic traits, allele frequencies or DNA sequences. For example, genetic distance between two populations having the same allele frequencies at a particular locus and based solely on the locus is zero.
- **Genetic diversity:** The variability present within a species, between individuals of a population or different population groups of the same species for one or a group of traits.
- **Genetic drift:** Tandom variation in gene frequency from one generation to another.
- **Genetic engineering:** *In vitro* DNA technologies used to isolate genes from an organism, manipulate them in laboratory as per desire, and insert them into another cell system for specific genetic trait. It is also called gene cloning.

- **Genetic equilibrium:** Condition in a group of interbreeding organisms in which the allele frequencies remain constant over time.
- **Genetic fingerprinting:** A technique of analyzing DNA of an individual to reveal the pattern of repetition of particular nucleotide sequences through the genome. The unique pattern of DNA is identified by a PCR or Southern hybridization technique.
- **Genetic heterogeneity:** The situation in which different mutant genes produce the same phenotype.
- **Genetic immunization:** Use of DNA for immunization.
- **Genetic information:** Information contained in a nucleotide base sequence in chromosomal DNA or RNA.
- **Genetic instability:** Origin of genetic variation in a relatively high frequency, usually, much higher than that ascribable to spontaneous mutations.
- **Genetic Manipulation Advisory Committee (GMAC):** A body that advises the Australian government on matters pertaining to genetic engineering (e.g. new rDNA product approvals). The GMAC is analogous to Germany's ZKBS (Central Commission on Biological Safety), Brazil's CTNBio (National Technical Biosafety Commission), and the Kenya Biosafety Council.
- **Genetic map (linkage map):** The linear array of gene on a chromosome based on recombination frequencies.
- **Genetic markers:** Alleles used as experimental probes to keep track of an individual a tissue, a cell, a nucleus, a chromosome, or a gene.
- **Genetic material:** The chemical that contains the genetic information, i.e. of which genes are composed; in most of the organisms, DNA is the genetic material; in only some viruses, RNA serves this purpose.
- **Genetic modification (GM):** Any process that alters the genetic material of living organism. This includes duplicating, deleting or inserting one or more new genes or altering the activities of an existing gene. It can be performed on microbes, plants or animals (humans included). Where this is done in humans, it is gene therapy, and only human genes are used.
- **Genetic resource:** Sum total of all the genes and their alleles present in a species and its wild relatives.
- **Genetic screening:** Testing a population for alterations in the activity (mutations) of particular genes.

- **Genetic selection:** The process of selecting genes, cells, clones, etc. within populations or between populations or species.
- **Genetic slippage:** The loss of an actually potential genotype due to its failure to reach an optimum level of phenotype as a consequence of G × E interaction.
- **Genetic targeting:** The insertion of antisense DNA molecules *in vivo* into selected cells of the body in order to block the activity of undesirable genes. These genes might include oncogenes, or genes crucial to the life cycle of parasites such as trypanosomes (which cause sleeping sickness).
- **Genetic transformation:** Introduction of DNA or recombinant DNA into a suitable cell/organism.
- **Genetic use restriction technologies (GURTs):** A general term refering to several different technologies intended to control the expression (or nonexpression) of the gene(s) for specific (e.g. valuable) traits.
- **Genetic variation:** Differences between individuals attributable to differences in genotypes.
- **Genetically engineered microbial pesticides (GEMP):** One or more microbes that have been genetically engineered to be effective in combatting pest(s) that attack crops or livestock. For example, a microbe that naturally attacks a crop pest could be genetically engineered to make the microbe more potent, or more durable in field environments when applied via selected method of microbe application.
- **Genetically engineered microorganism:** Microorganism, which has one or more genetically engineered traits.
- **Genetically modified crops:** A crop variety expressing a transgene; produced by genetic engineering.
- **Genetically modified food:** Foods are additives obtained from genetically modified organisms.
- **Genetically modified organism (GMO):** An organism with a unique gene combination that does not occur naturally, and is produced either by using genetic engineering or protoplast fusion.
- **Genetically modified pest protected (GMPP) plants:** Plants that have been genetically engineered so they resist (or are more tolerant to) attacks by pests (e.g. insects).
- **Genetics:** The branch of biology concerned with the transmission, expression and evolution of genes- the molecules which

control the function, development and ultimate appearance of individuals.

- **Genistein (Gen):** One of the several phytochemicals produced by the soybean plant as a defense against certain plant diseases; and to signal *Rhizobium japonicum* bacteria to produce nitrogen for the soybean plant via colonization of its roots, followed by nitrogen fixation from the air. Genistein can also be produced as a by-product of mycobacterium fermentation (the process used to produce commercial amounts of certain antibiotics). Genistein is an isoflavone, a steroid-like compound that can be lethal to certain animal cells via its kinase-inhibiting properties. Genistein fights cancer (tumor cells) by inhibiting protein tyrosine kinase and topoisomerase II. Genistein also exhibits the property of antiangiogenesis (i.e. inhibition of tumor growth via prevention of the formation/development of new blood vessels in tumors). Attached to a pharmaceutical "guided missile" such as a monoclonal antibody or the CD4 protein, genistein is potentially useful for treatment against some tumors and has been investigated as a possible treatment against B-cell precursor leukemia. A human diet containing a large amount of genistein has been shown to increase bone density and to decrease total serum (blood) cholesterol, thereby lowering risk of osteoporosis and coronary heart disease. Research also indicates that human consumption of genistein can help to prevent breast cancer, prevent adverse increases in blood platelet aggregation, and inhibit the proliferation of smooth-muscle cells in plaque deposits (inside blood vessels).

- **Genistein:** The α-glycoside form (isomer in which glucose is attached to the molecule at the 7 position of the A ring) of the isoflavone known as genistein (aglycone form).

- **Genome analysis:** Analysis of chromosome pairing relationships among genomes of different species.

- **Genome compaction:** Reduction in genome size achieved by reducing sequences not involved in genetic functions.

- **Genome:** The complete set of sequences in the genetic material of an organism. It includes the sequence of each chromosome and any DNA in organelles.

- **Genome map:** A detailed schematic description of the structural and functional organization of the complete genome of an organism.

- **Genomic (chromosomal):** DNA clones are sequences of the genome carried by a cloning vector.
- **Genomic library:** A collection of clones containing sequences of genomic DNA of an organism. These molecules are propagated in bacteria or viruses.
- **Genomic sciences:** An encompassing term utilized to refer to the knowledge of, and attempts to decipher/understand, the structure and function of the genomes of organisms.
- **Genomics:** The study of genomes, including nucleotide sequence, gene content, organization and gene number. Cloning and molecular characterization of whole genomes. Categorized into two basic areas: 1. Structural genomics-characterizing; 2. The physical nature of whole genomes; functional genomics-characterizing the proteome and overall patterns of gene expression.
- **Genosensors:** Biosensors (electronic) that can detect the individual nucleotides that comprise a genome (DNA) molecule. Automated genosensors enable rapid, nondestructive sequencing of DNA molecules.
- **Genotoxic carcinogens:** Compounds that act directly on the genetic material (i.e. DNA) of an organism, thus causing cancer in that organism. Of the numerous chemicals that have been documented to be human carcinogens, the majority of them are genotoxic.
- **Genotoxic:** Refers to compounds that interfere with normal functioning of genetic material (i.e. DNA). For example, the antitumor antibiotic family of duocarmycin drugs.
- **Genotype:** The genetic constitution (genetic make-up) of an organism with respect to a trait. Complete set of genes inherited by an individual. For a single trait on an autosome, an individual can be homozygous for the dominant trait or homozygous for the recessive trait, or heterozygous. Yellow seeds are dominant, but yellow seeded plants could have a genotype of either YY or Yy.
- **Gentechnik gesetz (gene technology law):** The 1990 law that governs recombinant DNA research and development in the country of Germany. It was amended on January 1, 1994, to make it less restrictive.
- **Genus:** A group of closely related species.
- **GEO:** Genetically engineered organism.
- **Geomicrobiology:** Applications of microbiological knowledge to an understanding of geological phenomena.

- **Geotropism:** A growth curvature induced by gravity aka graitropism.
- **Germ:** In botany, a common name for a plant embryo and in colloquial, a disease-causing microorganism.
- **Germ cell:** The sex cell (sperm or egg). It differs from other cells in that it contains only-half (haploid) the usual number of chromosomes.
- **Germ layers:** The layers of cells in an animal embryo at the gastrula stage from which the various organs of the animal's body will be derived.
- **Germ line cells:** The cells that produce gamete.
- **Germ plasm:** The total genetic variability to an organism, represented by the total available pool of germ cells or seed.
- **Germicide:** Any chemical agent used to control or kill any pathogenic and nonpathogenic microorganisms.
- **Germinal epithelium:** A layer of epithelial cells on the surface of the ovary that is continuous with the mesothelium.
- **Germination:** The initial stages in the growth of a seed to form a seedling.
- **Gestation:** The period in animals bearing live young (especially mammals) from fertilization of the egg to birth of the young (parturition).
- **Ghost gene:** A vertical resistance gene has succumbed to the corresponding virulence gene of the pathogen.
- **Gibberellins:** Plant hormones that, regulate the growth of grass species, including rice (after the relevant gibberellin is activated by an enzyme). In 1996, Lew Mander and Richard Pharis discovered an analogue (i.e. a chemical that is similar) to grass gibberellin that does not cause grass to grow. When this analogue is sprayed onto grass, it mixes into the naturally occurring grass gibberellin and significantly slows grass growth (thus potentially reducing the amount of mowing required for lawns, golf courses, etc.) (Fig. 2).

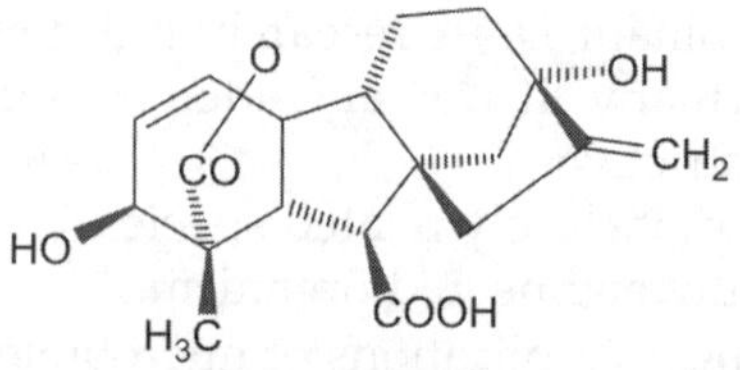

Fig. 2: Gibberellins

- **Gland:** A group of cells or a single cell in animals or plants that is specialized to secrete a specific substance.
- **Glaucus:** A surface with a waxy, white coating. In most cases this waxy covering can be rubbed off.
- **GleevecTM:** A pharmaceutical (imatinib mesylate, also known as STI571), developed and trademarked by Novartis AG, used to treat the blood cancer known as chronic myelogenous leukemia or chronic myeloid leukemia or chronic myelocytic leukemia (CML). CML results from a genetic defect (single nucleotide polymorphism) that causes excessive production of white blood cells in the body of the affected (human) and the excessive production of white blood cells results when the defective gene (i.e. SNP) causes excessive production of the enzyme Bcr-Abl tyrosine kinase. Because Gleevec™ is a protein tyrosine kinase inhibitor, it arrests excessive production of white blood cells (and induces apoptosis — cell death —in the cells that have the Bcr-Abl gene/SNP).
- **Glial derived neurotrophic factor (GDNF):** A neurotrophic factor that assists the survival and functional activity of the brain's dopaminergic neurons. Because dopaminergic neurons typically deteriorate and die in brains of the victims of Parkinson's disease, it is possible that GDNF may someday be used in treatment of Parkinson's disease.
- **Globular protein:** A soluble protein in which the polypeptide chain is tightly folded in three dimensions to yield a globular (roughly oval, circular) shape.
- **Globulins:** Common proteins in blood, eggs and milk and as a reserve protein in seeds. Globulins are insoluble in water but soluble in salt solutions.
- **Glomalin:** A "sticky" protein molecule naturally produced by certain fungi which grow on most plant roots (in the soil). Glomalin acts sort of like glue, thereby improving soil stability by "gluing" soil into clumps. Proper soil "clumping" (i.e. glomming together) allows air and water to pass through that soil more easily, increases the amount of carbon contained within the soil (thereby removing that "greenhouse gas" carbon dioxide from the atmosphere), increases the number of ("healthy") bacteria in that soil, and improves that soil's overall

fertility (i.e. its ability to produce high-yield crops or a large amount of biomass per hectare/acre). The glomalin (and thus carbon) content of soil in a field is increased by farmer utilization of low-tillage or "no-tillage" methods of crop production.

- **Glucagon:** A hormone produced by the pancreas that causes the breakdown of glycogen in the liver. Glycogen is a form of storage sugar and its breakdown releases glucose for energy production.

- **Glucocerebrosidase (trade name ceredase):** An enzyme used in treatment of inherited Gaucher's disease in which there is abnormal deposition of glucocerebrosides (hydrophobic lipid molecules that contain a hydrophilic sugar head group). Gaucher's disease is an enzyme deficiency disease that may be amenable to cure by incorporation of the gene coding for glucocerebrosidase into the patient's genome via gene delivery techniques.

- **Glucocorticoid response element (GRE):** A sequence in a promoter or enhancer that is recognized by the glucocorticoid receptor, which is activated by glucocorticoid steroids.

- **Glucogenic amino acid:** Amino acids whose carbon chains can be metabolically converted by cells into glucose or glycogen.

- **Gluconeogenesis:** The net biosynthesis (formation) of new glucose from noncarbohydrate precursors such as pyruvate, lactate, glycerol, acetyl-CoA (in plants), certain amino acids, and intermediates of the citric acid cycle.

- **Glucose (GLc):** A prime fuel for the generation of energy by organisms. It is broken down (to obtain energy) via a metabolic process called glycolysis. Glucose is a hexose, a sugar possessing six carbon atoms in its molecule. The six carbon atoms are connected to each other to form a closed ring structure known as a hexose (6) ring. Animal cells store glucose in the form of glycogen (sometimes called animal starch), a large branched polymer of glucose units. Plant cells store glucose in the form of starch, a large polymer of glucose units. Yeasts and bacteria store glucose in the form of dextran, a polymer of glucose units. The difference between the forms of storage glucose is; 1. in the size (molecular weight) of the final polymer formed; 2. in the type of linkages that connect the single glucose units together in the branched molecule, and; 3. in the degree of branching which occurs in the polymer (Fig. 3).

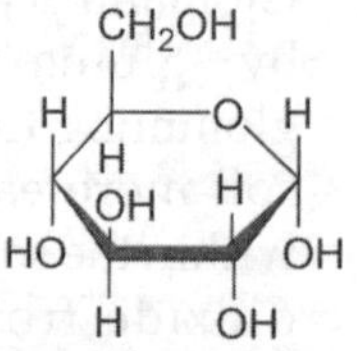

Fig. 3: Glucose

- **Glucose isomerase:** An enzyme that catalyzes the conversion of glucose to fructose. A molecule of fructose contains the same atoms as a molecule of glucose (but in a different arrangement).
- **Glucose oxidase:** An enzyme that breaks down sugar molecules (causing oxygen consumption in an organism). Industrial uses include removing dissolved oxygen from certain food products (e.g. sugar-containing drink products).
- **Glucose repression (Catabolite repression):** It describes the decreased expression of many bacterial operons that results from addition of glucose.
- **Glucosinolates:** Toxins (neurotoxic phytotoxins) naturally produced in the seeds of some plants (e.g. rapeseed, wild mustard (*Brassica juncea/Brassica rapa*), grass pea (*Lathyrus sativus*), etc.) in order to dissuade wild animals from eating those plants' seeds. For example, when large amounts of grass pea (*Lathyrus sativus*) are consumed by humans, the glucosinolates build up in the body and can cause lathyrism (i.e. an irreversible spastic paralysis of the legs). The glucosinolates in rapeseed (*Brassica rapa*) oil have been linked to heart damage in humans who consume rapeseed (high erucic acid) oil; plus those glucosinolates impart a bitter taste to such plant oils. The rapeseed glucosinolate 5-vinyl oxazolidine I cyano-2-hydroxy-3-butene causes poultry livers to hemorrhage (bleed internally) if it is fed via rapeseed meal or rapeseed oil to poultry for several weeks (at 20% of total diet).
- **Glutamate dehydrogenase:** An enzyme found naturally in certain soil bacteria, which helps those bacteria to utilize soilborne nitrogen. When its gene (GDH gene) is inserted into corn plant via genetic engineering, the resultant plant production of glutamate dehydrogenase enables that corn plant to better utilize soilborne nitrogen. As a result, such genetically engineered corn [*Zea mays* (L)] has a protein yield increase of approximately 10%, according to research begins in 1991 by David Lightfoot.
- **Glutamic acid:** A dicarboxylic amino acid of the α-ketoglutaric acid family.
- **Glutamine:** An amino acid; the monamide of glutamic acid. Glutamine is of fundamental importance for amino acid biosynthesis in all forms of life.
- **Glutamine synthetase:** An enzyme that catalyzes the synthesis of glutamine (which is crucial for amino acid biosynthesis).

- **Glutathione:** A tripeptide that is found in all cells of higher animals, which acts to help protect against oxidative stress. Composed of the amino acids glutamic acid, cysteine, and glycine. The cysteine possesses a sulfhydryl group that makes glutathione a weak reducing agent.
- **Gluten:** A term used to refer to a naturally occurring mixture of two different proteins—glutenin and gliadin—in the seeds of bread wheat (*Triticum aestivum*). In flour made from traditional varieties of wheat, glutenin proteins constitute approximately 50% of the total gluten. The relative content of those two proteins determines one of the most commercially important properties of the wheat (strength and elasticity of the flour made from that particular wheat). For example, more of the high molecular weight glutenin (which is "stretchy" and imparts physical strength to a dough made from such flour, so that dough holds together while rising) results in a flour that is better suited to manufacture higher-quality yeast-raised bread products.
- **Glutenin:** A protein naturally present in the gluten within seeds of wheat (*Triticum aestivum*).
- **Glyceraldehyde (D- and L-):** One of the smallest monosaccharides, it is called an aldose because it contains an aldehyde group. Glyceraldehyde has a single asymmetric carbon atom; thus there are two stereoisomers (D-glyceraldehyde and L-glyceraldehyde).
- **Glycine (gly):** The simplest (and smallest) of the amino acids found in proteins. It is the only amino acid that does not have an asymmetric carbon atom within its molecule. Thus, it is not optically active (Fig. 4).

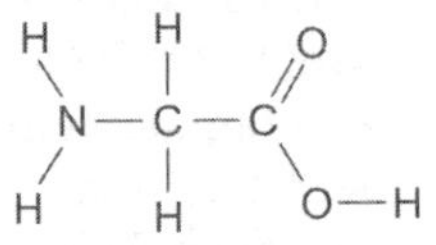

Fig. 4: Glycine

- **Glycinin:** One of the (structural) categories of proteins that are produced within seeds of legumes. In general, glycinins contain 3–4 times more cysteine (cys) and methionine (met) per unit of protein than does α-conglycinin.
- **Glycitin:** The α-glycoside form (isomer in which glucose is attached to molecule at the 7 position of the A ring) of the isoflavone known as glycitin (aglycone form).
- **Glycobiology:** The study of the involvement (function) of sugars in biological processes.
- **Glycocalyx:** A polysaccharide matrix involved (in some microorganisms) in firm attachment of the organism to a solid surface.

- **Glycocalyxation:** Addition of sugar residues to proteins after translation.
- **Glycoform:** One of the several molecular arrangements that a given glycoprotein can possess [varieties are determined by the attachment of various oligosaccharide(s)]. Some glycoforms of a given glycoprotein may exhibit greater or lesser biological activity (e.g. pharmaceutical effectiveness for biotherapeutic glycoproteins) because the oligosaccharide units of the glycoprotein molecule mediate interactions of the glycoprotein with the cells of the body.
- **Glycogen:** A polymer of glucose with a branching, tree-like molecular structure. It is the chief storage form of carbohydrates in animals. In mammals, glycogen is stored mainly in the liver and muscles. Its molecular weight may be several million.
- **Glycolipid:** A lipid containing at least one carbohydrate group within its molecule. It has a head consisting of an oligosaccharide, linked to a fatty acid tail.
- **Glycolysis:** A metabolic process in which sugars are broken down into smaller compounds with the release of energy. This series of chemical reactions is found in plant and animal cells as well as in many microorganisms. Except for the final reaction in the series, the chemical reaction pathway of glycolysis is the same as that for fermentation.
- **Glycoprotein:** A conjugated protein containing at least one carbohydrate (oligosaccharide) group within its molecule. A commonly occurring category of glycoproteins found in nature is called mucoproteins. These are protein—polysaccharide compounds that occur in the tissues, particularly in mucous secretions. Other glycoproteins include lymphokines (e.g. interleukins), hormones (e.g. somatotropins), receptors (e.g. GP120), enzymes (e.g. tissue plasminogen activator), and some therapeutics (e.g. CD4PE40).
- **Glycoprotein remodeling:** The use of restriction endoglycosidases to (enzymatically) remove sugar (i.e. oligosaccharide) "branches" from glycoprotein (i.e. part of protein, part of oligosaccharide) molecules. One reason to perform such glycoprotein remodeling would be to remove one or more oligosaccharide branches so that the glycoprotein is less or no longer antigenic (i.e. triggers an immune response). This allows the glycoprotein to be injected into the body (e.g. for pharmaceutical purposes) without incurring an unwanted immune response.

G

- **Glycosidases:** Enzymes that catalyze the cleavage (hydrolysis) of glycosidic molecular bonds. For example, lysozyme (an enzyme found in human tears) lyses (cuts up) certain bacteria by cleaving the (α, β-configuration) glycosidic linkages (bonds) between the monosaccharide units that (when linked) comprise the polysaccharide component of the bacterial cell walls. A bacterial cell devoid of a cell wall usually bursts.
- **Glycoside:** Any of a group of compounds that yield sugar molecules on hydrolysis. All parts of a glycoside compound may be sugar molecules, so that sucrose, raffinose, starch, and cellulose—all of which hydrolyze into sugar molecules—may all be considered to be glycosides. However, the name (glycoside) is usually applied to a compound in which part of the molecule is not a sugar. This nonsugar component is called the aglycon.
- **Glycosylation (to glycosylate):** Addition of oligosaccharide units (e.g. to protein molecules). The oligosaccharide units are linked to either asparagine side chains by N-glycosidic bonds or to serine and threonine side chains by O-glycosidic bonds.
- **Glycosyltransferases:** A class of enzymes (transferases) that catalyze the addition (chemical reaction) of specific sugars (molecular groups) to oligosaccharides, glycoproteins, or glycosides.
- **Glyphosate:** An active ingredient in some herbicides, it kills plants (e.g. weeds) by inhibiting the crucial plant enzyme EPSP synthase.
- **Glyphosate isopropylamine salt:** One of the several forms of an active ingredient utilized in some glyphosate-based herbicides.
- **Glyphosate oxidase:** An enzyme that (via catalysis) chemically breaks down glyphosate (i.e. the active ingredient in some herbicides). Glyphosate oxidase is produced in nature by acclimated microorganisms. In 1988, Michael Heitkamp discovered a strain of *Pseudomonas* bacteria which possessed a gene (GO) that caused those particular *Pseudomonas* bacteria to produce unusually large amounts of glyphosate oxidase. That glyphosate oxidase (GO) gene can be incorporated into a variety of crop plants (soybean, cotton, etc.) in order to help enable those plants to survive post-emergence applications of glyphosate-containing herbicides. Additionally, a plant can be genetically engineered to survive post-emergence applications of glyphosate-containing and/or

sulfosate-containing herbicides via insertion of gene (cassette) for plant production of the enzyme CP4 EPSPS.

- **Glyphosate oxidoreductase:** An enzyme naturally produced in one strain of the microorganism *Ochrobactrum anthropi*. This enzyme (by catalysis) chemically breaks down glyphosate (the active ingredient in some herbicides). If a gene (called goxv247) that codes for the production of glyphosate oxidoreductase is inserted via genetic engineering into crop plants, that would help enable such plants to survive post-emergence applications of glyphosate- and/or sulfosate-containing herbicides. Additionally, a plant can be genetically engineered to survive post-emergence applications of glyphosate and/or sulfosate-containing herbicides via insertion of gene (cassette) for plant production of the enzyme CP4 EPSPS.
- **Glyphosate-Trimesium:** One of several forms of active ingredient utilized in some glyphosate- based herbicides.
- **Gm Fad2–1:** A (plant) gene that codes for delta 12 desaturase (Δ12).
- **GMAC:** Acronym for the Genetic Manipulation Advisory Committee of the Country of Australia, which advises the Australian government on matters pertaining to genetic engineering (e.g. new rDNA product approvals). The GMAC is analogous to Germany's ZKBS (central commission on biological safety), Brazil's CTNBio (national technical biosafety commission), and the Kenya biosafety council.
- **GMO:** Genetically manipulated organism, or genetically modified organism.
- **GMP-PCP** is an analog of GTP that cannot be hydrolyzed. It is used to test which stage in a reaction requires hydrolysis of GTP.
- **GMS:** Genetically modified soya.
- **GNE:** Group of national experts on safety in biotechnology. The group of people within the OECD that developed OECD's guidelines for nations to utilize their safety evaluations of foods derived from biotechnology.
- **Golden rice:** A biotechnology-derived rice (*Oryza sativa*) created in the 1990s by Ingo Potrykus and Peter Beyer, which contains large amounts of beta carotene (precursor of vitamin A) in its seeds. The human body converts beta carotene into vitamin A. Potrykus and Beyer utilized *Agrobacterium tumefaciens* bacteria to genetically engineer rice plants (by inserting the following

genes from daffodil and from the bacterium *Erwinia uredovora*: 1. Phytoene synthase—from daffodil (*narcissus*) which converts geranylgeranyl- diphosphate into phytoene; 2. "CRTL" gene—from *Erwinia uredovora*, which codes for phytoene desaturase, which causes the rice plant to convert phytoene (a "light harvesting" carotenoid involved in photosynthesis) into lycopene (a carotenoid which is then utilized by the rice plant in the production of β-carotene); 3. Lycopene beta-cyclase—from daffodil, which converts lycopene into β-carotene (Fig. 5).

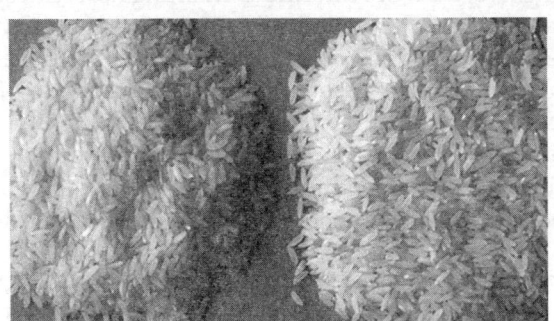

Fig. 5: Golden rice

- **GoldenRice™:** A registered trademark now owned by the company Syngenta AG.
- **Golgi apparatus:** Individual stacks of membrane near the endoplasmic reticulum; involved in glycosylating proteins and sorting them for transport to different cellular locations.
- **Golgi bodies (also known as Golgi complexes):** First described by Camillo Golgi in 1898, these are the primary "sorting centers" of cells, and the mechanism for glycosylation of (i.e. adding oligosaccharide and polysaccharide branches onto) proteins, before those proteins are transported by transfer vesicles to lysosomes, secretory vesicles, or the plasma membrane. In plant cells, Golgi complexes are where, these complex polysaccharides are "sorted" and assembled in preparation for making the cell wall (located just outside the cell's plasma membrane). Visually, a Golgi complex is a stack of flattened membranous sacs (usually 6 sacs in mammal cells and 20 sacs in plant cells).
- **Gonad:** Any of the usually paired organs in animals that produce reproductive cells (gametes).

- **Gonad ridge:** Within an embryo, the area of cells that will develop into the gonads of fetus. This usually develops around 32 days after fertilization.
- **Good laboratory practice for nonclinical studies (GLPNC):** The good laboratory practice (GLP) that is required by the US food and Drug Administration (FDA) for studies of the safety and toxicological effects of new drugs for livestock.
- **Good laboratory practices (GLP):** A set of rules and regulations issued by the Food and Drug Administration (FDA) that establishes broad methodological guidelines for procedures and record keeping. They are to be followed in laboratories involved in the testing and/or preparation of pharmaceuticals. GLPs also apply to the Environmental Protection Agency (EPA) (e.g. in toxicity testing of new herbicides).
- **Good manufacturing practices (GMP):** The set of general methodologies, practices, and procedures mandated by the Food and Drug Administration (FDA) which is to be followed in the testing and manufacture of pharmaceuticals. The purpose of GMPs is essentially to provide for record keeping, and in a wider context to protect the public. GMP guidelines exist instead of specific regulations due to the newness of the technology, and may later be superceded (modified) due to further advances in technology and understanding (*See also cGMP*).
- **Gossypol:** A yellow pigment produced in glands and seeds of the cotton plant (*Gossypium* spp.), and some other plants. When consumed by monogastric animals (e.g. swine, poultry, etc.), gossypol is somewhat toxic to those animals.
- **GP120 protein:** An adhesion molecule (glycoprotein) on the envelope (surface membrane) of HIV (i.e. AIDS-causing) viruses that directly interacts with the CD4 protein on helper T cells; enabling the HIV viruses to bind to and infect helper T cells. In 1994, a group at America's Scripps Research Institute led by Dennis Burton and Carlos Barbas III announced that they had generated a recombinant human antibody to the GP120 protein; which neutralized more than 75% of HIV isolates against which it was tested. This advance holds the potential to someday lead to a vaccine against AIDS.
- **GPA1:** A gene, found in most plants, responsible for controlling water retention and cell division in those plants. The GPA1 gene codes for a G-protein, which transmits/regulates signals (light,

temperature, phytohormones, nutrients, etc.) controlling the plant's development. During 2001, Alan Jones and colleagues discovered that "knocking out" (silencing) the GPA1 gene caused the (then-resultant) G-protein to be insensitive to abscisic acid. Because abscisic acid is a phytohormone (plant hormone) utilized by plants to control the size of stomatal pores [i.e. the openings in leaves through which plants exchange oxygen and carbon dioxide (and also water inadvertently) with the atmosphere], the "knocked-out GPA1" plants wilted due to uncontrolled water loss to the atmosphere.

G

- **GPCRs:** Acronym for G-Protein-Coupled receptors.
- **G-Proteins:** (guanyl-nucleotide binding proteins) Discovered by Rodbell and coworkers at America's National Institutes of Health (NIH), and Alfred G Gilman and coworkers at the American University of Virginia-Charlottesville, during the 1970–1980s. These are proteins embedded in the surface membrane of cells. G-proteins "receive chemical signals" from outside the cell (e.g. hormones) and "pass the signal" into the cell, so that cell can "respond to the signal". For example, a hormone, drug, neurotransmitter, or other "signal" binds to a receptor molecule on the surface of the cell's exterior membrane. That receptor then activates the G-protein, which causes an effector inside cell to produce a second "signal" chemical inside the cell, which causes the cell to react to the original external chemical signal. The G-proteins are called thus, because they become GTP and GDP forms alternately, as part of their reaction cycle (i.e. in "passing the signal"). Dysfunction of G-proteins in humans causes the salt and water losses inherent in cholera (the body's compromised immune defense inherent in pertussis), and is believed responsible for some symptoms of diabetes and alcoholism. Dysfunction of G-proteins in plants causes rapid water loss (wilting).
- **Gradient elution:** An elution system where the solvent composition is varied during the run.
- **Graft:** To place a detached branch (scion) in close cambial contact with a rooted stem (rootstock) in such a manner that scion and rootstock unite to form a single plant.
- **Graft inoculation test:** A test based on the use of a suspected viral carrier which is grafted to an indicator plant. If symptoms appear in the indicator for plant the viral assay is positive.

- **Graft union:** The point at which a scion from one plant is joined to a stock from another plant.
- **Graft-versus-host disease (GVHD):** The rejection of transplanted organs by the recipient's immune system. Also known as hyperacute rejection. It is caused by the attack of the recipient's T lymphocytes (T cells, a certain class of white blood cells) on the transplanted organ. The recipient's T cells are able to distinguish between self and foreign cells, and are hence able to recognize the foreign (nonself) cells of the transplanted organ. They then, naturally, try to destroy the "foreign invaders" in the body. This constitutes rejection of the transplanted organ. From this it should be understood that there is nothing wrong with the body, but that it is behaving exactly as it should.
- **Gram molecular weight:** The weight in grams of a compound that is numerically equal to its molecular weight; the weight of one mole (6.023×10^{23} molecules).
- **Gram stain:** Devised by Hans Christian Joachim Gram in 1884, this is a test that illuminates the composition/makeup of the physical structure of the cell wall of bacteria being tested. It is utilized to judge the effectiveness of a given chemical compound (e.g. an antibiotic) against bacteria types. The test consists of a differential staining procedure, which allows most bacteria to be visually separated into two groups, known as Gram- positive (G⁺) and Gram-negative (G⁻). An antibiotic is defined in terms of the group of (pathogenic) bacteria that it is effective against, which is known as that antibiotic's "spectrum of activity". An antibiotic is said to have a spectrum of activity against Gram-positive bacteria, Gram-negative bacteria, or the bacteria of both groups. An antibiotic that is effective against both groups of bacteria is termed "broad spectrum" or "wide spectrum".
- **Gram-negative (G⁻):** Pertaining to one of the most important ways of classifying bacteria by means of the differences in the way they stain. The set of bacteria that are not able to be stained (blue) when treated with the gram staining procedure. Gram negativity (and gram positivity) is conferred not by the chemical constituents of the bacteria, but rather by the physical structure of the bacteria cell wall. The staining procedure involves the staining of all cells in a sample with a blue dye. Gram-negative bacteria have a very thin peptidoglycan cell wall (capsule). Hence, the washing procedure, which is an integral part of the

overall staining procedure, washes out the blue dye (known as crystal violet). This leaves the Gram-negative bacteria colorless. The cells are then stained with a red acidic counterstain (dye) such as acid fuchsin or safranine. After treatment with counterstain, the Gram-negative cells are red and the Gram-positive cells are blue.

- **Gram-positive (G⁺):** Pertaining to bacteria, holding the color of the primary stain (blue) when treated with Gram's stain (a commercial staining agent), or Gentian violet solution. In contrast to the Gram-negative bacteria, the Gram-positive bacteria possess a much thicker peptidoglycan cell wall (capsule). Because of this, the blue crystal violet dye (with which the bacteria were stained) does not wash out of the cell and the bacteria appear blue under the microscope.

- **Grana:** Structures within chloroplasts seen as green granules with the light microscope and as a series of parallel lamellae with the electron microscope. Disk or sac like structures found in chloroplasts composed of stacked membranes and containing the chlorophyll and carotenoid pigments directly involved in photosynthesis (singular: Granum).

- **Granulation tissue:** A mixture of proteins and cells produced by the fibroblast growth that results from a wound.

- **Granulocidin:** A protein produced by white blood cells, which has demonstrated (in the laboratory) an ability to kill a broad-spectrum of pathogens.

- **Granulocyte colony stimulating factor (G-CSF):** A colony stimulating factor (CSF; a protein) that stimulates production of granulocytes, particularly neutrophils.

- **Granulocyte-macrophage colony stimulating factor (GM-CSF) (or Granulocyte-monocyte colony stimulating factor):** A colony stimulating factor (CSF; a protein) that stimulates production of granulocytes/macrophages/monocytes.

- **Granulocytes (Polymorphonuclear granulocytes):** Phagocytic (scavenging, ingesting) cells that are part of the immune system. When their cell nucleus is segmented into lobes and they have granule-like inclusions within their cytoplasm (the neutrophils, eosinophils, and basophils), they are collectively known as polymorphonuclear granulocytes.

- **GRAS list:** A list of food additives/ingredients considered to be Generally Recognized as safe, by the US Food and Drug

Administration (FDA). This list of additives is judged to be safe by a panel of FDA pharmacologists and toxicologists, who base their judgment upon data that is available for each ingredient. In practice, those additives for which extensive experience of common use in foods (without known ill effects) has been accumulated over time (e.g. common table salt) are often approved by the FDA due more to the "common use factor" than to any toxicology data, *per se*.

- **Gratuitous inducers:** A authentic inducers of transcription but are not substrates for the induced enzymes.
- **Green fluorescent protein:** A protein that is naturally present within the jellyfish *Aequorea victoria*. Green fluorescent protein (GFP) is utilized by scientists to "mark" certain endpoints in experiments (at which point the green light signals that endpoint was reached).
- **Green manuring:** A farming practice where a leguminous plant which has derived benefits from its association with appropriate species of *Rhizobium* is ploughed in the soil and then nonlegume is grown and allowed to take the benefits of the already fixed nitrogen.
- **Green revolution:** Advances in genetics, petrochemicals and machinery that culminated in a dramatic increase in crop productivity during the third quarter of the 20th century.
- **Growth (microbial):** An increase in the number of cells.
- **Growth cabinet:** A cupboard used for incubating tubes or culture vessels under controlled environmental conditions. The degree of control over temperature, light and humidity is a function of the equality of the cabinet.
- **Growth curve:** The change in the number of cells in a growing culture as a function of time.
- **Growth factor:** A ligand, usually a small polypeptide, that activates a receptor in the plasma membrane to stimulate growth of the target cell. Growth factors were originally isolated as the components of serum that enabled cells to grow in culture.
- **Growth hormone (GH):** A hormone produced by the anterior pituitary gland. This hormone is a protein (somatotropin) and can be obtained from the bodies of animals, or produced by genetically engineered microorganisms. Its major action in humans (human growth hormone) is a generalized stimulation of skeletal growth. However, human growth hormone (hGH)

is also known to affect the growth of other tissues, to be important in fat, protein, and carbohydrate metabolism, and to enhance the effects of various other hormones.

- **Growth hormone-releasing factor (GRF or GHRF):** Also termed growth hormone releasing hormone (GRH). A factor that causes the release of growth hormone, it is 44 amino acids in length.
- **Growth inhibitor:** Any substance inhibiting the growth of an organism. The inhibitory effect can range from mild inhibition (growth retardation) to serve inhibition or death (toxic reaction). Two plant growth regulators that may act as inhibitors are ethylene and abscisic acid.
- **Growth rate:** Increase in mass per unit of time.
- **Growth regulator:** A synthetic or natural compound that at low concentrations elicits and controls growth responses in a manner similar to hormones.
- **Growth retardant:** A chemical that selectively interferes with normal hormonal promotion of growth and other physiological processes but without appreciable toxic effects.
- **Growth ring:** Any of the rings that can be seen in a cross-section of a woody stem such as a tree trunk. It represents the xylem formed in one year as a result of fluctuating activity of the vascular cambium.
- **Growth substance:** Any organic substance other than a nutrient that is synthesized by plants and regulates growth and development. They are usually made in a particular region such as the shoot tip and transported to other regions where they take effect.
- **GT/PT correlation:** Abbreviation for genotype/phenotype correlation.
- **GT-AG rule:** The presence of these constant dinucleotides at the first two and last two positions of introns of nuclear genes.
- **GTO:** Abbreviation for gene technology office.
- **GTPases:** Guanosine triphosphatases. These are G-proteins (enzymes) which are crucial for growth, movement, and maintenance of the cell's shape. When active, GTPases are bound to cell membranes (surfaces) by an isoprene molecule (receptor).
- **GTS:** Glyphosate tolerant soybean.
- **Guanine:** One of the two purines (nine membered double ringed nitrogenous bases) in DNA or RNA (Fig. 6).

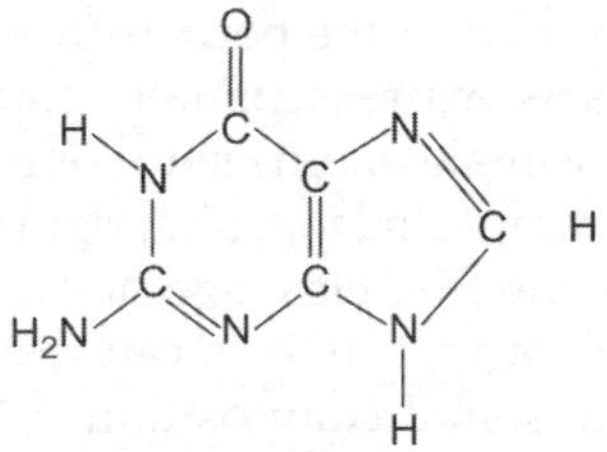

Fig. 6: Guanine

- **Guanosine:** A nucleoside consisting of one guanine molecule linked to a D-ribose sugar molecule. The derived nucleotides, guanosine mono-, di-, and triphosphate (GMP, GDP and GTP, respectively) are important in various metabolic reactions.

- **Guard cell:** Specialized epidermal cell that occurs as a pair around a stoma and controls opening and closing of the stoma through changes in turgor.

- **Guide RNA:** A small RNA whose sequence is complementary to the sequence of a correctly edited RNA. It is used as a template for the insertion of nucleotides into the pre-edited RNA.

- **Guide sequence:** An RNA molecule (or a part of it) which hybridizes with eukaryotic mRNA and aids in the splicing of intron sequences. Guide sequences may be either external (EGS) or internal (IGS) to the RNA being processed and may hybridize with either intron or exon sequences close to the splice junction.

- **GUS gene:** A gene that codes for production of α-glucuronidase (i.e. GUS protein) in *Escherichia coli* bacteria. The GUS gene is commonly utilized as a marker gene for genetically engineered plants. α-glucuronidase causes a color change, in the presence of the chemical 5-bromo-4-chloro-3-indoyl-beta-dyglucuronic acid, by cleaving ('cutting') a glucuronic acid molecule off the 5-bromo-4- chloro-3-indoyl-beta-D-glucuronic acid. The (remaining) molecule is an insoluble blue dye.

- **Gut-associated lymphoid tissues (GALT):** A variety of specialized lymph-reticular tissues that line the inside of an animal's digestive system. GALT include Peyer's Patches, the appendix, and small solitary lymphoid tissues in the gut. They constitute the intestinal immune system (response to antigens).

- **Gymnosperm:** Any plant whose ovules and the seeds into which they develop are borne unprotected rather than enclosed in ovaries as are those of the flowering plants (the term gymnosperm means naked seed).

- **Gynandromorphs:** Part of the body expresses male characters whereas other parts express female characters. A bilateral gynanadromorph is male on one side (right or left) and female on the other. For example in *Drosophila* right and left body halves are determined at the first cleavage of the zygote. Lagging of the X chromosome at first mitosis can result in two daughter cells of the chromosomal composition AAXX giving normal female, AAXO developing into the male (sterile).
- **Gynogenesis:** Female parthenogenesis after fertilization of the ovum the male nucleus is eliminated and the haploid individual (described as gynogenetic) so produced possesses the maternal genome only of androgenesis parthenogenesis anther culture.
- **Gyrase:** A type II topoisomerase of *E.coli* with the ability to introduce negative supercoils into DNA.

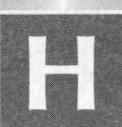

- **3'-Hydroxyl end:** The hydroxyl group attached to 3' carbon atom of sugar of the terminal nucleotide of a nucleic acid.
- **H. pylori:** A bacteria that has been linked (e.g. cause) to gastric ulcers and other gastric problems in humans. This link was first announced by Barry Marshall in the early 1990s.
- **H₂ locus:** The mouse major histocompatibility complex, a cluster of genes on chromosome 17. The genes encode proteins for antigen presentation, cytokines, and complement proteins.
- **HA:** Abbreviation for the word hemagglutinin.
- **Habitat:** The natural environment of an organism within an ecosystem. The place, in an ecosystem, where an organism lives.
- **Habitutation:** The acquired ability of cells to grow and divide independently of growth regulators.
- **Hair:** A single or multicellular absorptive (root hair) or secretory (grandular hair) and sometimes only a superficial outgrowth (covering hair) of the epidermal cells. The term trichome is often used but includes outgrowths from tissue below the epidermal layer. Distinguishing between hairs and trichomes can be difficult. Trichomes are usually connected to the vascular system whereas hairs lack a vascular connection.
- **Hairpin loop:** A region of double helix formed by base pairing within a single strand of DNA or RNA which folds itself.
- **Hairpin:** A double-helical region formed by base pairing between adjacent (inverted) complementary sequences in a single strand of RNA or DNA.
- **Hairy root culture:** A fairly recent development in plant culture consisting of highly branched roots of a plant.
- **Hairy root disease:** A disease of broad-leaved plants where a proliferation of root-like tissue is formed from the stem. Hairy root disease is a tumorous state similar to crown-gall and is induced by the bacterium *Agrobacterium rhizogenes* containing a Ri plasmid.

- **Halophile:** Microorganisms that require NaCl (salt) for growth (they are called obligate halophiles). Those, that do not require it, but can grow in the presence of high NaCl concentrations, are called facultative halophiles. Natural habitats containing high salt concentrations are, for example, the Great Salt lake in Utah, the Dead sea in Israel, and the Caspian sea in Russia.
- **Halophyte:** A plant that can tolerate a high concentration of salt in the growing medium.
- **Halothane:** A volatile anaesthetic.
- **Haploid:** A cell with one set of chromosomes; half as many chromosomes as the normal somatic body cells contain. A characteristic of sex cells.

H

- **Haplophase:** A phase in the life cycle of an organism in which it has only one copy of each gene. The organism is then said to be haploid. Yeast can exist as true haploids. Humans are haploid for only a few genes and cannot exist as true haploids.
- **Haplotype:** A group of alleles of different genes (as of the major histocompatibility complex) on a single chromosome that are closely enough linked to be inherited usually as a unit.
- **Hapten:** A small molecule that acts as an antigen when conjugated to a protein.
- **Haptoglobin:** A protein which is a component in human blood; that can occur in one of two different molecular forms (i.e. "large" version or "small" version of that molecule). The "small" version of haptoglobin is very effective at capturing and removing free radicals (high-energy oxygen atoms which bear an "extra" electron) from the bloodstream before they damage tissues (e.g. in the eye, kidneys, and/or arteries). The "large" version of haptoglobin, which is the only haptoglobin molecule in the bloodstream of one particular haplotype (genetic subgroup) of people, is not effective at capture/removal of those free radicals (e.g. generated at a high rate in people with diabetes disease), so diabetics within that particular haplotype tend to suffer extreme damage to eyes, kidneys, and arteries (sometimes necessitating limb amputation).
- **Hardening:** Gradual acclimatization of *in vitro* grown plants to *in vivo* conditions just to adapt the outdoor conditions.
- **Hardy Weinberg equilibrium:** The frequencies of genotypes at a locus resulting from random mating that locus for two alleles A_1 and A_2, with respective to frequencies p and q.

- **Harpin:** A protein naturally produced by the *Erwinia amylovora* bacteria (which usually causes the plant disease known as fire blight in apple trees, pear trees, and some ornamental plants of the rose family). Discovered in 1992 by Zhong-Min Wei and colleagues, harpin causes numerous species of plants to initiate a protective/defensive response (cascade) against bacteria, viruses, fungi, and some insects and nematodes. Harpin also causes plants (i.e. that it is sprayed onto) to increase photosynthesis and root growth/proliferation; which can lead to greater crop yields.
- **Harvesting:** A term used to describe the recovery of microorganisms from a liquid culture (in which they have been grown by man). This is usually accomplished by means of filtration or centrifugation.
- **Harvesting enzymes:** Enzymes that are used to gently dissociate (break apart) cells in living tissues in order to produce single, separate cells that can then be established and propagated in a cell culture reactor. Harvesting enzymes are also used to dissociate cells that have been grown for sometime in a cell culture reactor.
- **HAT (Histone acetyl transferase):** Enzymes modify histones by addition of acetyl groups; some transcriptional coactivators have HAT activity.
- **Hazard analysis and critical control points (HACCP):** A quality control program (for food processing) to systematically prevent hazards (e.g. pathogens) from entering the production process. HACCP was initially developed in the 1950s by the Pillsbury Company to supply food products for astronauts in America's space program. Under HACCP, food processors/handlers must analyze and identify in advance the points where hazards are most likely to occur, and eliminate them. For example, because melons lie in pathogen-contaminated dirt while growing, a "critical control point" for restaurants serving sliced melon is cleansing of the knife after each melon is cut (to prevent the knife carrying pathogens from one infected melon to other melons).
- **Hb anti-lepore:** A fusion gene produced by unequal crossing-over that has the N-terminal part of α-globin and the C-terminal part of β-globin.
- **Hb Kenya:** A fusion gene produced by unequal crossing-over between the A7 and β-globin genes.

- **Hb Lepore:** An unusual globin protein that results from unequal crossing-over between the 3rd and 8th genes. The genes become fused together to produce a single β-like chain that consists of the N-terminal sequence of 8 joined to the C-terminal sequence of β.
- **HbH:** Disease results from a condition in which there is a disproportionate amount of the abnormal tetramer β-4-relative to the amount of normal hemoglobin (a2P2).
- **HDAC (Histone de acetyl transferase):** Enzymes remove acetyl groups from histones; they may be associated with repressors of transcription.
- **Head piece:** The DNA-binding domain of the *lac* repressor.
- **Heat pump:** An apparatus that extract heat from a fluid or gas that is marginally above ambient temperature. Heat pump are commonly used to heat (or cool) greenhouses and laboratories.
- **Heat shock:** Genes are a set of loci that are activated in response to an increase in temperature (and other abuses to the cell). They occur in all organisms. They usually include chaperones that act on denatured proteins.
- **Heat shock protein (HSP):** Protein whose rate of synthesis increases after an increase in temperature or any other stress.
- **Heat shock response element (HSE):** A sequence in a promoter or enhancer that is used to activate a gene by an activator induced by heat shock.
- **Heavy chain:** The immunoglobulin heavy chain is one of two types of polypeptides in an antibody. Each antibody contains two heavy chains. The N-terminus of the heavy chain forms part of the antigen recognition site, whereas the C-terminus determines the subclass (isotype).
- **Heavy strands and light strands of a DNA:** Duplex refer to the density differences that result when there is an asymmetry between base representation in the two strands, such that one strand is rich in T and G bases and the other is rich in C and A bases. This occurs in some satellite and mitochondrial DNAs.
- **Heavy-chain variable (VH) domains:** The regions (domains) of the antibody (molecule's) "heavy chain" that vary in their amino acid sequence. The "chains" (of atoms) comprising the antibody (immunoglobulin) molecule consist of a region of variable (V) amino acid sequence and a region in which the

amino acid sequence remains constant (C). An antibody molecule possesses two antigen binding sites, and it is the variable domains of the light (VL) and heavy (VH) chains which contributes to the antigen binding ability.

- **Hedgehog proteins:** Signaling molecules (consisting of "signaling protein" with cholesterol molecule attached to it), that direct/control tissue differentiation during mammal embryo development (into various organs, limbs, etc.). The signaling protein (within an embryo cell) cleaves itself into two peptides, one of which then acts as a transferase (i.e. enzyme that catalyzes the addition of a functional group to a given molecule — in this case to the other "hedgehog peptide"). When the cell secretes the cholesterol/peptide molecule, the cholesterol (functional group) "anchors" it to the cell surface, while the "signaling protein" end of the cholesterol/peptide directs differentiation of nearby cells.

- **Helicase:** An enzyme that uses energy provided by ATP hydrolysis to separate the strands of a nucleic acid duplex.

- *Helicoverpa zea* **(*H. zea*):** Known as the corn earworm (when it is on corn plants), and known as the tomato fruitworm (when it is on tomato plants), this is one of three insect species that is called "bollworms" (when on cotton plants). *H. zea* chews on those crop plants, and is one of the insects that can act as a vector (carrier) of *Aspergillus flavus* fungus. In 1997, scientists at the US Department of Agriculture created/optimized a monoclonal antibody against *Helicoverpa zea* vitellin, which thus holds potential to be used as a means to control that insect.

- *Heliothis virescens* **(*H. virescens*):** Known as the tobacco budworm (when it is on tobacco plants), this is one of three insect species that is called "bollworms" (when they are on cotton plants). As part of Integrated Pest Management (IPM), farmers can utilize the parasitic *Euplectrus comstockki* wasp to help in controlling the tobacco budworm/cotton bollworm. When that wasp's venom is injected into *Heliothis* larva, it stops the larva from molting (and thus maturing).

- **Helix:** A spiral, staircase-like structure with a repeating pattern described by two simultaneous operations (rotation and translation). It is one of the natural conformations exhibited by biological polymers.

- **Helix-loop-helix (HLH):** Motif is responsible for dimerization of a class of transcription factors called HLH proteins. A basic helix loop helix protein has a basic sequence close to the dimerization motif that binds to DNA.

- **Helix-turn-helix:** Motif describes an arrangement of two a helices that form a site that binds to DNA, one fitting into the major groove of DNA and other lying across it.

- **Helper T cell:** A T lymphocyte that activates macrophages and stimulates B cell proliferation and antibody production. Helper T cells usually express cell surface CD4 but not CD8.

- **Helper plasmid:** A plasmid that provides a function or functions to another plasmid in the same cell.

- **Helper virus:** It provides functions absent from a defective virus, enabling the latter to complete the infective cycle during a mixed infection.

- **Hemagglutinin (HA):** A special protein that some viruses utilize to gain entry into the cells, they have "targeted". The HA protein helps the virus adhere to the cell it targets. Hemagglutinin is also utilized to refer to specific plant cell proteins (lectins) that are naturally produced by certain plants such as the soybean plant (*Glycine max* (L) Merrill). The presence of those lectin molecules (e.g. on surfaces of root cells of the soybean plant) help nitrogen fixing *Rhizobium japonicum* bacteria to adhere to soybean plant roots, where they begin to "fix nitrogen" (i.e. create natural nitrate fertilizer, which improves the soil and helps plants to grow).

- **Hematologic growth factors (HGF):** A class of colony stimulating factors (proteins) that stimulates bone marrow cells to produce certain types of red and white blood cells. Some colony stimulating factors are: 1. Granulocyte-macrophage colony stimulating factor (GM-CSF) 2. Granulocyte-monocyte colony stimulating factor 3. Granulocyte colony stimulating factor (GM-CSF) 4. Erythropoietin (EPO) 5. Interleukin-3 (IL-3) 6. Macrophage colony stimulating factor (M-CSF).

- **Hematopoietic growth factors:** Growth factors that stimulate the body to produce blood cells.

- **Hematopoietic stem cells:** Certain stem cells present (e.g. in infants' bodies, and in the umbilical cord of newborn infants), that can be differentiated (via chemical signals in the growing body) to give rise to red blood cells and the infection-fighting cells of the immune system.

- **Heme:** The iron-porphyrin prosthetic group of a class of proteins called "heme proteins".
- **Hemicellulase:** An enzyme that degrades hemicellulose to galactose. Hemicellulose is available as a commercial product.
- **Hemimethylated:** Duplex DNA where only one of the two strands are methylated and is important for regulating and protecting DNA.
- **Hemizygote:** A diploid individual that has lost its copy of a particular gene (e.g. because a chromosome has been lost) and which therefore has only a single copy.
- **Hemizygous:** If there is only one copy of a gene for a particular trait in a diploid organism, the organism is hemizygous for the trait, and can display a recessive phenotype. X-linked genes in fly or human males are hemizygous.
- **Hemoglobin:** An oxygen-transporting respiratory pigment; it is present in humans, animals, and some plants (e.g. land plants that withstand occasional immersion/flooding). In humans, hemoglobin is carried in the red blood cells (erythrocytes), and is responsible for the red color of the blood. It is composed of two pairs of identical polypeptide chains and iron-containing heme groups, comprising the (total) hemoglobin molecule. The molecular structure of hemoglobin was determined by Max Perutz in 1959. A human disease known as sickle-cell anemia is caused by small change in the hemoglobin molecule's (genetically induced) structure (in victims of that disease).
- **Hemolymph:** The mixture of blood and other fluids in the body cavity of an invertebrate.
- **Hemophilia:** An inherited disease that is due to a deficiency or lack of certain compounds, such as factor VIII or IX, in the blood. This results in excessive internal or external bleeding due to impaired blood clotting.
- **Heparin:** A polysaccharide; sulfuric acid ester found in the liver, lung, and other tissues that prolongs the clotting time of blood by preventing the formation of fibrin. Used in vascular surgery and in treatment of post-operative thrombosis and embolism.
- **HER-2 gene:** Abbreviation for Human Epidermal growth factor Receptor-2 gene, an oncogene that is responsible for approximately 30% of breast cancers (i.e. in those women whose body

over-expresses that particular oncogene, and it spreads via meta-staticism). In addition to conventional treatments (mastectomy, chemotherapy, etc.), the US Food and Drug Administration (FDA) in 1998 approved use of a humanized monoclonal antibody (trastuzumab) to be utilized alone, or in combination with, certain chemotherapy agents (e.g. paclitaxel) against such metastatic breast cancers. That monoclonal antibody attaches to the extracellular domain (i.e. portion of the Her-2 receptor sticking out of the surface of breast tissue cells) and down regulates the Her-2 gene, i.e. resulting in fewer Her-2 receptors. being produced on the plasma membrane surface of that woman's breast tissue cells.

H

- **HER-2 receptor:** An epidermal growth factor receptor (protein molecule embedded in the surface of cells) that is present in abundance attached to the plasma membrane surface of breast tissue cells in humans possessing the HER-2 gene.
- **Herbicide:** Any substance that is toxic to plants usually applied to agrochemicals intended to kill specific unwanted plants such as weeds.
- **Herbicide resistance:** The ability of a plant to withstand herbicide. Herbicide resistance has been one of the early targets of plant genetic engineering.
- **Herbicide-tolerant crop:** Crop plants that have been developed to survive application(s) of one or more commercially available herbicides by the corporation of certain gene(s) via biotechnology methods such as genetic engineering or traditional breeding methods (such as natural, chemical, or radiation mutation).
- **Heredity:** Transfer of genetic information from parent cells to progeny.
- **Heritability:** In genetics, a statistical term used to denote the proportion of phenotypic variance due to variance in genotypes that is genetically determined, denoted by h^2.
- **Hermaphrodite:** Animal that has both male and female reproductive organs or a mixture of male and female attributes.
- **Hetero:** A chemical nomenclature prefix meaning "different". For example, a heterocyclic compound is one with a (ring) structure made up of more than one kind of atom. A heterokaryon refers to a cell containing nuclei of different species.
- **Heteroalleles:** Mutations that are functionally allelic but structurally non-allelic; that occurs at different sites of a gene.

- **Heterochromatin:** It describes regions of the genome that are permanently in a highly condensed condition, are not transcribed, and are late-replicating; May be constitutive or facultative.
- **Heterocysts:** The modified vegetative cells in cyanobacteria associated with N_2 fixation.
- **Heterodimer:** A protein consisting of two polypeptide chains encoded by different genes.
- **Heteroduplex (hybrid) DNA:** DNA generated by base pairing between complementary single strands derived from the different parental duplex molecules; it occurs during genetic recombination.
- **Heterogametic sex:** The sex that produces gametes containing different sex chromosomes.
- **Heterogeneous:** Large RNA molecules which are nonedited mRNA transcripts found in nucleus of an eukaryotic cell nuclear RNA (hnRNA).
- **Heterogeneous (catalysis):** Catalysis occurring at a phase boundary, usually a solid fluid interface.
- **Heterogeneous (chemical reaction):** A chemical reaction in which the reactants are of different phases: like gas with liquid, liquid with solid, or a solid catalyst with liquid or gaseous reactants.
- **Heterogeneous (mixture):** One that consists of two or more phases such as liquid-vapor, or liquid-vapor-solid.
- **Heterogeneous nuclear (HN) RNA:** Comprises transcripts of nuclear genes made by RNA polymerase II; it has a wide size distribution and low stability.
- **Heterokaryon:** A somatic cell containing nuclei from two different sources.
- **Heterologous DNA:** Refers to a DNA molecule in which each of the (double) strands is from different sources (e.g. different species).
- **Heterologous probe:** A DNA probe desired for one species and used to screen for a similar DNA sequence from another species.
- **Heterologous proteins:** Those proteins produced by an organism that is not the wild type source of those proteins. For example, bacteria have been genetically engineered to produce human growth hormone and bovine (i.e. cow) somatotropin.
- **Heterology:** A sequence of amino acids in two or more proteins that are not identical to each other.

- **Heteromultimeric proteins:** It consists of non-identical subunits (coded by different genes).
- **Heteroplasmy:** A cellular condition in which two genetically different types of organelles are present.
- **Heteroploid:** Term given to a cell culture when the cells comprising the culture possess nuclei containing chromosome numbers other than the diploid number.
- **Heteropycnosis:** Property of certain chromosomes, or of their parts, to remain more dense and to stain more intensely than other chromosomes or parts during the cell cycle.
- **Heterosis:** The observation that in some circumstances, the heterozygotes in a population have higer fitness than the homozygotes, for example, they grow better, are better able to survive, and more fertile than the homozygotes. Also known as "hybrid vigor".
- **Heterotroph:** An organism that obtains nourishment from the ingestion and breakdown of organic matter.
- **Heterozygote:** An individual with different alleles at some particular locus.
- **Heterozygous:** Differing alleles for a trait in an individual, such as Yy. A zygote is said to be heterozygote, if the two members of an allelic pair are unlike.
- **HETP- (Height equivalent to a theoretical plate):** The number obtained by dividing the column length by the theoretical plate number.
- **Hexadecyltrimethylammonium bromide (CTAB):** A solvent that is widely utilized to dissolve plant DNA samples (e.g. when a scientist wants to sequence that sample of plant DNA). CTAB solvent helps the scientist to separate out contaminants that are commonly present in samples from plant tissues (polysaccharides, quinones, etc.) because DNA molecules are much more soluble in CTAB than are the contaminant molecules.
- **HF (hydrofluoric) cleavage:** A research process in which hydrofluoric acid is used to sequentially remove side-chain protective groups from peptide chains; Also used to remove the resin support from peptides that have been prepared via solid-phase peptide synthesis. The HF cleavage reaction is a temperature dependent process.
- **Hfr strain (high frequency recombination):** A bacterial stain with chromosomally integrated plasmid that helps in transfer of part of chromosome to a recipient F cell during conjugation.

- **High mannose oligosaccharide:** An N-linked oligosaccharide that contains N-acetylglucosamine linked only to mannose residues. It is covalently added to transmembrane proteins in rough endoplasmic reticulum and is trimmed and modified in the Golgi apparatus.
- **High-amylose corn:** Refers to those corn (maize) hybrids that produce kernels in which the starch that is contained within those kernels is atleast 50% amylose, versus the average of 24–28% amylose in traditional corn starch.
- **High-density lipoproteins (HDL):** So called "good" cholesterol, it consists of lipoproteins that can help move excess low-density lipoproteins ("bad" cholesterol, which can clog arteries) out of the human body by binding to the low-density lipoproteins (LDL) (also known as LDL cholesterol) in the blood and then attaching to special LDL receptor molecules in the liver. The liver then clears those (bound) low-density lipoproteins out of the body as a part of regular liver functions. Studies have shown that humans having high bloodstream levels of HDL will offset high levels of LDL (e.g. the HDL can still help lower the risk of developing coronary heart disease). Since cholesterol does not dissolve in water (which constitutes most of the volume of blood), the body makes HDL cholesterol into little "packages" surrounded by a hydrophilic ("water loving") protein. That protein "wrapper" is known as apolipoprotein A-1, or apo A-1, and it enables HDL cholesterol to be transported in the bloodstream because the apolipoprotein A-1 is attracted to water molecules in the blood.
- **High-isoflavone soybeans:** Developed in the US in the 1990s, these soybean varieties contain greater content of isoflavones than do traditional soybean varieties (i.e. isoflavones constitute 0.15–0.3% of a traditional variety soybean's dry weight). Consumption of isoflavones helps to reduce the blood level of low-density lipoproteins ("bad cholesterol") in humans. A human diet containing a large amount of isoflavones helps prevent osteoporosis, causes reduced risk of certain cancers (breast cancer, prostate cancer, endometrial cancer, etc.), and decreases risk of prostate enlargement.
- **High-lactoferrin rice:** Refers to rice plants (*Oryza sativa*) which have been genetically engineered to produce substantial amounts of lactoferrin in the grain they yield. Lactoferrin is a compound that is naturally produced in human breast milk.

Consumption of lactoferrin by infants helps to strengthen their immune system. Consumption of lactoferrin (e.g. from genetically engineered rice) by old humans helps their immune systems to resist some infectious diseases. Lactoferrin "binds" free iron (e.g. in body fluids), thereby denying that iron to pathogenic bacteria (which need free iron to grow/infect). Lactoferrin also promotes intestinal cell growth in humans.

- **High-laurate canola:** Refers to canola (*Brassica napus/campestris*) varieties genetically engineered (e.g. via insertion of gene for lauroyl-ACP thioesterase) to produce atleast 40% laurate (lauric acid) in their oil (in seed).

H

- **Highly repetitive DNA:** A first component to reassociate and is equated with satellite DNA.

- **Highly unsaturated fatty acids (HUFA):** Refers to a number of unsaturated fatty acids (e.g. that the human body forms from polyunsaturated fatty acids it consumes in diet) containing four or more double (molecular) bonds; i.e. arachidonic acid, docosa-hexanoic acid, eicosapentaenoic acid. These HUFAs are utilized (by the human body) to make prostaglandins and other eicosanoids.

- **High-lysine corn:** Developed in the US in the mid-1960s, these were initially corn (maize) varieties possessing the opague-2 gene. The opague-2 gene causes such corn to contain 0.30–0.55% lysine (i.e. 50–80% more than traditional No. 2 yellow corn). Other genes have subsequently been discovered, when inserted into the corn/maize genome (e.g. via genetic engineering techniques), cause production of larger amounts of lysine than in traditional corn/maize varieties. High-lysine corn is particularly useful for feeding of swine, since traditional No. 2 yellow corn does not contain enough lysine for optimal swine growth.

- **High-methionine corn:** Developed in the US in the mid-1960s, these were initially corn (maize) varieties possessing the floury-2 gene. The floury-2 gene causes such corn to contain slightly higher levels of methionine than traditional No. 2 yellow corn. Other genes have subsequently been discovered that, when inserted into corn/maize genome (e.g. via genetic engineering techniques), cause production of larger amounts of methionine than in traditional corn/maize varieties. High-methionine corn is particularly useful for feeding of poultry, since traditional No. 2 yellow corn does not contain enough methionine for optimal poultry (especially feather) growth.

- **High-oil corn:** Conceived in 1896 at the University of Illinois in the US, high-oil corn (HOC) is defined to be corn (maize) possessing a kernel oil content of 5.8% or greater. Traditional No. 2 yellow corn varieties tend to contain 4.5% or less oil content.
- **High-oleic oil soybeans:** Soybeans from plants which have been genetically engineered to produce soybeans bearing oil that contains more than 70% oleic acid, instead of the typical 24% oleic acid content of soybean oil produced from traditional varieties of soybeans. Co-suppression, via inserted gene for $\Delta 12$ desaturase (an enzyme that normally converts oleic acid to linoleic acid as part of the oil creation process in traditional varieties of soybean plants), causes the higher amount of oleic acid in the soybean oil than traditional one. High-oleic soybean oil would tend to have greater oxidative stability (especially at elevated temperatures) than soybean oil from traditional varieties of soybeans. Because of that, nuts that were fried in high-oleic oil have been shown to possess a longer shelf-life than nuts fried in traditional oils. A human diet containing a large amount of oleic acid causes lower blood cholesterol level, and thus lower the risk of coronary heart disease (CHD).
- **High-phytase corn and soybeans:** Crop plants that have been genetically engineered to contain in their grain/seed high(er) levels of the enzyme phytase (which aids digestion and absorption of phosphate in that grain/seed). High-phytase grains or oilseeds are particularly useful for the feeding of swine and poultry, since traditional No. 2 yellow corn (maize) or traditional soybean varieties do not contain phytase in amounts needed for complete digestion/absorption of phosphate naturally contained in those traditional soybeans and corn (maize) in the form of phytate.
- **High-stearate canola:** Canola varieties which have been genetically engineered so their seeds contain a higher percentage of stearate (also called stearic acid) in the canola oil than the typical stearate content in canola oil produced from traditional canola varieties. Co-suppression, via inserted gene for D-stearoyl-ACP desaturase (i.e. enzyme that normally converts stearic acid to to oleic acid in the oil creation process in traditional varieties of canola), causes the higher amount of stearic acid in the canola oil than traditional one.
- **High-stearate soybeans:** Soybean plant varieties which have been bred or genetically engineered so their beans contain at least

12% stearate (also known as stearic acid) within their soybean oil (i.e. more than four times the typical 3% stearic acid content in the soybean oil produced from traditional soybean varieties). Some high-stearate soybeans contain more than 20% stearate. Cosuppression, via inserted gene for D-stearoyl-ACP desaturase (i.e. enzyme that normally converts stearic acid to oleic acid in the oil creation process in traditional varieties of soybeans), is the primary way to cause the higher amount of stearic acid than traditional in the resultant soybean oil. A human diet containing stearate instead of alternative saturated fatty acids, does not cause an increase in blood cholesterol levels (whereas human consumption of the other saturated fatty acids causes bloodstream cholesterol levels to increase, which increases the risk of coronary heart disease).

- **High-sucrose soybeans:** Another name for low-stachyose soybeans because the soybeans replace the (reduced) stachyose with (additional) sucrose.

- **High-throughput identification:** Determination of the identification of a given chemical compound (e.g. within a mixture), the desired impact (cell apoptosis, etc.), a specific segment (sequence) of DNA (i.e. a specific gene), a specific ligand or receptor (e.g. "attaching" itself to a given molecule), etc. within the overall process known as high throughput screening.

- **High-throughput screening (HTS):** A methodology utilized to quickly screen large numbers of compounds for use as pharmaceuticals or agrochemicals (e.g. herbicides). HTS allows a researcher to quickly conduct million of chemical, genetic or pharmacological tests.

- **Histamine:** A base that is naturally present in ergot (a fungus) and plants; it is also naturally produced by basophils (basophilic leukocytes) in the human body. It is formed from histidine by decarboxylation, and is held to be responsible for the dilation and increased permeability of blood vessels which play a major role in allergic reactions.

- **Histidine (his):** A basic amino acid that is essential in the nutrition of the rat. It is formed by the decomposition of most proteins (as globin) (Fig. 1).

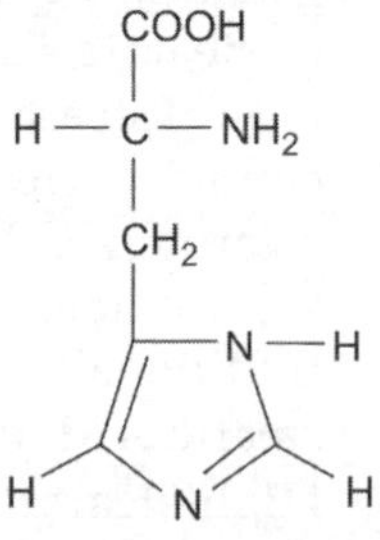

Fig. 1: Histidine

- **Histocompatibility:** The degree to which tissue from one organism will be tolerated by the immune system of another organism.
- **Histology:** Science that deals with the study of microscopic structure of animal and plant tissues.
- **Histone fold:** A motif found in all four core histones in which three α-helices are connected by two loops.
- **Histones:** Five kinds of proteins form complexes with eukaryotic DNA.
- **Histopathologic:** Refers to changes in tissue caused by a disease. For example, certain diseases (e.g. jaundice) cause the skin to turn yellow.
- **HIV:** Human immunodeficiency virus. The retrovirus that causes AIDS in humans.
- **HLA:** Locus is the human major histocompatibility complex, a cluster of genes on chromosome 6. The genes encode proteins for antigen presentation, cytokines, and complement proteins.
- **HNE:** The common chemical (by)product of lipid oxidation, known as 4-hydroxy-2-nonenal, which is an aldehyde.
- **HNGF:** Human nerve growth factor. A protein whose hormone like action affects differentiation, growth, and maintenance of neurons.
- **hnRNP:** It is the ribonucleoprotein form of hnRNA (heterogeneous nuclear RNA), in which the hnRNA is complexed with proteins.
- **Holandric:** In humans the genes present on Y chromosomes, transmitted from males to males.
- **Holliday:** An intermediate structure in homologous recombination, where the two duplexes of DNA are connected by the genetic material exchanged between two of the four strands, one from each duplex. A joint molecule is said to be resolved when nicks in the structure restore two separate DNA duplexes.
- **Hollow fiber separation (of proteins):** The separation of proteins from a mixture by means of "straining" the mixture through hollow, semipermeable fibers (e.g. polysulfone fibers) under pressure. The hollow fibers are constructed in such a way that they have very tiny (molecular size) holes in them. In this way, large molecules are retained in the original liquid while smaller molecules, which are able to pass through the holes, are filtered out.

H

- **Holoenzyme (Complete enzyme):** It is the complex of five sub-units including core enzyme $(\alpha\beta_2\beta')$ and σ factor that is competent to initiate bacterial transcription.
- **Holometabolous:** An insect that undergoes complete metamorphosis to the adult from a morphologically distinct larval stage.
- **Homeobox:** Describes the conserved sequence that is part of the coding region of *D. melanogaster* homeotic genes; it is also found in amphibian and mammalian genes expressed in early embryonic development.
- **Homeobox:** A sequence of about 180 nucleotides that encodes 60-amino acid sequence called a homeodomain, which is part of a DNA-binding protein that acts as a transcription factor.
- **Homeodomain:** A DNA-binding motif that specifies a class of transcription factors. The DNA sequence that codes for it is called the homeobox.
- **Homeostasis:** A tendency toward maintenance of a relatively stable internal environment in the bodies of higher animals through a series of interacting physiological processes. An example is the mammal's maintenance of a constant body temperature despite extremes in weather temperature.
- **Homeotic genes:** It is defined as mutations that convert one body part into another; for example, an insect leg may replace an antenna.
- **Homeotic mutation:** A mutation that causes a body part to develop into an inappropriate position in an organism such as the mutation in Drosophila that causes legs to develop on the head in place of antennae.
- **Homing receptor:** Specific adhesion molecules expressed on leukocytes that serve to direct leukocyte migration towards specific tissues in association with tissue-expressed ligand counter parts (addressins).
- **Homoalleles:** Mutations that are both functionally and structurally allelic mutations at the same site in the same gene.
- **Homodimer:** A protein consisting of two identical polypeptide chains encoded by the same gene.
- **Homogametic sex:** The diploid chromosome constitution, 2A + XX.
- **Homogeneously staining region (HSR):** Region produced by the tandem amplification of a chromosomal sequence. As a result, it does not have a banded pattern.

- **Homogenotisation:** A genetic technique used to replace one copy of a gene or other DNA sequence, within a genome, with an altered copy of that sequence.
- **Homokaryon:** A cell with two or more identical nuclei as a result of fusion.
- **Homologous chromosomes:** The pair of chromosomes in a diploid individual that have the same overall genetic content, centromere placement and pair during meiosis. One member of each homologous pair of chromosomes is inherited from each parent.
- **Homologous recombination (generalized recombination):** Involves a reciprocal exchange of sequences of DNA, e.g. between two chromosomes that carry the same genetic loci.
- **Homology:** A sequence of amino acid in two or more proteins that are identical to each other. Nucleic-acid homology refers to complementary strands that can hybridize with each other.
- **Homomultimeric protein:** Protein consisting of more than two identical subunits.
- **Homoplasmy:** A cellular condition in which all copies of an organelle are genetically identical.
- **Homopolymer:** A nucleic acid strand composed of one kind of nucleotide.
- **Homotropic enzyme:** An allosteric enzyme whose own substrate functions as an activity modulator.
- **Homozygote:** An individual with the same allele at corresponding loci on the homologous chromosomes.
- **Homozygous:** When both alleles for a trait are the same in an individual. They can be homozygous dominant (YY), or homozygous recessive (yy). A zygote is said to be a homozygote, if the two members of an allelic pair are alike.
- **Horizontal gene transfer:** Transmission of DNA between species, involving close contact between the donor's DNAs and the recipient, uptake of DNA by the recipient, and stable incorporation of the DNA into the recipient's genome.
- **Hormone:** A type of chemical messenger (peptide), occurring in both plants and animals, that acts to inhibit or excite metabolic activities (in that plant or animal) by binding to receptors on specific cells to deliver its "message." A hormone's site of production is distant from the site of biological activity (i.e. where the message is delivered).

- **Host cell:** A cell whose metabolism is used for growth and reproduction by a virus; also the cell into which a plasmid is introduced (in recombinant DNA experiments).
- **Host specific toxin:** A metabolite produced by a pathogen which has a host specificity equivalent to that of the pathogen. Such toxins are utilized for *in vitro* selection experiments to screen for tolerance or resistance to the pathogen.
- **Host vector (HV) system:** The host is the organism into which a gene from another organism is transplanted. The guest gene is carried by a vector (i.e. a larger DNA molecule, such as a plasmid, or a virus into which that gene is inserted) which then propagates in the host.
- **Hot spot:** A region in DNA that is more prone to mutagenesis by a particular mutagen.
- **Housekeeping (constitutive) genes:** Those (theoretically) expressed in all cells because they provide basic function needed for sustenance of all cell types.
- **Hox:** Genes are clusters of mammalian genes containing homeoboxes; the individual members are related to the genes of the complex loci ANT-C and BX-C in *D. Melanogaster*.
- **HPLC:** High-performance liquid chromatography. A system for separating and/or measuring components in a chemical mixture.
- **Human artificial chromosomes (HAC):** Chromosomes that have been synthesized (made) from chemicals that are identical to chromosomes within human cells.
- **Human chorionic gonadotropin:** A human hormone. In 1986, Mark Bogart discovered that elevated levels of human chorionic gonadotropin in pregnant women are correlated with babies (later) born with Down syndrome.
- **Human colon fibroblast tissue plasminogen activator:** A second generation tissue plasminogen activator (tPA), which has the clot-sensitive activation of plasminogen with potentially greater selectivity and (clot) specificity.
- **Human EGF-receptor-related receptor (HER-2):** A gene that appears to be directly related to human breast cancer mortality. The more copies of the HER-2 gene (in a patient's breast tumor cells), the more dismal that patient's prospects for survival.

H

- **Human embryonic stem cells:** Those cells (in the early embryo's inner cell mass) from which each of the human body's 210 different types of tissues arise via differentiation, proliferation, and growth processes.
- **Human genome project:** An international research project to map each human gene and to completely sequence human DNA.
- **Human gamma-glutamyl transpeptidase:** A glycoprotein that is thought to possess a different oligosaccharide when it is produced by a (liver) tumor cell instead of a healthy cell. Thus, it is a possible early warning marker for liver cancer.
- **Human growth hormone:** A protein produced in the pituitary gland that stimulates the liver to produce somatomedins, which stimulate growth of bone and muscle.
- **Human immunodeficiency virus (HIV):** It is a retrovirus, RNA containing virus that replicates by making a DNA intermediate. It consists of an outer lipid envelope derived from the host cell.
- **Human leukocyte antigens (HLA):** A very complex array of six proteins that cover the surface of leukocytes (and the bone marrow cells that produce leukocytes). These HLA are usually different (i.e. a nonmatch) for individuals that are not genetically related to each other (e.g. a father-son or a father-daughter), so have been used in the past to prove paternity. HLA must also be matched (as nearly as possible) for successful bone marrow transplants, to prevent the donated bone marrow (and the narrow recipient) from "rejecting" each other.
- **Human protein kinase C:** An enzyme that is involved in the control of blood coagulation and fibrinolysis.
- **Human superoxide dismutase (hSOD):** An enzyme that "captures" oxygen free radicals (oxygen atoms bearing an extra electron, thus high in energy: e.g. sometimes generated in a biological system such as within the body of an organism). Oxygen free radicals are generated within occluded blood vessels when a blood clot blocks arteries in the heart, causing a heart attack. These oxygen free radicals are highly energized and can cause damage to blood vessel walls after the clot is dissolved (e.g. with tissue plasminogen activator), so hSOD may profitably be administered in conjunction with clot-dissolving pharmaceuticals to minimize damage when occluded arteries are reopened. Research indicates that hSOD may help protect elderly patients from the lethal effects of

influenza (flu), because influenza often causes overproduction of free radicals in the victim's body. Recent research indicates that hSOD may be made more effective when administered in combination with certain copper/zinc compounds to bolster its efficacy.

- **Human thyroid-stimulating hormone (hTSH):** A naturally occurring hormone that causes the thyroid gland to develop.

- **Humoral immune response:** Refers to the rapid manufacture and secretion by the body of the soluble blood serum components—e.g. antibodies (by B cells), complement proteins, cecropins, etc.—in response to an infection.

- **Humoral immunity:** The immune system response consisting of the soluble blood serum components that fight an infection (antibodies, complement proteins, cecropins, etc.).

- **Humoral response:** An immune response that is mediated primarily by antibodies. It is defined as immunity that can be transferred from one organism to another by serum antibody.

- **HuSNPs:** Abbreviation for Human SNPs (single-nucleotide polymorphisms).

- **Hybrid dysgenesis:** It describes the inability of certain strains of *D. Melanogaster* to interbreed, because the hybrids are sterile (although otherwise they may be phenotypically normal).

- **Hybrid:** Heterozygous, usually referring to the offspring of two true-breeding (homozygous) individuals differing in the traits of interest.

- **Hybrid-arrested translation:** A technique that identifies the cDNA corresponding to an mRNA by relying on the ability to base pair with RNA *in vitro* to inhibit translation.

- **Hybrid cell:** The mononucleosis cell which results from the fusion of two different cells leading to the formation of a synkaryon.

- **Hybrid dysgenesis:** A syndrome of abnormal germline traits including mutation chromosome breakage and sterility which results from activity of transposable elements.

- **Hybrid seed:** Seed produced by crossing genetically dissimilar parents.

- **Hybrid selection:** The process of choosing individuals possessing desired characteristics from among a hybrid population.

- **Hybridization (molecular genetics):** The pairing (tight physical bonding) of two complementary single strands of RNA and/or DNA to give a double-stranded molecule.

- **Hybridization (plant genetics):** Production of a hybrid by pairing complementary ribonucleic acid (RNA) and deoxyribonucleic acid (DNA) strands.

- **Hybridization surfaces:** Various physical substrates (surfaces) onto which have been "attached" genetic materials (DNA, RNA, oligonucleotides, etc.). Relevant complementary genetic materials (DNA, RNA, oligonucleotides, etc.) then are hybridized onto those attached-to-surface genetic materials for various specific purposes (e.g. detection of the presence of those unattached genetic materials, in the case of biosensor's hybridization surface). One of the technologies that can be utilized to assay (evaluate) DNA from hybridization surfaces is Matrix-Assisted Laser Desorption Ionization Time of Flight Mass Spectrometry (MALDI-TOF-MS).

- **Hybridoma:** A cell line produced by fusing a myeloma with a lymphocyte; it continues indefinitely to express the immuno-globulins of both parents.

- **Hydrate:** A compound formed by the incorporation of water.

- **Hydrazine:** A chemical with formula N_2H_4; Used as a rocket fuel, and in the hydrazinolysis of glycoproteins.

- **Hydrazinolysis:** A technique that used the chemical hydrazine to separate and isolate the oligosaccharide portion from the protein portion of a glycoprotein. The hydrazine chemically "chews up" the polypeptide (i.e. protein) portion of a glycoprotein molecule, leaving the intact oligosaccharides behind. It can subsequently be analyzed (after chromatographic separation from the peptide pieces and other chemical components).

- **Hydrogen bond:** A relatively weak bond formed between a hydrogen atom (which is covalently bound to a nitrogen or oxygen atom) and a nitrogen or oxygen atom with an unshared electron pair.

- **Hydrogen uptake (Hup) gene:** A gene found in N_2 fixing microbes that converts H_2 to $2H^+$ and harvests energy of the organisms.

- **Hydrogenation:** A chemical reaction/process in which hydrogen atoms are added to molecules (e.g. of unsaturated fatty acids) in edible oils. In the case of fatty acids, the fraction of each isomeric form (*trans* vs. *cis* fatty acids) and the molecular chain length (of the fatty acids present) have a large impact on the melting characteristics of each (fat or oil), with shorter-chain fats melting at lower temperature. Hydrogenation is the most common chemical reaction utilized in the edible oils (processing) industry. Hydrogenation increases the solids (i.e. crystalline fat) content of edible fats/oils, and improves their resistance to thermal and atmospheric oxidation (e.g. for frying of foods). Those increases in solids and resistance to oxidation result from the reduction in the fat/oil relative unsaturation, plus increased geometric and positional isomerization of the fat/oil molecules. The edible oil/fat hydrogenation reaction is accomplished by treating fats/oils with pressurized hydrogen gas in the presence of a catalyst. As a result, the (usually) liquid oils are converted to more saturated fats, which are semisolid at an ambient temperature of 72°F (22°C). The presence of *trans* fatty acids in hydrogenated edible oils can be reduced significantly via changes in catalyst, temperature, pressure, etc. used in the hydrogenation reaction. In general, natural oils and fats possessing melting points lower than 121°F (50°C) are nearly completely absorbed in the digestive system of typical humans.

- **Hydrolysis:** Literally, means "cleaved by water". It is used for a chemical reaction in which the chemical bond attaching an atom, or group of atoms to the (rest of the) molecule is cleaved, followed by attachment of a hydrogen atom at the same chemical bond.
- **Hydrolytic cleavage:** A chemical reaction in which a portion (e.g. an atom or a group of atoms) of a molecule is "cut" off the molecule via hydrolysis.
- **Hydrolytic reaction:** The reaction in which a covalent bond is broken down with the incorporation of a water molecule.
- **Hydrolyze:** To "cut" a chemical bond (with a molecule) via hydrolysis.
- **Hydropathy plot:** A measure of the hydrophobicity of a protein region and therefore of the likelihood that it will reside in a membrane.
- **Hydrophilic:** Hydrophilic groups interact with water, so that hydrophilic regions of protein or the faces of a lipid bilayer reside in an aqueous environment.
- **Hydrophobic:** Hydrophobic groups repel water, so that they interact with one another to generate a non-aqueous environment.

- **Hydroponics:** The growing of plants in aerated water containing all the essential mineral nutrients with no soil. Also called soil less gardening or cultivation.

- **Hydrops fetalis:** A fatal disease resulting from the absence of the hemoglobin in a gene.

- **Hydroxyl end:** The hydroxyl group that is attached to the 3' carbon atom of the sugar (ribose or deoxyribose) of the terminal nucleotide of a nucleic acid molecule.

- **Hydroxylation reaction:** A chemical reaction in which one or more hydroxyl groups (the –OH group) is introduced (i.e. is chemically attached) to a molecule.

- **Hyperchromicity:** The increase in optical density that occurs when DNA is denatured.

- **Hypermutation:** Describes the introduction of somatic mutations in a rearranged immunoglobulin gene. The mutations can change the sequence of the corresponding antibody, especially in its antigen-binding site.

- **Hyperploid:** A genetic condition in which a chromosome or a segment of a chromosome is over-represented in the genotype.

- **Hypersensitive response:** A protective/defensive response by certain plants to "infection" by plant pathogens (bacteria, fungi, etc.), in which those plant cells that are immediately adjacent (to the infected area of plant) are "instructed" to self-destruct via apoptosis, in order to cordon off the infected area (to prevent further spread of the infection). The initiation of the hypersensitive response is often triggered by signaling molecules that are produced by the pathogens themselves. For example, one particular protein produced by the soil fungus triggers a hypersensitive response that often is so severe that the entire plant dies.

- **Hypersensitive site:** A short region of chromatin detected by its extreme sensitivity to cleavage by DNAase I and other nucleases; it comprises an area from which nucleosomes are excluded.

- **Hypertonic:** A solution with an osmotic potential greater than that of living cells leading to water loss from shrinkage or plasmolysis of cells in a hypertonic situation.

- **Hypervariable regions:** An immunoglobulin are the parts of the variable region that show maximum alteration when different antibodies are compared.

- **Hypochlorite:** Generic term for aqueous solutions of sodium hypochlorite, potassium hypochlorite or calcium hypochlorite which are oxidizing agents and used for disinfecting surfaces and surface sterilizing tissues and for bleaching.
- **Hypocotyl:** Portion of an embryo or seedling below the cotyledons which is a transitional area between stem and root.
- **Hypomorph:** A mutation that reduces but does not completely abolish gene expression.
- **Hypoplastic:** Reduction in plant growth or development (dwarfing, stunting) resulting from an abnormal condition associated with a disease or nutritional stress.
- **Hypoploid:** A genetic condition in which a chromosome or segment of a chromosome is under represented in the genotype.
- **Hypostasis:** Interaction between nonallelic genes in which one gene will not be expressed in the presence of a second.
- **Hypothalamic peptides:** Peptides generated in the vertebrate forebrain and is concerned with regulating the body's physiological state.
- **Hypothalamus:** A part of the brain structure, lying near the base of the brain, it regulates a number of hormones. As a part of the brain, it constantly receives (neurochemical) signals from nerve cells (neurons). The hypothalamus monitors those signals, and converts them into hormonal signals [e.g. it generates a "burst" of hormones in response to certain visual stimuli, certain physical (e.g. sexual) stimuli, etc.]. Also, the hypothalamus is able to monitor and detect changes in the blood levels of hormones coming from endocrine glands. For example, the metabolic hormone insulin (from the pancreas) and the reproductive hormone estrogen (from the ovaries) both trigger changes in function in the hypothalamus. The hypothalamus regulates biological processes (metabolic rate, appetite, etc.). A major function of the hypothalamus is to control reproduction, via secretion of gonadotropin- releasing hormone (GnRH) from the tips of hypothalamic nerve fibers that extend downward toward (into) the pituitary gland. Similarly, hypothalamus also helps to control the body's growth (from birth until the end of puberty) via secretion of growth hormone-releasing factor (GhRF) to the pituitary gland.

- **Hypothesis:** A tentative theory or supposition, provisionally adopted to explain certain facts and to guide in the investigation of other facts. Once proven by rigorous scientific investigation it becomes a theory or a law.
- **Hypotonic:** Osmotic potential less than that of living cells. Cells placed in a hypotonic solution display swelling and turgidity.

H

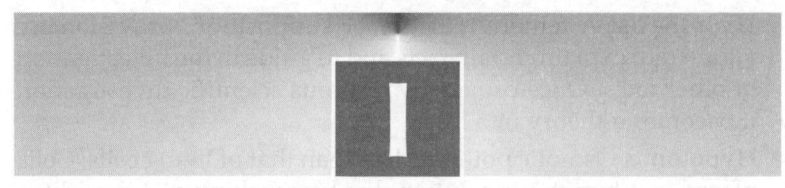

- **IAPs** are inhibitors of apoptosis. They function by antagonizing the actions of caspases.
- **ICAM:** Intercellular adhesion molecule.
- **Icosahedral symmetry:** It is typical of viruses that have capsids that are polyhedrons.
- **IDA:** Acronym for Iron Deficiency Anemia.
- **IDE:** "Investigational device exemption" application to the Food and drug administration (FDA) seeking approval to begin clinical studies of a new medical device.
- **Ideal protein concept:** A concept where the amino acids pattern (defined as a percentage of lysine) maximizes growth, nitrogen retention or another response criterion. In this profile, all inter-dispensable amino acids are equally limiting for performance, just covering the requirements for all physiological functions.
- **Ideogram:** A diagrammatic representation of the G-banding pattern of a chromosome.
- **Idiotype:** The region of the antibody molecule that enables each antibody to recognize a specific foreign structure (i.e. epitope or hapten) is said to have an idiotype (for that epitope or hapten). An identifying characteristic (or property) of the epitope or hapten that one is talking about.
- **Idling reaction:** The production of pppGpp and ppGpp by ribosomes when an uncharged tRNA is present in the A site; triggers the stringent response.
- **IF-1:** A bacterial initiation factor that stabilizes the initiation complex.
- **IF-2:** A bacterial initiation factor that binds the initiator tRNA to the initiation complex.
- **IF-3:** A bacterial initiation factor required for 30S subunits to bind to the initiation sites in mRNA. It also prevents 30S subunits from binding to 50S subunits.
- **IFN-alpha:** Alpha-interferon.

- **IFN-beta:** Beta-interferon.
- **Illuminate:** To supply or brighten with light. Illumination is an absolute requirement for tissue culture. Fluorescent lights are commonly employed. The light intensity is dependent on the light source and the requirements of the culture.
- **Imaginal disk:** A mass of cells in the larvae of *Drosophila* and other holometabolous insects that gives rise to particular adult organs such as antennae eyes or wings.
- **Imbibition:** The absorption of liquid or vapour into the ultramicroscopic spaces or pores found in materials.
- **Immediate early phage genes:** A viral gene in lambda phage is equivalent to the early class of other phages. They are transcribed immediately upon infection by the host RNA polymerase.
- **Immobilization:** Attachment of cells or protoplasts into a matrix.
- **Immobilized cells:** Cells entrapped in matrices such as alginate, polyacrylamide and agarose designed for use in membrane and filter bioreactors.
- **Immobilized enzymes:** An enzyme physically localized in a defined region enabling it to be reused in a continuous process.
- **Immortalization:** It describes the acquisition by a eukaryotic cell line the ability to grow through an indefinite number of divisions in culture.
- **Immortalizing oncogene:** A gene that upon transfection enables a primary cell to grow indefinitely in culture.
- **Immune response:** An organism's reaction, mediated by components of the immune system, to an antigen.
- **Immunity region:** A segment of the phage genome that enables a prophage to inhibit additional phage of the same type from infecting the bacterium. This region has a gene that encodes for the repressor, as well as the sites to which the repressor binds.
- **Immunity:** The ability of organism to resist diseases, either through the activities of specilized blood cells or antobaloes produced by them in response to nature eryosure or inocalation.
- **Immunization:** The production of immunity in an individual by artificial means. Active immunization involves the introduction either orally or by infection of specially treated bacteria, viruses or their toxins so as to stimulate the production of antibodies.
- **Immunoaffinity chromatography:** A purification technique in which an antibody is bound to a matrix and is subsequently used to bind and separate a protein from a complex mixture.

- **Immunoassay:** The use of antibodies to identify and quantify (measure) substances by a variety of methods. The binding of antibodies to antigen (substance being measured) is often followed by tracers, such as fluorescence or (radioactive) radioisotopes, to enable measurement of the substance.
- **Immunochemical control:** Use of immune agents to combat infections.
- **Immunoconjugate:** A molecule that has been formed by attachment of two originally different molecules. One of these is generally an antibody; hence, the word "immunoconjugate". Classic organic drug molecules such as methotrexate, adriamycin chlorambucil, etc. radionuclides; enzymes; toxins; and ribosome-inhibiting proteins may be conjugated to antibodies. The salient point is that the antibody portion of the conjugate is there to "steer" the biologically active molecule to its target.
- **Immunocontraception:** Any process or procedure in which an organism's immune system is utilized to attack or inactivate the reproductive cells (like sperm) within the organism.
- **Immunodiagnostics:** The use of certain antibodies to detect and measure a substance. Useful in diagnosing infectious diseases and could be used to detect tumor cells in the future.
- **Immunogenicity:** The ability to elicit an immune response.
- **Immunoglobulin (IgA, IgE, IgG, and IgM):** A class of (blood) serum proteins representing antibodies. Often used, alongwith the more specific monoclonal antibodies, in health diagnostic reagents. In certain people genetically predisposed to foodborne allergies, immunoglobulin-E (IgE) initiates an immune system response to antigen(s) present on protein molecule(s) in the particular food to which that person is allergic. Severe allergic reactions to foods may lead to death.
- **Immunosensor:** A biosensor having an antibody as biological part.
- **Immunosuppression:** The suppression of immune response. Immune suppression is necessary following organ transplants in order to prevent the host rejecting the grafted organ.
- **Immunosuppressor:** A substance, an agent or a condition that prevents or diminishes the immune response.
- **Immunosuppressive:** That suppresses the immune system response (e.g. certain chemicals).
- **Immunotherapy:** The concept of using the immune system to treat disease. For example, developing a vaccine against cancer.

Immunotherapy may also refer to the therapy of diseases caused by the immune system, for example allergies.

- **Immunotoxin:** A conjugate formed by attaching a toxic molecule (e.g. ricin) to an agent of the immune system (e.g. a monoclonal antibody), that is specific for the pathogen or tumor to be killed. The immune system-agent portion (of the conjugate) delivers the toxic chemical directly to the specified (disease) site, thus sparing other healthy tissues from the effect of the toxin.
- **Impeller:** An agitator that is used for mixing the contents of a bioreactor.
- **Importins:** Transport receptors that bind cargo molecules in the cytoplasm and translocate into the nucleus, where they release the cargo.
- **Imprecise excision:** Occurs when transposon removes itself from the original insertion site, but leaves behind some of its sequence.
- **Imprinting:** A cellular process in which certain genes within an organism's cells are "disabled" during the earliest stage(s) of the organism's development. For example, the embryo of a female mammal (which receives two copies of the X chromosome—one from each parent) disables one of those copies, at random, in each of its cells, so the female becomes a genetic mixture of its two parents.
- **Imprinting:** It describes a change in a gene that occurs during passage through the sperm or egg with the result that the paternal and material alleles have different properties in the very early embryo. May be caused by methylation of DNA.
- *In silico* **biology:** Refers to computational models of biology. In *silico* is an expression used to mean performed on a computer or via computer simultation. It is used in system biology.
- *In silico* **screening:** Computationl approach which have the potential to increase the global R and D productivity in pharmaceutical industry, in particular to speed up the identification of targets, hits, and decrease the attrition rate.
- *In situ* **hybridization:** The use of a DAN or RNA probe to detect complementary genetic material in cells or tissue. *In situ* hybridization involves hybridizing a labeled nucleic acid to suitably prepared cells or tissues on microscope slides to allow visualization *in situ* (in normal location).
- *In situ*: It means 'in original or natural place'.

- *In vitro* **complementation assay:** It consists of identifying a component of a wild-type cell that can confer activity on an extract prepared from a mutant cell. The assay identifies the component rendered inactive by the mutation.
- *In vitro* **mutagenesis:** The production of either random or specific mutations in a piece of cloned DNA. Typically, the DNA will then be repackaged and introduced into a cell or an organism to assess the results of the mutagenesis.
- *In vitro* **selection:** A search process (e.g. for a new pharmaceutical) that first involves the construction of a large "pool" of polynucleotide sequences (at least some of which are likely to possess the desired pharmaceutical properties), synthesized by a totally random process. This is followed by repeated cycles of screening (for those sequences possessing desired properties) and/or enriching, and amplification (of the screened/enriched sequences). Common amplification techniques include polymerase chain reaction (PCR), ligase chain reaction (LCR), selfsustained sequence replication (SSR), Q-beta replicase technique, and strand displacement amplification (SDA).
- *In vitro* **translation:** Protein synthesis directed by purified DNA with bacterial extracts or mRNA that provide ribosomes, tRNA and protein synthesis factors. The reaction mixture is supplemented with ATP, GTP and amino acids.
- *In vitro*: In glass, as in a test tube. An *in vitro* test is one that is done in glass or plastic vessels in the laboratory.
- *In vivo*: The natural conditions in which organisms live.
- **Inactivated agent:** A virus, bacterium or other organism that has been treated to prevent it from causing a disease.
- **Inbred line:** The product of inbreeding i.e. the mating of individuals that have ancestors in common.
- **Inbreeding:** Mating between individuals that have one or more ancestors in common. The extreme condition being self-fertilization which occurs in many plants and some primitive animals.
- **Inbreeding depression:** Reduction in vigour, yield, etc. of a population that is commonly seen as the level of inbreeding increases. The traits that shows greatest inbreeding depression are those that are most closely associated with viability and reproductive ability.
- **Incision:** It is a step in a mismatch excision repair system. An endonuclease recognizes the damaged area in the DNA, and isolate it by cutting the DNA strand on both sides of the damage.

- **Inclusion body:** Protein that is overproduced in a recombinant bacterium and forms a crystalline array inside the bacterial cell.
- **Incompatibility:** The inability of certain bacterial plasmids to coexist in the same cell. It is a cause of plasmid immunity.
- **Incomplete dominance:** Intermediate phenotype in F_1, one allele of a heterozygous pair only partially dominates the expression of its partner, red (RR) and white (rr) flowered snapdragon plants produce pink-flowered (Rr) offspring, this does not support a blending theory, parental phenotypes reappear in F_2 generation, color is determined at a single locus, level of gene-directed protein production may be between that of the two homozygotes.
- **Incomplete linkage:** Occasional separation of two genes on the same chromosome by a recombination event.
- **Incomplete penetrance:** When some individuals in a population have a specific genotype that causes an abnormality, but are not affected.
- **Incubation:** The hatching of eggs by means of heat either natural or artificial.
- **Incubator:** An apparatus in which environmental conditions (light, photoperiod, temperature, humidity, etc.) are fully controlled and used for hatching eggs, multiplying micro-organisms, culturing plants, etc. of culture room growth cabinet.
- **IND:** "Investigational new drug" application to the Food and Drug Administration (FDA) seeking approval to begin clinical studies of a new pharmaceutical.
- **Indehiscent:** Describing a fruit or fruiting body that does not open to release its seeds or spores when ripe.
- **Independent assortment:** The random distribution of alleles (from different loci) to the gametes that occurs when genes are located in different chromosomes or far apart on large chromosomes. The distribution of alleles at one locus is independent of the distribution of alleles at another locus.
- **Indeterminate growth:** Unlimited growth potential for a definite or indefinite period. Some apical meristems can produce unrestricted number of lateral organs. In legumes, used to describe plant architecture.
- **Indian department of biotechnology:** The governmental body in India that regulates all recombinant DNA research. It is the Indian counterpart of the American government's recombinant DNA advisory committee (RAC), the Australian government's

Gene technology regulator (GTR), and the French government's Commission of biomolecular engineering.

- **Indirect embryogenesis:** Embryo formation on callus tissues derived from zygotic or somatic embryos, seedling plant or other tissues in culture.
- **Indirect end-labeling:** A technique for examining the organization of DNA by making a cut at a specific site and isolating all fragments containing the sequence adjacent to one side of the cut; it reveals the distance from the cut to the next break(s) in DNA.
- **Indirect organogenesis:** Organ formation on callus tissues derived from explants.
- **Induced fit:** A substrate-induced change in the shape of an enzyme molecule that causes the catalytically functional groups of the enzyme to assume positions that are optimal for catalytic activity to occur.
- **Induced mutations:** A mutation that is produced by treatment with a physical or chemical agent that affects the deoxyribonucleic acid molecules of a living organism.
- **Inducer exclusion:** Describes the inhibition of uptake of other carbon sources into the cell that is caused by uptake of glucose.
- **Inducer:** A small molecule (for example lactose) whose introduction into the medium increases the transcription of an operon (lac operon).
- **Inducible enzymes:** Enzymes whose rate of production can be increased by the presence of certain chemical molecules.
- **Inducible:** Operon is expressed only in the presence of a specific small molecule (the inducer).
- **Induction of prophage:** The mechanism by which latent viruses, such as genetically transmitted tumor viruses (proviruses) or prophages of lysogenic bacteria are induced to replicate and then released as infectious viruses.
- **Induction:** It refers to the ability of bacteria (or yeast) to synthesize certain enzymes only when their substrates are present; applied to gene expression, refers to switching on transcription as a result of interaction of the inducer with the regulator protein.
- **Induction media:** Media used to induce the formation of organs or other structures.
- **Industrial Biotechnology Association (IBA):** An American trade association of companies involved in biotechnology.

Formed in 1981, the IBA tended to consist of the larger firms involved in biotechnology. In 1993, the industrial biotechnology association (IBA) was merged with the association of biotechnology companies (ABC) to form the Biotechnology Industry organization (BIO).

- **Inert:** A support structure that makes no chemical contribution and whose only function is to support physiologically. It is a neutral or immobile unit.

- **Infection:** The invasion of any living organisms by disease-causing microorganisms which proceed to establish themselves, multiply and form tissues of particular structure and function.

- **Informational molecules:** Molecules containing information in the form of specific sequences of different building blocks. They include protein and nucleic acids.

- **Ingestion:** Taking a substance into the body. For example, amoeba surrounds a food particle, then ingests the particle.

- **Inhibition:** The suppression of the biological function of an enzyme or system by chemical or physical means.

- **Initiation codon:** AUG-three base sequence in mRNA which specifies methionine, the first amino acid.

- **Initiation complex:** Complex is in bacterial protein synthesis contains a small ribosome subunit, initiation factors, and initiator aminoacyl-tRNA bound to mRNA at an AUG initiation codon.

- **Initiation:** Describe the stages of transcription up to the synthesis of the first bond in RNA. This includes binding of RNA polymerase to the promoter and melting a short region of DNA into single strands.

- **Initiation factors (If in prokaryotes, eIF in eukaryotes):** Proteins that associate with the small subunit of the ribosome specifically at the stage of initiation of protein synthesis.

- **Innate immunity:** It is the rapid response mediated by cells with nonvarying (germline-encoded) receptors that recognize pathogen. The cells of the innate immune response act to eliminate the pathogen and initiate the adaptive immune response.

- **Inner core:** It is an intermediate in the synthesis of N-linked oligosaccharides. It is produced upon the removal of mannose residues from a high mannose oligosaccharide in the *cis* golgi and is resistant to degradation by endoglycosidase H.

- **Inoculate:** Deliberately introduce something into. The process is inoculation. Not the same as contamination. In bacteriology, tissue culture etc. placing inoculum into (or onto) medium to initiate a culture. In immunology, to immunize.
- **Inoculation cabinet:** Small room or cabinet for inoculation (of tissue or microorganism cultures) operations often with a current of sterile air to carry contaminations away from the work area.
- **Inoculum:** A culture containing viable cells of microorganism. A small piece of tissue cut from callus or an explant from a tissue or organ or a small amount of cell material from a suspension culture transferred into or onto fresh medium for continued growth of the culture.
- **Inorganic compound:** A chemical compound that generally is not derived from living process compounds that do not contain carbon.
- **Inositol:** A cyclic acid that is constituent of certain cell phosphoglycerides. A water soluble nutrient frequently referred to as a 'vitamin' in plant tissue culture. Also acts as a growth factor in some animals and microorganisms.
- **Inositol liquid:** A membrane anchored phospholipid that transduces hormonal signals by stimulating the release of any of several chemical messengers.
- **Inr:** The sequence of a pol II promoter between −3 and +5 and has the general sequence Py2CAPy5. It is the simplest possible pol II promoter.
- **Insecticide:** A substance that kill insects.
- **Insert DNA:** A DNA molecule incorporated into a cloning vector.
- **Insertion element:** Genetic term for DNA sequences found in bacteria capable of genome insertion. Postulated to be responsible for site-specific phage and plasmid integration.
- **Insertion mutations:** Changes in the base sequence of a DNA molecule resulting from the random integration of DNA from another source.
- **Insertion sequence:** A small DNA sequence carrying gene for transposase enzyme for its transposition. A mobile piece of bacterial DNA (several hundred nucleotide pairs in length) that is capable of inactivating a gene into which it inserts.
- **Insertion site:** A unique restriction site in a vector DNA molecule into which foreign DNA can be be inserted.

- **Insertions:** A rare non-reciprocal translocation involving three breaks in which a segment in removed from one chromosome and then inserted into a broken region of a non-homologous chromosome.
- **Instability:** A random type variation or a lack of steadiness. Due to genetic instability, cell lines lose certain characteristics or functions in culture.
- **Instructive:** A gene or protein that plays an **instructive** role in development is one that gives a signal telling the cell what to do.
- **Insulator:** A sequence that prevents an activating or inactivating effect passing from one side to the other.
- **Insulin:** A peptide hormone secreted by the Langerhans islets of the pancreas, and regulates the level of sugar in the blood.
- **Insulin-dependent diabetes mellitus (IDDM):** An autoimmune disease in which the insulin-producing cells of the pancreas (i.e. beta (β) cells, also known as Islets of Langerhans) are attacked and destroyed by the cytotoxic T-cells of the body's immune system.
- **Insulin-like growth factor-1 (IGF-1):** A protein hormone produced by the body's bone cells (when stimulated by parathyroid hormone and/or estrogen), that is a promoter of bone formation and follicle development (in ovaries). Another function of IGF-1 is to facilitate the transport of amino acids into cells, and further inhibit protein breakdown in cells. If the body is injured, IGF-1 works with platelets derived growth factor (PDGF) to stimulate fibroblast and collagen cell division/metabolism to cause healing of wounds and bones. IGF-1 also occurs naturally in cow's milk.
- **Intasome:** A protein-DNA complex between the phage lambda integrase (Int) and the phage lambda attachment site *(attP).*
- **Integral membrane protein:** A protein (non-covalently) inserted into a membrane; it retains its membranous association by means of a stretch of ~ 25 amino acids that are uncharged and/or hydrophobic.
- **Integrant (stable transfectant):** A cell line in which a gene introduced by transfection has become integrated into the genome.
- **Integrase:** An enzyme that is responsible for a site-specific recombination hand inserts one molecule of DNA into another.
- **Integrated pest management (IPM):** An ecosystem-based strategy that focuses on long- term prevention of pests or their

damage through a combination of techniques such as biological control habitat manipulation, modification of cultural practices and use of resistant varieties.

- **Integrating vector:** A vector that is designed to integrate cloned DNA into the host cell chromosomal DNA.
- **Integration:** Incorporation of the genetic material of a virus into the host genome.
- **Integrins:** A class of proteins found on the surface (membranes) of cells, and that function as cellular adhesion receptors. For example, integrin avb3 is a receptor on the surface of endothelial cells in tumors. It binds angiogenic endothelial cells, enabling them to form new blood vessels.
- **Integument:** One of the layers that enclosed the ovule and is the precursor of the seed coat.
- **Inteins:** Selfish DNA elements (genetic elements) found within coding regions (protein coding sequences). They are translated with their host protein, but then catalyze their own excision and the formation of a peptide bond between their flanking protein regions. The intein protein domain is approximately 140 amino acid long and is sufficient for carrying out the protein splicing reaction.
- **Intellectual property rights:** Patents, copyrights and trademarks.
- **Intensifying screen:** A plastic sheet impregnated with a rare earth compound such as calcium tungstate which absorbs radiation and emits light.
- **Interaction:** In statistics, an effect that cannot be explained by the additive action of contributing factors, a departure from strict additively.
- **Interallelic complementation:** It describes the change in the properties of a heteromultimeric protein brought about by the interaction of subunits coded by two different mutant alleles; the mixed protein may be more or less active than the protein consisting of subunits only of one or the other type.
- **Interbands:** Relatively dispersed regions of polytene chromosomes that lie between the bands.
- **Intercalary:** Growth between the upper branches and the lower branchesorbracts on a stem.
- **Intercalary growth:** A pattern of stem elongation, typical of grasses. Elongation proceeds from the lower internodes to the

upper internodes through the differentiation of meristematic tissue at the base of each internode.

- **Intercalating agent:** A chemical capable of inserting between adjacent base pairs in a DNA molecule.

- **Intercellular space:** Pore space between cells especially typical of leaf tissues.

- **Intercistronic region:** Any of the DNA in between gene-coding DNA, including untranslated regions, 5' and 3' flanking regions, introns, non-functional pseudogenes, and non-functional repetitive sequences. This DNA may or may not encode regulatory functions.

- **Interfascicular cambium:** Cambium that arises between vascular bundles.

- **Interference:** A measure of the degree to which one crossover interferes with the chances of another crossover in an adjacent region of the same chromatid. Positive interference reduces the probability of another crossover; negative interference increases the chances of a second crossover event.

- **Interferon:** A glycoprotein produced by a virus-infected cells which protect another cell from attack of the virus.

- **Intergeneric:** A cross between two different genera.

- **Intergenic regions:** DNA sequences located between genes that comprise a large percentage of the human genome with no known function.

- **Interim office of the gene technology regulator (IOGTR):** The regulatory body of Australia's government that was responsible for approvals of new rDNA products (e.g. new genetically engineered crops) before they could be introduced in Australia, during 1999–2001. IOGTR replaced/superceded Australia's Gene Technology Office (in this role) in 1999, and was itself scheduled to be replaced by the Gene Technology Regulator (GTR) in 2001.

- **Interleukin-1 (IL-1):** A cytokine (glycoprotein) released by activated macrophages, during the inflammatory stage of immune system response to an infection, which promotes the growth of epithelial (skin) cells and white blood cells. Recent research has indicated that too much IL-1 is linked to the development of rheumatoid arthritis, diabetes, inflammatory bowel disease, and other autoimmune diseases.

- **Interleukin-1 receptor antagonist (IL-1ra):** A glycoprotein (produced by macrophages in response to presence of Interleukin-1, and endotoxin in tissues) that preferentially binds to those cell receptors in the body that typically bind the lymphokine, Interleukin-1(IL-1). When manufactured by man (via genetic engineering) and injected into the body in large quantities, IL-1ra can block the deleterious effects of (too much) Interleukin-1.

- **Interleukin-2 (IL-2):** Known as T-cell growth factor. A cytokine (glycoprotein) secreted by (immune system response) stimulated helper T-cells which promotes the proliferation/differentiation of more helper T-cells, and promotes the growth of lymphocytes to combat an infection. Interleukin-2 also stimulates the lymphocytes to produce gamma interferon. It is gamma interferon that prompts the cytotoxic T-cells to attack virus-infected cells and kill the virus within them. The structure of the gene that codes for synthesis of IL-2 (by immune system cells) was determined by Tadatsugu Taniguchi in 1983.

- **Interleukin-3 (IL-3):** A hematologic growth factor (glycoprotein) cytokine that stimulates the proliferation of a wide range of white blood cells (to combat an infection).

- **Interleukin-4 (IL-4):** A cytokine (glycoprotein) that stimulates production of antibody producing B cells, immunoglobulin-E (IgE), and promotes cytotoxic T-cell (i.e. killer T-cells) growth.

- **Interleukin-5 (IL-5):** A cytokine (glycoprotein) that stimulates eosinophil growth.

- **Interleukin-6 (IL-6):** A cytokine (glycoprotein) that is pleiotropic (i.e. stimulates several different types of immune system cells), and is a hematopoietic growth factor.

- **Interleukin-7 (IL-7):** A cytokine (glycoprotein) synthesized in the bone marrow that stimulates early (fetal) proliferation and differentiation of B-cells and T-cells. May be useful in regenerating lymphoid cells in patients whose immune systems have been devastated by cancer chemotherapy.

- **Interleukin-8 (IL-8):** A basic polypeptide (glycoprotein) with heparin-binding activity. Endogenous endothelial IL-8 appears to regulate transvenular traffic during acute inflammatory responses.

- **Interleukin-9 (IL-9):** A cytokine (glycoprotein) that is released at sites in the body where inflammation has occurred.

- **Intermediary metabolism:** The chemical reactions that take place in the cell and transform the complex molecules derived from food into the small molecules, needed for the growth and maintenance of the cell.

- **Intermediate component (s):** A reassociation reaction, those reacting between the fast (satellite DNA) and slow (non-repetitive DNA) components; contain moderately repetitive DNA.

- **Internalization:** A process through which a ligand-receptor complex is brought into the cell.

- **International Food Biotechnology Council (IFBC):** An organization that was established in 1988 by the Industrial Biotechnology Association (IBA) and the International Life Sciences Institute (ILSI), in order to "produce a (recommended) set of guidelines that could be used to assess the safety of genetically altered foods."

- **International Life Sciences Institute (ILSI):** A nonprofit foundation established in 1978 to advance the understanding of scientific issues relating to nutrition, food safety, toxicology, risk assessment, and the environment. ILSI is headquartered in Washington, D.C. and has branches in Argentina, Australia, Brazil, Europe, India, Japan, Korea, Mexico, Africa, Thailand, Singapore, China, and other nations.

- **International office of epizootics (OIE):** One of the three international SPS standard setting organizations recognized by the World Trade Organization (WTO), the OIE is an International Veterinary Organization Headquartered in Paris. The OIE was established in 1924, originally as part of the League of Nations, and is the worldwide authority for development of animal health and zoonoses standards, guidelines, and recommendations.

- **International plant protection convention (IPPC):** One of the three international SPS standard-setting organizations recognized by the World Trade Organization (WTO), the IPPC is the worldwide authority for development of plant health standards, guidelines, and recommendations (e.g. to prevent transfer of a plant disease or plant pest from one country to another). The treaty establishing the IPPC was signed in 1952 (amended in 1979 and 1997), and currently has 107 member countries (i.e. signatories to the 1979 text). The IPPC Secretariat is within the United Nations' Food and Agriculture Organization (FAO). IPPC standards are set (and enforced) via regional SPS institutions such as North American Plant Protection Organization (NAPPO), European Plant Protection Organization (EPPO), etc. There are currently nine RPPOs (i.e. regional plant protection organizations) under Article VIII of the 1979 IPPC text.

- **International society for the advancement of biotechnology (ISAB):** A nonprofit organization of individuals that was started in 1994 "to advance and promote the general welfare of science and commercialization of genetic engineering and industrial biotechnology".
- **Internode:** The region of a stem between two successive nodes.
- **Interphase:** The period of mitotic cell division; divided into G1, S, and G2.
- **Intersex:** An organism displaying a mixture of male and female attributes.
- **Interspecific:** An interspecific cross is a cross between two different species.
- **Interspersed repeats:** Originally defined as short sequences that are common and widely distributed in the genome. They are now known to consist of transposable elements.
- **Intervening:** Intervening sequence is an intron.
- **Intracellular:** Occuring within a cell.
- **Intracytoplasmic sperm injection (ICSI):** The injection using micromanipulation of a single sperm into the cytoplasm of a mature oocyte.
- **Intrageneric:** Within a genus such as hybrid resulting from a cross between species within one genus.
- **Intragenic complementation:** Complementation that occurs between two mutant alleles of a gene common only when the product of the gene functions as a homomultimer.
- **Intraspecific:** Within a species or its population including subspecies such as an intraspecific cross or variation.
- **Intrinsic terminators:** These are able to terminate transcription by bacterial RNA polymerase in the absence of any additional factors.
- **Introgression:** The incorporation of exotic (i.e. wild type) genes into elite germplasm (i.e. domesticated breeding lines), or of transgenes (i.e. genes from transgenic organisms) into a wild type's genome.

- **Intron:** Describes the process when a pair of splicing sites are recognized by interactions involving only the 5' site and the branch point/3' site.
- **Intron homing:** Describes the ability of certain introns to insert themselves into a target DNA. The reaction is specific for a single target sequence.
- **Intron:** A portion of DNA between coding regions in a gene that is transcribed, but does not appear in the final mRNA product.
- **Inulin:** A fructose oligosaccharide (FOS) that is naturally produced in more than 30,000 plants. Like many other FOS, consumption of inulin by humans results in several health benefits (helps prevent coronary heart disease, promote growth of bifidobacteria in the intestines, reduce likelihood of developing diabetes, promote absorption of calcium from foods, etc.). Need consideration to be a part of meaning.
- **Invariant:** Base positions in tRNA have the same nucleotide virtually in all (>95%) of tRNAs.
- **Invasin:** A transmembrane (through the membrane of the cell) protein that enables bacterial cells to invade normal (body) cells.
- **Inversion:** A segment that gets separated from the chromosome and is reinserted at the same place but in reverse order; the position and sequence of the genes are altered.
- **Invasiveness:** Ability of a plant to spread beyond its introduction site and become established in new locations, where it may have a deleterious effect on organisms already existing there.
- **Inverted repeat:** Two nearby DNA sequences in opposite strands are same when read in 5' to 3' direction.
- **Inverted terminal repeats:** The short related or identical sequences present in reverse orientation at the end of some transposons.
- **Ion channel:** A transmembrane protein which selectively allows the passage of one type of ion across the membrane. Ion channels are usually oligomers with a central aqueous pore through which the ion passes.
- **Ion:** From the Greek *ion*, means something that goes. An ion is an atom or molecule possessing a positive or a negative electrical charge. Ions are produced by the dissociation (coming apart) of a (electrolyte) molecule resulting from an electrolyte dissolving in a solution. One example is the dissociation of common table salt (sodium chloride) in water, which results in positively charged sodium ions (called cations) and negatively charged

chloride ions (called anions). Ions play critically important roles in many biological processes such as nerve activity.

- **Ion selectivity:** The specificity of an ion channel for a particular type of ion.
- **Ion-exchange chromatography:** Separation of ionic compounds (which include nucleic acids and proteins) in a chromatographic column containing a polymeric resin (i.e. the stationary phase) having fixed charge groups. The process works in that the charges of the column (stationary phase) interact with the opposite charges of the material dissolved in the solution that is flows through the column (mobile phase). The charge interaction between the column material, i.e. the protein, has the effect of slowing down the rate of movement of the protein through the column. The other molecules, meanwhile, which do not interact with the column, flow right on through. This constitutes the separation process.
- **Ionic bonds:** Attractions between oppositely charged chemical groups.
- **Ionizing radiation:** The portion of the electromagnetic spectrum that results in the production of positive and negative charges (ion pairs) in molecules; X-rays and gamma rays are examples of ionizing radiation.
- **IP-6:** Inositol hexaphosphate.
- **IPTG:** An inducer of the lac (lactose) operon. In recombinant DNA technology. IPTG is often used to induce cloned genes that are under the control of the lac-repressor lac-promoter system.
- **Iron deficiency anemia (IDA):** A disease caused by lack of iron in an organism's body, due to shortfall in diet or due to dietary iron not being bioavailable (digestible) to that organism's body. For example, the phytate naturally present in traditional varieties of corn (maize) inhibits absorption of the iron in that corn (maize) by humans, swine, and poultry. IDA is a major cause of childhood diseases and maternal death (i.e. death of the mother following childbirth) in many developing countries. IDA also makes people more susceptible to diphtheria.
- **Irradiation:** Exposure to any form of radiation. Treatment with a ray such as ultraviolet rays etc.
- **IS element:** An abbreviation for insertion sequence (IS), a small bacterial transposon carrying only the genetic functions involved in transposition.

- **Islets of Langerhans:** (also called beta cells) Cells in the pancreas that produce insulin in response to the presence of glucose (sugar) in the bloodstream. The failure of insulin production results in the disease called diabetes.
- **Isoaccepting tRNAs:** Isoaccepting tRNAs represent the same amino acid.
- **Isoalleles:** Different forms of a gene that produce the same phenotype or very similar phenotypes.
- **Isochromosome:** A chromosome with two identical arms and identical genes. The arms are mirror images of each other.
- **Isocratic elution:** Elution with a solvent mixture of constant composition.
- **Isodiametric:** Term commonly used to describe cells with equal diameters.
- **Isoelectric focussing:** The ordering and concentration of substances according to their isoelectric points.
- **Isoelectric point:** The pH at which a substance has a zero net charge.
- **Isoflavones:** 3-phenychromone; isomeric form of flavonoids in which the benzene group is attached to the 3 position of the benzopyran ring instead of the 2-position.
- **Isoform:** A member of a family of closely related proteins that have some amino acid sequences in common and some different.
- **Isogamy:** Sexual reproduction involving the fusion of gametes that are similar in size and structure.
- **Isogenic stocks:** Strains of organisms which are genetically identical.
- **Isolating mechanism:** Any of the biological properties of organisms that prevent interbreeding (and therefore exchange of genetic material) between members of different species inhabiting the same geographical area.
- **Isolation medium:** An optimum medium suitable for explants survival, growth and development.
- **Isoleucine (Ile):** A monocarboxylic amino acid occurring within most dietary proteins.
- **Isomer:** One of the two or more chemical substances having the same elementary percentage composition (i.e. same atoms) and molecular weight, but differing in structure and therefore in properties. There are many ways in which such structural differences (between the two or more isomeric molecules) occur.

One example is n-butane $[CH_3(CH_2)_2CH_3]$ and isobutane $[CH_3CH(CH_3)_2]$.

- **Isomerase:** An enzyme-catalyzing transformation of a compound into its positional isomer.
- **Isoprene:** The five-carbon hydrocarbon molecule, 2-methyl-1,3 butadiene. It is a recurring structural unit of the terpenoid molecules, which are either linear or cyclic. There exists a very large number of terpenes and many are major components of essential plant oils (Fig. 1).

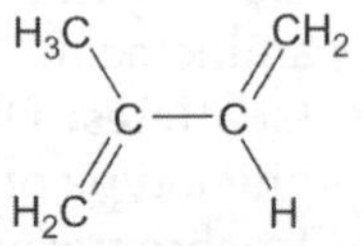

Fig. 1: Isoprene

- **Isoschizomers:** Restriction enzymes that cleave the same DNA sequence but are affected differently by its state of methylation.
- **Isotonic:** Solutions having the same osmotic potential and the same molar concentration. For protoplasts to survive the medium they are suspended in must be isotonic.
- **Isotope:** Refers to one of the several "varieties" of atoms that exist, of the same element, that differ from each other in the number of neutrons in the atom's nucleus. For example, the element chlorine exists primarily in two forms (isotopes) in nature, with 18 neutrons (76% of the time) and with 20 neutrons (24% of the time). The chemical properties of isotopes of a given element are virtually identical.
- **Isotype:** A group of closely related immunoglobulin chains.
- **Isozyme:** Multiple molecular forms of an enzyme that exhibit similar catalytic properties.
- **ISPM:** Acronym for International standards for pest management.

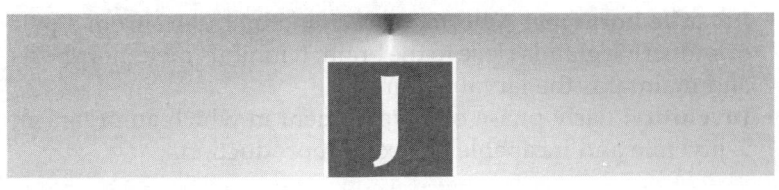

- **J segment:** It is a polypeptide that is integral to the assembly of dimeric IgA and pentameric IgM. It forms disulfide bonds with the immunoglobulin heavy chain.
- **Japan bioindustry association:** An association of the largest Japanese companies that are engaged in atleast some form of genetic engineering research or production. Similar to America's Biotechnology Industry Organization (BIO), it is headquartered in Tokyo.
- **Jasmonic acid:** Jasmonic acid is a signaling molecule in systemic acquired resistance (SAR) when SAR is triggered in plants (via spray application of harpin protein to various plants, via chewing of insects on the leaves of certain plants, and/or via the entry into plant of certain pathogenic bacteria/fungi, etc.).
- **Jiffy pot:** Pots made from wood pulp and peat commonly used for transplanting tissue culture derived plants into soil medium.
- **Joint molecule:** It is a pair of DNA duplexes that are connected together through a reciprocal exchange of genetic material.
- **Joule:** The amount of energy needed to apply a force of 1 newton over a distance of 1 metre.
- **Jumping genes:** Genes that move (change positions) within the genome. These genes are associated with transposable elements, a segment fragment of deoxyribonucleic acid (DNA) that can move from one position in the genome to another.
- *Juncea*: Refers to a group of related plants; often commonly called "wild mustard".
- **Junk DNA:** A term historically utilized, to refer portions of an organism's DNA that were not obviously genes (i.e. not transcribed into mRNA; thus not part of the DNA "tagged" with ESTs, etc.). However, it has recently been discovered that at least some was formerly called "junk DNA" (e.g. introns) helps enable more than one specific protein molecule to be expressed from certain genes.

- **Juvenile hormone:** A hormone secreted by insects from a pair of endocrine glands close to the brain. It inhibits metamorphosis and maintains the larval features.
- **Juvenility:** Early phase of development in which an organism is juvenile and incapable of sexual reproduction.

J

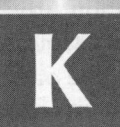

K

- **Kanamycin:** An antibiotic of aminoglycoside family that poisons translation by binding to the ribosomes.
- **Kanr:** Kanamycin resistance gene.
- **Kappa chain:** One of the two classes of antibody light chain.
- **Karnal bunt:** A plant disease that is caused by the smut fungus *Tilletia indica* in wheat.
- **Karyogamy:** The fusion of nuclei or nuclear material, that occurs during sexual reproduction.
- **Karyogram:** A diagram representing the characteristic features of the chromosomes of a species.
- **Karyokinesis:** The division of a cell nucleus.
- **Karyotype:** A size-order alignment of an organism's chromosome pairs in the form of a chart. It enables the correlation of chromosomes to symptoms of diseases (e.g. of genetic diseases in the organism) and traits.
- **Karyotyper:** A scientist (or more frequently an automated analytical machine) that 1. Takes a video picture of a given cell under a microscope 2. Digitizes that picture within a computer 3. "Cuts out" the individual chromosomes contained within that cell's genome 4. Arranges the cell's chromosomes in pairs by size order into a chart (called a karyotype).
- **kb:** Kilobase pairs.
- **K_{cat}:** The catalytic rate constant that characterizes an enzyme catalyzed reaction. The larger the k_{cat} value the faster the conversion of substrate into product.
- **Kefauver rule:** A 1962 US law that mandates that the food and drug administration (FDA) requires proof of pharmaceutical efficacy for drugs to be sold in the US.
- **Kenya Biosafety Council:** The country of Kenya's national regulatory body for granting approval to a new genetically engineered plant (e.g. a new genetically engineered crop to be planted). The Kenya Biosafety Council is analogs to Germany's

ZKBS (Central Commission on Biological Safety), Australia's GMAC (Genetic Manipulation Advisory Committee), or Brazil's CTNBio (National Biosafety Commission).

- **Keratins:** Insoluble protective or structural proteins consisting of parallel polypeptide chains arranged in an α-helical or β-conformation.
- **Ketose:** A simple monosaccharide having its carbonyl groups other than a terminal position.
- **Killer T cells:** T cells that carry T-cell receptors which kill cells, this displaying the recognized antigens.
- **Kilobase (kb):** A unit of length of DNA consisting of 1000 nucleotides.
- **Kilobase pairs (Kbp):** A unit of DNA equals to 1,000 base pairs.
- **Kilocalorie (kcal):** It is equal to 1,000 cal.
- **Kilodalton (Kd):** A unit of mass equal to 1,000 daltons.
- **Kinase:** An enzyme that phosphorylates (add a phosphate group to a substrate), the substrates for protein.
- **Kinases:** Amino acids in other proteins, and there are divided into two specific groups one for tyrosine and other specific for threonine/serine (and histidine in prokaryotes).
- **Kinetics:** The branch of chemistry or biochemistry concerned with measuring and studying the rate of reactions.
- **Kinetic complexity:** The complexity of a DNA component measured by the Kinetics of DNA reassociation.
- **Kinetic proofreading:** Describes a proofreading mechanism that depends on incorrect events proceeding more slowly than correct events, so that incorrect events are reversed before a subunit is added to a polymeric chain.
- **Kinetin:** One of the cytokinins, a group of growth regulators that acteristically promote cell division in plants.
- **Kinetochore:** Structure formed at centromere during mitosis for binding microtubules.
- **Kinetosomes:** Granular cytoplasmic structure which forms the base of a cilium or flagellum of basal body.
- **Kinin (in plant):** A compound that promotes cell division and inhibits ageing in plants (in animals). Any of a group of substances formed in body tissue in response to injury. They are polypeptides and cause vasodilation and smooth muscle contraction.

K

- **Kirromycin:** An antibiotic that inhibits protein synthesis by acting on EF-Tu.
- **Klenow fragment:** A part of bacterial DNA polymerase with polymerase activity but lacks exonuclease acitivity.
- **K_m:** A dissociation constant that characterizes the binding of an enzyme to a substrate. The smaller the value of K_m the tighter the binding of the enzyme to the substrate, also called Michaelis constant.
- **Knockout:** An animal resulting from an embryonic stem cell in which a normal functional gene has been replaced by a non functional form of the gene. This technique is used extensively in mice and much can be learned about the function of a gene by studying the phenotype of animals that lack the peptide product of that gene.
- **Knot in DNA:** An entangled region that cannot be resolved without cutting and rearranging the DNA.
- **Konzo:** A term used in some countries to refer lathyrism.
- **Koseisho:** The Japanese government agency that must approve new pharmaceutical products for sale with Japan. It is equivalent to the US Food and Drug Administration.
- **Kuru:** A human neurological disease caused by prions. It may be caused by eating infected brains.

K

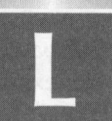

- **Label:** A radioactive compound attached with DNA/RNA to indicate the presence of a complementary DNA strand in a sample.
- **Labeling:** The process of replacing a stable atom in a compound with a radioactive isotope of the same element to enable it to be detected by autoradiography or other techniques. Increasingly, radioactive labeling is being replaced by fluorescent labeling. The method is used to trace the path of the labeled compound through a biological or chemical system.
- **Lac operon:** An operon in *Escherichia coli* (*E. coli*) that codes for three enzymes involved in the metabolism of lactose.
- **Lachrymal fluid (tears):** A salty solution produced by the tear glands to bathe.
- **Lactoferricin:** A protein compound that acts to inhibit pathogenic (disease-causing) bacteria and yeasts (e.g. in the human body).
- **Lactonase:** An enzyme that "breaks open" the lactone ring (molecular structure) in the mycotoxin zearalenone.
- **Lactose:** Milk sugar, a disaccharide with one unit each of glucose and galactose.
- **Lactoperoxidase:** A protein compound (enzyme) that acts to inhibit pathogenic bacteria (e.g. in human body).
- **Lag phase:** Time required by inoculated cells in fresh medium to adapt the new environment before the start of cell division.
- **Lagging strand:** DNA must grow overall in the 3′–5′ direction and is synthesized discontinuously in the form of short fragment (5′–3′) that are later connected covalently.
- **Lambda chain:** Although light chains are found in many multimeric proteins, lambda (λ) chain usually refers to the light chains of immunoglobulins. These are of 22 kd and of one of two types, kappa or lambda. A single immunoglobulin has identical light chains (2 kappa and 2 lambda). Light chains have

one variable and one constant region. There are isotype variants of both kappa and lambda.

- **Lambda phage:** A bacteriophage that infects *Escherichia coli* (*E. coli*). It is commonly used as a vector in recombinant DNA (deoxyribonucleic acid) research.
- **Lamella:** A double membrane plate or vesicle that is formed by two membranes lying parallel to each other.
- **Lamina:** Blade or expanded part of a leaf.
- **Laminar air flow cabinet/hood:** Cabinet for inoculation of cultures. The working area is kept sterile by a continuous non-turbulent flow of sterilizer.
- **Laminarin:** A storage polysaccharide of the brown algae.
- **Lampbrush chromosomes:** The large meiotic chromosomes found in amphibian oocytes.
- **Landrace:** An early cultivated form of a crop species evolved from a wild population.
- **Large subunit (of ribosome):** Involved in peptide bond formation through peptidyl transferase activity (50S in bacteria, 60S in eukaryotes).
- **Lariat:** An intermediate in RNA splicing in which a circular structure with a tail is created by a 5′–2′ bond.
- **Larva:** The active immature form of an insect, forming the stage between egg and pupa.
- **Late endosome:** It is the part of the endosomal compartment in which endocytosed molecules appear after 5 to 10 minutes. Late endosomes are located close to the nucleus, function in delivering molecules to lysosomes, and are more acidic than early endosomes.
- **Late genes:** They are transcribed when phage DNA is being replicated. They code for components of the phage particle.
- **Late infection:** It is the part of the phage lytic cycle from DNA replication to lysis of the cell. During this time, DNA is replicated and structural components of the phage particle are synthesized.
- **Late period:** Part of a phage infective cycle. After the onset of replication, is known as late period of lytic development.
- **Latent agent:** Usually, a virus that is present in a host organism without producing any symptoms.
- **Latent bud:** An inactive bud not held back by rest or dormant period but it may start growth if stimulated.
- **Lateral bud:** A bud produced at the base of a leaf petiole.

- **Lateral element:** A structure in the synaptonemal complex. It is an axial element that is aligned with the axial elements of other chromosomes.
- **Lateral meristem:** A meristem giving rise to secondary plant tissues such as the vascular and cork cambia. The term is sometimes used to refer to an ancillary meristem.
- **Late-replicating:** Material does not replicate until the end of S phase. Typically, it consists of the heterochromatin.
- **Laurate:** A medium chain length (i.e. C12) fatty acid that is naturally produced by coconut trees, oil palm trees, and certain species of wild plants. In 1992, some canola varieties were genetically engineered so that they could also produce (desirable) laurate in their seeds.
- **Lauroyl-ACP thioesterase:** The enzyme that is required for the synthesis (manufacturing) of laurate in plants. For example, the presence of this enzyme in the California bay tree (*Umbellularia californica*) causes its seed oil to contain as much as 45% laurate.

L

- **Law of independent assortment of alleles:** Alleles of different genes are assorted independently of one another during the formation of gametes (genes for different characters are inherited independently of one another). The different pairs of homologous chromosomes arrange themselves on the metaphase I equator in an independent manner and remain independent throughout meiosis. As a consequence, genes that are located on nonhomologous chromsomes (in other words, genes that are not linked) undergo independent assortment in meiosis.
- **Law of segregation:** Alleles segregate from one another during the formation of gametes. When two different alleles are brought in a hybrid, both of them coexist without contaminating each other and are separated in meiosis as pure as brought from the parents. During the formation of gametes, the paired unit factors separate or segregate randomly so that each gamete receives one or the other. The principle of segregation applies to homologous chromosomes during meiosis.
- **Lawn:** In biotechnology, a uniform and uninterrupted layer of bacterial growth in which individual colonies cannot be observed.
- **Layering:** Technique for vegetative propagation in which new plants produce adventitious roots before being severed from the parent plant.

- **Lazaroids:** A class of drugs being developed to "bring back from the dead" tissues that have been (almost) killed due to lack of oxygen (e.g. Krebs cycle L caused by a clot blocking a vital artery).
- **LD50 (Lethal dose 50%):** The amount of a chemical required to kill 50% of the test population. The higher the LD50 the lower the presumed toxicity of the chemical.
- **Leader (5' UTR):** Of a mRNA is the nontranslated sequence at the 5' end that precedes the initiation codon.
- **Leader:** Of a protein is a short N-terminal sequence responsible for initiating passage into or through a membrane.
- **Leader peptide:** The product that would result from translation of a short coding sequence used to regulate expression of the tryptophan by controlling ribosome movement.
- **Leader sequence:** A protein is a short N-terminal sequence responsible for passage into or through a membrane.
- **Leading strand:** DNA is synthesized continuously in the 5'-3' direction.
- **Leaf blade:** The usually flattened portion of the leaf.
- **Leaf bud cutting:** A cutting that includes a short section of stem with attached leaf.
- **Leaf margin:** The edge of a leaf.
- **Leaf primordium:** A lateral outgrowth from the apical meristem which will become a leaf when fully developed and expanded.
- **Leaf roll:** Virus diseases characterized by symptomatic curling of the host's leaves.
- **Leaf scar:** Mark left on a stem after leaf abscission.
- **Leaflet:** Expanded leaf like part of a compound leaf.
- **Leaky mutants:** A mutant in which the mutated gene product, such as an enzyme, still possesses a fraction of its normal biological activity.
- **Leaky mutations:** One in which the amino acid substitution only partially disrupts the functions of protein, in bacteria this is usually manifested by reduced growth rate.
- **Lecithin (crude, mixture):** A mixture of phospholipids (i.e. lecithin-phosphatidylcholine, cephalin, inositol phosphatides, glycerides, tocopherols, glucosides, and certain pigments). Historically, crude (mixture) lecithin has often been utilized commercially in food processing as an emulsifier, instantizing agent, and lubricating agent. Because lecithin-phosphatidylcholine naturally contains a high content of linoleic acid, consumption

of lecithin-phosphatidylcholine by humans results in similar impact (e.g. lowered cholesterol levels in blood) as consumption of linoleic acid. Because dietary fats are generally not absorbed directly through the intestinal wall (when eaten), they must first be emulsified, to form micelles that can pass through the intestinal wall and thus be absorbed by the body. That emulsification/micelle-formation is aided by lecithin, since it is an emulsifier.

- **Lecithin (refined, specific):** A byproduct of the refining process for soybean oil (deoiled lecithin from processed soybeans is composed of approximately 20–25% phosphatidyl choline by weight). The lecithin molecule (i.e. phosphatidyl choline) naturally contains a high content of linoleic acid, so consumption of lecithin by humans results in similar impact (e.g. lowered cholesterol levels in blood) as consumption of linoleic acid (Fig. 1). Because dietary fats are generally not absorbed directly through the intestinal wall (when eaten), they must first be emulsified to form micelles that can pass through the intestinal wall and be absorbed by the body. The emulsification/micelle-formation is aided by lecithin, since it is an emulsifier. Lecithin (also known as phosphatidylcholine) is a source of choline when digested, and is a critical component of the lipoproteins that transport fat and cholesterol molecules in the bloodstream (e.g. from the digestive system, to body cells, to the liver, etc.). Lecithin (phosphatidylcholine) promotes synthesis of high-density lipoproteins (HDLP, also known as "good" cholesterol) by the liver, when it is consumed by humans. Phosphatidylcholine (PC) is involved in cell signal transduction (e.g. via which a cell reacts to an external chemical "signal"). Some other common dietary sources of lecithin includes egg, red meat, spinach, and nuts.

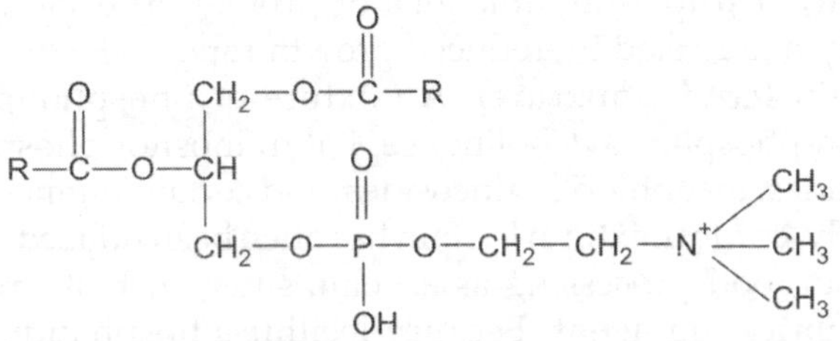

Fig. 1: Lecithin (refined, specific)

- **Lectins:** A class of proteins that have the capability to rapidly (and reversibly) combine with specific sugar molecules (e.g. those sugar molecules or glycoproteins on the surface of adjacent cells, within an organism). Lectins are a common component of the surface (membranes) of plant and animal cells, and are so specific (regarding sugar molecules that they will or won't combine with/attach to) that they discriminate between different monosaccharides and different oligosaccharides (i.e. on the surface of adjacent cells within an organism). This capability to reversibly combine with sugar (i.e. carbohydrate) molecules (on the surface of adjacent cells) is utilized by: 1. Bacteria and other microorganisms, to adhere to (sugar molecules on surface of) host cells, as the first step in the process of infecting those host cells; 2. White blood cells (lymphocytes), to adhere to the walls of blood vessels (endothelium), the first step to leav the bloodstream to fight infection (pathogens, trauma) in tissues adjacent to the blood vessel. The lectin (glycoprotein) that adheres to the endothelial sugar molecule on blood vessel wall is called L-selectin, or the homing receptor. The two sugar molecules (glycoproteins) on the blood vessel wall (endothelium) are called P-selectin and E-selectin (also known as ELAM-1); 3. Cancerous tumor cells, to adhere to the walls of blood vessels (endothelium) as part of the tumor-proliferation process known as metastasis (i.e. new tumors are "seeded" throughout the body via this process). Separate and apart from the above impacts, some plant lectins (e.g. in the seeds of certain plants) are toxic to some of the animals that consume those seeds.
- **Left splicing junction:** The boundary between the right end of an exon and the left end of an intron.
- **Leghaemoglobin:** A globular protein containing heme expressed in legume root nodules.
- **Legume:** A member of the pea family that possesses root nodules containing nitrogen-fixing bacteria.
- **Leptin:** A protein hormone that is produced by fat cells (adipose tissue) in the body. When leptin is produced and travels to cell whose surface bears leptin receptors (e.g. in the brain), those (brain) cells receive signal (transduction) indicating fullness/satiety. Leptin has been found to be present in the bloodstream of obese humans at a concentration of approximately four times the concentration found in bloodstreams of lean humans. High

levels of leptin present in the bloodstream disrupt some of the activities of insulin (hormone which regulates blood sugar levels), and may possibly lead to diabetes.

- **Leptin receptors:** Cellular receptors which are specific to leptin. In 1996, H Ralph Snodgrass discovered that leptin receptors are involved in the "sorting" of immature blood cells (from bone marrow) to create subpopulations.
- **Leptonema:** Stage during meiosis immediately precedes synapsis in which the chromosomes appear as single, fine, threadlike structures (but they are really double because DNA replication has already taken place).
- **Lethal alleles:** Mutated genes that are capable of causing death.
- **Lethal locus:** Any gene in which a lethal mutation can be obtained (usually by deletion of the gene).
- **Lethal mutation:** Mutation of a gene to yield no, or a totally defective, gene product (protein), thereby making it unable to function, and hence unable to sustain the life of the organism.
- **Leucine (leu):** A monocarboxylic essential amino acid.
- **Leucine zipper:** A dimerization motif adjacent to a basic DNA-binding region that is found in a class of transcription factors.
- **Leucine-rich region (LLR):** It is a motif found in the extracellular domains of some surface receptor proteins in animal and plant cells.
- **Leukocytes (white blood cells):** A diverse family of nucleated cells that has many immunological functions.
- **Leukotrienes:** Lipid mediator molecules (synthesized from arachidonic acid) released by certain cells (T cells), which "signal" leukocytes (white blood cells) during the initial stages of an infection or an allergic reaction. When thus activated, the leukocytes migrate to the site of infection to combat the pathogens (or allergens), and mediate the inflammation.
- **Levorotary (L) isomer:** An isomer of an optically active compound; rotates (when illuminated) the plane of plane-polarized light to the left.
- **Library:** A set of cloned fragments together representing the entire genome.
- **Licensing factor:** It is something in the nucleus that is necessary for replication, and is inactivated or destroyed after one round of replication. New licensing factors must be provided for further rounds of replication to occur.

- **Life cycle:** The series of stages in form and functional activity through which an organism passes between successive recurrences of a specified primary stage.
- **Ligand (in biochemistry):** In general, a molecule or ion that can bind to (interact with) a protein molecule. For example, a drug that binds to a receptor protein molecule on the surface of a cell may be called a ligand.
- **Ligand (in chromatography):** A term used to describe a substance (the ligand) that has the capacity for specific and noncovalent (reversible) binding to some protein. A ligand may be a coenzyme for a specific enzyme. The ligand can be covalently attached (immobilized) by means of the appropriate chemical reaction to the surface of certain porous column material. When a mixture of proteins containing the enzyme to be isolated is passed through the column, the enzyme, which is capable of tightly binding to the ligand, does so, and is in this manner held to the column. The other proteins present, which have no specific affinity for the ligand, pass on through the column. The protein/ligand complex is then dissociated and the enzyme eluted from the column, which may be accomplished by passing more free (unbound) coenzymes through the column. The ligand may be hormones (i.e. used to isolate receptor molecules) or any other type of molecule that is capable of binding specifically and reversibly to the desired protein or protein complex.
- **Ligand-gated:** Channels open or close in response to the binding of a specific molecule.
- **Ligase:** An enzyme used by a genetic engineer to join the cut ends of the double stranded DNA.
- **Ligate:** The process of joining two or more DNA fragments.
- **Ligation:** The formation of a phosphodiester bond to link two adjacent bases separated by a nick in one strand of a double helix of DNA (the term can also be applied to blunt-end ligation and joining of RNA).
- **Light chain:** The immunoglobulin light chain is one of two types of polypeptides in an antibody. Each antibody contains two light chains. The N-terminus of the light chain forms part of the antigen recognition site.
- **Light-chain variable (VL) domains:** The regions (domains) of the antibody (molecule's) "light chain" that vary in their amino

acid sequence. The "chains" (of atoms) comprising the antibody (immunoglobulin) molecule consist of a region of variable (V) amino acid sequence and a region in which the amino acid sequence remains constant (C). An antibody molecule possesses two antigen binding sites, and it is the variable domains of the light (VL) and heavy (VH) chains which contribute to this (antigen binding ability).

- **Lignans:** A category of phytochemicals that play defensive roles (e.g. against infections by bacteria, fungi, etc.) within land plants (e.g. those grown by man for crops). Lignans are also sometimes referred "phytoestrogens", and are typically beneficial to the health of humans that consume them. Lignans are found virtually in all fruits, vegetables, and cereals (grains) generally within the seed coat, stem, leav, or flower. One of the beneficial lignans commonly consumed by humans is sesamin, found in seeds of the sesame plant (*Sesamum indicum*) which acts as an antioxidant.

L

- **Lignification:** Impregnation of a cell wall with lignin.
- **Lignins:** A category of phenolic ("ring-shaped" molecules) polymeric (composed of more than one molecular unit) compounds produced by land plants within the cell walls (i.e. exterior of cell's plasma membrane) to reinforce/strengthen those cell walls.
- **Lignocellulose:** A complex biopolymer comprising the bulk of woody plants. It consists of polysaccharides and polymer phenols.
- **Lineage:** Several individuals originating from a common descent such as the production of a cell line from a single cell plated *in vitro*.
- **Linear phase:** When cell number constantly increases. The linear phase is located between the exponential growth and the deceleration phase.
- **Lines:** A long-period interspersed sequences in mammalian genomes that are retroposons generated from RNA polymerase II transcripts.
- **Linkage:** Describes the tendency of genes to be inherited together as a result of their location on the same chromosome; measured by percent recombination between loci.
- **Linkage disequilibrium:** The occurrence in a population of two linked alleles at a frequency higher or lower than expected on the basis of the gene frequencies of the individual genes.

- **Linkage groups:** All genes on a single chromosome form one linkage group. Number of linkage groups is equal to the haploid chromosome number except in sexes with dissimilar sex chromosomes. Fruit flies have four pairs of chromosomes to hold thousands of genes.
- **Linkage map:** A map showing the linear order of genes on a chromosome and the relative distances between them in recombinational units.
- **Linkage:** The association of genes having loci on the same chromosome, which results in the tendency of a group of such nonallelic genes to be associated in inheritance.
- **Linked genes/markers:** Genes and/or markers that are so closely associated on the chromosome that they are coinherited in 80% or more of cases.
- **Linker DNA:** All DNA contained on a nucleosome in excess of the 146 bp core DNA.
- **Linker fragment:** A short synthetic duplex oligonucleotide containing the target site for some restriction enzyme; may be added to the ends of a DNA fragment, prepared by cleavage with some other enzyme during reconstruction of recombinant DNA.
- **Linker scanner mutations:** Introduced by recombining two DNA molecules *in vitro* at a restriction fragment added to the end of each; the result is to insert the linker sequence at the site of recombination.
- **Linkers:** A synthetic double stranded oligonucleotide carrying the sequence for one or more restriction sites.
- **Linking number paradox:** It describes the discrepancy between the existence of 2-supercoils in the path of DNA on the nucleosome compared with the measurement of 1-supercoil released when histones are removed.
- **Linking number:** The number of times that two strands of a closed, circular DNA duplex cross-over each other.
- **Linking:** The process of "attaching" a drug or a toxin to a monoclonal antibody, or another homing molecule of the immune system. This attachment should be reversible, so that the homing molecule can release the drug or toxin after delivering that drug or toxin to the desired site in the body (e.g. delivery of a toxin to a tumor, to kill the tumor), linking is a difficult process to reliably achieve.

- **Linoleic acid:** One of the so-called "omega-6" (n-6) polyunsaturated fatty acids (PUFA), historically comprised approximately 53% of the total fatty acid content of soybean oil. It is an essential fatty acid for humans. When consumed by humans, linoleic acid causes LDLP cholesterol levels in the blood to decrease, which reduces risk of coronary heart disease (CHD). The human body converts linoleic acid to the n-6 highly unsaturated fatty acid (HUFA) arachidonic acid.

- **Lipase:** An enzyme (one of a class of enzymes) that catalyzes the hydrolytic cleavage of lipid molecules (triglycerides) to yield free fatty acids. Lipase was the first enzyme to be produced via genetic engineering and marketed, also occurs naturally in cow's milk, and in the intestines of many animals (where it aids/assists digestion of fats that an animal consumes).

- **Lipid bilayer:** The form taken by concentration of lipids in which the hydrophobic fatty acids occupy the interior, and the polar heads faces the exterior.

- **Lipid trafficking:** The movement of lipids among the various membranes of a eukaryotic cell.

- **Lipids:** Lipids have polar heads, containing phosphate (phospholipid), sterol (such as cholesterol), or saccharide (glycolipid) connected to a hydrophobic tail consisting of fatty acid(s).

- **Lipofection:** Delivery into eukaryotic cells of DNA, RNA or other compounds that have been encapsulated in an artificial phospholipid vesicle.

- **Lipophilic:** A "fat loving" molecule, or portion of a molecule. Relating to, or having strong affinity for fats or other lipids.

- **Lipopolysaccharide (LPS):** A molecule containing both lipid and sugar components. It is present in the outer membrane of Gram-negative bacteria. It is also an endotoxin responsible for inducing septic shock during an infection.

- **Lipoprotein:** A conjugated protein containing a lipid or a group of lipids. For example, low-density lipoproteins (also known as "bad" cholesterol) are a "package" of cholesterol (lipid) surrounded by a hydrophilic protein. Low-density lipoproteins (LDLPs) and very low-density lipoproteins (VLDLs) are the specific lipoproteins that are most likely to deposit cholesterol (plaque) on artery walls, which increases the risk of coronary heart disease (CHD).

- **Lipoprotein-associated coagulation (clot) inhibitor (LACI):** A protein that prevents formation of blood clots. This occurs because LACI inhibits the controlled series of zymogen activations (enzymatic cascade) which causes the formation of fibrinogen (precursor to fibrin), leading subsequently to clot formation.
- **Liposomes:** Artificial vesicles of phospholipis.
- **Lipoxygenase (LOX):** A "family" of enzymes that is naturally produced within its seeds (soybeans) by the soybean plant (*Glycine max* (L.) Merrill). In the presence of moisture and certain other conditions, lipoxygenase enzymes catalyze a chemical reaction in which objectionable "beany" flavor can be produced from certain components of the soybean. That "beany" flavor decreases the suitability of resultant soybean raw materials for manufacture of human foods in some countries. Prevention of the reactions that create the "beany" flavor can be accomplished via heat denaturation (of lipoxygenases present in the soybeans) or via creation of soybeans that do not contain any lipoxygenase enzymes (known as "LOX null" soybeans). Lipoxygenase enzymes also catalyze a reaction in which certain volatile chemicals are produced that inhibit growth of any *Aspergillus flavus* fungus.
- **Liquefaction:** Enzymatic digestion (α-amylase) of gelatinized starch to form low molecular weight polysaccharides.
- **Liquid (solution) hybridization:** A reaction between complementary nucleic acid strands performed in solution.
- **Liquid media:** Media without a solidifying agent.
- **Liquid membranes:** Thin films made up of liquid (solids) which are stable in another liquid (usually water). Thus, the liquid must not dissolve in the water but nevertheless must be prevented from collapsing into a lot of small droplets.
- **Liquid nitrogen:** Nitrogen gas condensed to a liquid with a boiling point of about $-196°C$. Very commonly the medium in which container of genetic material are stored.
- *Listeria monocytogenes:* Refers to the "family" (numerous strains) of *Listeria monocytogenes* bacteria, that can grow in many different foodstuffs (e.g. meats) under specific conditions, and can cause food poisoning (Listeriosis) in humans who subsequently consume those foodstuffs. When consumed by humans, certain strains/serotypes of *Listeria monocytogenes* can

cause fever, severe headaches, stiffness, nausea, diarrhea, and possibly miscarriages in pregnant women. On January 19, 2001, all meat processed in the US is required to be tested for the presence of *Listeria monocytogenes*.

- **Litmus:** A pH indicator paper (range 4.5–8.3) impregnated with an extracted lichen pigment. It turns red in acidic medium and blue in alkaline solutions. However, the use of litmus paper as an indicator is not a precise method of pH measurement.
- **Live vaccine:** A living, or nonliving form of microorganism or virus that is used to elicit an antibody response that will protect the inoculated organism against infection by a virulent form of the microorganism or virus.
- **Loci:** The plural of locus see locus.
- **Locus control region (LCR):** That is required for the expression of several genes in a domain.
- **Locus:** Position on a chromosome at which the gene for a particular trait resides; a locus may be occupied by any one of the alleles for the gene.
- **LOD score:** A measure of genetic linkage, defined as the $\log_{10}$ ratio of the probability that the data would have arisen if the loci are linked to the probability that the data could have arisen from unlinked loci. The conventional threshold for declaring linkage is a LOD score of 3.0, that is, a 1000:1 ratio (which must be compared with the 50:1 probability that any random pair of loci will be unlinked).
- **Long template:** A DNA strand that is synthesized during the polymerase chain reaction, and has a primer sequence at one end but is extended beyond the site that is complementary to the second primer at the other end.
- **Long day plant:** Plant requiring short nights before flowering is initiated.
- **Long terminal repeat (LTR):** is the sequence that is repeated at each end of the integrated retroviral genome.
- **Long-period interspersion:** A pattern in which long stretches of moderately repetitive and nonrepetitive DNA alternate.
- **Loop:** A single-stranded region at the end of a hairpin in RNA (or single-stranded DNA); corresponds to the sequence between inverted repeats in duplex DNA.
- **Loop bioreactors:** Fermenters in which the fermenting material is cycled between a bulk tank and a smaller tank or loop of pipes.

- **Loose binding site:** Any random sequence of DNA that is bound by the core RNA polymerase when it is not engaged in transcription.
- **LOSBM:** Low-oligosaccharide soybean meal.
- **Loss-of-function:** Mutation inactivates a gene. It is recessive.
- **Low-density lipoproteins (LDLP):** So-called "bad" cholesterol (i.e. LDL cholesterol), which carries cholesterol molecules from the digestive system (e.g. intestine) to body cells and can sometimes clog arteries over time (a disease called atherosclerosis, or coronary heart disease). Since cholesterol does not dissolve in water (which constitutes most of the volume of blood), the body makes LDL cholesterol (derived from the digestion of fatty foods) into little "packages" surrounded by a hydrophilic ("water loving") protein. That protein "wrapper" is known as apolipoprotein B-100, or apo B-100, and it enables LDL cholesterol to be transported in the bloodstream because the apolipoprotein B-100 is attracted to water molecules in the blood.
- **Low-linolenic oil soybeans:** Soybeans from soybean (*Glycine max*) plant varieties which have been bred specifically to produce soybeans bearing oil that contains less than 4% linolenic acid, instead of the typical 8% linolenic acid content of soybean oil produced from traditional varieties of soybeans. Low linolenic soybean oil would tend to have greater flavor stability (especially at elevated temperatures utilized in frying foods) than soybean oil from traditional varieties of soybeans.
- **Low-phytate corn:** Developed in the US during the 1990s, these are corn (maize) hybrids possessing the Lpa1 gene, the Lpa2 gene, or the (HAP) highly available phosphorous gene (which was discovered by Victor Raboy). That gene causes corn (maize) hybrids possessing it to produce much less phytate than the 0.15% typically present in traditional varieties of corn (maize). Because phytate is not digestible in humans and other monogastric animals (swine, poultry, etc.), substituting low phytate corn in place of traditional corn varieties in those animals' diets helps lessen adverse environmental impact of animal feeding (e.g. phosphorous emissions in excess of annual cropland requirements).
- **Low phytate soybeans:** Developed in the US during the 1990s, these are soybean varieties possessing less than 0.30% (of total

L

soybean weight) phytate, vs. the typical 0.45% phytate content of soybeans from traditional soybean varieties. Because phytate is not digestible in humans and other monogastric animals (swine poultry, etc.), substituting lowphytate soybeans in place of traditional soybean varieties in those animals' diets helps to lessen adverse environmental impact of animal feeding (e.g. manure phosphorous emissions in excess of cropland requirements).

- **Low-stachyose soybeans:** Those soybean varieties that contain lower than 1% levels of the relatively indigestible stachyose carbohydrate (and thus higher levels of easily digestible other nutrients) than traditional varieties of soybeans (which typically contain 1.4–4.1% stachyose in traditional soybean varieties). Compared to traditional varieties of soybeans, low-stachyose soybeans have approximately 10% more metabolizable (i.e. useable by animals) energy content and a 3% increase in amino acid digestibility. Low-stachyose soybeans are particularly useful for feeding of monogastric animals (swine, poultry, etc.), since their single stomach cannot digest stachyose. Thus, stachyose tends to "ferment" (promote excess bacterial growth) in their intestines, causing them to feel prematurely full.

- **Low-Tillage crop production:** A methodology of crop production in which the farmer utilizes a minimum of mechanical cultivation (i.e. only two to four passes over the field with tillage equipment instead of the conventional five passes per year utilized for traditional crop production). This reduced mechanical tillage leaves more carbon in the (less disturbed) soil, leaves more earthworms (*Eisenia foetida*) per cubic foot or per cubic meter living in the topsoil, and reduces soil compaction (i.e. the reduction in interstitial spaces between individual soil particles); thereby increasing the fertility of "low till" farm fields.

- **LOX null soybeans:** Refers to soybeans that do not contain any of the three lipoxygenase enzymes (thus, they result in a "null" test reading).

- **LOX-1:** One of the isozymes (enzyme molecule variations) of the lipoxygenase (LOX) enzyme "family".

- **LOX-2:** See LOX-1.

- **LOX-3:** See LOX-1.

- **LPAAT protein:** A protein consisting of lysophosphatidic acid acyl transferase (enzyme), which (when present in a plant) causes production of triglycerides (in the seeds) possessing saturated fatty acids in the "middle position" of the triglycerides' molecular (glycerol) "backbone". For example, canola (rapeseed) plants genetically engineered to contain LPAAT protein are able to produce high levels of saturated fatty acids (including laurate) in their oil.
- **L-selectin:** Also known as the homing receptor.
- **LTR:** An abbreviation for long-terminal repeat, a sequence directly repeated at both ends of a retroviral DNA.
- **Luciferase:** Refers to a group of enzymes that can catalyze a chemical reaction that results in the production of light (i.e. bioluminescense) within certain living oganisms. For example, the common firefly is able to emit light from its tail (photophores) via luciferase-catalyzed bioluminescence. The ocean jellyfish known as the sea pansy (*Renilla reniformis*) is able to emit light via similar use of a slightly different luciferase molecule.
- **Lumen:** The interior of a compartment bounded by membranes, usually the endoplasmic reticulum or the mitochondrion.
- **Luminescent assays:** Refers to assays (i.e. tests/test techniques) which detect or measure the presence of a specific substance (e.g. bacteria ATP on surfaces in a slaughterhouse) and the efficacy (i.e. effectiveness) of a specific substance via the enzyme (e.g. luciferase) catalyzed production of light. For example, one (rapid) luminescent assay utilizes two chemical reagents which first breakdown bacteria cell membranes, then cause ATP from those broken-open cells to luminesce. Subsequent measurement of that light is the assay's proof (e.g. that bacteria had been present on the tested surface in a slaughter house).
- **Lupus:** An autoimmune disease of the body, in which anti-DNA antibodies bind to DNA. The resulting complexes (of DNA and antibodies) travel to the kidneys via the bloodstream, and become lodged in the kidneys, where they cause inflammatory reactions (that can lead to kidney failure). Sometimes joints, blood vessels, bone marrow, and the liver are also damaged by this disease.
- **Lutein:** A carotenoid (i.e. "light harvesting" compound utilized in photosynthesis) that is naturally produced in carrots, summer squash, broccoli, dark lettuce, and green peas. Lutein is a

phytochemical/nutraceutical conducive to good eye health, and regular consumption of large amounts of lutein has been shown to reduce the risk of the disease age-related macular degeneration, a leading cause of blindness in elderly people. Research indicates that consumption of lutein by humans also reduces risk of prostate cancer and breast cancer.

- **Luteinizing hormone (LH):** A reproductive hormone that acts upon the ovaries to stimulate ovulation. It is secreted by the pituitary gland.
- **Lux:** The unit of measurement for illuminance (i.e. the amount of illumination) impinging upon a surface. 1 lx is the illuminance impinging upon a surface of 1 m, each point of which is at a distance of 1 m away from a uniform point source of light of 1 cd (candela). It supersedes the foot-candle.
- **Luxury consumption:** Nutrient absorption by an organism in excess of that required for optimum growth and productivity.
- **Luxury genes:** Those coding for specialized functions synthesized (usually) in large amounts in particular cell types.
- **Lyase:** A class of enzymes that catalyze either the cleavage of a double bond and the addition of new groups to a substrate or the information of a double bond.
- **Lycopene:** An acyclic carotenoid occuring in tomatoes and some other ripe fruit as a red pigment. As an antioxidant its consumption can reduce the risk of some cancers like prostate (Fig. 2).

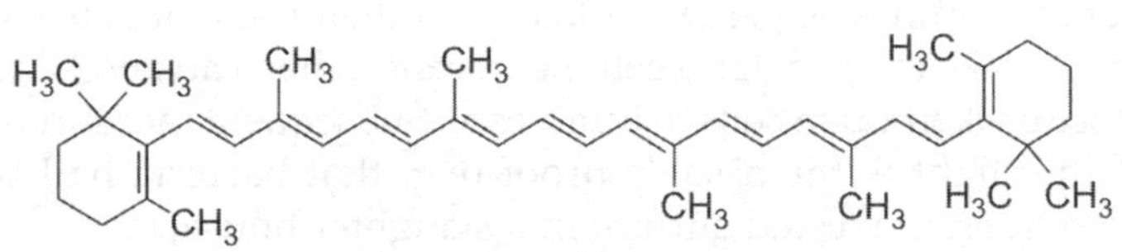

Fig. 2: Lycopene

- **Lymphocyte:** A type of cell found in the blood, spleen, lymph nodes, etc. of higher animals. They are formed very early in fetal life, arising in the liver by the sixth week of human gestation. There exist two subclasses of lymphocytes: B lymphocytes and T lymphocytes. B lymphocytes make antibodies (immunoglobins) of which there are five classes: IgM, IgA, IgG, IgD and IgE. The antibodies circulate in the bloodstream. T lymphocytes recognize and reject foreign tissue, modulate B cell activity, kill tumor cells, and kill host cells infected with virus. T-lymphocytes are also called T cells.

- **Lymphokines:** Peptides and proteins secreted by (immune system response) stimulated T cells. These hormone-like (peptide and protein) molecules direct the movements and activities of other cells in the immune system. Some examples of lymphokines are interleukin-1, interleukin-2, tumor necrosis factor (TNF), gamma interferon, colony stimulating factors, macrophage chemotactic factor, and lymphocyte growth factor. The suffix "-kine" comes from the Greek word *kinesis*, meaning movement.

- **Lymphoma:** Cancer originating in the lymph nodes, spleen and other lympho-reticular sites.

- **Lyophilize:** Rapid freezing followed by dehydration under high vacuum. The process is lyophilization.

- **Lyophilization:** The process of removing water from a frozen biomaterial (e.g. a microbial culture or an aqueous protein solution) via application of a vacuum. It is a drying method for long-term preservation of proteins in the solid state, and for long-term storage of live microbial cultures.

- **Lyse:** To rupture a membrane (cell). The act of lysis (rupturing a membrane).

- **Lysine (lys):** An essential amino acid that can be obtained from many proteins by hydrolysis (i.e. cutting apart the protein molecule).

- **Lysis:** The dissolution of cells such as blood cells or bacteria, as by the action of a specific lysin that disrupts the cell membrane.

- **Lysogen:** A bacterial cell or strain that has been infected with a temperate virus.

- **Lysogenic immunity:** The ability of a prophage to prevent another phage genome of the same type from becoming established in the bacterium.

- **Lysogenic life cycle:** The life cycle of a temperate bacteriophage in which the virus can either replicate via the lytic life cycle or become a latent prophage within the infected host bacterium and does not replicate.

- **Lysogenic repressor:** The protein responsible for preventing a prophage from re-entering the lytic cycle.

- **Lysogeny:** The ability of a phage to survive in a bacterium as a stable prophage component of the bacterial genome.
- **Lysophosphatidyl ethanolamine (LPE):** Also known as phosphatidyl ethanolamine. It is one of the lipids (phospholipids) naturally found in soybean oil. In plants, it functions as a signaling molecule (e.g. speeding the ripening process).
- **Lysosomes:** Small bodies, enclosed by membranes that contain hydrolytic enzymes in eukaryotic cells.
- **Lysozyme:** An enzyme, naturally produced by some animals, which possesses antibacterial (bacteria-killing) properties. Discovered in 1922 by Alexander Fleming, in his nasal mucus, Mr. Fleming named it from the Greek "*lyso*"—due to its ability to lyse (cut) bacteria—and "*zyme*"—due to its being an enzyme. Lysozyme lysis certain kinds of bacteria, by dissolving the polysaccharide components of the bacteria's cell wall. When that cell wall is weakened, the bacterial cell bursts because osmotic pressure (inside that bacteria cell) is greater than the weakened cell wall can contain. Tears and egg whites both contain significant amounts of lysozyme, as agent to prevent bacterial infections (e.g. against bacteria entering the body via eye openings; against bacteria entering the chicken embryo through the egg shell).
- **Lytic infection:** Infection of a bacterium by a phage which replicates uncontrollably, destroying its host and eventually releasing many copies into the medium.

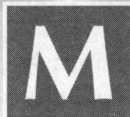

- **M phase kinase (MPF):** It was originally called the maturation promoting factor (or M phase-promoting factor). It is a dimeric kinase, containing the p34 catalytic subunit and a cyclin regulatory subunit, whose activation triggers the onset of mitosis.
- **M13:** A single stranded DNA bacteriophage used as vector for DNA sequencing.
- **Marketing authorization application (MAA):** It is the European Union (EU) equivalent to a US-NDA (New Drug Application). An MAA is an application to the EU's committee for proprietary medicinal products (CPMP) seeking approval of a new drug that has undergone phase 2 and phase 3 clinical trials.
- **Macerate:** To disintegrate tissues to obtain a cell dissociation. Cutting, soaking or enzymatic actions are commonly used.
- **Macromolecules:** Large molecules with molecular weights ranging from a few thousand to hundreds of millions.
- **Macronutrient:** For growth media an essential element normally required in concentrations > 0.5 millimole/liter.
- **Macrophage:** Cell of the mononuclear phagocyte system. Derived from blood monocytes which migrate into tissues and differentiate there.
- **Macrophage colony stimulating factor (M-CSF):** A CSF that stimulates production of macrophages in the body.
- **Macropropagation:** Production of plant clones from growing parts (traditional method of farming).
- **MACS:** Acronym for magnetic cell sorting.
- **Magainins:** Discovered within frog skin tissues by Michael Zasloff in 1987, magainins are antimicrobial, amphopathic peptides that lyse (burst) certain cells upon contact by "worming" their hydrophobic portion into the cell's membrane, which creates a transmembrane (i.e. through the surface) pore (allowing ions to flow into the cell, causing osmotic bursting).

Magainins are selective against bacteria, fungi and protozoa cells. The word magainin comes from the Hebrew word "shield".

- **Magic bullet:** When this term was first coined by Paul Ehrlich in 1905, it initially referred only to antibodies (e.g. because antibodies seek their own target, without damaging other nearby tissues). However, over time, this term has come to be applied to immunotoxins and other immunoconjugates (i.e. toxic or pharmacological molecules which are "attached" to an antibody that "steers/guides" the toxic or pharmacological molecule to the intended "target" in the body such as a tumor).

- **Magnetic particles:** Refers to various tiny pieces of natural magnetic materials, that are bonded (attached) to antibodies (e.g. monoclonal antibodies that are specific to a particular type of cell). These can then be mixed with a large population of many cell types (crude tissue samples, cells grown in a vat/reactor, etc.), where the magnetic antibodies will attach themselves to only the desired cells, then the desired cells are separated out using a magnetic field (the magnetic particles/antibodies are subsequently removed from those cells).

- **Main band (of genomic DNA):** A broad peak on a density gradient, excluding any visible satellite DNAs that form separate bands.

- **Maintenance methylase:** Adds a methyl group to a target site that is already hemimethylated.

- **Major grooves:** Grooves of DNA is 22Å across.

- **Major histocompatibility complex (MHC):** A chromosomal region containing genes that are involved in the immune response. The genes encode proteins for antigen presentation, cytokines, and complement proteins. The MHC is highly polymorphic.

- **Major histocompatibility locus:** A large chromosomal region containing a giant cluster of genes that code for transplantation antigens and other proteins found on the surface of lymphocytes.

- **MALDI-TOF-MS:** Acronym for matrix-associated laser desorption ionization time of flight mass spectrometry. A mass spectrometry methodology/technology that can establish, in seconds, the identity, purity, etc. of a sample of proteins, oligonucleotide, or (poly)peptides. Also the identification of gram-positive microorganisms, or characterization of genetic materials (DNA, RNA, etc.) on hybridization surfaces. MALDI–TOF utilizes measurement of the time for particles (e.g. proteins) to transit a specific distance after being "dislodged" from ("adhered") surface by specific amount of energy to precisely determine the molecular weight (of proteins, etc.).

- **Malignant:** Having the properties of cancerous growth.
- **Malt extract:** A mixture of organic compounds from malt used as a culture medium adjunct.
- **Malting:** A process of generating starch degrading enzymes in grain by allowing it to germinate in a humid atmosphere.
- **Mammalian:** Describes the group of vertebrates that have internal development of the embryo, mammary glands that can produce milk, live-born young, a body covering of hair or fur, a four chambered heart, a well developed cerebral cortex, the ability to maintain a constant body temperature and in most adults a permanent set of teeth.
- **Mammalian cell culture:** Technology to cultivate cells, artificially of mammal origin, in a laboratory or production-scale device (i.e. *in vitro*). Can be either a batch or continuous process device. The first mammalian cell culture was performed by a neurobiologist named R. G. Harrison in 1907, when he added chopped-up spinal cord tissue to clotted (blood) plasma in a humidified growth chamber. The nerve cells from the spinal cord tissue successfully grow, divide, and extendeds long fibers into the clot.
- **Mammary glands:** The milk producing organs of female mammals which provide feed for the young one.
- **Mammary tumors:** Tumors of the milk glands.
- **Mannanoligosaccharides (MOS):** A family of oligosaccharides that can be produced by man in commercial quantities via certain yeast cells. Consumption of mannanoligosaccharides by mammals also causes macrophages to move toward the gastrointestinal tract (in body's tissues), where those macrophages eliminate some pathogens (i.e. growing/reproducing in the gastrointestinal tract).
- **Mannitol:** A sugar alcohol widely distributed in plants. It is commonly used as a nutrient and osmoticum in suspension medium for plant protoplasts.
- **Mannose:** A hexose component of many polysaccharides and mannitol. Mannose is occasionally used as a carbohydrate source in plant tissue culture media.

M

- **Map distance:** Measured as cM (centiMorgans) = percent recombination (sometime subject to adjustments).
- **MAP kinase (MAPK):** A Ser/Thr protein kinase named for its original identification as a mitogen-activated kinase. There is a large group of cytosolic Thr/Ser protein kinases that form several signaling pathways. The name reflects their original isolation as mitogen-activated protein kinase.
- **Map unit:** A distance between genetic markers corresponding to 1% recombination frequency between the markers.
- **Mapping:** Determine the location of a locus (gene of genetic marker) on a chromosome.
- **Mapping function:** A mathematical expression relating observed recombination fraction to map distance expressed in centi morgans.
- **MAR (matrix attachment site):** (also known as SAR for scaffold attachment site) A region of DNA that attaches to the nuclear matrix.
- **Marker (DNA):** A fragment of known size used to calibrate an electrophoretic gel.
- **Marker (genetic):** Any allele of interest in an experiment.
- **Marker assisted selection:** The utilization of DNA sequence "markers" by commercial breeders to select the organisms (crops, livestock, etc.) that possess gene(s) for a particular performance trait (rapid growth, high yield, etc.) desired, for subsequent breeding/propagation. Marker Assisted Selection has been utilized in many plant (e.g. crop) breeding programs since the mid-1970s.
- **Marker peptide:** A portion of fusing protein that facilitates its identification or purification.
- **Mass selection:** As practiced in plant and animal breeding the choosing of individuals for reproduction from the entire population on the basis of individual phenotypes.
- **Mass spectrometer:** An analytical device that can be used to determine the molecular weight (mass) of proteins and nucleic acids, the sequence of (composition and order of amino acids comprising) protein molecules, the chemical composition of virtually any material, and the rapid identification of intact Gram-negative and Gram-positive microorganisms (the latter, using matrix assisted laser desorption ionization time of flight mass spectrometry).

M

- **Mast cells (also known as mastocyte and labrocyte):** A resident cell of several types of tissues and contains many granules rich in histamine and heparin. They play an important protective role as well, being intimately involved in wound healing and defense.
- **Maternal effect:** An effect attributable to some aspect of performance of the mother of the individual being evaluated.
- **Maternal gene:** A gene from the mother's genome in which its expression on the phenotype of the zygote is determined from the mother's genotype, not from the zygote's.
- **Maternal inheritance:** The preferential survival in the progeny of genetic markers provided by one parent.
- **Mating type:** A group of individuals, within a species, which cannot breed among themselves but which are able to breed with individuals of other such groups.
- **Matrix metalloproteinases (MMP):** A family of enzymes that contain zinc metal ion (Zn^{2+}) at their active sites. Among this family are the collagenases.
- **Maturation:** The formation of gametes or spores.
- **Maximum residue level (MRL):** The maximum amount of residue legally permitted on food. Once residuces are demonstrated to be safe for consumers, MRLs are set by independent scientists, based on rigorous evalution of each pesticide legally authorised.
- **Mda:** Multiple drop away.
- **M-dominant:** Site or mutation affects the properties only of its own molecule of DNA. Co-dominance is taken to indicate that a site does not code for a diffusible product. (A rare exception is that a protein is cis-dominant when it is constrained to act only on the DNA or RNA from which it was synthesized.)
- **MEA:** Acronym for multilateral environmental agreement; an agreement (treaty) between a number of nations intended to protect/benefit the environment.
- **Mean:** In statistics, the arithmetic average is the sum of all measurements or values in a sample divided by the total number of sample size.
- **Median:** In a set of measurements, the central value above and below which there are an equal number of measurements.
- **Mediator:** A large protein complex associated with yeast bacterial RNA polymerase II. It contains factors that are necessary for transcription from many or most promoters.

- **Medicines control agency (MCA):** The British Government Agency, that, in concert with the committee on safety in medicines, regulates the approval and sale of pharmaceutical products in the United Kingdom.
- **Medium:** A substance used to provide nutrients for cell growth. It may be liquid (e.g. broth) or solid (e.g. agar).
- **Megabase (Mb):** A length of DNA consisting of 10^6 bp (1 Mb = 10^3 kb = 10^{-6} bp).
- **Megabase cloning:** The cloning of very large DNA fragments.
- **Megadalton (Mda):** One megadalton is equal to 10^6 daltons.
- **Megakaryocyte stimulating factor (MSF):** A colony stimulating factor (protein) involved in the regulation of platelet production, white blood cell production, and red blood cell production from stem cells in bone marrow.
- **Megaspores macrospore:** A haploid (n) spore developing into a female gametophyte in heterosporous plants.
- **Mega-Yeast artificial chromosomes (mega YAC):** A large (greater than 500 base pairs in length) piece of DNA that has been cloned (made) inside a living yeast cell. While most bacterial vectors cannot carry DNA pieces that are larger than 50 base pairs, and "standard" YACs typically cannot carry DNA pieces that are larger than 500 base pairs, mega YACs can carry DNA pieces (chromosomes) as large as one million base pairs in length.
- **Meiosis:** Occurs in two successive divisions (meiosis I and II) that reduce the number of 4n chromosomes to 1n in each of four product cells. Products may mature to germ cells (sperm or eggs) (Fig. 1).

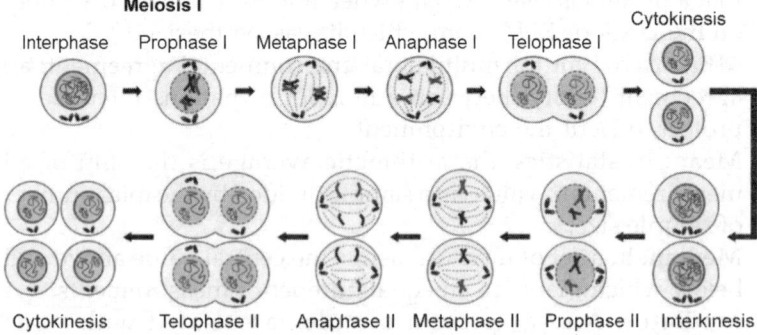

Fig. 1: Meiosis

- **Meiotic analysis:** A technique used to analyse chromosome pairing relationships.
- **Meiotic drive:** Any mechanism that causes alleles to be recovered unequally in the gametes of a heterozygote.
- **Melanin:** Pigment as typically produced by specialized epidermal cells called melanocytes.
- **Melting (of DNA):** Melting DNA means to heat-denature it. When this happens, the hydrogen bonds holding the DNA molecule together in the normal way are disrupted, allowing a more random polymer structure to exist.
- **Melting (of substance other than DNA):** To change from a solid to a nonsolid (e.g. liquid) state by the addition of heat (to the solid substance).
- **Melting temperature (T_m):** The midpoint of the temperature range over which DNA is denatured.
- **Melting:** DNA denaturation.
- **Membrane proteins:** Proteins have hydrophobic regions that allow part or all of the protein structure to reside within the membrane; the bonds involved in this association are usually noncovalent.
- **Membrane transport:** The facilitated transport of a solute across a membrane, usually by a specific membrane protein (e.g. adhesion molecule).
- **Membrane transporter protein:** A class of transmembrane proteins (i.e. protein molecules embedded in a cell's membrane, extending through both sides of the membrane) that function to transport certain molecules through the cell's membrane. Such molecules which are "transported" include: sugar molecules (utilized by the cell as "fuel"); inorganic ions (which catalyze certain cellular processes); polypeptides ["manufactured" in the cell's ribosome(s) and then secreted from the cell to perform some function elsewhere in the body of the organism]; anticancer drugs; antibiotics.
- **Membranes (of a cell):** A thin sheet-like structure, composed characteristically of a bimolecular leaflet of lipid and protein, enclosing a cell, an organelle or a vacuole. It is selectively permeable to ions and organic molecules and controls the movement of substances in and out of the cells.
- **Memory cell:** A lymphocyte that has been stimulated during the primary immune response to antigen and that is rapidly

activated upon subsequent exposure to that antigen. Memory cells respond more rapidly to antigen than naive cells.

- **MEMS (nanotechnology):** Acronym utilized by Americans to refer to "microelectromechanical systems" (which Europeans tend to refer to as "microsystems technology"— MST).

- **mEPSPS:** The "m" variant (of the many forms) of the enzyme 5-enolpyruvyl-shikimate-3-phosphate synthase. mEPSPS is unaffected by glyphosate- or sulfosate-containing herbicides, so introduction of the gene (coding for mEPSPS) into crop plants (e.g. corn/maize) makes those crop plants essentially impervious to glyphosate- or sulfosate containing herbicides.

- **Mendelian population:** A natural interbreeding unit of sexually reproducing plants or animals sharing a common gene pool.

- **Mendelism:** The theory of heredity that forms the basis of classical genetics, proposed by Gregor Mendel in 1866, and formulated in two laws.

- **Meristem:** Undifferentiated but determined tissue, the cells of which are capable of active cell division and differentiation into specialized and permanent tissue such as shoot and root.

- **Meristem culture:** A tissue culture containing meristematic dome tissue without adjacent leaf primordia or stem tissue. The term may also imply the culture of meristemoidal regions of plants or meristematic growth in culture.

- **Meristem tip:** An explant comprising the meristem (meristematic dome) and usually one pair of leaf primordial. Also refers to explants originating from apical meristem tip.

- **Meristem tip culture:** Cultures derived from meristem tip explants.

- **Mericlinal:** Refers to a chimera with tissue of one genotype partly surrounded by that of another genotype.

- **Mericloning:** A propagation method using shoot tips in culture to proliferate multiple buds which can then be separated, rooted and planted out.

- **Meristele:** The vascular cylinder to the stem.

- **Meristemoid:** A localized group of cells in callus tissue characterized by an accumulation of starch, RNA and protein and giving rise to adventitious shoots or roots.

- **Merozygote:** Partial zygote produced by a process of partial genetic exchange such as transformation in bacteria.

- **Mesoderm:** The middle germ layer that forms in the germinal layer in the early animal embryo and gives rise to parts such as bone and connective tissue.

- **Mesodermal adult stem cells:** Certain stem cells present within (adult) bodies of organisms, that can be differentiated (via chemical signals) to give rise to bone, muscle, and/or fat cells.

- **Mesophile:** An organism that grows best in the temperature range of 25°C (77°F) to 40°C (104°F).

- **Messenger RNA (mRNA):** It is the intermediate that represents one strand of a gene coding for protein. Its coding region is related to the protein sequence by the triplet genetic code.

- **Metabolic cell:** A cell that is not dividing.

- **Metabolic engineering:** The selective, deliberate alteration of an organism's metabolic pathway(s) via genetic engineering of the genes that define/control the organism's metabolism. Some reasons to do metabolic engineering of an organism include: altering cell "behavior" and organism metabolic patterns to induce production of proteins/polypeptides and/or metabolites that are desired by mankind (e.g. "golden rice"). Altering cell "behavior" and organism metabolic patterns to induce a given organism to consume or accumulate toxic wastes or valuable materials (e.g. gold) that are present at a site in low concentration or highly dispersed. Altering cell "behavior" and organism metabolic patterns to cure disease.

- **Metabolic pathway:** Refers to a particular pathway [i.e. series of chemical reactions, each of which is dependent on previous one(s)] within the overall process of metabolism in an organism. For example, when humans consume the herb known as Saint John's Wort (*Hypericum perforatum*), certain components in that herb induce a (new) metabolic pathway—catalyzed by cytochrome P450 enzymes—that (more) rapidly metabolizes (i.e. breaks down) a number of commercial pharmaceuticals (thereby lowering the effectiveness of a given dose of that particular pharmaceutical).

- **Metabolism:** The entire set of enzyme-catalyzed transformations of organic nutrient molecules (to sustain life) in living cells. Conversion of food and water molecules into nutrients that can be used by the body's cells, and the use of those nutrients by those cells to sustain life, grow, etc.

- **Metabolite:** A chemical intermediate in the enzyme-catalyzed chemical reactions of metabolism.

- **Metacentric chromosome:** A chromosome with the centromere near the middle and consequently two arms of about equal length.

- **Metalloenzyme:** An enzyme having a metal ion as its prosthetic group.

- **Metalloproteins:** A term that is utilized to refer to any protein molecule that contains within it (i.e. in "peptide chain") a metal atom (zinc, iron, copper, etc.). Approximately, one-third of all proteins are metalloproteins. Those that contain a zinc atom (Zn^{2+}) are generally enzymes (thus called metalloenzymes), because that metal acts as a catalyst.

- **Metallothionein:** A protective protein that binds heavy metals such as cadmium and lead.

- **Metamodel methods (of bioinformatics):** These refer to methods utilized to integrate data that has been independently generated/created (and generally stored in separate database models) via independent genomics research projects, combinatorial chemistry projects, high-throughput screening projects (e.g. via biochip use), etc. Metamodel methods sometimes reveal important interrelationships that were not apparent in the individual models (i.e. created solely for the genomics project data, or for the combinatorial chemistry project data, or for the high-throughput screening project data, etc.).

- **Metaphase:** Stage of mitosis during which the chromosomes or atleast the kinetochores lie in the central plane of the spindle. It is the stage following prophase and preceding anaphase.

- **Metastasis:** The ability of tumor cells to leave their sites of origin and migrate to other locations in the body, where a new colony is established.

- **Meter:** A unit of measurement, contrived by French scientists during the 1670s. It was initially defined to be one ten-millionth of the distance from the earth's equator to its poles.

- **Methionine (met):** An essential amino acid, furnishes (to organism) both labile methyl groups and sulfur necessary for normal metabolism.

- **Methotrexate:** A drug that inhibits the enzyme dihydrofolate reductase (DHFR).

- **Methyl jasmonate:** The volatile chemical compound that results when methyl groups (CH_3) are chemically added to a molecule of jasmonic acid.
- **Methyl salicylate:** The volatile chemical compound that results when methyl groups (CH_3) are added to a molecule of salicylic acid. During 1997, Ilya Raskin showed that methyl salicylate emitted by one tobacco plant (e.g. under 'attack' by insects, fungi, bacteria, or viruses) could cause other nearby tobacco plants to "turn on" their self defense mechanism (systemic acquired resistance).
- **Methylated:** Refers to a DNA molecule that is saturated with methyl groups (i.e. methyl submolecule groups, $-CH_3$, have attached themselves to the DNA molecule at all possible locations). Generally, when a DNA molecule is methylated, the genes comprising that DNA molecule are "turned off" (inactivated).
- **Methylation:** The addition of a methyl group ($-CH_3$) to a macromolecule such as the addition of a methyl group to specific cytosine and occasionally adenine residues in DNA.
- **Methyltransferase (methylase):** An enzyme that adds a methyl group to a substrate, which can be a molecule, protein, or a nucleic acid.
- **MHC class I:** Protein mostly presents, to CD8+ T cells, peptides that are produced by proteolytic degradation in the cytosol.
- **MHC class II:** Protein mostly presents, to CD4+ T cells, peptides that are produced by proteolytic degradation in the endocytic pathway.
- **Micelle:** The spherical structure formed by the association of a number of amphiphilic molecules dissolved in water. Structurally, the outer surface of the micelle (sphere) is covered with the polar domains (head groups) which are directed toward (stick into) the water while the interior of the micelle contains the nonpolar domains (tails), which self-associate to create an "oil droplet" microenvironment. Micelles may be used to solubilize nonwater (oil) soluble or sparingly water soluble molecules in water. They may be formed by ionic or non-ionic surfactants.
- **Micro total analysis systems (μTAS):** A flowing stream based analysis system that integrates one or several laboratory functions on a single microchip of a few square centimeters in size.

- **Microaerophile:** An organism that grows best in the presence of a small amount of oxygen.
- **Microalgal culture:** Culture in bioreactors of microalgae that include seaweeds.
- **Microarray (testing):** Refers to a piece of glass, plastic, or silicon onto which a large number of biosensors are placed. These microarrays (sometimes called "biochips" or "DNA chips") can then be utilized to test a single biological sample for a variety of attributes or effects.
- **Microbe:** A microscopic organism; applied particularly to bacteria. The word "microbe" was coined by Monsieur Sedillot, a colleague of Louis Pasteur.
- **Microbial mats:** Layered groups or communities in microbial populations.
- **Microbial physiology:** An understanding of cell structure, growth factors, metabolism and genetic composition of micro-organisms.
- **Microbial source tracking (MST):** The process of systematically determining the original source (in a specific environment) of a microbe (e.g. the one that has caused a given disease outbreak). Some of the technologies utilized in MST include genetic fingerprinting, polymerase chain reaction (PCR), serotyping, etc.
- **Microbicide:** Any chemical that kills microorganisms, used synonymously with the terms biocide and bactericide.
- **Microbody:** A cellular organelle always bound by a single membrane, spherical in shape, 20 to 60 nm in diameter containing a variety of enzymes.
- **Microbiology:** Study of Microbes; The science dealing with the structure, classification, physiology, and distribution of microorganisms, and their technical and medical significance.
- **Microcarriers:** Small particles used as a support carrier material for cells and particularly mammalian cells which are too fragile to be pumped and stirred, as bacterial cells are in a large scale culture.
- **Micrococcal nuclease:** An enzyme, produced by a member of the genus *Micrococcus*, which cleaves nucleic acids to oligonucleotides terminating in 3′–phosphates.
- **Micrococcal nuclease:** An endonuclease that cleaves DNA; in chromatin, DNA is cleaved preferentially between nucleosomes.
- **Microelement:** An element required in very small quantities.

- **Microencapsulation:** A process of enclosing a substance in very small sealed capsules from which material is released by heat, solutions or other means.
- **Microenvironment:** The local environment close enough to the surface of a living or non-living object to be influenced by it.
- **Microfibrils:** Exceedingly small fibre visible only at high magnification of the electron microscope.
- **Microfilaments:** Very thin filaments found in the cytoplasm of cells.
- **Microfluidics:** Refers to the science and properties of fluids when flowing through very small passages (e.g. micron or nanometer dimensions) and/or in very small amounts (e.g. femtogram quantities). For example, to move fluid (samples), microfluidic chips utilize either capillary action or else they "pump" fluid (through microchannels in those chips) electrokinetically (i.e. cause the flow to occur by applying a controlled electrical field, so liquid is attracted to electrical charge, and thereby flows). Such "pumping" could also be utilized to deliver certain medicines in very small, precisely timed and metered doses (e.g. if the microfluidic chip is embedded into diseased tissue within the body). Another potential application of such "pumping" could be to perform multiple chemical analysis (e.g. body fluids within diseased tissues), in which case such microfluidic chips are known as "lab-on-a-chip"/laboratory-on-a-chip analytical devices.
- **Microgram:** 10^{-6} gram, 2.527×10^{-8} ounce (avoirdupoir).
- **Microinjection:** A technique of injecting DNA or RNA into the nucleus of protoplast of cell with the help of a micropipette.
- **Micromachining:** Refers to the technology and tools or methods utilized to create the very small parts, grooves (in chips/arrays), etc. in nanoelectromechanical systems (NEMs), biochips, microarrays, and other devices of the field of nanotechnology.
- **Micron:** Also called micrometer; A unit of length convenient for describing cellular dimensions; the Greek letter ì is used as its symbol. A micron is equal to 10^{-3} mm (millimeter) or 10^{4}Å (Angstrong) or 0.00003937 inch.
- **Micronutrient:** Added in growth media; the essential element which are required in concentrations < 0.5 millimole/litre.
- **Microorganism:** Any organism of microscopic size (i.e. requires a microscope to be seen by man). First viewed by Antoni Lie

Van Leeuwenhoek in 1676. Some microorganisms are pathogenic (disease-causing) and some are not.

- **Microparticles:** Particles between 0.1 μm and 100 μm in size. These are immunologically unique to their cells of origin and may play a role in antigen presentation.
- **Microplasts:** Vesicles produced by subdivision and fragmentation of protoplasts or thin-walled cells.
- **Microprojectile bombardment:** A procedure for modifying cells by shooting DNA-coated metal (tungsten or gold) particles into them.
- **Micropropagation:** The technique of small piece of tissue, such as meristem, grown in culture to produce large number of plants.
- **Micropyle:** A small opening on the surface of a plant ovule through which the pollen tube passes prior to fertilization.
- **MicroRNAs:** Very short RNAs that may regulate gene expression.
- **Microsatellite DNA:** Pieces of the same small segment (a DNA sequence) which are "repeated" (appear repeatedly in sequence within the DNA molecule) adjacent to a specific gene within the DNA molecule. Thus, these "microsatellites" are linked to that specific gene.
- **Microsomes:** Fragmented pieces of endoplasmic reticulum associated with ribosomes.
- **Microspore:** The smaller sized spore of the two kinds of meiospores produced by heterosporous plants in the course of microsporogenesis in seed plants. Microspores give rise to the pollen grain, the male gametophyte.
- **Microtuber:** Miniature tuber, produced in tissue culture, which is readily regenerable into a normal tuberous plant.
- **Microtubule associated proteins (MAPs):** Proteins associated with microtubules and responsible for influencing their stability and organization.
- **Microtubule organizing center (MTOC):** A structure from which microtubules may be extended. The major MTOCs in a mitotic cell are the chromosomes.
- **Microtubules:** Filaments consisting of dimers of tubulin; interphase microtubules are recognized into spindle fibers at mitosis, when they are responsible for chromosome movement.

M

- **Midbody:** The last connection between two cells, separated at the end of cytokinesis. A parallel array of microtubules derived from the mitotic spindle enters the midbody from each cell, and the two arrays interdigitate across its whole width.

- **Middle genes:** Phage genes that are regulated by the proteins coded by early genes. Some proteins coded by middle genes catalyze replication of the phage DNA; others regulate the expression of a later set of genes.

- **Middle lamella:** Original thin membrane separating two adjacent protoplasts and remaining as a distinct cementing layer between adjacent cell walls.

- **Mid-Oleic sunflowers:** Refers to sunflower (crop) plant varieties which have been breeded so that their seeds contain 50–75% oleic acid within the oil in those seeds; vs. historical average of 20% oleic acid in the oil of traditional sunflower (crop) plant varieties.

- **Mid-Oleic vegetable oils:** Refers to any vegetable oils (other than sunflower oil) that contain 50–70% oleic acid. The range of oleic acid content is slightly different for mid-oleic sunflower oil definition.

- **Mid-parent value:** In quantitative genetics, the average of the phenotypes of two mates.

- **Minicell:** An anucleated bacterial (*E. coli*) cell produced by a division that generates a cytoplasm without a nucleus.

- **Minichromosome (of SV 40 or polyoma):** The nucleosomal form of the viral circular DNA.

- **Minimized proteins:** The domain/active site of a native protein (former) after all or most of its extraneous (unneeded) portions (peptides) have been removed. In 1995, Brian Cunningham and James A. Wells reduced the 28-residue (peptide) protein (hormone) Atrial Natriuretic Factor to 15-residues (peptides) size without reducing its potency (biological activity). Minimized proteins that retain their potency hold the potential for medicines possessing a greater serum lifetime (when injected into a patient's body), and as "models" for the creation of organichemical-synthesized mimetic drugs possessing the same therapeutic effect as the native protein did.

- **Miniprep:** A small scale (mini-1) preparation of plasmid or phage DNA; used to analyse DNA in a cloning vector after a cloning experiment.
- **Minisatellite:** A section of DNA that consists of a short series of bases 10–160 base pairs (bp). These occur at more than 1,000 locations in the human genome.
- **Minituber:** Small tubers (5–15 mm in diameter) formed by shoot cultures or by cutting of tuber forming crops, such as potato.
- **Minor groove:** In helix of DNA it is 12Å across.
- **Minus strand DNA:** The single-stranded DNA sequence that is complementary to the viral RNA genome of a plus strand virus.
- **Mismatch repair:** A DNA repair mechanism that fixes bases that do not pair properly. The mechanism preferentially corrects the sequence of the daughter strand, by distinguishing the daughter strand and parental strand on the basis of their states of methylation.
- **Mismatch:** When normal base pairing is not observed in DNA, say for example pairing between T and G.
- **Missense mutation:** A mutation that alters a codon so that it encodes a different amino acid.
- **Missense:** When mutation change lead to in a single codon and may cause the replacement of one amino acid by another in a protein sequence.
- **Missense suppressor:** Codes for a tRNA that has been mutated so as to recognize a different codon. By inserting a different amino-acid at a mutant codon, the tRNA suppresses the effect of the original mutation.
- **Mist propagation:** Application of fine droplets of water to leafy cuttings rooting stage to reduce transpiration.
- **Mites:** Free-living and parasitic animals belonging to the order Acarina, class Arachnida (with spiders). Mites may infest plant crops reducing their harvest.
- **Mitochondria:** Granular or rod-shaped body (organelles) in a cell's cytoplasm, that contain enzyme systems required in the citric acid cycle, electron transport, beta-oxidation of fatty acids, and synthesis of ATP via oxidative phosphorylation (Fig. 2).

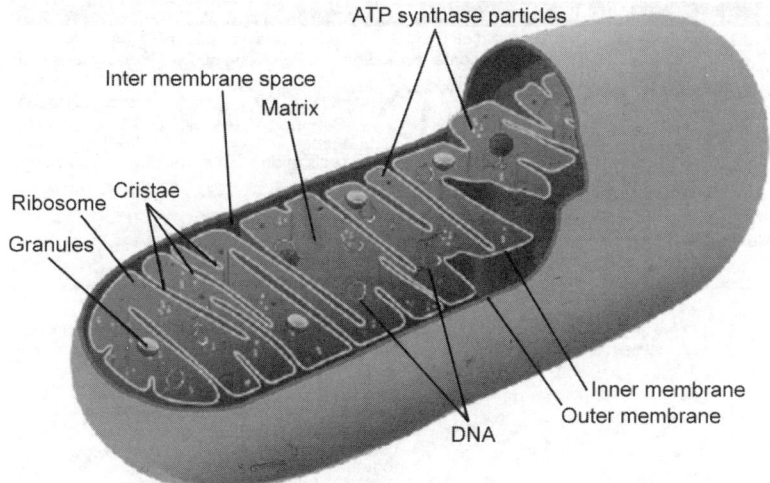

Fig. 2: Mitochondria

- **Mitochondrial DNA (mtDNA):** An independent DNA genome, usually circular, located in the mitochondria.
- **Mitogen:** A substance (growth factor, hormone, etc.) that initiates cell division or mitosis within the body. For example, most angiogenic growth factors (e.g. fibroblast growth factor) stimulate cell division of the endothelial cells which line blood vessel walls.
- **Mitosis (M phase):** The process by which the cell nucleus divides, resulting in daughter cells that contain the same genetic material as that of parent cell (Fig. 3).
- **Mitotic cyclin (G2 cyclin):** It is a regulatory subunit that partners a kinase subunit to form the M phase inducer.
- **Mixed bud:** A bud containing both rudimentary leaves and flowers.
- **Mixed-function oxygenase:** Enzymes catalyzing simultaneous oxidation of two substances by oxygen, one of which is usually NADPH or NADH.
- **Mixoploid:** Cells with variable (euploid, aneuploid) chromosome numbers. Mosaics or chimeras differ in chromosome number as a result of a variety of mitotic irregularities.
- **Mobile phase:** The mixture of solvents that is percolated through the column.

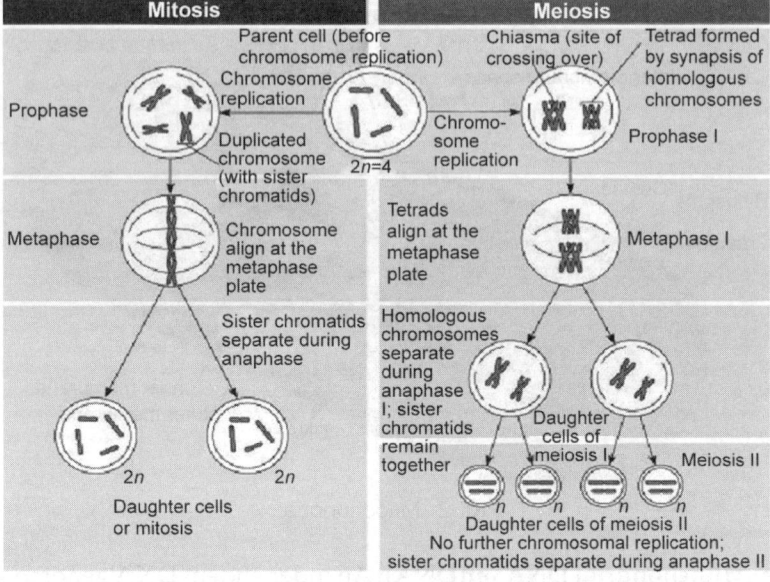

Fig. 3: Mitosis and meiosis

- **Mobility:** The velocity of a particle or ion attains for a given voltage. A relative measure of how quickly an ion moves in an electric field.
- **Mobilization:** The transfer of a non-conjugative plasmid by a conjugative plasmid between the bacteria.
- **Mobilizing function:** The genes on a plasmid that give the ability to facilitate the transfer of either a non-conjugative or a conjugative plasmid from one bacterium to another.
- **Model class mode:** In a frequency distribution the class having the greatest frequency.
- **Model organism:** Refers to an organism that is utilized (e.g. in scientific experiments) to conduct tests, etc. in an attempt to infer results applicable to larger, more complex organisms. For example, the use of the microscopic roundworm *C. elegans* in high through put screening to attempt to find pharmaceuticals that will be useful for humans.
- **Model:** A mathematical description of a biological phenomenon.
- **Modification (of DNA or RNA):** Includes the changes made to the nucleotides after initial incorporation into the polynucleotide chain.

- **Modified bases:** All those except the usual four from which DNA (T, C, A, G) and RNA (U, C, A, G) are synthesized; they result from post-synthetic changes in the nucleic acid.
- **Modifier modifying gene:** A gene that affects the expression of some other gene.
- **Moiety:** Referring to a part or portion of a molecule, generally complex, having a characteristic chemical or pharmacological property.
- **Molality:** The number of moles of solute per litre of solvent.
- **Molarity:** The number of moles of a substance contained in a kilogram of solution.
- **Mole:** An Avogadro's number (6.023×10^{23}) of whatever units are being considered. One gram molecular weight of an element or a compound (i.e. same number of grams of an element or a compound as that substance's molecular weight), equals to 6.023×10^{23} molecules.
- **Molecular beacon:** Term that is used to refer to specific oligonucleotides possessing a "hairpin loop" and bearing a fluorescent dye. A "quencher dye" located on a nearby portion of the hairpin loop prevents fluorescence until the hairpin loop is opened up. Molecular beacons (sometimes called fluorogenic probes) are utilized (e.g. in high-throughput screening or high-throughput identification) to detect the presence of a desired "target" molecule. When the "target" (i.e. a molecule possessing the desired functional group or desired property) is present within a given sample being evaluated, the "hairpin loop" opens up because a portion of it forms a stronger bond to the "target," than to the rest of the loop thereby allowing the fluorescent dye to emit light.
- **Molecular biology:** A term coined by Vannevar Bush during the 1940s, that eventually mean the study and manipulation of molecules that constitute, or interact with cells. Molecular biology as a distinct scientific discipline originated largely as a result of a decision to provide "support for the application of new physical and chemical techniques to biology", during the 1930s by Warren Weaver, director of the biology (funding) program at America's Rockefeller Foundation (a philanthropic organization).
- **Molecular breeding TM:** A trademarked term that refers to certain "molecular evolution" technologies developed by Maxygen Company. This term is also sometimes used to refer

M

to the utilization of molecular genetics and/or marker assisted selection in a breeding program (e.g. within a seed company or a university) to select the organisms (e.g. crop varieties) that possess gene(s) for a particular trait (higher yield, disease resistance, etc.).

• **Molecular chaperone:** A protein that is needed for the assembly of proper folding of some other protein, but which is not itself a component of the target complex.

• **Molecular cloning:** The biological amplification of a specific DNA sequence through mitotic division of a host cell, into which it has been transformed or transfected.

• **Molecular diversity:** Sometimes referred to as "irrational drug design," this refers to the drug design technique of generating large numbers of diverse candidate molecules (e.g. pieces of DNA, RNA, proteins, or other organic moieties) at random (via a variety of methods). These diverse candidate molecules are then tested to see which is best at working against a disease/condition (e.g. fitting a cell receptor, or category of receptors relevant to the disease in question). Molecular candidates that show promise (e.g. via a "pretty good fit" to receptor) are then produced in larger quantities (e.g. via Polymerase Chain Reaction techniques) alongwith additional molecules that are similar though slightly different in structure (e.g. via site-directed mutagenesis) in an attempt to create a molecule that is a "perfect fit" (e.g. to receptor).

• **Molecular farming:** Growing and harvesting genetically modified crops, with the object of producing not foodstuffs but pharmaceuticals. It refers to the use of genetic engineering putting specific genes from other organisms into a plant to create plants which will produce products such as drugs, chemicals, vaccines and even biodegradable plastics. More than 150 proteins and peptides (linked amino acids) have been produced using tobacco mosaic virus as vector. In the past, molecular farming of drugs from transgenic livestock such as pigs, sheep and cows required the death of the animal so the drug could be harvested from their blood. Now the focus has been shifted to producing useful proteins secreted into the mills of transgenic livestock (Fig. 4).

• **Molecular genetics:** The science dealing with the study of the nature and biochemistry of the genetic material and includes the technologies of genetic engineering.

Candidate protein

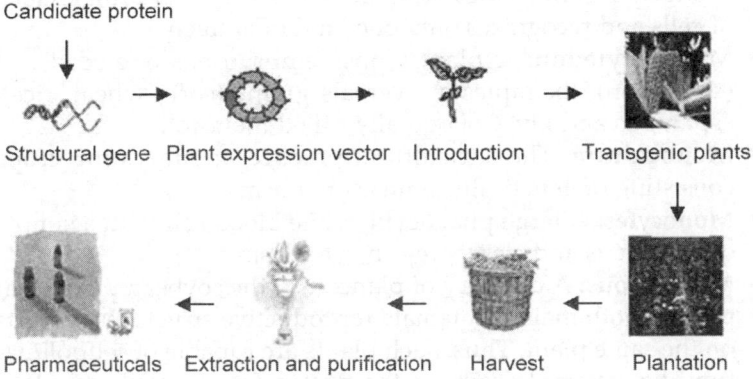

Structural gene   Plant expression vector   Introduction   Transgenic plants

Pharmaceuticals   Extraction and purification   Harvest   Plantation

Fig. 4: Molecular farming

- **Molecular machines:** Refers to nanometer dimension "machines" capable of doing various tasks.
- **Molecular markers:** The markers (DNA sequences) revealing variation at DNA level which can be detected and monitored in the subsequent generations e.g. RFLP, RAPD, SSR, etc.
- **Molecular pharming TM:** A trademark of the Groupe Limagrain company, refers to the production of pharmaceuticals and certain other chemicals (e.g. intermediates utilized to manufacture pharmaceuticals) in agronomic plants (which have been genetically engineered).
- **Molecular sieving:** Separation of molecules on the basis of their effective sizes.
- **Molecular weight:** The sum of the atomic weights of the constituent atoms in a molecule.
- **Molecule:** A unit of matter; the smallest portion of an element or a compound that retains chemical identity with the substances in mass. The molecule usually consists of a union of two or more atoms. Some organic molecules contain a very large number of atoms.
- **Monarch butterfly:** Refers to the insect (*Lepidoptera*: *Danaidae* or *Danaus plexippus*) whose pupae (caterpillars) feed exclusively on tissue of the plant known as common milkweed (*Asclepias syriaca*), and whose territory extends from northern Mexico to approximately Canada's southern border.
- **Monocistronic mRNA:** An mRNA that codes for single protein.

- **Monoclonal antibodies:** Antibodies derived from a single clone of cells and recognizes only one kind of antigen.
- **Monocotyledon:** A plant whose embryo has one seed leaf (cotyledon). Examples are cereals grains (corn, wheat, rice), asparagus and lily. Colloquially called monocot.
- **Monoculture:** The agricultural practice of cultivating crops consisting of genetically similar organisms.
- **Monocytes:** A large phagocytic white blood cell with a simple oval nucleus and clear, greyish cytoplasm.
- **Monoecious:** A category of plants (e.g. the soybean plant) that possess both male and female reproductive structures or parts on the same plant. Thus, such plants are capable of selfpollination. For example, 95% of the pollen from a soybean plant (*Glycine max*) does not leave the flower in which it was produced.
- **Monogastric animals:** Animals with simple stomach that do not ruminate.
- **Monogenic:** Controlled by a single gene as opposed to multigenic.
- **Monohybrid:** The offspring of two homozygous parents that differ from one another by the alleles present at only one locus.
- **Monohybrid cross:** A type of cross involving parents differing in only one trait or in which only one trait is considered.
- **Monolayer:** It describes the growth of eukaryotic cells in culture as a layer only one cell deep.
- **Monomer:** The basic molecular subunit from which, by repetition of a single reaction, polymers are made. For example, amino acids (monomers) link together via condensation reactions to yield polypeptides or proteins (polymers). A monomer is analogous to a link (monomer) in a metal chain (polymer).
- **Monophyletic:** Describing any group of organism that are assumed to have originated from the same ancestor.
- **Monosaccharides:** The chemical building blocks of carbohydrates, hence known as "simple sugars". They are classified by the number of carbon atoms in the (monosaccharide) molecule. For example, pentoses have five and hexoses have six carbon atoms. They normally form ring structures. The empirical formula for monosaccharides is $(CH_2O)n$.
- **Monosomy (2n-1):** Occurs when an individual has only one type of a particular chromosome.

- **Mono-unsaturated fatty acids (MUFA):** Refers to the category of those fatty acids (e.g. oleic acid) that possess one less than the maximum possible number of hydrogen atoms (e.g. possible to be attached to the molecular structure of oleic acid). Enzymes (e.g. $\Delta12$ desaturase) present in some oilseed plants (soybean, corn/maize, canola, etc.) convert some MUFAs to polyunsaturated fatty acids (PUFAs) within their developing seeds. Diets that are high in MUFA content have been shown to reduce low-density lipoproteins ("bad" cholesterol) blood content while simultaneously leaving blood levels of high density lipoproteins ("good" cholesterol) essentially unchanged. Soybean oil has historically averaged approximately 24.5% MUFA content by weight.
- **Monounsaturates:** Oil containing mono-unsaturated fatty acids.
- **Monozygotic twins:** One egg or identical twins derived from the splitting of a single fertilized ovum.
- **Monster:** Particles of bacteriophages form as the result of an assembly defect in which the capsid proteins form a head that is much longer than usual.
- **Morphogen:** A factor that induces development of particular cell types in a manner that depends on its concentration.
- **Morphogenesis:** The development of a structure from an unorganized state to a differentiated and organized state.
- **Morphogenetic:** An adjective referring to formation and differentiation of tissues and organs in an organism.
- **Morphology:** First used in print by the poet Johann Wolfgang von Goethe, this word is utilized to refer to the form/structure of an organism or any of its parts.
- **Mosaic:** An organism or part of an organism that is composed of cells with different origin.
- **MPF (maturation- or M phase-promoting factor):** A dimeric kinase, containing the p34 catalytic subunit and a cyclin regulatory subunit, whose activation triggers the onset of mitosis.
- **Mrus:** Minimum recognition units.
- **mtDNA:** Mitochondrial DNA.
- **Multicopy:** Describing plasmids which replicate to produce many plasmid molecules per host genome e.g. pBR322 is a multicopy plasmid.

- **Multicopy control:** A plasmid is said to be under multicopy control when the control system allows the plasmid to exist in more than one copy per individual bacterial cell.
- **Multicopy plasmids:** Plasmids present inside bacteria in quantity greater than one plasmid per (host) cell.
- **Multienzyme system:** A sequence of related enzymes participating in a given metabolic (chemical reaction) pathway.
- **Multiforked chromosome (in bacterium):** More than one replication fork, because a second initiation has occurred before the first cycle of replication has been completed.
- **Multigene family:** A group of genes that are similar in nucleotide sequence or that produce polypeptides with similar amino acid sequences.
- **Multigenic:** Controlled by several genes as opposed to monogenic.
- **Multilocus probe:** A probe that hybridizes to a number of different sites in the genome of an organism.
- **Multimeric proteins:** It consists of more than one subunit.
- **Multiple aleurone layer (MAL) gene:** A gene in corn (maize) that (when present in the DNA of a given plant) causes that plant to produce seed that contains higher than normal level of calcium, magnesium, iron, zinc, and manganese. These higher mineral levels are particularly useful for feeding of swine, since traditional No. 2 yellow (dent) corn does not contain enough for optimal pig growth.
- **Multiple alleles:** More than two alleles for one locus, but each individual inherits only two alleles, e.g. ABO system of human blood type.
- **Multiple sclerosis:** A disease in which the human body's immune cells attack myelin (the "insulation" that surrounds nerve fibers in the spinal cord and brain) and the body's acetylcholine receptors. That leads to recurrent muscle weakness, loss of muscle control, and (potentially) eventual paralysis.
- **Multipotent adult stem cell:** Certain stem cells present within (adult) body of an organisms, that can be differentiated (via chemical signals) to give rise to a variety of different cell/tissue types (bone, cartilage, fat, muscle, red blood cells, B cells, T cells, etc.).
- **Multivalent vaccine:** A single vaccine that is designed to elicit an immune response either to more than one infectious agent or to several different epitopes of a molecule.

M

- **Murine:** Of, or pertaining to, mice. For example, the first monoclonal antibodies were produced using cells from mice. This frequently caused adverse immune responses to monoclonal antibodies when they were injected into the human body (limiting their use in therapeutic purposes).

- **Muscular dystrophy (MD):** A genetic disease caused by a defect in the X chromosome (resulting in nonexpression of the Duchenne Muscular Dystrophy gene); first recognized by G. A. B. Duchenne in 1858. The disease afflicts males almost exclusively because males have only one X chromosome, whereas females inherit two copies of the X chromosome and have a "backup" in case one X chromosome is damaged (as is the case for MD victims). In 1981, Kay E. Davies used DNA probes (genetic probes) to discover that the Duchenne Muscular Dystrophy (DMD) gene must lie somewhere between two unique (to MD victims) segments on the upper, shorter arm of the X chromosome.

- **Mushrooms:** Edible fruiting bodies of ascomycetous and basidiomycetous fungi (Fig. 5).

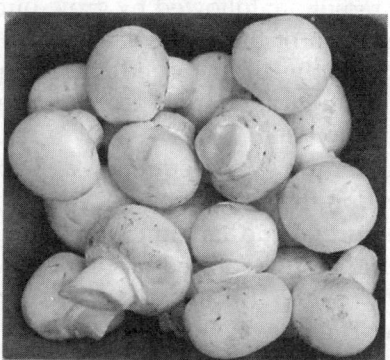

Fig. 5: Mushrooms

- **Mutable gene:** Genes with an unusually high mutation rate.
- **Mutagen:** Any agent that causes mutations by damaging DNA.
- **Mutagenesis:** Changes in the genetic constitution of a cell through alterations to its DNA.
- **Mutant:** An organism differing from the normal or wild type due to a change in its DNA sequence.

- **Mutase:** An enzyme catalyzing transposition of a functional group in the substrate (substance acted upon by the enzyme). Intramolecular transfer of a chemical group from one position (i.e. carbon atom) to another within the same molecule. An example of a mutase is phosphoglucomutase. It has a molecular weight of about 60,000 Daltons with about 600 amino acid residues (monomers). The mutase can interchange (move) a phosphate unit between the 1 and 6 position, where 1 refers to a carbon atom designated as "#1" and the 6 refers to a different carbon atom designated as "#6".

- **Mutation breeding:** Refers to several techniques, involving induced mutations, that were utilized by some crop plant breeders (primarily in the 1960s and 1970s) to introduce desirable genes into the plants with which they were working. For example, gene(s) to confer resistance to plant diseases, increased yield per acre/hectare or improvements in composition that were not present within the historic/natural germplasm of that plant species. These new-to-that-species genes were "created" via soaking its seeds or pollen in mutation-causing chemicals (i.e. mutagens), or via bombardment of seeds with ionizing radiation; followed by grow-out of the resultant plants and selection of the particular mutation (i.e. beneficial trait) desired by the plant breeder. That plant was then propagated via straightforward breeding to yield seeds that are still sown today.

- **Mutation frequency:** The frequency at which a particular mutant is found in the population.

- **Mutation pressure:** A constant mutation rate that adds mutant genes to a population. Repeated occurences of mutations in a population.

- **Mutation rate:** The rate at which a particular mutation occurs, usually given as the number of events per gene per generation.

- **Mutation:** Change in the DNA sequence of a gene to some new, heritable form generally, but not always a recessive allele. A forward mutation converts a wild-type allele to mutant allele.

- **Mutator:** A gene in which mutation results in an increase in the basal level mutation of the genome. Such genes often code for proteins that are involved in repairing damaged DNA.

- **Mutual recognition agreements (MRAs):** Legal agreements (treaties) between two or more nations, to recognize and respect each other's approval process (e.g. for new crops derived via biotechnology).

- **Mycelium:** Thread-like filament making up the vegetative portion of thallus fungi.
- *Mycobacterium tuberculosis*: The pathogen that causes tuberculosis, a human disease, in which lungs are destroyed as this bacteria grows (within lung tissue). In 1998, scientists completed sequencing of the genome of *Mycobacterium tuberculosis*. Recently, a new strain of *M. tuberculosis*, that is resistant to virtually all commercial antibiotics, has begun to infect some people.
- **Mycoherbicide:** Fungal preparations that kill the abnoxious weeds/herbs.
- **MycoRhiz®:** A commercial preparation of *Pisolithus tinctorius* mycelia produced by Abbott Lab (USA) used for raising tree seedling through tailoring of roots.
- **Mycorrhiza:** Fungi that form an association with or have a symbiotic relationship with roots of plants.
- **Mycotoxins:** Toxins produced by fungi. More than 350 different mycotoxins are known to man, but the first ones to be isolated and scientifically characterized (i.e. described) was the aflatoxins, in 1961. The second group was the ochratoxins, in 1965. Almost all mycotoxins are harmful and possess the capacity to alter the immune systems of animals. Consumption by animals (including humans) of certain mycotoxins (via eating infected corn/maize, wheat, certain tree nuts, peanuts, cotton seed products, etc.) can result in liver toxicity, gastrointestinal lesions, cancer, muscle necrosis, etc.
- **Myeloma:** A tumor cell line derived from a lymphocyte; usually produces a single type of immunoglobulin.
- **Myoelectric signals:** The nerve signals that are sent by the body in order to control muscle movement.
- **Myristoylation:** Transformation of proteins in cells in such a manner that these cells then cause cancer.
- **Myxoma:** The name of the virus that causes myxomatosis in rabbits. It is carried by mosquitoes and fleas.
- **Myxomatosis:** A disease of rabbits caused by the myxoma virus. It results in streaming eyes, swelling of the head, difficulty in breathing and eventually death.

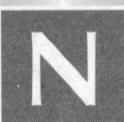

- **N₂:** Free nitrogen gas, in liquid form used as a cryopreservant.
- **N nucleotide sequence:** A short non-templated sequence that is added randomly by the enzyme at coding joints, during rearrangement of immunoglobulin and T cell receptor genes. N nucleotides augment the diversity of antigen receptors.
- **N-1 rule:** States that only one X chromosome is active in female mammalian cells; other(s) are inactivated.
- **n-3 fatty acids:** Also known as "omega-3" fatty acids. A family of long-chain polyunsaturated fatty acids, primarily eicosapentaenoic-C20:5 and docosahexanenoic acid–C22:6; dietary NFAs cardioprotective and have a positive impact on inflammation, interfering with production of inflammatory mediators–e.g. leukotrienes, PAF, IL-1, TNF.
- **n-6 fatty acids:** Also known as "omega-6" fatty acids. A polyunsaturated fatty acid whose carbon chain has its first double valence bond six carbons from the beginning.
- **NAD (NADH, NADP, NADPH):** Nicotinamide adeninedinucleotide, also known as diphosphopyridine nucleotide, codehydrogenase 1, coenzyme 1, and coenzymase by its discoverers, Harden and Young. $C_{21}H_{27}O_{14}N_7P_2$. An organic coenzyme (molecule) that functions as a distinct yet integral part of certain enzymes. NAD plays a role in certain enzymes concerned with oxidation/reduction reactions. Meanings: NADH, nicotinamide-adenine dinucleotide, reduced; NADP, nicotinamide-adenine dinucleotide phosphate; and NADPH, nicotinamide-adenine dinucleotide phosphate, reduced.
- **NADH:** Nicotine-adenine dinucleotide, reduced.
- **NADP:** Nicotine-adenine dinucleotide phosphate.
- **NADPH:** Nicotinamide-adenine dinucleotide phosphate, reduced.
- **Naked bud:** A bud not protected by bud scales.

- **Naked gene:** A purified DNA sequence with no associated proteins. An immune response can be evoked by directly injecting into the host DNA that encodes an immunogen of interest.
- **Nanobots:** Refers to very small "robots" whose dimensions could be measured in terms of nanometers (nm), and could perform specific tasks.
- **Nanocomposites:** A multiphase solid material where one of the phases has one, two or three dimensions of less than 100 nanometers (nm), or structures having nano-scale repeat distances between the different phases that make-up the material.
- **Nanocrystal molecules:** Double-standed DNA molecules that have attached to them several multi-atom clusters of gold.
- **Nanocrystals:** A term used to refer to any crystalline structure possessing dimensions (e.g. overall width) measured in terms of nanometers.
- **Nanoelectromechanical system (NEMS):** Refers to working (i.e. those with moving "mechanical parts") systems of a scale whose relevant dimensions are measured in terms of nanometers (nm). For example, in 2000, Carlo Montemagno and colleagues assembled a NEMS in which a tiny metal "propeller" was caused to spin within the domain of the enzyme ATP Synthase. The metal propeller was attached (via a biotinstreptavidin "molecular linkage") to one subunit (designated alpha) of ATP Synthase that rotates within the other (hollow) part of ATP Synthase molecule when ATP is "fed" to a free standing (i.e. not in cell) molecule of ATP Synthase.
- **Nanogram (ng):** 10^{-9} gram, or 3.5273×10^{-11} OZ (ounce) (avoirdupoir).
- **Nanometer (nm):** A unit of length equal to 1×10^{-9} meter.
- **Nanopore:** A nanopore is a very small hole. It may, for example, be created by a pore-forming protein or as a hole in synthetic materials such as silicon or graphene.
- **Nanoscience:** A term utilized to refer to the science underlying nanotechnology, nanocrystals, nanocrystal molecules, nanocomposites, "quantum dots", nanoelectromechanical systems (NEMS), etc. "Nanoscale" materials (i.e. those whose dimensions are approximately 1 – 100 nanometers) generally possess different chemical and physical properties than "bulk" materials. For example, when bulk gold metal is formed into

nanoscale rods, the intensity of its fluorescence increases by a factor of approximately 10 million. Another example is silicon nanocrystals (i.e. quantum dots) dispersed in a silicon dioxide matrix, emit larger than typical-for-silicon amounts of light, when stimulated (i.e. bombarded) with pulses of ultraviolet light.

- **Nanotechnology:** Derived from the Latin word *nanus*, means dwarf, so it literally means "dwarf technology". The word was originally coined by Norio Taniguchi in 1974, to refer to high precision machining. For example, enzyme molecules function essentially as jigs and machine tools to shape large molecules as they are formed in biochemical reactions. The technology also encompasses biochips, biosensors, and manipulating atoms and molecules in order to form (build) bigger, but still vanishingly small functional structures and machines.

- **Narrow host range plasmid:** A plasmid that can replicate in one or at most a few different bacterial species.

- **Narrow sense heritability:** In quantitative genetics the proportion of the phenotypic variance that is due to variation in breeding values.

- **Nascent RNA:** A ribonucleotide chain that is synthesized, so that its 3′ end is paired with DNA where RNA polymerase is elongating.

- **National Academy of Sciences (NAS):** A private, self-perpetuating society of distinguished scholars in scientific and engineering research, dedicated to the advancement of science and technology and their use for the general welfare. Under the authority of its congressional charter of 1863, the NAS has a working mandate that calls upon to advise the US Federal Government on scientific and technical matters.

- **National Cancer Institute (NCI):** One of the National Institutes of Health.

- **National Center for Biotechnology Information (NCBI):** It was established in 1988 for development of information system in molecular biology. It is the foremost repository of publically available genomic and proteomic data.

- **National Heart, Lung, and Blood Institute (NHLBI):** One of the National Institutes of Health.

- **National Institute of Allergy and Infectious Diseases (NIAID):** The main agency of the National Institutes of Health.

- **National Institute of General Medical Sciences (NIGMS):** One of the National Institutes of Health.
- **National Institutes of Health (NIH):** The major U.S. Government sponsor of biotechnology research. It is composed of a group of government institutes that each focus on specific medical areas.
- **National Science Foundation (NSF):** A non regulatory agency which has oversight of biotechnology research activities that funds the agency.
- **Native:** Refers to organisms that have not been recently introduced into an ecosystem.
- **Native conformation:** The normal, biologically active conformation (i.e. the three dimensional arrangement of its atoms) of a protein molecule.
- **Native protein:** The naturally occurring form of a protein.
- **Natural killer cells:** These cells are involved in tumor surveillance. They also kill virus laden cells.
- **Natural selection:** The differential survival and reproduction of organisms because of differences in characteristics that affect their ability to utilize environmental resources.
- **Near-infrared spectroscopy (NIR):** A spectroscopic method that uses the near-infrared region of the electromagnetic spectrum (from about 800 nm to 2500 nm).
- **Near-infrared transmission (NIT):** Refers to energy in the region of the electromagnetic radiation spectrum at wavelengths longer than those of visible light, but shorter than those of radio waves.
- **Necrosis:** Refers to cell death caused by physical injury to the cell (e.g. exposure to toxin, exposure to ultraviolet light, lack of oxygen, etc.).
- **Neem tree:** A tropical tree (*Azadirachta indica*) found in India, Somalia, Mauritania, Australia, and other tropical countries; that resists insect (e.g. whiteflies, mealybugs, aphids, mites) depravations and certain fungal diseases (rusts, powdery mildew, etc.) via secretions of liquids that contain Azadirachtin (an insect-repelling chemical).
- **Negative autogenous regulation/negative self regulation:** Inhibition of the expression of a gene or set of co-ordinately regulated genes by the product of the gene or of one of the genes.
- **Negative complementation:** Occurs when interallelic complementation allows a mutant subunit to suppress the activity of a wild-type subunit in a multimeric protein.

- **Negative control system:** A mechanism in which the regulatory protein(s) is required to turn off gene expression.
- **Negative regulation:** When an active protein inhibits or turns off transcription of an operon.
- **Negative regulator:** One molecule that controls the effect of another (or itself) by repressing or inactivating it.
- **Negative selection:** Selection of individuals that do not possess a certain character. A method by which growing cells that do not carry a DNA insert integrated at a specific chromosomal location are selected.
- **Negative supercoiling:** Comprises the twisting of a duplex of DNA in space in opposite sense to the turns of the strands in the double helix.
- **Nematodes:** Any of several worms of the phylum Nematoda, having unsegmented, cylindrical bodies, often narrowing at each end, and including parasitic forms such as the hookworm and pinworm. Also called roundworm.
- **Neo-formation:** Organogenesis; the production of newly formed structures such as tissues, meristems and embryos.
- **Neoplasia:** New growth.

N

- **Neoplasm:** Localised cell multiplication. Generally it designates a collection of cells which have undergone genetic transformation forming a tumor. Neoplasmic cells differ in structure and function from the original cell type.
- **Neoplastic growth:** A new growth of animal or plant tissue, resembling (more or less) the tissue from which it arises but having distinct biochemical differences from the parent cell. The neoplastic tissue is a mutant version of the original and appears to serve no physiological function in the same sense as did the original tissue. It may be benign or malignant (i.e. a cancerous tumor).
- **Neoteny:** The sexual maturity of an animal while it is in a mainly larval state, as in the axolotl. Also called paedogenesis.
- **Nerve growth factor (NGF):** A small secreted protein that is important for the growth, maintenance, and survival of certain target neurons (nerve cells). It also functions as a signaling molecule.
- **Nested PCR:** Refers to a specific polymerase chain reaction (PCR) technique of two consecutive-run PCRs, in which the

second PCR amplifies (makes multiple copies of) a DNA sequence within the product (amplicon) of the first PCR.

- **Net photosynthesis:** Photosynthesis activity minus respiratory activity as measured by carbon dioxide exchange.

- **Neuraminidase (NA):** A transmembrane (through the membrane) glycoprotein enzyme that appears in the (external) membrane of the influenza virus.

- **Neuron:** Cells of the body's nervous system, which transmit nerve impulses (electrical signals conducted by the flow of ions across the plasma membrane of neuron cells). Neurons are involved in controlling movement (known as motor control), emotions, and memory. There are approximately 100 billion neurons in the typical human brain. The nerve impulses within them move at a speed of approximately 400 kilometers per hour (300 miles per hour) (Fig. 1).

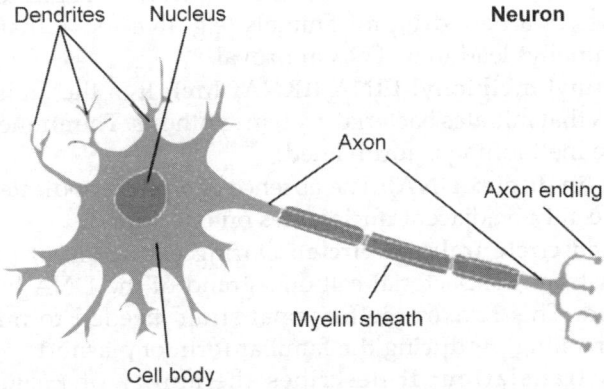

Fig. 1: Neuron

- **Neurotransmitter:** An organic, low molecular weight compound that is secreted from the axon (terminal) end of a neuron (in response to the arrival of an electrical impulse) into a liquid-filled gap that exists between neurons. The transmitter molecule then diffuses across the small gap and attaches to the next neuron. This attachment causes structural changes in the membrane of the neuron and initiates the conductance of an electrical impulse. In this way, an electrical impulse is transmitted (via this "cascade") along a neuron network in which the neurons themselves do not physically touch. A neurotransmitter serves to transmit a nerve impulse between different neurons. Examples of neurotransmitters include dopamine and norepinephrine. A shortage of dopamine in the brain causes the disease known as Parkinson's disease.

- **Neutral mutation:** Changes in DNA sequence that are neither beneficial nor detrimental to the ability of an organism to survive and reproduce.
- **Neutral substitutions:** Proteins are those changes of amino acids that do not affect activity.
- **Neutral theory:** The theory that much of evolution has been primarily due to random drift of neutral mutations.
- **Neutrophils:** Phagocytic (ingesting, scavenging) white blood cells produced in the bone marrow. They ingest and destroy invading microorganisms and facilitate post-infection tissue repair.
- **New animal drug application (NADA):** An application to the US Food and Drug Administration (FDA) to begin testing/ studies of a new drug for animals (e.g. livestock), that might (eventually) lead to its FDA approval.
- **N-formyl-methionyl-tRNA (tRNAf Me):** It is the aminoacyl-tRNA that initiates bacterial protein synthesis. The amino group of the methionine is formylated.
- **Nick (in duplex DNA):** The absence of a phosphodiester bond between two adjacent nucleotides on one strand.
- **Nicked circle (relaxed circle):** During extraction of plasmid DNA from the bacterial cell one strand of the DNA becomes nicked. This relaxes the torsional strain needed to maintain supercoiling producing the familiar form of plasmid.
- **Nick translation:** It describes the ability of *E.coli* DNA polymerase I to use a nick as a starting point from which one strand of a duplex DNA can be degraded and replaced by resynthesis of new material; is used to introduce radioactively labeled nucleotides into DNA *in vitro*.
- ***Nif* (Nitrogen fixing) genes:** A 24 kb long nucleotide sequence organized in 7 operons (transcriptional units) which take part in nitrogen fixation.
- **Ninhydrin reaction:** A color reaction given by amino acids and peptides on heating with the chemical ninhydrin. The technique is widely used for the detection and quantitation (measurement) of amino acids and peptides. The concentration of amino acid in a solution (of hydrochloric acid) is proportional to the optical

absorbance of the solution after heating it with ninhydrin. ?-Amino acids give an intense blue color, and amino acids (such as proline) gives a yellow color. One is able to determine the concentration of a protein or peptide and also obtain an idea of the type of protein or peptide that is present.

- **Nitrate reduction:** The reduction of nitrate to nitrite or ammonia by an organism.
- **Nitrates:** Refers to nitrogen compounds that exist in a chemical form which plant roots are able to take in (utilized by the plant to make nitrogen-containing molecules such as proteins). Nitrates are produced from nitrogen: • Taken out of the atmosphere by nitrogen- fixing bacteria (living in the roots of legume plants such as the soybean, etc.) • Taken out of nitrites (in soil) by nitrate bacteria • Taken out of the atmosphere by blue-green algae.
- **Nitric oxide NO:** A molecule produced in the body of an organism, which can act as a signaling molecule (e.g. to cause a firefly's tail to begin the chemical reaction of luciferin with luciferase that results in the light emission known as bioluminescence).
- **Nitric oxide synthase:** An enzyme that catalyzes the reaction which the body (of animals or plants) utilizes to make nitric oxide from L-arginine (via cleavage of that molecule). The cofactor for that reaction is nicotine - adenine dinucleotide phosphate (NADP).
- **Nitrification:** The oxidation of ammonia (e.g. from ammonia-containing substances such as liquid wastes excreted by animals, decomposed animals and plants, etc.) to nitrates by a microorganism.
- **Nitrilase:** An enzyme catalyse the hydrolysis of nitriles to carboxylic acids and ammonia, without the formation of "free" amide intermediates. Nitrilases are involved in natural product biosynthesis and post-translational modifications in plants, animals, fungi and certain prokaryotes.
- **Nitrites:** Refers to nitrogen compounds that exist in a chemical form which plant roots are unable to take in. A salt or ester of nitrous acid, containing the anion NO_2^- or the group $-NO_2$.
- **Nitrocellulose:** A membrane used to immobilize DNA, RNA or protein which can then be probed with a labeled sequence or antibody.

- **Nitrocellulose (cellulose nitrate):** A nitrate derivative of cellulose. It is made into membrane filters of defined porosity used immobilize DNA, RNA or protein which can then be probed with a labeled sequence or antibody. These filters have a variety of uses in molecular biology particularly in nucleic acid hybridization experiments extensively in the Southern and northern blotting procedures involving DNA and RNA.
- **Nitrogen assimilation:** The incorporation of nitrogen into organic cellular substances by living organisms.
- **Nitrogen cycle:** The cycling of various forms of biologically available nitrogen through the plant, animal, and microbial worlds (kingdoms), as well as the atmosphere and geosphere.
- **Nitrogen fixation:** Conversion of atmospheric nitrogen (N_2) into ammonia; a soluble, biologically available form (nitrates). The conversion is carried out by nitrogen-fixing organisms (e.g. *Rhizobium* bacteria) which live symbiotically in the roots of legume plants, e.g. alfalfa or soybeans.
- **Nitrogenase system:** A system of enzymes capable of reducing atmospheric nitrogen (N_2) to ammonia (NH_4^+) in the presence of ATP.
- **Nitrogenase:** An enzyme expressed by *nif* genes that converts N_2 to NH_4^+ under O_2-tense conditions in prokaryotes.
- **Nitrogenous bases:** The purines (adenine and guanine) and pyrimidines (thymine, cytosine and uracil) that form DNA and RNA molecules.
- **Nod box:** A DNA sequence that controls the transcriptional regulation of rhizobium nodulation genes.
- **Nod genes:** Genes that encodes nodulins.
- **Nodal culture:** The culture of a lateral bud and a section of adjacent stem tissue.
- **Node:** Slightly enlarged portion of the stem where leaves and buds arise and where branches originate. Stems have nodes but roots do not.
- **Nodular:** Term commonly used to describe a pebbly (rough) texture of a callus.
- **Nodulation:** Formation of root nodules in legumes by bacteria *Rhizobium*.
- **Nodule:** The enlargement or swelling on roots of nitrogen fixing plants. The nodules contain symbiotic nitrogen fixing bacteria (Fig. 2).

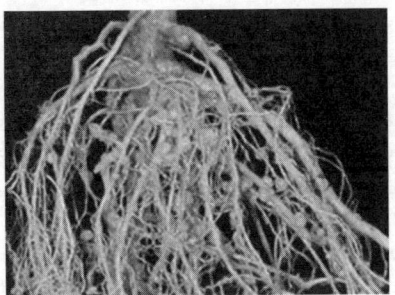

Fig. 2: Nodule

- **Nonrepetitive transposition:** It describes the movement of a transposon that leaves a donor site (usually generating a double-strand break) and moves to a new site.
- **Nonallelic:** Genes are two (or more) copies of the same gene that are present at different locations in the genome (contrasted with alleles which are copies of the same gene derived from different parents and present at the same location on the homologous chromosomes).
- **Nonautonomous:** A term ferering to biological units that cannot function by themselves. Such units require the assistance of another unit or "helper".
- **Nonautonomous controlling elements:** Defective transposons that can transpose only when assisted by an autonomous controlling element of the same type.
- **Nondefective virus:** Describes a transforming retrovirus that has all the normal capabilities in replication etc. Its ability to transform depends on its effects on expression of host genes at its site of insertion into the cellular genome.
- **Nondisjunction:** The failure of chromosomes to separate, it is more common during meiosis I than meiosis II; it can also occur in mitosis.
- **Nonessential amino acids:** Amino acids of proteins that can be made (biochemically synthesized within the body) by humans and certain other vertebrate animals from simple chemical precursors (in contrast to the essential amino acids). These amino acids are thus not required in the diet (of humans and those other vertebrates).
- **Nonheme-iron proteins:** Proteins containing iron but no porphyrin groups (within which iron atoms are held) in their structure.

- **Nonhistone:** Any structural protein found in a chromosome except one of the histones.
- **Nonhomologous end-joining (NHEJ):** Ligates blunt ends. It is common to many repair pathways and to certain recombination pathways (such as immunoglobulin recombination).
- **Nonpermissive:** Conditions do not allow conditional lethal mutants to survive.
- **Nonpolar group:** A hydrophobic ("water hating") group on a molecule; usually hydrocarbon (composed of hydrogen and carbon atoms) in nature.
- **Nonproductive rearrangement:** The recombination of V, (D), J gene segments results in a nonproductive rearrangement if the rearranged gene segments are not in the correct reading frame. A nonproductive rearrangement occurs when nucleotide addition or subtraction disrupts the reading frame.
- **Nonreciprocal recombination:** Results from an error in pairing and crossing-over in which nonequivalent sites are involved in the two reacting genomes. It produces one recombinant with a deletion of material and one with a duplication.
- **Nonrepetitive DNA:** Shows reassociation kinetics expected of unique sequences.
- **Nonreplicative transposition:** Describes the movement of a transposon that leaves a donor site (usually generating a double-strand break) and moves to a new site.
- **Nonsense codons:** UAA, UAG, UGA codons that do not specify any amino acid. Also known as termination or stop codons.
- **Nonsense mutation:** Any change in DNA that causes a codon (termination) to be replaced by a codon representing an amino acid.
- **Nonsense suppressor:** A gene coding for a mutant tRNA able to respond to one or more of the termination codons.
- **Nonsense-mediated mRNA decay:** A pathway that degrades an mRNA that has a nonsense codon prior to the last exon.
- **Nonstarch polysaccharide (NSP):** It refers to polysaccharide molecules (in plant seeds) other than starch. These include arabinoxylans, pectins, beta-glucans, and alpha-galactosides (e.g. raffinose, stachyose, verbascose).
- **Nontarget organism:** An organism which is affected by an interaction for which it was not an intended recipient.

- **Non-template strand:** In transcription the non-transcribed strand of DNA called as sense strand or coding strand. It will have the same sequence as the RNA transcript except that T is present at positions where U is present in the RNA transcript.
- **Nontranscribed spacer:** The region between transcription units in a tandem gene cluster.
- **Nonviral superfamily:** Of transposons originated independently of retroviruses.
- **Nopaline plasmid:** Ti plasmids of *Agrobacterium tumefaciens* that carry genes for synthesizing the opine, nopaline. They retain the ability to differentiate into early embryonic structures.
- **Normal phase:** A chromatographic mode in which the mobile phase is less polar than the stationary phase.
- **North American plant protection organization (NAPPO):** One of the international SPS standard-setting organizations that develops plant health standards, guidelines, and recommendations (e.g. to prevent transfer of a disease from one country to another). Subsidiary to the International Plant Protection Convention (IPPC), it covers the countries of North America. Its secretariat is located in Nepean, Canada.
- **Northern blot:** A technique used in molecular biology research to study gene expression by detection of RNA in a sample.
- **Northern blotting:** Hybridization of a labeled DNA probe to RNA fragments that have been transferred from an agarose gel to a nitrocellulose filter. It is also called northern hybridization (Fig. 3).
- **Northern corn rootworm:** A corn rootworm (*Diabrotica barberi* syn. *D. longicornis*) often destructive to Indian corn in the northern parts of the central and eastern United States.
- **NOS terminator:** A termination codon (sequence of DNA) frequently utilized in genetic engineering of plants to "terminate" expression of the inserted gene (i.e. to halt synthesis of desired protein in the plant, after the desired protein synthesis has occurred). The NOS terminator was originally extracted from the bacteria species *Agrobacterium tumefaciens*.
- **No-tillage crop production:** A methodology of crop production in which a farmer virtually utilizes no mechanical method cultivation (i.e. one only pass over the field, with a planter; instead of the conventional four passes per year with mechanical cultivator equipment plus one pass with planter, used for traditional crop production).

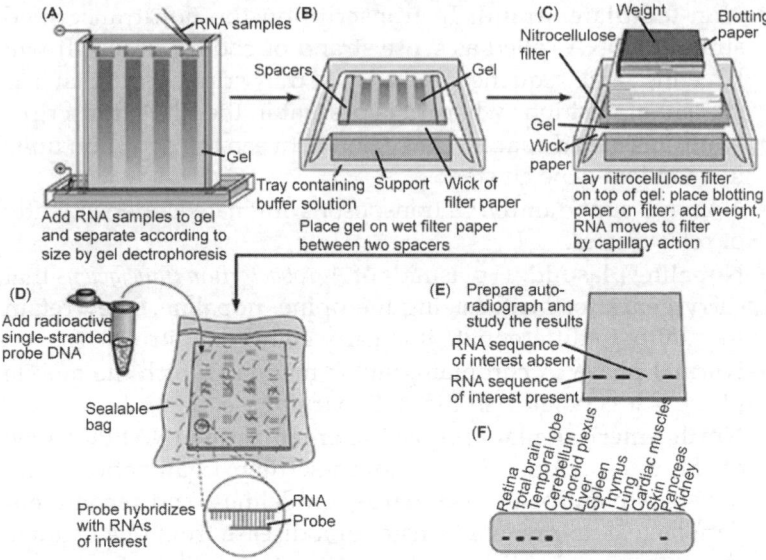

Fig. 3: Northern blotting

- **NPT II gene:** A marker gene that codes for (i.e. "causes manufacture of") the enzyme neomycin phosphotransferase II, which can inactivate the antibiotic kanamycin. The NPT II gene is commonly utilized as a "marker gene" for genetically engineered plants. Neomycin phosphotransferase confers kanamycin resistance to cells expressing it (i.e. cells that contain the NPT II gene in addition to the other gene(s) inserted along with it), so those (engineered) cells will live in a laboratory vessel containing kanamycin.

- **NT:** An acronym for Nuclear Transfer.

- **Nucellar embryo:** An embryo which has developed vegetatively from somatic tissue surrounding the embryo sac rather than by fertilization of the egg cell.

- **Nucellus:** Tissue composing the main part of the young ovule in which the embryo sac develops megasporangium (Fig. 4).

- **Nuclear DNA:** The DNA contained within the nucleus of a cell.

- **Nuclear envelope:** A layer of two membranes surrounding the nucleus. It is penetrated by nuclear pores. The inner membrane is bound on the interior by the nuclear laminin. The outer

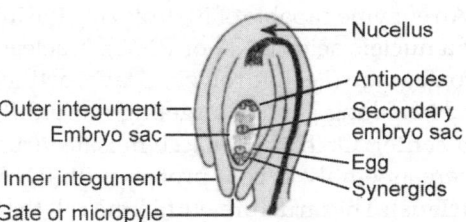

Fig. 4: Nucellus

membrane extends in the cytosol into the network of the endoplasmic reticulum.

- **Nuclear export signal (NES):** A domain of a protein, usually a short amino acid sequence, which interacts with an exportin, resulting in the transport of the protein from the nucleus to the cytoplasm.
- **Nuclear lamina:** It consists of a proteinaceous layer on the inside of the nuclear envelope. It consist of (up to) three lamin proteins.
- **Nuclear localization signal (NLS):** It is a domain of a protein, usually a short amino acid sequence, that interacts with an importin, allowing the protein to be transported into the nucleus.
- **Nuclear matrix proteins:** Protein molecules present in cancerous cells, but not in normal (non-mutated) cells.
- **Nuclear matrix:** A network of fibers surrounding and penetrating the nucleus.
- **Nuclear pore complex (NPC):** It is a very large, proteinaceous structure that extends through the nuclear envelope, providing a channel for bidirectional transport of molecules and macromolecules between the nucleus and the cytosol.
- **Nuclear pores:** Large structures that extend across the nuclear envelope and transport macromolecules both into and out of the nucleus.
- **Nuclear receptors:** Receptors in a cell's outer membrane that serve to convey a "signal" from outside the cell all the way into the cell's nucleus.
- **Nuclear transfer:** A method of cloning a living organism, in which that organism's entire genetic information is conveyed via transfer of an (adult) cell nucleus into an unfertilized egg (from another animal of the same species) whose nucleus had previously been removed.

- **Nuclease:** An enzyme capable of hydrolyzing the internucleotide linkages of a nucleic acid (DNA or RNA). Nucleases present in cells tend to degrade (i.e. hydrolyze, cleave) artificially inserted DNA strands, making genetic targeting more difficult.
- **Nucleation center:** Of TMV (tobacco mosaic virus) is a duplex hairpin where assembly of coat protein with RNA is initiated.
- **Nuclei (nucleus):** The structure within the cell that contains the chromosomes.
- **Nucleic acids:** A nucleotide polymer. A large, chain-like molecule containing phosphate groups, sugar groups, and purine and pyrimidine bases; two types are ribonucleic acid (RNA) and deoxyribonucleic acid (DNA). The bases involved are adenine, guanine, cytosine, and thymine (uracil in RNA). Nucleic acids are either the specific (genetic) informational molecule (DNA), or act as agent (RNA) in causing that information to be expressed (as a protein).
- **Nuclein:** The term used by Friedrich Miescher to describe the nuclear material he discovered in 1869 which today is known as DNA.
- **Nucleoid:** The compact body that contains the genome in a bacterium.
- **Nucleo-cytoplasmic ratio:** In a cell, the ratio of nuclear to cytoplasmic volume. This ratio is high in meristematic cells and low in differentiated cells.
- **Nucleolar organizer:** The region of a chromosome carrying genes coding for rRNA.
- **Nucleolar zone:** Any chromosomal region, irrespective of whether or not, it is a secondary constriction that is associated with the formation of the nucleus during telophase.
- **Nucleoplasm:** The non-staining or slightly chromophilic, liquid or semiliquid, ground substance of the interphase nucleus and fills the nuclear space around the chromosomes and the nucleoli.
- **Nucleolus:** A discrete region of nucleus created by the transcription of rRNA genes.
- **Nucleolytic:** The reactions involving the hydrolysis of a phosphodiester bond in a nucleic acid.
- **Nucleophilic group:** An electron-rich group with a strong tendency to donate electrons to an electron-deficient nucleus.
- **Nucleoporin:** was originally defined to describe the components of the nuclear pore complex that bind to the inhibitory lectins,

but now is used to mean any component of the basic nuclear pore complex.

- **Nucleoproteins:** Complexes made up of nucleic acid and protein. These two substances are apparently not linked by strong chemical bonds, but are held together by salt linkages and other weak bonds. Most viruses consist entirely of nucleoproteins, although some viruses also contain fatty substances. Nucleoproteins are also found in animal and plant cells, and in bacteria.
- **Nucleoside:** A hybrid molecule consisting of a purine (adenine, guanine) or pyrimidine (thymine, uracil, or cytosine) base covalently linked to a five-membered sugar ring (ribose in the case of RNA and deoxyribose in the case of DNA).
- **Nucleoside analog:** A synthetic molecule that resembles a naturally occurring nucleoside but it lacks a bond-site needed to link it to an adjacent nucleotide.
- **Nucleoside diphosphate sugar:** A coenzyme like carrier of a sugar molecule functioning in the enzymatic synthesis of polysaccharides and sugar derivatives.
- **Nucleosome positioning:** Describes the placement of nucleosomes at defined sequences of DNA instead of at random locations with regards to sequence.
- **Nucleosome:** Spherical particles composed of a special class of basic proteins (histone) in combination with DNA (146 bp of DNA are wrapped 1.75 times around a "core" of histone proteins). The particles are approximately 12.5 nm in diameter and are connected to each other by DNA filaments. Under an electron microscope they appear somewhat like a string of pearls.
- **Nucleotide:** An ester of a nucleoside and phosphoric acid. Nucleotides are nucleosides that have a phosphate group attached to one or more of the hydroxyl groups of the sugar (ribose or deoxyribose). In short, a nucleotide is a hybrid molecule consisting of a purine or pyrimidine base covalently linked to a 5-membered sugar ring which is covalently linked to a phosphate group. While (polymerized) nucleotides are the structural units of a nucleic acid, free nucleotides that are not an integral part of nucleic acids are also found in tissues and play important roles in the cell, e.g. ATP and cyclic AMP.
- **Nucleus:** Usually spherical body in each living cell that contains hereditary biological material (DNA, genes, chromosomes, etc.)

and controls the cell's life functions (e.g. metabolism, growth, and reproduction). The nucleus is a highly differentiated, relatively large organelle lying in the cytoplasm of the cell, that is surrounded by a (nuclear) membrane which is quite similar to the plasma (cell) membrane, except the nuclear membrane contains holes or pores. It is characterized by its high content of chromatin, which contains most of the cell's DNA. Chromatin is normally (when cell is not in process of dividing) distributed throughout the nucleus in a diffuse manner (Fig. 5).

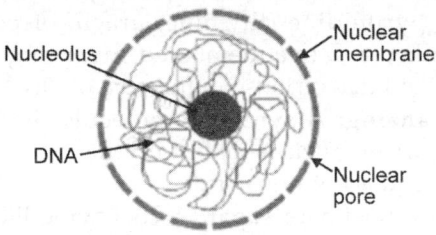

Fig. 5: Nucleus

- **Null mutation:** Completely eliminates the function of a gene, usually because it has been physically deleted.
- **Nullisomy:** Diploid cell or organism lacking both members of a chromosome pair (chromosome formula 2n-2).
- **Nurse culture:** Planting a cell from a suspension culture on a raft of filter paper above a callus tissue piece (nurse tissue). The filter paper serves to prevent tissue union but allows the flow of essential substances from the nurse to the isolated cell. In such culture a piece of callus is first placed on nutrient agar. Over this tissue is laid with strip of filter paper.
- **Nutraceuticals:** Coined in 1989 by Stephen DeFelice, this term is used to refer to either a food or portion of food (a vitamin, essential amino acid, etc.) that possesses medical or health benefits (to the organism that consumes that nutraceutical). For example, saponins (present in beans, spinach, tomatoes, potatoes, alfalfa, clover, etc.) possess some cancer-prevention properties. Also sometimes called pharma foods, functional foods, or designer foods, these are food products that have been designed to contain specific concentrations and/or proportions of certain nutrients (vitamins, amino acids, etc.) that are critical for good health.

- **Nutrient cycle:** The passage of a nutrient or element through an ecosystem including its assimilation and release by various organisms and its transformation into various organic or inorganic chemical forms.
- **Nutrient deficiency:** Absence or insufficiency of some factor needed for normal growth and development.
- **Nutrient enhanced™:** A phrase that is now a trademark of Garst Seed Company; it refers to plants that have been modified to possess novel traits that make those plants more economically valuable for nutritional uses (e.g. higher-than-normal protein content in certain feed grains).
- **Nutrient film technique (NFT):** Hydroponic technique used to grow plants. NFT delivers a film of water or nutrient solution either continuously or through on-off cycles (e.g. on-8 minutes and off-7 minutes).
- **Nutrient gradient:** A diffusion gradient of nutrients and gases that develops in tissues where only a portion of the tissue is in contact with the medium. Gradients are less likely to form in liquid media than in callus cultures.
- **Nutrient medium:** A solid, semi-solid or liquid combination of major and minor salts as energy source (sucrose), vitamins plant growth regulators and occasionally other defined or undefined supplements. Often made from stock solutions then sterilized by autoclaving or filtering through a microspore filter.

N

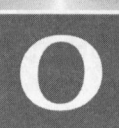

- **Occupational safety and health administration (OSHA):** One of the US agencies responsible for regulation of biotechnology. The major law under which the agency has regulatory powers is the Occupational Safety and Health Act.

- **Ochratoxins:** A term that refers to a group of related mycotoxins (i.e. toxic metabolites produced by fungi) that are produced by some *Aspergillus* species and some *Penicillium* species of fungi (e.g. *Penicillium viridicatum*). These particular fungi tend to produce ochratoxins when they grow in damaged grain (e.g. during grain storage), especially when grain temperature is above 4°C (40°F) and grain moisture content is above 18%. Ochratoxin A is very carcinogenic (cancer-causing) toxin when consumed by humans. When dairy cattle consume ochratoxin-A containing grain, the ochratoxin A soon appears in the milk produced by those cows.

- **Ochre codon:** The triplet UAA, one of three codons that cause termination of protein synthesis.

- **Ochre mutation:** A mutation yielding the termination codon UAA, resulting in premature termination of a polypeptide chain.

- **Ochre suppressor:** A gene that codes for an altered tRNA so that its anticodon can recognize the ocher codon and thus allows the continuation of protein synthesis. A suppressor of an ochre mutation is a tRNA that is charged with the amino acid corresponding to the original codon or a neutral substitute. Ochre suppressors will also suppress amber codons.

- **Octadecanoid/Jasmonate signal complex:** A chemical signal created and emitted by certain plants in response to those plants being wounded (e.g. via chewing) by insects. The octadecanoid/jasmonate signal complex then causes the production and also emission of volatile chemicals such as volicitin, which attract certain types of wasps that are natural enemies of those insects which initially wounded the plants. Thus, the octadecanoid/

jasmonate signal complex is a crucial part of an (indirect) defense mechanism of such plants.

- **Octopine:** Plasmids of *Agrobacterium tumefaciens* carry genes coding the synthesis of opines of the octopine type. The tumors are undifferentiated.
- **Octoploid:** Cell or organism with eight sets of chromosomes, i.e. 2n = 8x.
- **Odorant binding protein:** A protein that enhances people's ability to smell odorants in trace quantities much lower than those needed to activate olfactory (smelling) nerves. The protein accomplishes this by latching onto (odorant) molecules and enhancing their aroma. Hence, it acts as a kind of "helper" entity in bringing about the ability to smell certain odorants present in low concentration.
- **Oestrogen/estrogen:** The genetic term for a group of female sex hormones which control the development of sexual characteristics and control oestrus.
- **Oestrus:** In female mammals the period of sexual excitement and acceptance of the male aka rut, heat.
- **Office of agricultural biotechnology (OAB):** A unit of the US department of agriculture incharge of a part of the federal regulatory process for biotechnology (e.g. field tests of transgenic plants).
- **Offset:** Young plant produced at the base of a mature plant.
- **Offshoot:** Short usually horizontal stem produced near the crown of a plant.
- **Offspring progeny:** New individual organisms that result from the process of sexual or asexual reproduction.
- **OH43:** Gene in plants (e.g. corn/maize) that causes production of a seed coat more resistant to tearing. Greater tear-resistance results in a lower incidence of fungi infestation in seed, which results in less mycotoxin production in seed.
- **OIE:** Office International des Epizootics.
- **Okazaki fragments:** The short stretches of 1,000–2,000 bases produced during discontinuous replication; they are later joined into a covalently intact strand (Fig. 1).
- **Oleic acid:** A fatty acid naturally present in the fat of animals and also in oils extracted from oilseed plants (soybean, canola, etc.). For example, the soybean oil produced from traditional varieties of soybeans tends to contain 24% oleic acid.

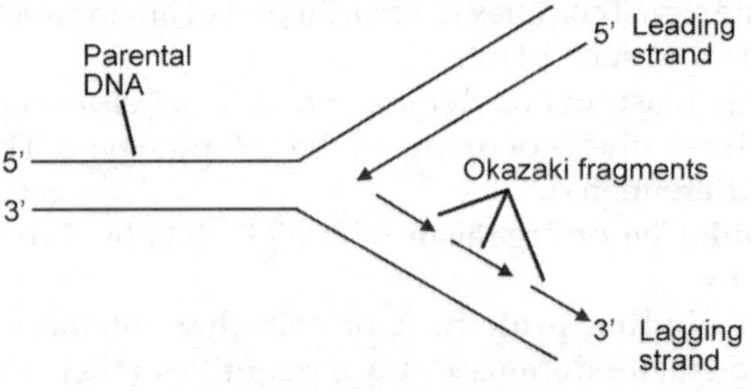

Fig. 1: Okazaki fragments

- **Oleosomes:** The storage bodies for lipids (fats) in the seeds of certain plants.
- **Oligomer:** A molecule formed from a small number of monomers.
- **Oligonucleotide probes:** Short chain fragments of DNA that are used in various gene analysis tests (e.g. the single base change in DNA that causes sickle-cell anemia).
- **Oligonucleotides:** A short synthetic single stranded DNA.
- **Oligopeptide:** A relatively short chain molecule made up of amino acids linked by peptide bonds.
- **Oligosaccharides:** A saccharide polymer containing a small number (typically two to ten) of simple sugars (monosaccharides). Oligosaccharides are commonly found on the plasma membrane of animal cells where they can play a role in cell-cell recognition.
- **Omega-3 fatty acids:** More properly called "n-3 fatty acids".
- **Omega-6 fatty acids:** More properly called "n-6 fatty acids".
- **Oncogene:** A gene that contributes to the production of cancer. Oncogenes are generally mutated forms of normal cellular gene.
- **Oncogenesis:** The progression of cytological, genetic and cellular changes that culminate in a malignant tumor.
- **Oncomouse:** A mouse that has been genetically modified to incorporate an oncogene. Oncogenes cause cells to undergo cancerous transformation.
- **Ontogeny:** Developmental life history of an organism.
- **Oocyte:** The egg mother cell. It undergoes two meiotic divisions (oogenesis) to form the egg cell. The primary oocyte is formed before completion of the first meiotic division, the secondary oocyte is formed after completion of the first meiotic division.

- **Oogenesis:** The formation and growth of the egg or ovum in an animal ovary.
- **Oogonium:** A germ cell of the female animal that gives rise to oocytes by mitotic division.
- **Oospore:** A resistant spore developing from a zygote resulting from the fusion of heterogametes in certain algae and fungi.
- **Opal codon:** UGA codon, also known as umber codon, stops proteins synthesis.
- **Open complex:** Describes the stage of initiation of transcription when RNA polymerase causes the two strands of DNA to separate to form the "transcription bubble".
- **Open continuous culture:** A continuous culture in which inflow of fresh medium is balanced by outflow of a corresponding volume of culture. Cells are constantly washed out with the out flowing liquid. In a steady state, the rate of cell washout equals the rate of formation of new cells in the system.
- **Open pollination:** Pollination by wind, insects or other natural mechanisms.
- **Open reading frame (ORF):** A series of triplets coding for amino acids without any termination codons; sequence is potentially translatable into protein.
- **Operational definition:** An operation or procedure that can be carried out to define or delimit something.
- **Operator:** The site on DNA at which a repressor protein binds to prevent transcription from initiating at the adjacent promoter.
- **Operon:** A unit of bacterial gene expression and regulation, including structural genes and control elements in DNA recognized by regulator gene product(s) (Fig. 2).
- **Opine:** The condensation product of an amino acid with *keto* acid or sugar.
- **Optical activity:** The capacity of a substance to rotate the plane of polarization of plane polarized light when examined in an instrument known as a polarimeter. All compounds that are capable of existing in two forms that are nonsuperimposable mirror images of each other, exhibit optical activity. Such compounds are called stereoisomers (or enantiomers or chiral molecules) and the two forms arise because compounds having asymmetric carbon atoms to which other atoms are connected may arrange themselves in two different ways.

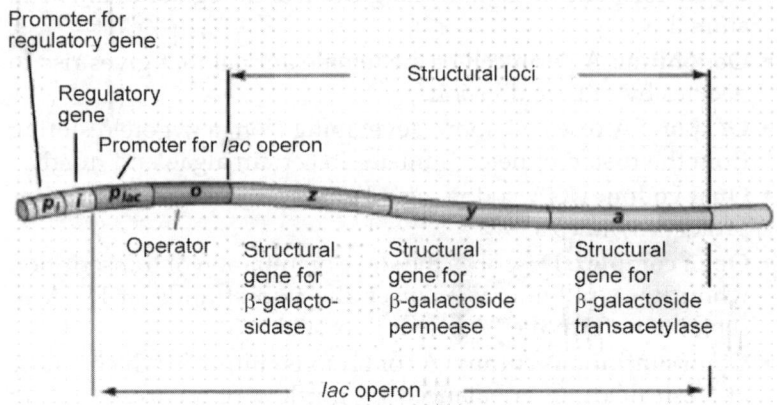

Fig. 2: Operon

- **Optical density (OD):** The absorbance of light of a specific wavelength by molecules normally dissolved in a solution. Light absorption depends upon the concentration of the absorbing compound (chemical entity) in the solution, the thickness of the sample being illuminated, and the chemical nature of the absorbing compound. An analytical instrument known as a spectrophotometer is used to (quantitatively) express the amount of a substance (dissolved) in a solution. Mathematically, this is accomplished using the Beer-Lambert law.
- **Optimum pH:** The pH at which an enzymatic or any other reaction or process is most effective under a given set of conditions.
- **Optimum temperature:** The temperature at which any operation such as the culture of any special microorganism is best carried on.
- **Optrode:** An optical sensor device that optically measures a specific substance usually with the aid of a chemical transducer.
- **Oral cancer:** Also sometimes known as "cancer of the mouth", involve the tissues lining the human mouth. Causes include consumption of carcinogens (tobacco products, certain mycotoxins, etc.) by humans. Oral cancerous cells arise from precancerous mouth lesions known as oral leukoplakia.
- **Ordinate:** The vertical axis of a graph. (Opp: abscises, abscissa).

- **Organ:** A tissue or group of tissues that constitute a morphologically and functionally distinct parts of an organism.
- **Organ culture:** Culture of an organ *in vitro*.
- **Organellar genes:** Genes located on organelle outside the nucleus.
- **Organelles:** Membrane-surrounded structures found in eukaryotic cells; they contain enzymes and other components required for specialized cell function (e.g. ribosomes for protein synthesis, or lysosomes for enzymatic hydrolysis). Some organelles such as mitochondria and chloroplasts contain DNA and can replicate autonomously (from the rest of the cell).
- **Organic:** Referring in chemistry, the compounds containing carbon, many of which have been in some manner associated with living organisms.
- **Organic compound:** Any member of a large class of gaseous, liquid, or solid chemical compounds whose molecules contain carbon.
- **Organic co-solvent:** A compound used to dissolve some neutral organic substances such as in media preparation. Organic co-solvents include alcohols (usually ethanol), acetone and dimethylsulphoxide (DMSO).
- **Organic molecule:** A molecule with a basic skeleton made up of a skeleton of carbon atoms plus hydrogen and oxygen atoms and, in proteins, nitrogen.
- **Organized growth:** Contributes towards the creation or maintenance of a defined structure. If occurs when plant organs such as the growing points of shoots or roots (apical meristems), leaf initials, young flower buds or small fruits, are transferred to culture and continue to grow with their structure preserved.
- **Organized tissue:** Composed of regularly differentiated cells.
- **Organizer:** An inductor, a chemical substance in a living system that determines the fate in the development of certain cells or groups of cells.
- **Organism:** Refers to any living plant, animal, bacteria, fungus, virus, etc. Also (e.g. in certain international treaties such as the Convention on Biological Diversity), this term includes things (e.g. seeds, spores, eggs) possessing the potential to become plants, animals, fungi, etc.
- **Organization for economic cooperation and development (OECD):** An international organization comprised of the world's

wealthiest (most developed) nations, originally established in 1960 to study trade and related matters. In 1991, the OECD's group of national experts on safety in biotechnology (GNE) completed a document entitled report on the concepts and principles underpinning safety evaluations of food derived from modern biotechnology. The "aim of that document was to elaborate the scientific principles to be considered (by OECD member nations' regulatory agencies) in evaluating the safety of new foods and food components" (e.g. genetically modified soybeans, corn/maize, potatoes, etc.).

- **Organogenesis:** The process of initiation and development of a structure which show natural organ form and/or function, the initiation of which is temporally separated from the initiation of other organs.
- **Organoid:** An organ like structure produced in culture such as leaves, roots or callus.
- **Organoleptic:** Having an effect on one of the organs of sense such as taste or smell.
- **Origin (*ori*):** A sequence of DNA at which replication is initiated.
- **Origin for replication (*ori*):** A site of nucleotide sequence from which replication begins (Fig. 3).

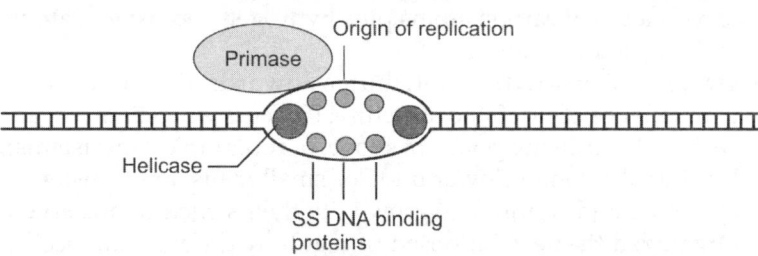

Fig. 3: Origin for replication

- **Orphan drug:** The name of the legal status granted by the food and drug administration's office of Orphan products development (to certain pharmaceuticals). This classification provides the sponsors of those pharmaceuticals with special tax and other financial incentives (e.g. market monopoly for a limited time). If companies feel that they possess a cure (drug) for a certain disease, but the number of potential patients is below a certain number and there is potential competition from rival companies, then the high cost of developing and shepherding the drug through the FDA would be such that the company would not be able to regain its development costs and make a profit. Hence, orphan drug status was designed to encourage drug development efforts for otherwise non-economic pharmaceuticals with less than 200,000 patients a year.

- **Orphan genes:** Genes within an organism's genome/DNA, that have no apparent function.
- **Orphan receptors:** Refers to cellular receptors (i.e. embedded in surface of cell membrane) that are not coupled to G-protein (cell) system complexes.
- **Orphans:** Isolated individual genes found in isolated locations, but related to membrane of a gene cluster.
- **Ortet:** The plant from which a clone is obtained.
- **Orthologs:** are corresponding proteins in two species as defined by sequence homologies.
- **Orthophosphate cleavage:** Enzymatic cleavage of one of the phosphate ester bonds of ATP to yield ADP and a single phosphate molecule is known as orthophosphate (designated as Pi). The cleavage of the phosphate bond is energy-yielding and is (except in the case of a futile cycle) coupled enzymatically to reactions that utilize the energy to run the cell. An orthophosphate cleavage reaction releases relatively less energy than does a corresponding pyrophosphate cleavage reaction.
- **Osmaticum:** Agents such as polyethylene glycol, mannitol, glucose, sucrose which maintains the osmotic potential of a nutrient medium equivalent to that of cultured cells.
- **Osmolarity:** The total molar concentration of the solutes. Osmolarity affects the osmotic potential of solution or nutrient medium.
- **Osmic acid:** A fixing agent commonly used to prepare tissue samples for electron microscopy.
- **Osmosis:** Movement of a solvent (as water) through a semipermeable membrane (as of a living cell) into a solution of higher solute concentration that tends to equalize the concentrations of solute on the two sides of the membrane (Fig. 4).
- **Osmotic pressure:** May be defined as the hydrostatic pressure which must be applied to a solution on one side of a semipermeable membrane (solution B in the example for osmosis) in

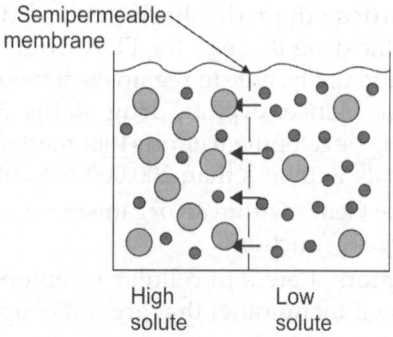

Fig. 4: Osmosis

order to offset the flow of solvent (water) from the other side (solution A in the example for osmosis). It is a measure of the tendency or "strength" of water to flow from a region of low salt concentration (and conversely high water concentration) to regions of high salt concentration (and conversely low water concentration).

- **Osmotins:** A category of proteins, which are produced by some organisms as a natural defense against pathogenic fungi.
- **Osteoarthritis:** A disease that affects primarily women older than 45, in which cartilage within the body's joint breaks down. Osteoarthritis encompasses approximately half of all cases of arthritis.
- **Osteoinductive factor (OIF):** A protein that induces the growth of both cartilage-forming cells and bone-forming cells (e.g. after a bone has been broken). When applied in the presence of transforming growth factor, beta type 2 (another protein), osteoinductive factor first causes connective tissue cells to grow together to form a matrix of cartilage (e.g. across the bone break), then bone cells slowly replace that cartilage. Osteoinductive factor also seems to thwart a type of cell that tears down bone formation, so OIF may someday be used to combat osteoporosis.
- **Osteoporosis:** A disease of humans in which the bones gradually weaken and become brittle. A diet containing a large amount of soy isoflavones (i.e. genistein) has been shown to increase bone density; thereby lowering the risk of osteoporosis. Groups that are especially at risk for osteoporosis include postmenopausal women (particularly of Caucasian or Asian

ethnicity), those who have undergone early menopause (i.e. prior to age 45), those who smoked, those who consumed excessive amounts of alcohol, and those who consumed excessive amounts of certain pharmaceuticals (e.g. steroids such as prednisone, thyroid hormone, etc.).

- **Outbreeding:** A mating system characterized by the breeding of genetically unrelated or dissimilar individuals. Since genetic diversity tends to be enhanced and since vigour or fitness of individuals can be increased by this process it is often used to counter the detrimental effects of continuous inbreeding.
- **Outcrossing:** The transfer of a given gene or genes (e.g. one synthesized by man and inserted into a plant via genetic engineering) from a domesticated organism (e.g. crop plant) to a wild type (relative of plant).
- **Outflow:** The volume of growing cells that is removed from a bioreactor during a continuous fermentation process.
- **Ovary:** Enlarged basal portion of the pistil of a plant flower that contains the ovules.
- **Overdominance:** That state in which the heterozygote has greater phenotype value and perhaps is more fit than the homozygous state for either of the alleles that it comprises.
- **Overlapping reading frames:** Start codons in different reading frames generate different polypeptides from the same DNA sequence.
- **Overwinding:** Overwinding of DNA is caused by positive supercoiling (which applies further tension in the direction of winding of the two strands about each other in the duplex).
- **Overwound:** A stretch of overwound DNA has more base pairs per turn than the usual average (10 bp = 1 turn). This means that the two strands of DNA are more tightly wound around each other, creating tension.
- **Ovulation:** In mammals the process of escape of the ovum (egg cell) from the ovary (Fig. 5).
- **Ovule:** A part of the reproductive organ in seed plants that consists of the nucellus, the embryo sac and integuments.
- **Ovum:** A gamete of female animals produced by the ovary.
- **Ovum pickup (opu):** The non-surgical collection of ova from a female.
- **Oxalate:** A salt or ester of oxalic acid.

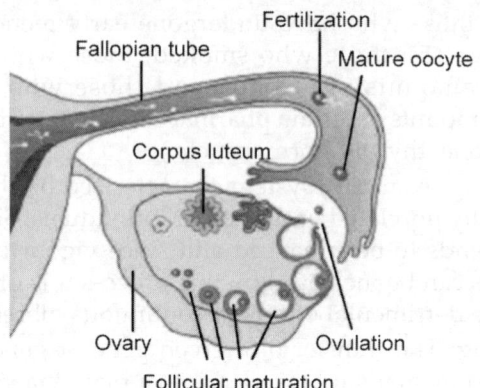

Fig. 5: Ovulation

- **Oxidation (chemical reaction):** Loss of electrons from a compound (or element) in a chemical reaction. When one compound is oxidized, another compound is reduced. That is, the other compound must "pick up" the electrons which the first has lost.
- **Oxidation:** A chemical transformation of fat/lipid molecules, in which oxygen (e.g. from air) is combined with those molecules. As a result of that (oxidation chemical reaction), various chemical entities are created (peroxides, aldehydes, etc.) which possess objectionable flavors/odors, and are harmful to animals that consume such (rancid) fats/oils.
- **Oxidation-reduction reaction:** A chemical reaction in which electrons are transferred from a donor to an acceptor molecule or atom.
- **Oxidative phosphorylation:** The enzymatic phosphorylation of ADP to ATP coupled to electron transport from a substrate to molecular oxygen. The synthesis (production) of ATP from the starting materials of ADP and inorganic phosphate (orthophosphate).
- **Oxidative stress:** A highly oxidized environment within cells that is thought to promote HIV replication because cells are forced into a highly activated state due to loss of control of their regulatory systems.
- **Oxidizing agent (oxidant):** The acceptor of electrons in an oxidation-reduction reaction. The oxidant is reduced by the end of the chemical reaction. That is, the oxidizing agent is the entity

that seeks and accepts electrons. Electron acceptance is, by definition, reduction.

- **Oxygenase:** An enzyme catalyzing a reaction in which oxygen is introduced into an acceptor molecule.
- **Oxygen electrode based sensor:** Sensor in which an oxygen electrode—a standard electrode chemical cell which measures the amount of oxygen in a solution is coated with a biological material that generates or absorbs oxygen. When the biological coating is active the amount of oxygen next to the electrode changes and the signal electrode from the electrode changes.

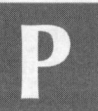

- **P element:** A transposon, whose genes (within this transposon) resist rearrangement during the process (i.e. transposition) of the P element being incorporated into a new location within an organism's genome (i.e. its deoxyribonucleic acid or DNA). In addition to "carrying" genes to a new location(s) in the genome, the P element itself codes for transposase (an enzyme that makes transposition possible).

- **P nucleotide:** Sequence is a short palindromic (inverted repeat) sequence that is generated during rearrangement of immunoglobulin and T cell receptor V, D, J gene segments. P nucleotides are generated at coding joints when RAG proteins cleave the hairpin ends generated during rearrangement.

- **P site:** The peptidyl tRNA binding site on the ribosome, the one to which the growing chain is attached, the incoming aminoacyl tRNA attaches to the A site.

- **P1 clones:** A cloning system for isolating genomic DNA that uses elements from phage P1 i.e. *loxP* and *pax* sites.

- **p53 gene:** A tumor-suppressor gene which controls passage (of a given cell) from the "GI" phase to the "s" (i.e. DNA synthesis) phase. The p53 protein that is coded for by the p53 gene is a transcription factor (i.e. it "reads" DNA to determine if damaged, then acts to control cell division, while the p53 gene codes for more production of additional p53 protein). Discovered in 1993 by Arnold J. Levine and colleagues, it is believed to be responsible for up to 50% of all human cancer tumors (when the p53 gene is damaged or mutated). Normally, the p53 gene codes for (i.e. causes to be manufactured in cell) the p53 protein, which acts to prevent cells from dividing uncontrollably when the cell's DNA has been damaged (e.g. via exposure to cigarette smoke or ultraviolet light). If, inspite of the presence of p53 protein, a cell begins to divide uncontrollably following damage to its DNA, the p53 gene can cause apoptosis, which is also known as "programed cell death" (to prevent tumors).

- **p53 protein:** A tumor-suppressor protein, sometimes called the master transcription factor, or the "guardian of the genome"; but whose amino acid sequence alterations (resulting from damage or mutation to the p53 gene) are believed to be responsible for up to 50% of all human cancer tumors. The p53 protein has four domains, one of which (i.e. the core domain) binds to a specific sequence(s) of the cell's DNA, in order to prevent the cell from dividing uncontrollably when the cell's DNA has been damaged (via exposure to cigarette smoke, ultraviolet light, or other carcinogen), until the damage to that DNA can be repaired. As the amount of DNA within a given (damaged) cell increases, the concentration of p53 protein also increases. Because p53 protein is a transcription factor (i.e. "reads" DNA to determine if damaged, then acts to control cell division, while p53 gene codes for more production), p53 is very efficient at preventing/ inhibiting tumors. However, if the cell's DNA cannot be repaired, the p53 protein can then causes apoptosis ("programed cell death") to prevent development of (cancerous) tumors.

- **Pachynema:** A mid-prophase stage in meiosis immediately following zygonema and preceding diplonema. In microscopic preparations the chromosomes are visible as long paired threads. Rarely four chromatids are detectable (Fig. 1).

P

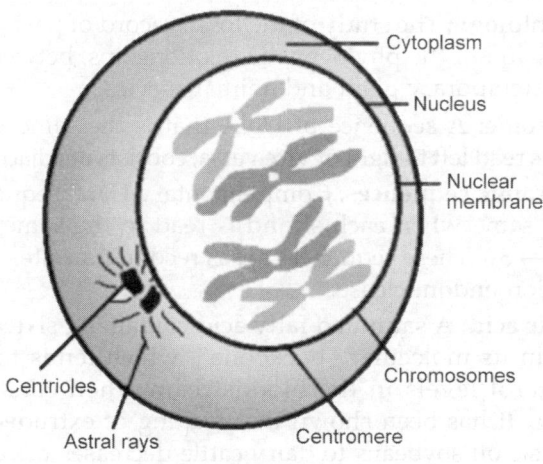

Fig. 1: Pachynema

- **Packing ratio:** The ratio of the length of DNA to the unit length of the fiber containing it.

- **Paclitaxel:** An anticancer compound (pharmaceutical) that was originally isolated from the Pacific yew tree (*Taxus brevifolia*), although it is made synthetically today. In 1966, Maurice Wall first identified antitumor effects in an extract from *Taxus brevifolia*. In 1992, the US food and drug administration approved paclitaxel for use to treat recurrent ovarian cancer. Other anticancer uses were later approved. When injected into the human body, paclitaxel also inhibits growth of the parasitic microorganism *Toxoplasma gondii* (which can cause loss of sight and neurological disease in humans, if not controlled).

- **PAF:** Acronym for platelet activating factor.

- **Pairing:** The lining up of the two homologous chromosomes or chromatids of each chromosome pair in meiosis or mitosis.

- **Pair-rule:** In *Drosophila* the pair-rule genes are a set of genes that help in setting up the segmentation of the embryo. They are expressed in a striped pattern with one stripe in every other future segment.

- **Pairing synapsis:** The pairing of homologous chromosomes during the prophase of the first meiotic division when crossing over occurs.

P

- **Pair rule gene:** A gene that influences the formation of body segments (in Drosophila).

- **Palaeontology:** The study of the fossil record of past geological periods and of the phylogenetic relationships, between extinct and contemporary plant and animal species.

- **Palindrome:** A sequence of DNA that is the same when one strand is read left to right or vice versa; consists of adjacent repeat.

- **Palindromic sequences:** Complementary DNA sequences that are the same when each strand is read in the same direction (e.g. $5' \rightarrow 3'$). These sequences act as recognition sites for type II restriction endonuclease.

- **Palmitic acid:** A saturated fatty acid containing sixteen carbon atoms in its molecular "backbone"; which tends to increase cholesterol levels in the bloodstream when consumed by humans. It has been shown that feeding of extruded (whole) high-oleic oil soybeans to dairy cattle decreases the content of palmitic acid in their milk (Fig. 2).

Palmitic acid
$C_{16}H_{32}O_2$

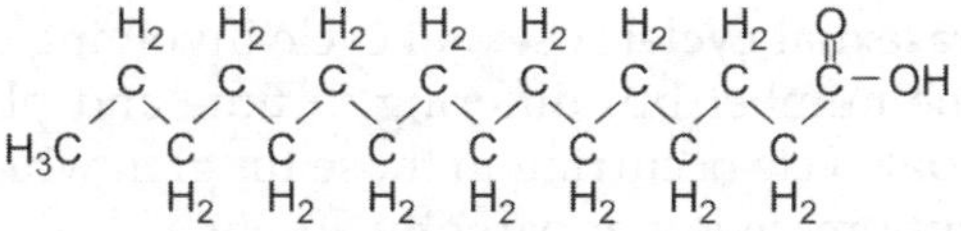

$$H_3C-C_{H_2}-C_{H_2}-C_{H_2}-C_{H_2}-C_{H_2}-C_{H_2}-C_{H_2}-C_{H_2}-C_{H_2}-C_{H_2}-C_{H_2}-C_{H_2}-C_{H_2}-C_{H_2}-C-OH$$

Fig. 2: Palmitic acid

- **Pancreas:** An organ (gland) located near the stomach that secretes insulin and glucagon into the bloodstream, and digestive fluids into the intestines.
- **Panicle:** An inflorescence, the main axis of which is branched. The branches bear loose racemose flower clusters.
- **Panicle culture:** Aseptic culture of grain panicle segments to induce microspore germination and development.
- **Panmictic population:** A population in which mating occurs at random.
- **Panmixis:** Random mating in a population.
- **Papovaviruses:** A class of animal viruses with small genomes, including SV 40 and polyoma.
- **Par gene:** A gene found in bacterial and plant cells and involved in partition of plasmids in cells.
- **Paracentric inversion:** An inversion that is entirely within one arm of a chromosome and does not include the centromere.
- **Paraffin (wax):** A translucent, white, solid hydrocarbon with a low meting point. Paraffin is used as an embedding medium to support tissue for sectioning for light microscopy observation.
- **Parafilm:** A stretchable film based on paraffin wax used to seal tubes and petridishes. Parafilm is a name which is applied colloquially to similar products.
- **Parahormone:** A substance with hormone like properties that is not a secreted product (e.g. ethylene carbon dioxide).
- **Parallel evolution:** The development of different organisms along similar evolutionary paths due to similar selection pressures acting on them.
- **Paralogs:** Highly similar proteins that are coded by the same genome.
- **Parameter:** A value or constant pertaining to an entire population.
- **Paranemic joint:** A region in which two complementary sequences of DNA are associated side by side instead of being intert-wined in a double helical structure.

- **Parasexual cycle:** A sexual cycle involving changes in chromosome number but differing in time and place from the usual sexual cycle occurring in those fungi in which the normal cycle is suppressed or apparently absent.
- **Parasite:** Organism that lives in or on another organism and uses it as a source of food and shelter and damages the host.
- **Parasitism:** The close association of two or more dissimilar organisms where the association is harmful to atleast one of the two.
- **Parasporal crystal:** Tightly packaged insect protoxin molecules that are produced by strains of *Bacillus thuringiensis* during the formation of resting spores.
- **Parasegment:** In *Drosophila,* a parasegment is a unit composed of the rear of one segment and the front of the adjacent segment.
- **Parenchyma:** A plant tissue consisting of spherical, undifferentiated cells frequently with air spaces between them.
- **Parenchymatous:** Adjective used to describe spherical and undifferentiated cells with primary cell walls capable of both cell division and differentiation.
- **Parental genotype:** The genotype that is identical to the genotype of one of the contributing parents.
- **Parental strand (of DNA):** The DNA strand that undergo replication and form a complementary daughter DNA strand.
- **Parental types:** Progeny of a genetic cross that is genetically identical to one or the other one of the parents.
- **Parkinson's disease:** A disease of the human brain, in which those nerve cells (neurons) associated with emotions and those neurons that are involved in controlling movement (motor control) die.
- **Poly ADP-ribose polymerase (PARP):** An enzyme naturally present in human cells that is involved in control of apoptosis, among other cellular processes. This enzyme can be commercially produced (e.g. to manufacture tests) by genetically engineered hamster cells grown in cell culture. This enzyme can be utilized by man in order to determine/test if a given substance (e.g. industrial chemical) is carcinogenic to humans.
- **Parthenocarpy:** The development of fruit without undergoing fertilization.
- **Parthenogenesis:** Production of an embryo from an unfertilized egg or androgenesis, apomixis, gynogenesis.

- **Partial digest:** Addition of a restriction enzyme to a DNA sample under particular conditions or for a limited period such that only a proportion of the target sites in any individual molecules are cleaved.
- **Partial diploid:** A bacteria with two copies of a part of its genome. It is due to the presence of plasmid or prophage carrying some part of bacterial DNA.
- **Particle radiation:** Refers to gamma (γ) particles (positively charged) and beta (β) particles (negatively charged) electrons, protons and neutrons. In plant tissue culture, these particles are used to produce mutant cells or organisms.
- **Partition coefficient:** A constant (number) that expresses the ratio in which a given solute will be partitioned (distributed) between two given immiscible liquids (e.g. oil and water) at equilibrium.
- **Partition:** Process by which a solute is distributed between two immiscible phases.
- **Parts per million (PPM):** Unit of any given substance per one million equivalent units such as the weight units of solute per million weight units of solution (i.e. 1 ppm = 1 mg/l).
- **Parturition:** The process or act of giving birth.
- **Passage:** The transfer or transplantation of cells from one culture vessel to another.
- **Passage number:** The number of times the cells in the culture have been sub-cultured. In descriptions of this process, the dilution ratio of the cells should be stated so that the relative cultural "age" can be ascertained.
- **Passage time:** Interval between successive sub-cultures.
- **Passive immunity:** An immune response (to a pathogen) that results from injecting another organism's antibodies into the organism that is being challenged by the pathogen.
- **Passive transport:** Describes movement of molecules along their electrochemical gradient; no energy is required.
- **PAT gene:** A dominant gene isolated from the *Streptomyces viridochromogenes* bacterium which codes for (causes production of) the enzyme phosphinothricin acetyl transferase (PAT). When the PAT gene is inserted into a plant's genome, it imparts resistance to glufosinate - ammonium containing herbicides. Because the glufosinate-ammonium herbicides act via inhibition of glutamine synthetase (an enzyme that catalyzes the synthesis

of glutamine), this inhibition of enzyme kills plants (e.g. weeds). That is because glutamine is crucial for plants to synthesize critically needed amino acids. The PAT gene is also often used by genetic engineers as a marker gene.

- **Patch recombinant:** DNA results from a holliday junction being resolved by cutting the exchanged strands. The duplex is largely unchanged, except for a DNA sequence on one strand that came from the homologous chromosome.
- **Patent:** A legal document issued by a government that permits the holder the exclusive right to manufacture, use of sell an invention for a defined period, which varies from country to country.
- **Paternal:** Pertaining to the father.
- **Pathogen:** Refers to a virus, bacterium, parasitic protozoan, or other microorganism that causes infectious disease by invading the body of an organism (animal, plant, etc.) known as the host. It should be noted that infection is not synonymous with disease because infection does not always lead to injury or harm the host.
- **Pathogen-associated molecular pattern (PAMP):** is a molecular structure on the surface of a pathogen. A given PAMP may be conserved across a large number of pathogens. During an immune response, PAMPs may be recognized by receptors on cells that mediate innate immunity.
- **Pathogen free:** Freedom from disease causing organisms (bacteria, fungi, viruses, etc.)
- **Pathogenesis related proteins:** Protective (i.e. disease-fighting) proteins that are produced within certain plants in response to the entry-into-plant of plant pathogens (bacteria, fungi, etc. that infect and cause disease in plants). One pathogenesis-related protein is chitinase, a protein enzyme that degrades (breaks down) the chitin within cell wall of pathogenic fungi. Production of pathogenesis-related proteins is often initiated by signaling molecules (e.g. harpin) produced by the pathogens.
- **Pathogenic:** Disease-causing.
- **Pathotoxin:** Very dilute substance synthesized and released by some pathogens and interacts with the host metabolism.
- **Pathovar:** In plant biotechnology strains of bacteria causing disease in specific plant cultivars.
- **Pathway:** A sequential series of chemical reactions, each of which is dependent on previous one in the pathway (e.g. the third reaction requires chemical product produced by first/

second chemical reactions), that overall yields a beneficial impact. For example, metabolism (i.e. the entire set of enzyme-catalyzed chemical reactions which converts food into nutrients that can be used by the body's cells and the use of these nutrients by the body's cells to sustain life, growth, etc.) occurs via a very specific metabolic pathway.

- **Pathway feedback mechanisms:** Chemically based mechanisms (e.g. series of chemical reactions) that hinder (or increase rate of) a given pathway. For example, when the body of bacteria need catabolism (i.e. energy production) to be slowed down, it uses the mechanism of catabolite repression (to slow down catabolism via chemical/reaction means).

- **PBR:** The intellectual property rights that are legally accorded to plant breeders by laws, treaties, etc. Similar to patent law for inventors.

- **pBR322:** An *Escherichia coli* (*E. coli*) plasmid cloning vector that contains the ampicillin resistance and tetracycline resistance genes. It consists of a circle of double-stranded DNA.

- **PC:** Phosphatidyl choline.

- **PCR (Polymerase chain reaction):** A technique in which cycles of denaturation, annealing with primer, and extension with DNA polymerase, are used to amplify the number of copies of a target DNA sequence by $>10^6$ times.

- **Peak:** A band or zone in a chromatogram showing a maximum concentration between two minima.

- **Pectin:** A white amorphous substance which when combined with acid and sugar yields a jelly substance cementing the cells together (the middle lamella) (Fig. 3).

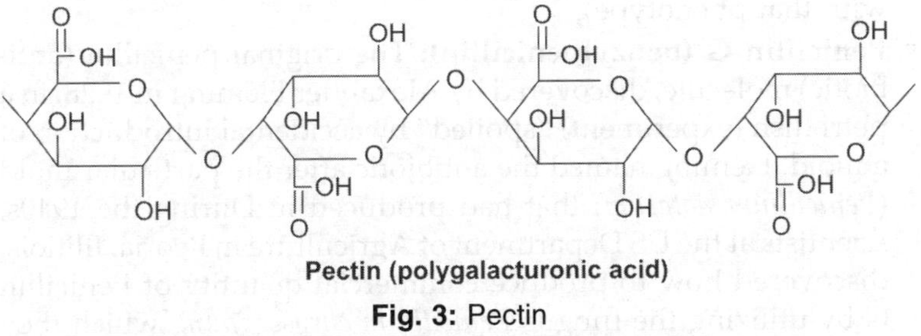

Pectin (polygalacturonic acid)

Fig. 3: Pectin

- **Pectinase:** Enzyme catalyzing the hydrolysis of pectins.

- **Pectinophora gossypiella:** Also known as the pink bollworm, this is one of three insect species that are called "bollworms" (when they are on cotton plants). The holes that they chew in cotton plants' bolls have been shown to enable the *Aspergillus flavus* fungus to infect those (chewed) cotton plants.

- **Pedicel:** Stalk or stem of the individual flowers of an inflorescence.
- **Pedigree:** A table, chart or diagram recording the ancestry of an individual.
- **Peduncle:** Stalk or stem of a flower that is born singly; the main stem of an inflorescence.
- **Polyethylene glycol superoxide dismutase (PEG-SOD):** A modified version of the enzyme human superoxide dismutase (hSOD), in which polyethylene glycol (a polymer made up of ethylene glycol monomers) is combined with the hSOD molecule. The PEG seems to wrap around or about the enzyme in such a way that the whole complex is able to exist in the blood for longer periods of time than the unmodified hSOD enzyme. This is because PEG effectively camouflages the hSOD molecule and hence protects it from being inactivated by the body's own defense mechanisms in the bloodstream. This technology is important in that hSOD is used to fight certain diseases by injecting it into the body. However, SOD must be present in the body for extended period of time in order to effectively work, and since the injected SOD is a foreign molecule, the body tries to destroy it (its function) as quickly as possible.
- **Penetrance:** The percentage of individuals in a population that shows a particular phenotype among those capable of showing it (i.e. among those that have the genotype normally associated with that phenotype).
- **Penicillin G (benzylpenicillin):** The original penicillin (antibiotic) molecule, discovered by Alexander Fleming in 1928, in a petri dish (experiment) "spoiled" by accidental introduction of a mold. Fleming named the antibiotic after the particular mold (*Penicillium notatum*) that had produced it. During the 1940s, scientists at the US Department of Agriculture in Peoria, Illinois, discovered how to produce commercial quantity of Penicillin G by utilizing the fungus *Penicillium chrysogenum*, which they found growing on a canteloupe in Peoria. Penicillin kills bacteria by blocking an enzyme which is crucial for growth and repair of the bacteria's cell wall (peptidoglycan layer), but penicillin

P

does not harm other species, so it is species-specific to pathogenic bacteria (e.g. Streptococcus, Meningococcus, and diphtheria bacillus).

- **Penicillinases (E.C. 3.5.2.6):** Also known as β-lactamases, these are enzymes that hydrolyze (break down) the β-lactam ring (portion) of the penicillin molecule's structure. Some microorganisms (e.g. pathogenic bacteria) have become able to produce these enzymes as a defense to penicillin and cephalosporin antibiotics (drugs).

- **Penicillium:** Refers to the genus of fungi (mold) that belongs to the category *Deutromycotina* and often causes (food) spoilage. Some of the genus have been utilized commercially to produce antiboiotics.

- **Pentose:** A simple sugar (monosaccharide molecule) whose backbone structure contains five carbon atoms. There exists many different pentoses. Some examples of pentoses are ribose, arabinose, and xylose.

- **Pepsin:** A crystallizable proteinase enzyme that in an acidic medium digests (breakdown) most proteins to polypeptides. It is secreted by glands in the mucous membrane of the stomach of higher animals. In combination with dilute hydrochloric acid, it is the chief active principle (component) of gastric juice. Also used in manufacturing peptones and in digesting gelatin for the recovery (i.e. recycling) of silver from photographic film.

- **Peptidase:** An enzyme that hydrolyzes (cleaves) a peptide bond.

- **Peptide bond:** A covalent bond between the amino (NH_2) group of one amino acid and the carboxyl (COOH) group of another amino acid (Fig. 4).

- **Peptide mapping (fingerprinting):** Refers to the characteristic pattern of peptides (i.e. pieces that make up a protein molecule) resulting from partial hydrolysis (cleavage, digestion) of a protein. The pattern (fingerprint) is obtained by separating the peptides via two-dimensional chromatography, in which the peptides are first subjected to chromatography using one solution which separates many, but not all, peptides. The chromatogram is then turned 90°, and is again chromatographed using a second solution, which then separates all of the peptides; thereby producing the final "fingerprint" of the protein.

- **Peptide vaccine:** A short chain of amino acids that can induce antibodies against a specific infections agent.

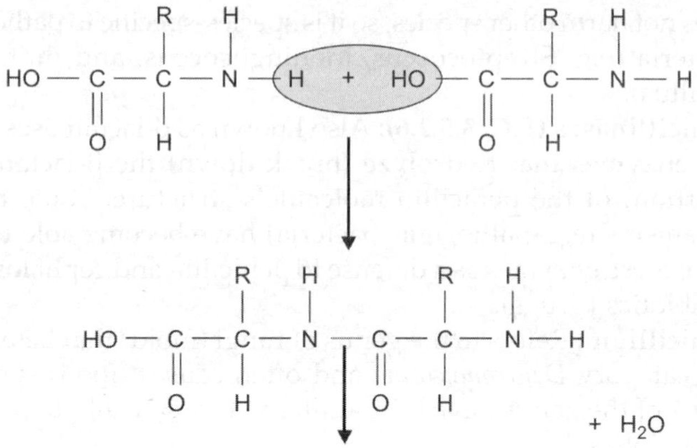

Fig. 4: Peptide bond

- **Peptide:** Two or more amino acids covalently joined by peptide bonds. An oligomer component of a polypeptide. A dipeptide, for example, consists of two (di) amino acids joined together by a peptide bond or linkage. By analogy, this structure would correspond to two joined links of a chain.

- **Peptidyl transferase:** The activity of the ribosomal 50S subunit that synthesizes a peptide bond when an amino acid is added to a growing polypeptide chain. The actual catalytic activity is a property of the rRNA.

- **Peptidyl-tRNA:** The tRNA to which the nascent polypeptide chain has been transferred following peptide bond synthesis, during protein synthesis.

- **Peptone:** A protein that has been partially hydrolyzed (cleaved) by the peptidase pepsin.

- **Perennial:** A plant that grows more or less indefinitely from year to year and once mature, usually produces seed each year.

- **Perforin:** A 70 Kd (kilodalton) protein that is instrumental in the lysis of infected cells. A series of reactions occurs on the surface of a cell which results in the polymerization of certain monomers to form transmembrane (through the membrane) pores 100 Å (Angstroms) wide, which allows ions to rush into the cell (due to osmotic pressure) and thus burst (lyse) that cell, so the (formerly) internal pathogens can be attacked by the body's immune system. Perforin is a protein that is akin to the C9 component of the complement.

- **Pericentric inversion:** Inversion in a chromosome of a single segment that includes the centromere.
- **Periclinal:** The plane of cell wall orientation or cell division parallel to the surface of the organ.
- **Periclinal chimera:** Genotypically or cytoplasmically different tissues arranged in concentric layers.
- **Pericycle:** Region of the plant bounded externally by the endodermis and internally by the phloem. Most roots and originate root hairs from the pericycle.
- **Perinuclear space:** Lies between the inner and outer membranes of the nuclear envelope.
- **Periodicity:** Periodicity of DNA is the number of base pairs per turn of the double helix.
- **Periodontium:** Tissue that anchors teeth in the jaw. Regrowth of periodontal tissue can be stimulated by a combination of platelet derived growth factor and insulin-like growth factor-1.
- **Periplasm:** The space between the cell membranes and the cell wall, in Gram-negative bacteria; contains proteins secreted by the cell.
- **Periseptal annulus:** A ring-like area where inner and outer membrane appear fused. Formed around the circumference of the bacterium, the periseptal annulus determines the location of the septum.
- **Peritoneal cavity/membrane:** The smooth, transparent, serous membrane that lines the cavity of the abdomen of a mammal.
- **Permafrost:** An area that is subjected to permanent ice and snow.
- **Permeable:** for a membrane, cell or cell system through which substances may diffuse.
- **Permissive:** A protein that plays a permissive role in development is one that sets up a situation where a certain activity can occur, but does not cause the occurrence itself.
- **Permissive conditions:** It allow conditional lethal mutants to survive.
- **Peroxidase:** An enzyme that catalyzes the oxidation of a substrate with hydrogen peroxide (as the electron acceptor, so the hydrogen peroxide is reduced). Peroxidase is naturally produced in soybeans by approximately half of all commercial soybean varieties. Peroxidase very effectively inhibits (stops) growth of *Aspergillus flavus* fungi that might be present (in the

P

soil). Peroxidase can be used to replace more toxic and environmentally problematic chemicals in certain industrial processes. Among other applications, peroxidase can replace formaldehyde use in paints, varnishes, glues, and computer chip manufacturing.

- **Peroxins:** The protein components of the peroxisome.
- **Peroxisome:** Is an organelle found in the cytoplasm, enclosed in a single membrane. It contains oxidizing enzymes.
- **Persistence:** The tendency of a compound (e.g. an insecticide) to resist degradation by biological means (e.g. metabolism by microorganisms), after that compound has introduced into the environment (e.g. sprayed onto a field) or by physical means.
- **Pesticide:** A toxic chemical product that kills harmful organisms or pests. (e.g. insecticides, fungicides, weedicides, rodenticides).
- **Petal:** One of the parts of the flower that make-up the corolla.
- **Petiole:** Stalk of leaf.
- **Petite:** A mutant first discovered in the yeast saccharomyces cerevisiae. Due to defect in the respiratory chain, 'petite' yeast are uanble to growth on media containing only non-fermentable carbon sources (such as glycerol or ethanol), and form small anaerobic colonies when grown in the presence of fermentable carbon sources (such as glucose). The petite phenotype can be caused by the absence of, or nutations in, mitochondrial DNA (termed "cytoplasmic petities"), or by mutations in nuclear encoded genes involved in oxidative phosphorylation.
- **Petite mutant:** A respiration deficient yeast mutant that produces small colonies when grown on glucose containing medium.
- **Petri dish:** Flat rounded dish with a matching lid made of glass or plastic material and used for culturing organisms aka plates hence termed to plate culture (Fig. 5).

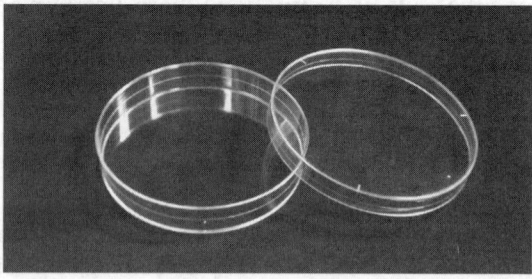

Fig. 5: Petri dish

- **Pfiesteria piscicida:** A single-celled microscopic algae which has a predator/prey relationship with fish in its ecosystem. During a large portion of its life cycle, *Pfiesteria piscicida* exists in a nontoxic cyst form at the bottom of a river. When those (cysts) detect certain substances (e.g. excreta) emitted by live fish, the *Pfiesteria piscicida* transform into an amoeboid or dinoflagellate form, which secretes a water-soluble neurotoxin into the water (which incapacitates nearby fish). The *Pfiesteria piscicida* next attach themselves to those fish, and excrete a lipid soluble toxin which destroys the epidermal layer of the fish's skin, allowing the *Pfiesteria piscicida* to begin "eating" the fish's tissue. Human exposure to the neurotoxin apparently causes short-term memory loss.
- **pH:** The negative logarithm of hydrogen ion concentration of any solution for measuring acidity or alkalinity.
- **Phage:** Abbreviation for bacteriophage. Another name for a specific type of virus. A virus that attacks bacteria is known as a bacteriophage. Bacteriophages are frequently used as vectors for carrying (foreign) DNA into cells by genetic engineers.
- **Phage T_4:** Phage T_4 is a virus that infects *E. coli* causing lysis of the bacterium.
- **Phage variation:** An alteration in the type of flagella produced by a bacterium.
- **Phagemid:** A cloning vector that contains components derived from both phage DNA and plasmid.
- **Phagocyte:** A cell such as a leukocyte that engulfs and digests cells, cell debris, microorganisms, and other foreign bodies in the bloodstream and tissues (phagocytosis). The ingested material is then degraded via enzymes. A whole class of cells is known to be phagocytic.
- **Phagocytosis:** The ingestion of a smaller cell or cell fragment, a microorganism, or foreign particles by means of the local infolding of a cell's membrane and the protrusion of its cytoplasm around the fold untill the material has been surrounded and engulfed by closure of the membrane and formation of a vacuole: characteristic of amebas and some types of white blood cells (Fig. 6).
- **Pharmacoenvirogenetics:** A word coined during 2000 by Tim Studt to describe the fact that environmental factors interact with a given individual's (human/animal/plant) genetic

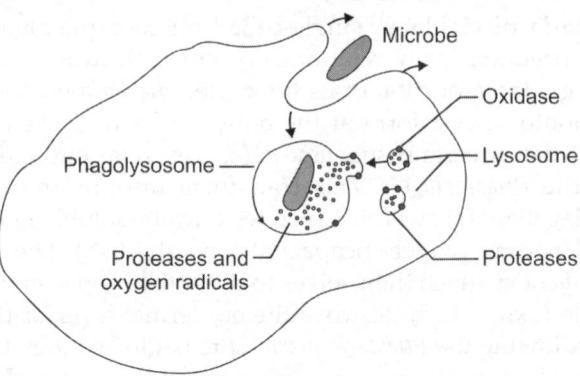

Fig. 6: Phagocytosis

makeup (i.e. genome) to determine those individual's (body's) response to a given pharmaceutical (and/or progression) of a disease. Those environmental factors include: 1. Foods eaten 2. The stress the individual is exposed to 3. Air and water pollution the individual is exposed to 4. Temperature and humidity the individual is exposed to 5. Geographical elevation the individual is exposed to 6. Bacteria or the individual is exposed to. For example, when *Rhizobium japonicum* bacteria grow in the soil near the roots of a soybean plant (*Glycine max* L.), that causes certain specific genes in the soybean plant to be expressed (i.e. "turned on") so that soybean plant's roots become more hospitable "home" for those *Rhizobium japonicum* bacteria to live symbiotically (in nodules) with the soybean plant.

- **Pharmacogenetics:** A branch of pharmacokinetics that deals with the reactions between drugs, or free radicals, or synthetic food ingredients, and specific individuals due to the genetics of those individuals. The subgroup of all those individuals whose DNA causes their bodies to respond in a specific way to a given drug or synthetic food ingredient, is known as a haplotype. For example, one haplotype (subgroup) of pediatric leukemia patients suffer severe and life-threatening reactions to some commonly used leukemia treatment drugs, due to the variation (i.e. SNP) in the thiopurine S-methyl transferase gene (allele) in their genome. Another example is that consumption of sodium-containing food ingredients tends to cause a dangerous increase in blood pressure (hypertension) among the African-American people living in the US, more often than among other ethnic groups living in the US.

- **Pharmacogenomics:** The study of association between genetics and drug response.
- **Pharmacokinetics (pharmacodynamics):** A branch of pharmacology dealing with the reactions between drugs or synthetic food ingredients and living structures (e.g. tissues, organs). The study of the: 1. Absorption—transport of the drug (pharmaceutical) or food ingredient into the bloodstream (e.g. from the intestinal tract, in the case of food ingredients). 2. Distribution—initial physical disposition/behavior of the substance in the body after the substance enters the body. For example, does the substance preferentially concentrate in the fat cells of the body? 3. Metabolism—breakdown of the substance (if breakdown does occur) into other compounds, and ultimate disposition of those compounds (or the original substance, if breakdown does not occur). For example, some pharmaceuticals break down into smaller compound(s); one of which then acts upon the relevant body cells (to relieve pain, lower blood pressure, etc.). 4. Elimination—the speed and thoroughness with which the substance is excreted or otherwise removed from the body. In short, pharmacokinetics deals with what happens to a substance that is introduced into a living system. For example, how quickly it is broken down, to what intermediates and metabolites it is broken down, and what the pathway of this breakdown is.
- **Pharmacology:** The study of chemicals (e.g. pharmaceuticals) and their effects on living organisms.
- **Pharmacophore:** The portion of a molecule (e.g. a pharmaceutical) that is responsible for its biological activity (i.e. therapeutic action on recipient's tissue, etc.).
- **Pharming:** The process of farming genetically engineered animals to be used as living pharmaceuticals factories.
- **Phase I clinical testing:** The first in a series of human tests of new pharmaceuticals, mandated by the US. Food and Drug Administration (US-FDA). The primary purpose of the Phase I clinical test is to detect if the new pharmaceutical is toxic or otherwise harmful to normal, healthy humans. The conclusion of phase I testing leads to phase II and phase III testing. During the 1990s, the FDA began to require the inclusion of ethnic minorities and women (in addition to men) as subjects in these

tests, to enable pharmacogenomics (i.e. the testing to determine if a given pharmaceutical causes nontypical response in the bodies of members of these subgroups).

- **Phase II clinical tests:** The second in a series of human tests of new pharmaceuticals, mandated by the US-FDA. The primary purpose of the phase II clinical tests is to determine the pharmaceutical's efficacy (i.e. does it work?). Successful conclusion of phase II tests allows phase III clinical tests to begin.

- **Phase III clinical tests:** The third in a series of human tests of new pharmaceuticals, mandated by the US-FDA. The primary purpose of phase III clinical tests is to verify proper dosage of a new pharmaceutical.

- **Phase state:** The coupling or repulsion of two linked genes.

- **Phenocopies:** The strength of environmental changes may modify several genes. In some instances specific environmental changes may modify the development of an organism so that its phenotype simulates the effect of a particular gene, although this effect is not inherited. Such individuals are known as phenocopies. The normal body color of the vinegar fly *(Drosophia melanogaster)* is light brown color. If larvae from normal flies are raised on food containing silver salts, they develop into yellow flies. The yellow-bodied but genotypically normal fly is a phenocopy of the yellow mutant. The offspring of a phenocopy have the normal brown body color unless raised again on food containing silver salts; however, the offspring of the yellow mutant have yellow bodies.

- **Phenolic hormones:** A category of compounds found in the human body, that are synthesized (manufactured) by the body from certain phenolic dietary substances (phytochemicals) such as isoflavones. Research indicates that phenolic hormones act to prevent a number of cancers such as those of the prostate, breast, large bowel, etc.

- **Phenolic oxidation:** Many plant species contain phenolic compounds that blacken through oxidation. The process is initiated after plants are wounded.

- **Phenols:** Compounds with hydroxyl group attached to the benzene ring forming esters, ethers and salts. Phenolic substances are produced from newly explanted tissues oxidizing to form coloured compounds visible in nutrient media.

- **Phenomics:** Utilized to refer to the relationship between genomics and phenotype/traits.
- **Phenotype:** The physical appearance of an organism with respect to a trait, e.g. yellow (Y) or green (y) seeds in garden peas. The dominant trait is normally represented with a capital letter, and the recessive trait with the same lower case letter.
- **Phenylalanine (*phe*):** An essential amino acid. L-Phenylalanine is one of the raw materials used to manufacture NutraSweet® (NutraSweet Co.) synthetic sweetener (Fig. 7).

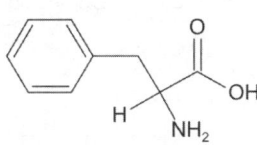

Fig. 7: Phenylalanine

- **Phenylketonuria (*pku*):** An inherited disorder that results in reduced production of phenylalanine hydroxylase. This substance is involved in the breakdown of phenylalanine in food or tyrosine.
- **Pheromone:** Pheromone a small molecule secreted by one mating type of an organism in order to interact or attract with a member of the opposite mating type of the same species.
- **Philadelphia chromosome:** Refers to a particular human chromosome that is (visibly) distorted by the mutated gene that results in the disease known as chronic myelogenous leukemia (CML, also known as chronic myeloid leukemia). That is because that gene codes for extensive production of the tyrosine kinase known as Bcr-Ab1—an enzyme which causes neoplastic (aberrant) cell growth and cell division. As a result, people with CML disease tend to have 10–25 times more white blood cells than normal. The pharmaceutical known as Gleevec™ induces apoptosis—"programed" (self destruct) cell death—in the cells that have the Philadelphia chromosome; thus leading to cessation of CML.
- **Phloem:** Food conducting tissue in plants consisting of sieve tubes, companion cells, phloem parenchyma and fibres (Fig. 8).
- **Phosphatase:** An enzyme that removes phosphate group from substrates.
- **Phosphate transporter genes:** Gene(s) within the genomes of at least some plants, which code for proteins that enable/ increase the ability of those plants to extract and utilize phosphate (form of phosphorous) from the soil. Since all plants require phosphorous for proper growth and functioning, yet most plants are not inherently very adaptable at extracting and

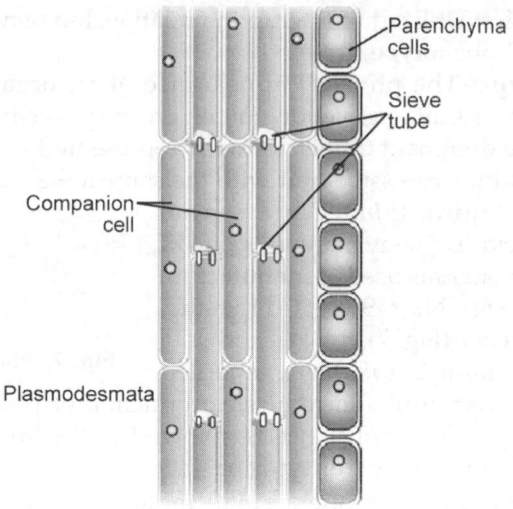

Fig. 8: Phloem

utilizing soil phosphate, adding (more) phosphate transporter genes to a given (crop) plant is likely to increase that plant's growth and yield (e.g. seeds).

- **Phosphate-group energy:** The decrease in free energy as one mole of a phosphorylated compound at 1.0 M concentration undergoes hydrolysis to equilibrium at pH 7.0 and 25°C (77°F). The energy that is available to do biochemical work. The energy arises from the breakage (cleavage) of a phosphate–phosphate bond.

- **Phosphinothricin acetyltransferase (PAT):** An enzyme which degrades (breakdown) phosphinothricin (also known as glufosinate), which is an active ingredient in some herbicides. PAT is naturally produced in some strains of soil bacteria (e.g. *Streptomyces viridochromogenes*). If a gene (called the "PAT gene") that codes for the production of phosphinothricin acetyltransferase is inserted via genetic engineering into a crop plant's genome, that would enable such plants to survive post-emergence applications of phosphinothricin-containing herbicides.

- **Phosphinothricin:** Another name for the herbicide active ingredient glufosinate.

- **Phosphodiesterases (PDE):** A category of enzymes that inhibit apoptosis.

- **Phosphodiester bond:** A bond in which a phosphate group joins adjacent carbon through ester linkages.
- **Phospholipase A2:** An enzyme which degrades type A2 phospholipids.
- **Phospholipid:** Phospholipid is a lipid that has a positively charged head that is linked by a phosphate group to the fatty acid tail.
- **Phosphorelay:** Describes a pathway in which a phosphate group is passed along a series of protein.
- **Phosphorolysis:** The cleavage of a bond by orthophosphate analogous to hydrolysis referring to cleavage by water.
- **Phosphorylation:** The introduction of a phosphate group into a molecule. Formation of a phosphate derivative of a biomolecule, usually by enzymatic transfer of a phosphate group from ATP.
- **Photon:** A single unit of light energy.
- **Photoperiod:** The optimum length or period of illumination required for the growth and maturation of a plant. The photo-period is distinct from photosynthesis.
- **Photoreactivation:** A type of direct repair that involves a light dependent enzyme (Fig. 9).
- **Photorhabdus luminescens:** A soil-dwelling bacterium that produces certain toxins (effective against a variety of insect pests), antibiotics, antifungal compounds, lipases, proteases, and bioluminescent (light-producing) compounds. *Photorhabdus luminescens* naturally colonizes the gut of the *Heterorhabditis*

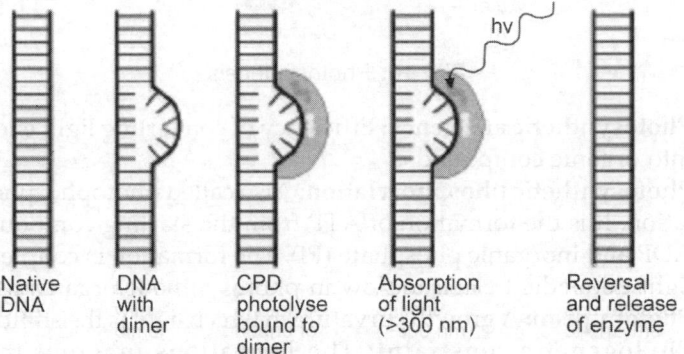

| Native DNA | DNA with dimer | CPD photolyse bound to dimer | Absorption of light (>300 nm) | Reversal and release of enzyme |

Fig. 9: Photoreactivation

nematode which attacks certain insect pests (tobacco hornworm, mealworm, cockroaches, etc.). When that nematode enters those insects, the *luminescens* is released inside the insect, which is subsequently killed via the toxins secreted by *P. luminescens.* synthesizes (manufactures) a protein that is high in amino acids content methionine and lysine; and there protein constitutes approximately 50% of the total protein content of *P. luminescens.*

- **Photosynthate:** The carbohydrates and other compounds produced in photosynthesis.
- **Photosynthesis:** A process by which plants, algae, and some bacteria containing chlorophyll synthesize organic compounds, chiefly carbohydrates, from atmospheric carbon dioxide and water, using light for energy and liberating oxygen in the process. (Fig. 10).

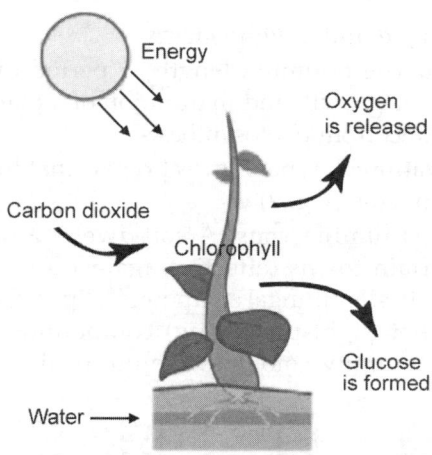

Fig. 10: Photosynthesis

- **Photosynthetic efficiency:** Efficiency of converting light energy into organic compounds.
- **Photosynthetic phosphorylation:** Also called photophosphorylation. It is the formation of ATP from the starting compounds ADP and inorganic phosphate (Pi). The formation is coupled to light-dependent electron flow in photosynthetic organisms.
- **Phototropism:** A growth curvature in which light is the stimulus.
- **Phylogenetic constraint:** The limitations inherent in an organism as a result of what its ancestors were. For example, a

horse will never fly and an ape will never speak, because the ancestors of neither possessed those capabilities.

- **Phylogeny:** A diagram illustrating the deduced evolutionary history of populations of related organisms.
- **Physical map (of genome):** A diagram showing the linear order of genes or genetic markers on the genome, with units indicating the actual distance between the genes or markers.
- **Physiology:** The branch of biology dealing with the study of the functioning of living things. The materials of physiology include all living organisms like animals, plants, microorganisms and viruses.
- **Phytase:** A digestive enzyme that is present in the digestive systems of many plant-eating animals to enable breakdown of phytate (also known as "phytic acid"). Phytase is sometimes present within the plant material consumed by animals. For example, phytase is naturally produced in the seed coat of wheat.
- **Phytate:** A salt or ester of phytic acid, occuring in plants, especially cereal grains, capable of forming insoluble complexes with calcium, zinc, iron, and other nutrients and interfering with their absorption by the body.
- **Phytic acid:** Also known as phytate or inositol hexaphosphate.
- **Phytoalexins:** Term utilized to refer to chemical compounds (enzymes, etc.) that are produced by certain plants in response to the presence of infectious agents (e.g. fungus, bacteria) or their products. From the Greek words (*phyton*, plant, and *alexein*, to defend) phytoalexins possess antimicrobial (fungus- killing, bacteria-killing) properties, so they can help plants to protect themselves against those microorganisms.
- **Phytochemicals:** Also called phytonutrient. Any of various bioactive chemical compounds found in plants, as antioxidants, considered to be beneficial to human health.
- **Phytochrome:** A protein plant pigment that serves to direct the course of plant growth and development and differentiation in a plant. The response is independent of photosynthesis, e.g. in the photoperiod (length of light period) response.
- **Phytoestrogens:** Compounds possessing molecular structures somewhat similar to that of estrogen and that are naturally found in all plants on earth. As a result every vegetable, fruit, cereal and legume contains at least one type of "phytoestrogen".

For example, flavones and flavonols are beneficial phytoestrogens (mostly red- and yellow-colored pigments) found in colored vegetables and fruits (red grapes, yellow grapefruit, oranges, etc.).

- **Phytohormone:** A substance that stimulates growth or other processes in plants. Phytohormones are chemical messengers that may pass through cells, tissues and organs and stimulate biochemical, physiological and morphological responses.
- **Phyto-manufacturing:** Refers to the production of valuable substances (e.g. polyhydroxybutylate biodegradable plastic, industrial-process enzymes, etc.) in plants (e.g. genetically engineered plants).
- **Phytoparasite:** Parasite on plants.
- **Phytopathogen:** An organism that causes disease in plants.
- **Phytophthora megasperma f. sp. glycinea:** A strain of *Phytophthora* fungus that can infect the soybean plant [*Glycine max* (L.) Merrill] under certain conditions, and thereby cause that soybean plant's stem and root to degrade (so-called "rot").
- ***Phytophthora* root rot:** A plant disease that is caused by a certain *Phytophthora* fungus (*Phytophthora sojae*). Some soybean varieties are genetically resistant to as many as 21 races/strains of *Phytophthora* fungi.
- **Phytoplankton:** Algae that floats or are freely suspended in the water.
- **Phytoremediation:** Refers to the use of specific plants to remove contaminants or pollutants from either soils (e.g. polluted fields) or water resources (e.g. polluted lakes). For example, the Brazil water hyacinth (*Eichhornia crassipes*) naturally accumulates in its tissues toxic metals such as lead, arsenic, cadmium, mercury, nickel, copper, etc., and so has been utilized as a "biofilter" (e.g. in India). Insertion of the *Escherichia coliform* bacteria gene known as glutathione 11 into the plant known as Indian mustard causes that plant to accumulate 40–90% higher amounts of cadmium (from cadmium-tainted soil) in its tissues than before; such genetically engineered plants could be utilized to extract cadmium from polluted sites.
- **Phytosanitary:** Relating to, or being measures for the control of plant diseases especially in agricultural crops.
- **Phytostat:** The name adopted by Tulecke in 1965 for an apparatus designed for the semicontinuous chemostat culture of plant cells.

- **Phytosterols:** A group of phytochemicals (i.e. solid alcohols consisting of ring-structured molecules) that are present in seeds produced by certain plants (e.g. the soybean plant *Glycine max* L.). Evidence shows that human consumption of certain phytosterols can help to prevent certain types of cancers, and lower total serum cholesterol and low-density lipoproteins (LDLP) levels; thereby reducing the risk of coronary heart disease (CHD). Evidence indicates that those phytosterols (e.g. campesterol, stigmasterol, β-sitosterol) interfere with absorption of dietary cholesterol by the intestines, and decrease the body's recovery and reuse of cholesterol-containing bile salts, causing more cholesterol to be excreted from the body than previously. In 2000, the researcher Joseph Judd fed phytosterols extracted from soybeans (*Glycine max* L.) to human volunteers that were consuming a "low-fat" diet. Their total blood serum cholesterol and low-density lipoprotein (LDLP) levels decreased by more than 10% in a short time.
- **Phytotoxin:** Any toxic compound produced by a plant.
- **Picogram (PG):** A unit of measure equal to one trillionth of a gram, or 10^{-12} gram.
- *Picorna*: A "family" of the smallest known viruses. The viruses of this family are a cause of the common cold and Hepatitis A in humans, one form of hoof and mouth disease in animals, and at least one disease in corn (maize). In 1994, Dr. Asim Dasgupta discovered a cellular molecule within ordinary baker's yeast that prevents *Picorna* virus reproduction. This advancement could lead to the creation of a treatment, in the future, to cure one or more of the above-mentioned diseases after infection has begun.
- **Pigments:** Any substance whose presence in the tissues or cells of animals or plants colors them.
- **Pilin:** Is the subunit that is polymerized into the pilus in bacteria.
- **Pilus (Pili):** is a surface appendage on a bacterium that allows the bacterium to attach to other bacterial cells. It appears like a short, thin, flexible rod. During conjugation, pili are used to transfer DNA from one bacterium to another.
- **Pink pigmented facultative methylotroph (PPFM):** A type of bacteria that is naturally present in virtually all plants. PPFM produces cytokinin, which aids cell division (growth) process in plants. PPFM also produces a chemical substance similar to

P

vitamin B_{12}. In 1996, Joe Polacco discovered that impregnation of aged seeds with PPFM improved the germination (sprouting) rate of those aged seeds.

- **Pinocytosis:** The process by which a living cell engulfs minute droplet of liquid.
- **Pipette:** A slender graduated tube into which small amounts of liquids are taken up by suction for measuring and transferring.
- **Pistil:** Central organ of the flower typically consisting of ovary, style and stigma. The pistil is usually referred the female part of a perfect flower.
- **Pituitary gland:** One of the endocrine glands, lies beneath the hypothalamus (at the base of the brain). Alongwith the other endocrine glands, the pituitary helps control long-term bodily processes. This control is accomplished via interdependent secretion of hormones alongwith the other glands comprising the total endocrine system. For example, the pituitary helps controlling the body's growth from birth until the end of puberty by secreting growth hormone (GH). Secretion of GH by the pituitary is itself governed by the hormone known as growth hormone-releasing factor (GHRF), received by the pituitary gland from the hypothalamus. The pituitary gland also helps in control reproduction (development and growth of ovaries, timing of ovulation, maturation of oocytes, etc.) by secreting two gonadotropic (reproductive) hormones named luteinizing hormone (LH) and follicle-stimulating hormone (FSH). Secretion of LH and FSH by the pituitary is itself governed by the hormones gonadotropin-releasing hormone (GnRH, received by the pituitary from the hypothalamus) and estrogen/progesterone (received by the pituitary from the ovaries).
- **Plant breeder's rights (PBR):** The intellectual property rights that are legally accorded to plant breeders by various laws, international treaties, etc. Similar to patent law for inventors.
- **Plant cell culture:** Growth of plant cells or roots of plants in bioreactors.
- **Plant growth promoting rhizobacteria (PGPR):** The soil bacteria inhabiting around/on the root involved in promoting plant growth and development via production and secretion of various regulatory chemicals in the vicinity of rhizosphere.
- **Plant hormone:** An organic compound synthesized in minute quantities by certain plants. It influences and regulates plant

physiological processes. Also called phytohormone. The four general types of hormones that together influence cell division, enlargement, and differentiation are the auxin, gibberellin, kinin, and abscisic acid.

* **Plant protection act:** A law passed by the US Congress in 1930 that enabled intellectual property protection via patents for new plants (developed by scientists) which are propagated asexually (e.g. via grafting).

* **Plant variety protection act (PVP):** A law passed by the US Congress in 1970 that enables intellectual property protection (analogous to copyright protection) for new seed plants and seeds in America.

* **Plant variety rights (PVR):** Rights granted to the breeder of a new variety of plant that give the breeder exclusive control over the propagating material (including seed, cuttings, divisions, tissue culture) and harvested material (cut flowers, fruit, faliage) of a new variety for a number of years.

* **Plant's novel trait (PNT):** The new (novel) trait added to a plant (e.g. crop plant such as cotton, corn/maize, soybean, etc.). Examples of novel traits are herbicide-tolerance (via inserted CP4 EPSPS gene, PAT gene, etc.), insect resistance (via inserted *Bt* gene, *Photorhabdus luminescens* gene, etc.), and resistance to aluminum toxicity (via inserted CSb gene, etc.).

* **Plantibodies™:** A trademark owned by EPIcyte Pharmaceutical, Inc. A type of antibody first produced in tobacco, plantibodies have the advantage of being less immunogenic than mouse antibodies; they have been used in research and have potential therapeutic value.

* **Plantigens:** Antigens (e.g. of pathogenic bacteria) produced in plants which are genetically engineered to produce those (specific) antigens. That process (i.e. genetically engineering plants to cause them to produce specific antigens) can be utilized to produce edible vaccines for the pathogenic bacteria possessing those antigens. Then people could be "vaccinated" against disease merely by eating the genetically engineered plant (e.g. banana).

* **Plantlet:** A small rooted shoot developed from seed or from cultured cells either by embryogenesis or organogenesis.

* **Plaque:** Clear zone in a bacterial culture resulting due to killing of bacterial cells by phage.

- **Plasma:** A pale, amber-colored fluid constituting the fluid portion of the blood in which are suspended the cellular elements. Plasma contains 8–9% solids. Of these, 85% are proteins consisting of three major groups, which are: fibrinogen, albumin and globulin. The other components are the lipids, which include the neutral fats, fatty acids, lecithin, and cholesterol. Also present are sodium, chloride and bicarbonate, potassium, calcium, lycopene and magnesium. A most essential function of plasma is the maintenance of blood pressure and the exchange (with tissues) of nutrients for waste.
- **Plasma cells:** Antibody producing white blood cells, derived from B lymphocytes.
- **Plasmalemma:** A delicate cytoplasmic double membrane found on the outside of the protoplast adjacent to the cell wall.
- **Plasma membrane:** A thin structure that completely surrounds the cell as a "skin." It may be seen with the aid of an electron microscope. The entire membrane appears to be about 100 Angstroms (Å; 0.1 mm) thick and is composed of two dark lines, each about 30 Å thick which are, however, separated by a lighter area. This trilaminar "sandwich" structure is referred to as the unit membrane. The plasma membrane is composed of lipoidal (fat-like) material in which proteins and protein complexes and whole functional systems are embedded (Fig. 11). In the plasma membrane various systems are incorporated such as energy-dependent transport systems Na^+ and K^+ transporting ATPase

P

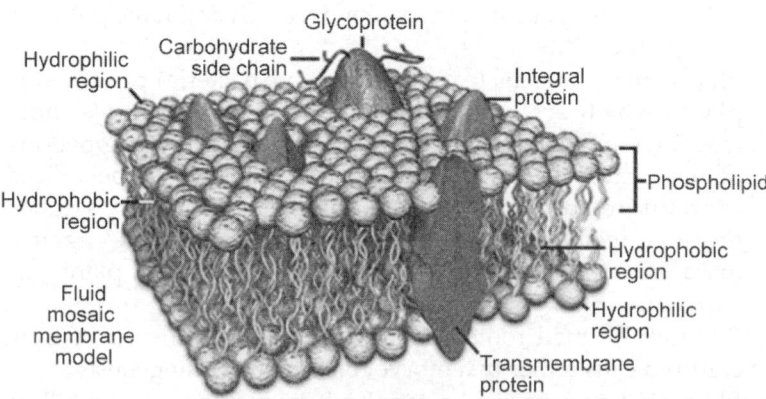

Fig. 11: Plasma membrane

and amino acid transport systems. Besides the cell, membranes also surrounds some such organelles as endoplasmic reticulum, vacuoles, lysosomes, Golgi bodies, mitochondria, chloroplasts and the nucleus, to mention just a few. The plasma membrane and membranes, in general, function as a permeability barrier to the free movement of substances between the interior and exterior of the cell or organelles that they surround.

- **Plasmid:** A small circular DNA molecule, which can replicate independently of the bacterial chromosome.
- **Plasmocyte:** Same as plasma cells.
- **Plastid:** An independent, stable, self-replicating piece of DNA inside a plant cell that is not part of the reproduction cell genome (i.e. in nucleus). Because there can exist up to 10,000 plastids in a given plant cell, the insertion of a gene (e.g. via genetic engineering) into plastids can result in a higher yield (of the specific protein coded for by that gene) than is achieved via insertion of the gene into the cell's nuclear DNA.
- **Plastoquinone:** A quinone which is one of a group of compounds involved in the transport of electrons in photosynthesis in chloroplasts.
- **Platelet-derived growth factor (PDGF):** A substance in platelets that is mitogenic for cells at the site of a wound, causing endothelial proliferation.
- **Platelets:** Disk-shaped blood cells that stick to the (microscopically "jagged") edges of wounds. The aggregation of platelets at the wound site leads to blood clotting, forming a temporary wound covering. During this blood clotting process, the platelets release platelet-derived growth factor (PDGF) which attracts fibroblasts to the wound area (for subsequent healing process).
- **Plating efficiency:** The percentage of cells plated on medium which develops colonies.
- **Playback:** Playback experiment describes the retrieval of DNA that has hybridized with RNA to check that it is nonrepetitive by further reassociation reaction.
- **Plectonemic:** A joint region that consists of one molecule of wound around another molecule, e.g. DNA strands in a double helix.
- **Plectonemic winding:** The inter twinning of the two strands in the classical double helix of DNA.

- **Pleiotropic:** Gene which affects more than one (apparently unrelated) characteristic of the phenotype.
- **Pleiotropy:** The phenomenon where a single gene is responsible for number of unrelated phenotypic effects (multiplies or manifold effects of a gene). For example in garden peas, the gene which controls the flower color also controls the color of the seed coat and the presence of red spots in the leaf axils. It is not essential that the traits are equally influenced.
- **Ploidy:** The number of copies of the chromosome set present in a cell; a haploid has one copy, a diploid has two copies, etc.
- **Plumule:** The first bud of an embryo or the protion of young shoot above the cotyledons.
- **Pluripotent stem cells:** Refers to those stem cells from which each of the human body's 210 different types of tissues could arise.
- **Plus strand DNA:** The strand of the duplex sequence representing a retrovirus that has the same sequence as that of the RNA.
- **Plus strand virus:** A single-stranded nucleic acid genome whose sequence directly codes for the protein products.
- **Point mutation:** A mutation consisting of a change of only one nucleotide in a DNA molecule. At "hot spots" (i.e. certain locations on the DNA within some organisms), numerous point mutations can occur. In the case of single-nucleotide polymorphisms (SNPs), the same point mutation occurs at the same location (on the DNA within some organisms) across a population of individuals of that organism.
- **Polar bodies:** In female animals, the products of a meiotic division that do not develop into an ovum.
- **Polar group:** A hydrophilic ("water loving") portion of a molecule; it may carry an electrical charge. A group that "likes" to be in the presence of water molecules or other polar compounds.
- **Polar molecule (dipole):** A molecule in which the center of positive and negative (electrical) charge do not coincide, so that one end of the molecule carries a positive (or partial positive) charge and the other end a negative (or partial negative) charge.
- **Polar mutation:** A mutation in one gene which, because transcription occurs only in one direction, reduces the expression of subsequent genes in the same transcription unit further down the line.

- **Polar nuclei:** Two centrally located nuclei in the embryo sac that unite with a second sperm cell in a triple fusion. In certain seeds, the product of this fusion develops into the endosperm.
- **Polar transport:** The directed movement within plants of compounds (usually endogenous plant growth regulators) mostly in one direction. Polar transport overcomes the tendency for diffusion in all directions.
- **Polarimeter:** An instrument used for measuring the degree of rotation of plane-polarized light by an optically active compound/solution.
- **Polarity (chemical):** The degree to which an atom or molecule bears an electrical charge or a partial electrical charge. In general, the more polar (i.e. separation or partial separation of charge) a molecule is, the more hydrophilic ("water loving") it is. Polarity results from an uneven distribution of electrons between the atoms comprising a molecule.
- **Polarity (genetic):** Having to do with the one way or unidirectionality of gene transcription in an operon unit. That is, the region near the operator is always transcribed before the more distant regions. By analogy, transcription begins at the left end of an operon unit and proceeds (reads, transcribes) toward the right end of the operon unit. The distinction between the 5' and the 32' ends of nucleic acids.
- **Polarity:** The effect of a mutation in one gene in influencing the expression (at transcription or translation) of subsequent genes in the same transcription unit.
- **Pole cells:** A group of cells in the posterior of *Drosophila* embryos that are precursors to the adult germ line.
- **Pollen:** The mass of germinated microspores or partially developed male gametophytes of seed plants.
- **Pollen culture:** The *in vitro* culture and germination of pollen grains. Callus cultures thus obtained will form shoots or embryoids which develop into monoploid plants.
- **Pollen grain:** A microspore produced in the pollen sac of angiosperms or the microsporangium of gymnosperms. Unicellular with variable shape and size and usually ovoid from 25–250 mm.
- **Pollination:** Transfer of pollen from anther to stigma in the process of fertilization in angiosperms. The transfer of pollen from male to female in the process of fertilization in gymnosperms.

- **Poly(A):** It is a stretch of-200 bases of adenylic acid that is added to the 3′ end of mRNA following its synthesis.
- **Poly(A) polymerase:** The enzyme that adds the stretch of polyadenylic acid to the 3′ of eukaryotic mRNA. It does not use a template.
- **Poly(A)-binding protein (PABP):** The protein that binds to the 3′ stretch of poly(A) on a eukaryotic mRNA.
- **Polyacrylamide gel:** A "sieving" gel, that is used in electrophoresis.
- **Polyacrylamide gel electrophoresis (PAGE):** A method for separation of nucleic acids or protein molecules according to their size. The molecules migrate through the inert gel matrix under the influence of an electric field.
- **Polyadenylation:** The addition of a sequence of polyadenylic acid to the 3′ end of a eukaryotic RNA after its transcription.
- **Polycistronic mRNA:** mRNA with more than one translational region so that same RNA can be translated into more than one polypeptide chains.
- **Polyclonal antibodies:** A serum containing antibodies that binds to different antigenic determinants of an antigen.
- **Polyclonal response (of immune system to a given pathogen):** Because a given pathogen generally has several antigenic sites on its surface, the B lymphocytes (activated by helper T cells in response to a pathogen invading the body) synthesize several (subtly different) antibodies against that pathogen. And since antibodies are made by different cells, the response is known as poly (many) clonal.
- **Polyembryony:** In the ordinary course of event one embryo is formed in each ovule and is derived from the fertilization of the ovum in the solitary embryo sac. However two or more embryos could start development even though only one may reach maturity.
- **Polyethylene glycol (PEG):** A polymer having the general formula $H-(O-CH_2-CH_2)_n-OH$ and available in a range of molecular weights from ca 1,000 to ca 6,000.
- **Polygalacturonase (PG):** An enzyme (e.g. present in tomatoes) that starts the breakdown (softening) of the fruit tissue. Recent advances make it possible to significantly delay the softening (i.e. spoilage) process by reducing the production of polygalacturonase through genetic engineering of the plant. In 1986,

William Hiatt of the American company Calgene discovered the gene for polygalacturonase. That led to the company commercializing a tomato variety that had been genetically engineered to reduce production of polygalacturonase in that variety's tomatoes (1994).

- **Polygene:** One of many genes of small effect influencing the development of a quantitative trait results in continuous variation and in quantitative inheritance.

- **Polygenic:** A trait or end product (e.g. in a grain-produced crop) that requires simultaneous expression of more than one gene. For example, the level of protein produced in soybeans is controlled by five genes.

- **Polygenic inheritance:** When a trait is controlled by several allelic pairs at different loci on a chromosome or on different chromosomes, contributing alleles have additive intermediate phenotypes; so they produce continuous variations whose frequency distribution forms a normal (bell-shaped) curve, e.g. kernel color in wheat and skin color and height in humans.

- **Polyhydroxyalkanoic acid (PHA):** A class of polyesters stored in inclusion bodies and found in many bacteria and in some archaea.

- **Polyhydroxylbutyrate (PHB):** One of the PHAs, polyhydroxyl-butyrate is an "energy storage" substance that is naturally produced by certain bacteria, yeasts, and plants. When removed from the bacteria and purified, this substance has physical properties quite similar to thermoplastics like polystyrene. PHB can quickly be broken down by soil microorganisms, so PHB is a biodegradable plastic.

- **Polylinker:** A segment of DNA that contains several restriction sites. It is also called multiple cloning sites.

- **Polymer:** A molecule possessing a regular, repeating, covalently bonded arrangement of smaller units called monomers. By analogy, a chain (polymer) that is composed of links (monomer) hooked together.

- **Polymerase:** An enzyme that catalyzes the assembly of ribonucleotides into RNA (RNA polymerase) and of deoxynucleotides into DNA (DNA polymerase).

- **Polymerase chain reaction (PCR) (Fig. 12):** A reaction that uses the enzyme DNA polymerase to catalyze the formation of multiple DNA strands from an original one by the execution of repeated cycles of DNA synthesis. Functionally, this is

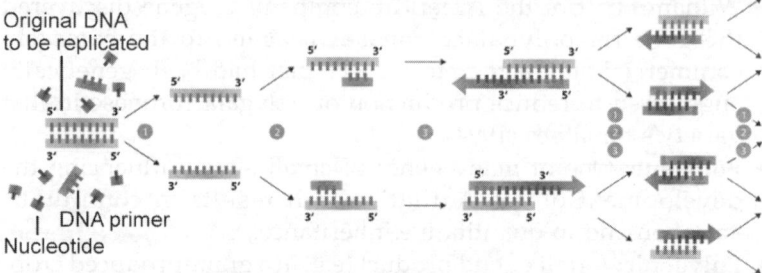

Original DNA
to be replicated

DNA primer

Nucleotide

❶ **Denaturation** at 94–96°C
❷ **Annealing** at ~68°C
❸ **Elongation** at ca. 72°C

Fig. 12: Polymerase chain reaction (PCR)

accomplished by heating and melting double-stranded (hydrogen bonded) DNA into single-stranded (nonhydrogen bonded) DNA and producing an oligonucleotide primer complementary to each DNA strand. The primers bind to the DNA and mark it in such a way that the addition of DNA polymerase and deoxynucleoside triphosphates cause a new strand of DNA to form which is complementary to the target section of DNA. The process described previously is repeated (trait, product, etc.) again and again to produce millions of copies (amplicons) of the desired strand of DNA. PCR and its registered trademarks are the property of F. Hoffmann-La Roche and Co. AG, Basel, Switzerland.

- **Polymerization:** Chemical union of two or more molecules of the same kind such as glucose or nucleotides to form a new compound (starch or nucleic acid) having the same elements in same proportions but have a higher molecular weight and different physical properties.
- **Polymery:** The phenomenon whereby a number of genes at different loci (which may be polygenes) can act together to produce a single effect.
- **Polymorphism (chemical):** The property of a chemical substance crystallizing (or simply existing) in two or more forms having different structures. For example, diamond and graphite are two different structures (manifestations) of the element carbon. Deoxyribonucleic acid (DNA) is a polymorphic compound because the polymer can take on different forms.

- **Polymorphism (genetic):** A name applied to a condition in which a species of plant or animal is represented by several distinct, non-integrating forms or types unrelated to age or sex. The differences are often in coloration, though any characteristic of the organism may be involved (e.g. nuclei shape for polymorphonuclear leukocytes).

- **Polymorphonuclear granulocytes:** Neutrophils, eosinophils, and basophils are collectively known as polymorphonuclear granulocytes. This is due to the fact that collectively their nuclei are segmented into lobes and they have granule-like inclusions within their cytoplasm.

- **Polymorphonuclear leukocytes (PMN):** Formerly named microphages, they are phagocytic (i.e. foreign particle-ingesting) white blood cells that have a lobed nucleus. For example, during an attack of the common cold (when virus first invades mucous membranes of the human nose), the body responds by making Interleukin-8 (IL-8); a glycoprotein that attracts large quantities of polymorphonuclear leukocytes to the mucous membranes of the nose (to try to combat the infection). Another example is when polymorphonuclear leukocytes (PMN) migrate into a female pig's uterus within 6 hours after semen is introduced via breeding. PMN remove excess sperm and bacteria, resulting in a "friendly" environment for embryos to develop in the uterus.

- **Polynucleotide:** A chain of nucleotides in which each nucleotide is linked by a phosphodiester bond to the next nucleotide in the chain. They can be double- or single-stranded. The term is used to describe DNA or RNA.

- **Polypeptide (Protein):** A molecular chain of amino acids linked by peptide bonds. Synonymous with protein. Via the synthesis (of this "chain") performed by ribosomes, each polypeptide (protein) in nature is the ultimate expression product of a gene. All of the amino acids commonly found in proteins have an asymmetric carbon atom, except the amino acid glycine. Thus, the polypeptide is potentially chiral in nature.

- **Polyphenols:** Phytochemicals (e.g. naturally found in coffee, certain types of grapes, certain red wines, green tea, cocoa, etc.) that act as antioxidants when consumed by humans. For example, polyphenols are naturally produced within the beans of the cocoa (cacao) tree (*Theobroma cacao*), and thus are present in chocolate made from those beans. Polyphenols naturally produced in apples have been shown to inhibit certain bacteria in the human mouth from producing the particular glucans that lead to a buildup of plaque on teeth; prevention of such plaque build-up may help prevent cavities from forming in teeth.

- **Polyploid cell:** It has more than two sets of the haploid genome.
- **Polyploidy:** Offspring with more than two complete sets of chromosomes. Polyploidy is a major evolutionary mechanism in plants; probably involved in 47% of flowering plants including major crops.
- **Polyprotein:** A gene product that is cleaved into several independent proteins.
- **Polyribosome (polysome):** A complex of a messenger RNA (mRNA) molecule on which ribosomes (ribosomal RNA; rRNA) are anchored. A number of ribosomes bound to only a single mRNA molecule. One mRNA molecule hence functions as a template for a number of polypeptide chains at one time.
- **Polysaccharides:** Linear and/or branched (structure) macromolecules (large molecules) composed of many monosaccharide units (monomers such as glucose) linked by glycosidic bonds.
- **Polysome (polyribosome):** An mRNA associated with a series of ribosomes engaged in translation.
- **Polyspermy:** The entry of several sperm into the egg during fertilization, although only one sperm nucleus actually fuses with the egg nucleus.
- **Polytene chromosomes:** Generated by successive replications of a chromosome set without separation of the replicas.
- **Polyunsaturated fatty acids (PUFA):** An unsaturated fatty acid whose carbon chain has more than one double or triple valence bond per molecule; found chiefly in fish, corn, soybean oil and sunflower oil.
- **Polyvalent vaccine:** A recombinant organism into which antigenic determinants have been cloned from a number of different disease causing organisms and used as a vaccine.
- **Polyvinylpyrrolidone (PVP):** An occasional constituent of plant tissue culture isolation media. PVP is of variable molecular weight and has an antioxidant properties so is used to prevent oxidative browning of explanted tissues. PVP is less frequently used as an osmoticum in culture media.
- **Population:** A local group of organisms belonging to the same species and interbreeding.

- **Population density:** Number of cells or individuals per unit. The unit could be an area or volume of medium.
- **Porcine somatotropin (PST):** A hormone, produced in the pituitary gland of pigs, that increases a swine's muscle tissue production efficiency. Injecting this hormone causes a faster growing, leaner pig.
- **Porphyrins:** Any of a group of pigments occurring widely in animal and plant tissues and having a heterocyclic structure formed from four pyrrole rings linked by four methylene groups.
- **Position effect:** A change in the expression of a gene brought about by its translocation to a new site in the genome. For example, a previously active gene may become inactive if placed on a new site in the genome.
- **Position effect variegation:** The consequences when a gene is inactivated in some cells but not in others as a result of variable spread of inactivity from heterochromatin.
- **Positional candidate gene:** A gene known to be located in the same region as a DNA marker that has been shown to be linked to a single locus trait or to a quantitative trait locus (QTL) and whose function suggests that it could be the source of genetic variation in the trait in question.
- **Positional cloning:** A technique used by researchers to zero the gene (s) responsible for a given trait or disease. A genetic map of the organism's genome is used to make an educated guess to the precise location of the gene of interest (e.g. near marker "x" or "y", etc.). Then those guessed genes are cloned, inserted into living organisms or cells, and tested to see if the guessed gene causes expression of the protein of interest (e.g. a protein that causes the disease that the researcher is attempting to cure).
- **Positional information:** Describes the localization of macro-molecules at particular places in an embryo. The localization may itself be a form of information that is inherited.
- **Positive and negative selection (PNS):** A strategy used in making gene knockouts designed to enrich for homologous recombinants and select against random integration of the targeting vector.
- **Positive control system:** A mechanism in which the regulatory protein is required to turn on gene expression.
- **Positive regulation:** Expression of a gene in the presence of an active regulatory protein.

- **Positive regulator proteins:** Required for the activation of a transcription unit.
- **Positive selection:** A method by which cells that carry a DNA insert integrated at a specific chromosomal location are selected.
- **Positive supercoiling:** The coiling of the double helix in space in the same direction as the winding of the two strands of the double helix itself.
- **Posterior system:** In *Drosophila,* the posterior system is one of the maternal systems that establishes the polarity of the oocyte. The set of genes in the posterior system play a role in the proper formation of the pole plasm and the abdomen.
- **Postmeiotic segregation:** The segregation of two strands of a duplex DNA that bear different information (created by heteroduplex formation during meiosis) when a subsequent replication allows the strands to separate.
- **Postreplication complex:** Postreplication complex is a protein-DNA complex in *S. cerevisiae* that consists of the origin recognition complex (ORC) bound to the origin.
- **Postreplication repair:** A recombination dependent mechanism for repairing damaged DNA.
- **Post-transcriptional processing (modification) of RNAs:** The enzyme-catalyzed processing or structural modifications of RNAs such as mRNAs, rRNAs, and tRNAs must undergo before they are functionally finished products. For example, in eukaryotes a block of poly A containing at least 200 AMP residues is enzymatically attached to the 3^1 end of mRNA in the nucleus of the cell. The mRNAs with the "tail" are then transferred to the cytoplasm and the tail enzymatically removed to form the functional mRNAs. It is believed that the poly A tail aids in the transfer of the complex and/or targets the complex to the cytoplasm.
- **Post-transcriptional regulation:** Regulation of gene expression after synthesis of mRNA from the gene.
- **Post-translational modification of protein:** Enzymatic processing of a polypeptide chain after its translation from its mRNA, i.e. addition of carbohydrate moieties to the protein or the removal of a portion of the polypeptide chain in order to produce a functional protein in the correct environment.

- **Post-translational translocation (post-translational):** The movement of a protein across a membrane after the synthesis of the protein is completed and it has been released from the ribosome.
- **Potato late blight:** A fungal disease of the potato plant (*Solanum tuberosum*) caused by the fungus *Phytophthora infestans*. During the 1840s, this plant disease struck the potato crops of Ireland and Europe, leading to the starvation of more than one million people (principally in Ireland, because that nation was very dependent on potatoes for food) (Fig. 13).

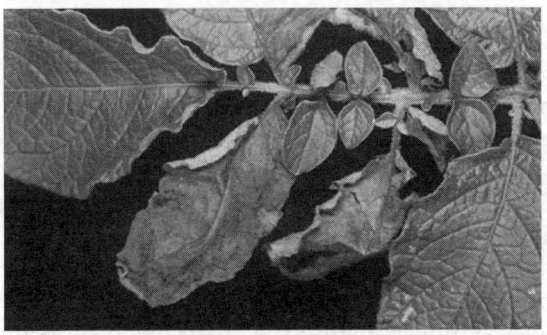

Fig. 13: Potato late blight

- **ppGpp:** ppGpp is guanosine tetraphosphate. Diphosphate groups are attached to both the 5' and 3' positions.
- **PPO:** Acronym for protoporphyrinogen oxidase.
- **pppGpp:** pppGpp is a guanosine pentaphosphate, with a triphosphate attached to the 5' position and a diphosphate attached to the 3' position.
- **ppm:** Parts per million.
- **Prebiotics:** Chemical compounds or microorganisms (e.g. yeasts) administered alone or in combination (e.g. in the feed rations of animals) that (generally) act to stimulate growth of beneficial types of bacteria within the digestive system of animals (e.g. livestock). Those compounds can include some organic acids (propionic acid, malic acid, etc.). For example, adding certain strains of yeast (culture) and malate (malic acid) to cattle feed rations has been shown to stimulate *S. ruminantium* bacteria (growth) in the rumen (i.e. the "first stomach" in cattle).

Selenomonas ruminantium tend to constitute 22–51% of the total bacteria in a typical rumen, and are important for optimal digestion (e.g. of the grass eaten by that animal). Inulin, and several fructose oligosaccharides, etc. act as prebiotics in the human digestive system (e.g. by stimulating growth of *Bifidus* species of bacteria in the digestive system). For animal feed rations, in addition to fructose oligosaccharides, transgalacto-oligosaccharides may be added, also act as prebiotics.

- **Precise excision:** Describes the removal of a transposon plus one of the duplicated target sequences from the chromosome. Such an event can restore function at the site where the transposon is inserted.
- **Precocious germination:** Premature germination of the embryo prior to completion of embryogenesis.
- **Predator:** Animal that kills another animal for food.
- **Prefilter:** A coarse filter used to screen out large particles before air is forced through a much finer filter.
- **Preinitiation complex:** Preinitiational complex in eukaryotic transcription describes the assembly of transcription factors at the promoter before RNA polymerase binds.
- **Premature termination:** Describes the termination of protein or of RNA synthesis before the chain has been completed. In protein synthesis it can be caused by mutations that create termination codons within the coding region. In RNA synthesis it is caused by various events that act on RNA polymerase.
- **Pre-mRNA:** It used to describe the nuclear transcript that is processed by modification and splicing to give an mRNA.
- **Preprotein:** A protein to be imported into an organelle or secreted from bacteria is called a "preprotein" until its signal sequence has been removed.
- **Prereplication complex:** It is a protein-DNA complex at the origin in *S. cerevisiae* that is required for DNA replication. The complex contains the origin recognition complex (ORC) complex, Cdc6, and the MCM proteins.
- **Pressure potential:** The pressure generated within a cell. It is the difference between the osmotic potential within the cell and the water potential of the external environment, provided the cell volume is constant.
- **Pretransplant:** Stage III in tissue culture micropropagation. The rooting, hardening stage prior to transfer to soil.

- **Preventive immunisation (vaccination):** Infection with an antigen to elicit an antibody response that will protect the organism against future infections.
- **Pribnow box:** The consensus sequence TATAATG centered about 10 base pairs before the starting point of bacterial genes. It is a part of the promoter and is especially important in binding of RNA polymerase.
- **Primary antibody:** In an ELISA or other immunology assay the antibody that binds to the target molecule.
- **Primary cells:** Eukaryotic cells taken into culture directly from the animal.
- **Primary cell wall:** The cell wall layer formed during cell expansion. Plant cells possessing only primary walls may divide or undergo differentiation.
- **Primary culture:** A culture started from cell, tissue, organ taken directly from an organism. It is regarded as such until sub-cultured for the first time. Then it becomes cell line.
- **Primary growth:** Growth that occurs as a result of cell division at the tips of stems and roots, and that give rise to primary tissue.
- **Primary immune response:** It is an organism's immune response upon first exposure to a given antigen. It is characterized by a relatively shorter duration and lower affinity antibodies than in the secondary immune response.
- **Primary meristem:** Meristem of the shoot or root tip giving rise to the primary plant body.
- **Primary structure:** The sequence of amino acids in a polypeptide chain.
- **Primary tissue:** A tissue that has differentiated from a primary meristem.
- **Primary transcript:** The original unmodified RNA product corresponding to a transcription unit.
- **Primase:** It is a type of RNA polymerase that synthesizes short segments of RNA that will be used as primers for DNA replication.
- **Primer:** A short sequence (often of RNA) that is paired with one strand of DNA and provides a free 3′ – OH end at which DNA polymerase starts synthesis of a deoxyribonucleotide chain.
- **–10 sequence:** The consensus sequence TATAATG centered about 10 bp before the startpoint of a bacterial gene. It is involved in the initial melting of DNA by RNA polymerase.

- **–35 sequence:** The consensus sequence centered about 35 bp before the startpoint of a bacterial gene. It is involved in the initial recognition by RNA polymerase.
- **Primer DNA polymerase:** DNA polymerase that provides primers for the DNA polymerization. Unlike RNA polymerase DNA polymerase is unable to initiate the *de novo* synthesis of a polynucleotide chain.
- **Primer walking:** A method for sequencing long (> 1 kb) cloned pieces of DNA.
- **Primordium:** A group of cells which gives rise to an organ.
- **Primosome:** The complex of proteins involved in the priming action that initiates synthesis of each Okazaki fragment during discontinuous DNA replication; the primosome may move along DNA to engage in successive priming events.
- **Prion:** A proteinaceous infectious agent, which behaves as an inheritable trait, although it contains no nucleic acid. Examples are PrP^{Sc}, the agent of scrapie in sheep and bovine spongiform encephalopathy, and Psi, which confers an inherited state in yeast.
- **Proanthocyanidins:** The chemical components within North American cranberries (*Vaccinium macrocarpon*) and blueberries (genus *Vaccinium*) that impart health benefits to humans who consume those cranberries/blueberries. For example, when humans consume cranberries, these chemical compounds prevent *Escherichia coli* bacteria from adhering to the cells lining the human urinary tract (thereby helping to prevent some urinary tract infections).
- **Probability:** The frequency of occurrence of an event.
- **Proband:** The individual in a family in whom an inherited trait is first identified.
- **Probe:** A relatively small molecule that can be used to sense the presence and condition of a specific protein, DNA fragment, RNA fragment, or nucleic acid by a unique interaction with that macromolecule.
- **Probiotics:** Compounds that (generally) act to stimulate growth of beneficial types of bacteria within the digestive system of animals (e.g. livestock). For example, organic acids (propionic acid, acetic acid, lactic acid, citric acid, etc.) act to inhibit the growth/multiplication of pathogens (disease-causing micro-organisms) in the digestive system of monogastric (single-stomach)

animals such as poultry and swine. Those acids are able to pass through the outer cell membrane (plasma membrane) of pathogenic bacteria and fungi. Once inside those pathogens' cells, the acids dissociate, and acidify the cells' interior (which disrupts the cells' protein synthesis, growth, and replication of the pathogen).

- **Procambium:** A primary meristem that gives rise to primary vascular tissues and in most woody plants to the vascular cambium.
- **Prokaryotes:** Simple organisms that lack a distinct nuclear membrane and other organelles. Many structural systems are different between prokaryotes and eukaryotes, including the DNA arrangement, composition of membranes, the respiratory chain, the photosynthetic apparatus, ribosome size, the presence or lack of cytoplasmic streaming, the cell wall, flagella, the mode of sexual reproduction, and the presence or lack of vacuoles. Some representative prokaryotes are the bacteria and blue-green algae.
- **Procentriole:** An immature centriole, formed in the vicinity of a mature centriole.
- **Process validation (for production of a pharmaceutical):** It is defined by the US Food and Drug Administration (US FDA) as "establishing documented evidence which provides a high degree of assurance that a specific process will consistently produce a (pharmaceutical) product meeting predetermined specifications and quality characteristics".
- **Processed pseudogene:** An inactive gene copy that lacks introns, contrasted with the interrupted structure of the active gene. Such genes presumably originate by reverse transcription of mRNA and insertion of a duplex copy into the genome.
- **Processing:** Processing of RNA describes changes that occur after its transcription, including modification of the 5' and 3' ends, internal methylation, splicing, or cleavage.
- **Processive enzymes:** Enzymes continue to act on a particular substrate, that is, do not dissociate between repetitions of the catalytic event.
- **Processivity:** Describes the ability of an enzyme to perform multiple catalytic cycles with a single template instead of dissociating after each cycle.
- **Proembryo:** A group of cells arising from the division of the fertilized egg cell or somatic embryo, before those cells which have to become the embryo are recognizable.

- **Production environment:** All input-output relationships over time at a particular location. The relationships will include biological, climatic, economic, social, cultural and political factors which combine to determine the productive potential of a particular livestock enterprise.
- **Production traits:** Characterized of animals such as the quantity or quality of the milk, meat, fibre, eggs, draught etc. they (or their progeny) produce, which contribute directly to the value of the animals for the farmer and also identifiable or measurable at the individual level.
- **Productive rearrangement:** The recombination of V, (D), J gene segments results in a productive rearrangement if all the rearranged gene segments are in the correct reading frame.
- **Productivity:** The amount of product that is produced within a given period of time from a specified quantity of resources.
- **Progeny testing:** For a single locus, the practice of ascertaining the genotype of an individual from its offspring, such as by mating it to other individuals and examining the progeny.
- **Progesterone:** A female sex hormone, secreted by the ovaries, that supports pregnancy and lactation (milk production).
- **Programmed frameshifting:** It is required for expression of the protein sequences coded beyond a specific site at which +1 or -1 frameshift occurs at some typical frequency.
- **Prokaryotic:** Organisms (bacteria) that lacks nuclei.
- **Prolactin:** A hormone produced by the anterior pituitary gland that stimulates and controls lactation in mammals.
- **Proliferation:** Increase by frequent and repeated reproduction or growth by cell division.
- **Promeristem:** The embryonic meristem that is the source of organ initials or foundation cells.
- **Promoter sequence:** A regulatory sequence of DNA that initiates the expression of a gene.
- **Promoter:** The region on DNA to which RNA polymerase binds and initiates transcription (of RNA). The promoter "promotes" the transcription (expression) of that gene, but the promoter's impact on the timing/degree of gene expression is itself regulated by the molecules that bind to the promoter. For example, the "binding" of RNA polymerase causes transcription of RNA to begin, and the "binding" to promoter of other STATs (i.e. signal transducers and activators of transcription) can

regulate the degree to which a given gene is expressed. A promoter is a region of DNA (deoxyribonucleic acid) which lies "upstream" of the transcriptional initiation site of a gene. The promoter controls where (which portion of a plant, which organ within an animal, etc.) and when (which stage in the lifetime of an organism) the gene is expressed. For example, the promoter named "Bce4" is "seed-specific" [i.e. it only "promotes" the expression of a given gene's product (protein, fatty acid, amino acids, etc.) within a plant's seed].

- **Pronucleus:** Either of the two haploid gamete nuclei just prior to their fusion in the fertilized ovum.
- **Proofreading:** Any mechanism for correcting errors in protein or nucleic acid synthesis that involves scrutiny of individual units after they have been added to the chain.
- **Propagation:** The multiplication of plants by numerous types of vegetative material. An ancient practice dating from the dawn of agriculture carried out in a nursery or directly in the field (vegetative propagation) and now in *in vitro* culture (micropropagation).
- **Propagule:** A part of plant that serve for propagation.
- **Prophage:** A bacteriophage that has intergrated its DNA into the nucleoid of a host bacterium.
- **Prophase:** An early stage in nuclear division characterized by the shortening and thickening of the chromosomes and their movement to the metaphase plate. It occurs between interphase and metaphase.
- **Prostaglandin endoperoxide synthase:** An enzyme that can exist in several different forms within the human body to catalyze the production of prostaglandins.
- **Prostaglandins:** A group of cyclic (circle shaped) fatty acids that act as hormones in the body (promote inflammation during infections, help promote maintenance of the tissues of the stomach/kidney/intestines, etc.). Originally isolated from sheep and human prostates, prostaglandins are synthesized (manufactured) by the body via chemical reactions catalyzed by the enzymes cyclo-oxygenase/prostaglandin endoperoxide synthase; usually from arachidonic acid (also docosahexanoic acid).
- **Prostate:** The gland in the body of males that produces the liquid which carries sperm into the females (during mating). In older

human males, the prostate will often become enlarged (e.g. by "antagonism" when estrogen molecules circulating in the blood contact its surface). Via the selective estrogen effect, isoflavones (e.g. from soybeans) consumed by such males can displace and replace those estrogen molecules from the surface of the prostate (thereby preventing enlargement).

- **Prostate-specific antigen (PSA):** An antigen whose concentration increases significantly 5–10 years prior to the (clinical) diagnosis of prostate cancer. This means that PSA level measurements can be utilized in diagnosis of prostate cancer before symptoms appear. However, a series of tests is required in order to accurately gauge the probability of cancer because PSA levels can also be elevated when a man develops a noncancerous enlarged prostate.

- **Prosthetic group:** A heat-stable metal ion or an organic group (other than an amino acid) that is covalently bonded to the apoenzyme protein. It is required for enzyme function. The term is now largely obsolete.

- **Protamines:** Small basic proteins that replace the histones in the chromosomes of some sperm cells.

- **Protease:** An enzyme that catalyzes the hydrolytic cleavage (breakdown) of proteins. By analogy, the enzyme breaks the link (peptide bond) holding a chain together. Proteases represent a whole class of protein-degrading enzymes.

- **Protease nexin I (PN-I):** A protein that acts as an inhibitor of protease.

- **Protease nexin II (PN-II):** A protein that is thought to regulate important activities in the body and brain by inhibiting specific enzymes and interacting with certain body cells. PN-II is formed from a precursor molecule known as beta–amyloid, via metabolic processing of the beta-amyloid. Recent research indicates that incorrect metabolic processing of beta-amyloid by the body results in amyloid plaques in the brain. The amyloid plaques are generally found in victims of Alzheimer's disease, and directly correlate (in number) with the degree of dementia.

- **Proteasome:** A large complex with an interior cavity that degrades cytosolic proteins, previously marked by covalent addition of ubiquitin.

- **Proteasomes:** Refers to enzymatic/catalytic bodies present within all mammal cells that activate certain transcription

P

factors, are involved in causing the cell to "present" antigens (from pathogens that invaded that cell) on the cell's surface, and perform various other cellular functions. For example, the 26S proteasome degrades (breakdown) all ubiquinated (ubiquitin-"tagged") proteins in that cell.

- **Protein C:** An anticlotting (glyco) protein that prevents post-operative arterial clot formation when administered intra-venously. May be synergistic (in its anticlotting effect) with tissue plasminogen activator (tPA).

- **Protein:** Coined in 1838 by Jons Berzelius. From the Greek word *proteios*, meaning the first or the most important or of the first rank. Any of a class of high molecular weight polymer compounds composed of a variety of β-amino acids joined by peptide linkages. Via the synthesis (of this "chain") performed by ribosomes, each protein is the ultimate expression product of a gene. More than one protein can be expressed from a given gene (the particular protein expressed is determined by factors such as the cell's temperature or other environmental variable, presence of STATs—some of which themselves are proteins, presence of certain bacteria, etc.). During their synthesis (after emerging from the cell's ribosome), proteins may also be phosphorylated (a "phosphate group" is added to the protein molecule), glycosylated (one or more oligosaccharides is added the protein molecule), acetylated (one or more "acetyl groups" is added to the protein molecule), farnesylated (a "farnesyl group" is added to the protein molecule), ubiquinated (a ubiquitin "tag" is added to the protein molecule), sulfated (a "sulfate group" is added to the protein molecule), or otherwise chemically modified. Proteins are the "workhorses" of living systems and include enzymes, antibodies, receptors, peptide hormones, etc. Proteins in living organisms respond to changing environmental and other conditions by changing their location within cells, by getting cut into (specific) pieces, by changing which (other) molecules they will bind (adhere) to, etc. All of the amino acids commonly found in (each and every one of the) proteins have an asymmetric carbon atom, except the amino acid glycine. Thus the protein is potentially chiral in nature.

- **Protein crystallisation:** Making crystals of a protein as a key part of most methods used for determining a protein's three-dimentional structure.

- **Protein digestibility-corrected amino acid scoring (PDCAAS):** A method of expressing the quality of a given (food) protein source, in terms of its digestible protein (amino acid constituents') ability to support growth in young growing humans (i.e. if that protein supplies all needed essential amino acids in their proportions required by humans, that protein scores 1.00). For example, the complete ("ideal") protein source soya protein (concentrate) has a PDCAAS of 0.99. PDCAAS has been recommended by the US Food and Drug Administration (FDA), and the Food and Agricultural Organization of the United Nations/World Health Organization (FAO/WHO).
- **Protein engineering (enzyme engineering):** Generation of protein with subtly modified structure that confer special properties (as present before) such as high pH stability, thermal stability, high catalytic specificity, etc.
- **Protein engineering:** The selective, deliberate (re)designing and synthesis of proteins. This is done in order to cause the resultant proteins to carry out desired (new) functions. Protein engineering is accomplished by changing or interchanging individual amino acids in a normal protein. This may be done via chemical synthesis or recombinant DNA technology (genetic engineering). "Protein engineers" (actually genetic engineers) use recombinant DNA technology to alter a particular nucleoside or triplet (codon) in the DNA (genes) of a cell. In this way it is hoped that the resulting DNA codes for the different or new amino acid in the desired location in the protein produced by that cell.
- **Protein folding:** The process by which a protein structure assumes its functional shape or conformation.
- **Protein interaction analysis:** Refers to a number of different analysis/technologies utilized to determine if a given (e.g. new) protein molecule interacts with a protein molecule whose function is already known (e.g. from previous research, or its use as a pharmaceutical). Through that analysis (e.g. inferring the "new" protein's function by its action vis à vis the "old"/known protein), useful information about the "new" protein can be gathered.
- **Protein kinases:** Enzymes capable of phosphorylating (covalently bonding a phosphate group to) certain amino acid residues in specific proteins. Protein kinases play crucial roles in the regulation of signaling within and between cells.

- **Protein metabolic step:** One step in the chain of reactions that take place in an organism and dictate the composition of that organism.

- **Protein microarrays:** Refers to a piece of glass, plastic, or silicon onto which has been placed a number of proteins (or molecules of other chemical compounds that interact with proteins in a specific manner). These microarrays (sometimes called "biochips") can then be utilized to test (e.g. a single sample) for a wide variety of attributes or effects (on or by the protein molecules in the sample that is exposed to that microarray).

- **Protein sequencing:** The process of determining the amino acid sequence of a protein or its polypeptides component.

- **Protein serine/threonine kinase:** Phosphorylates cytosolic proteins on either their serine or threonine residues.

- **Protein signaling:** The "communication" by protein molecules (e.g. to cells) that governs their transport and localization (i.e. destination in the cell). Discovered and delineated by Guenter Blobel during the 1970s, protein signaling (e.g. via a short sequence of amino acids attached to end of newly synthesized protein molecules) results in proteins traveling to the appropriate cell compartments (e.g. organelles) and/or out of the cell (i.e. secretion).

- **Protein sorting (targeting):** The direction of different types of proteins for transport into or between specific organelles.

- **Protein splicing:** Is the autocatalytic process by which an intein is removed from a protein and the exteins on either side become connected by a standard peptide bond.

- **Protein structure:** A polypeptide chain may take on a certain structure in and of itself because of the amino acid monomers it contains, and their location within the chain (Fig. 14). The chain may furthermore interact with other polypeptide chains to form larger proteins known as oligomeric proteins. In the following, the levels of protein structure normally encountered will be highlighted: 1. Primary structure—refers to the backbone of the polypeptide chain and to the sequence of the amino acids of which it is comprised. 2. Secondary structure—refers to the shape (recurring arrangement in space in one dimension) of the individual polypeptide chain. In some cases, because of its primary structure, the chain may take on an extended or

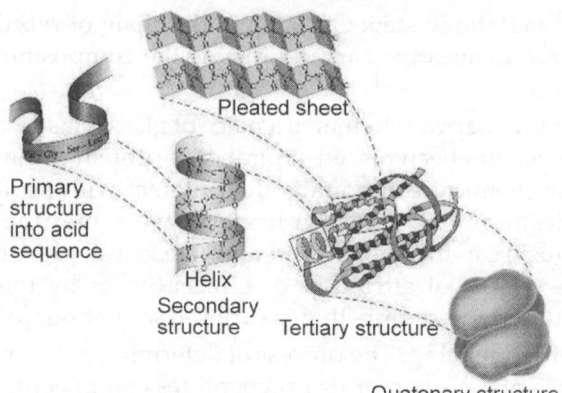

Fig. 14: Protein structure

longitudinally coiled conformation. 3. Tertiary structure—refers to how the polypeptide chain (the primary structure) is bent and folded in three-dimensional space in order to form the normal tightly folded and compact structure. 4. Quaternary structure—refers to how, in larger proteins made up of two or more individual polypeptide chains, the individual polypeptide chains are arranged relative to each other. These large multi-polypeptide proteins are called oligomeric proteins and the individual chains are called subunits. An example of such a protein is hemoglobin.

- **Protein synthesis:** The creation of proteins from their constituent amino acids in accordance with the genetic information carried in the DNA of the chromosomes.
- **Protein tyrosine kinase inhibitor:** Any compound (e.g. genistein, Gleevec™, etc.) that inhibits the action of the enzyme tyrosine kinase.
- **Protein tyrosine kinase:** A kinase enzyme whose target is a tyrosine amino acid in a protein.
- **Proteolysis:** Enzymatic degradation of a protein.
- **Proteolytic:** The ability to breakdown protein molecules.
- **Proteolytic enzymes:** Enzymes which catalyze the hydrolysis (breakdown) of proteins or peptides. Proteins (enzymes) that destroy the structure (by peptide bond cleavage) and hence the function of other proteins. These other proteins may or may not be enzymes.

- **Proteome chip:** A microarray ("biochip") developed by Michael Snyder et al., during 2001 which: 1. Has a large number of known sequence protein molecules (e.g. all proteins present in a given organism) attached to its surface at known locations (i.e. specific "addresses" on the microarray). 2. Utilizes specific bioactive agents such as certain lipids or biotinylated calmodulin (i.e. calmodulin molecules to which a molecule of biotin is "attached") in order to determine which of the protein molecules in #1 interacts with relevant bioactive agents. Because calmodulin is a well known and very well-characterized calcium-binding protein (i.e. bioactive agent) involved in (known) cellular processes, the binding of calmodulin to specific protein molecules attached to the microarray/biochip provides critical information about the (cellular, protein-protein, etc.) functions and interactions of those protein molecules in the organism. 3. Reveals a large amount of data concerning protein-protein interactions (e.g. via subsequent application to the microarray of dye-labeled streptavidin to identify the protein molecules via their addresses on the biochip) and protein- lipid interactions, all of which are needed, in order to determine the organism's proteome.
- **Proteome:** It is the complete set of proteins that is expressed by the entire genome. Because some genes code for multiple proteins, the size of the proteome is greater than the number of genes.
- **Proteomics:** The study of proteome or the array of proteins that an organism produce.
- **Protoclone:** Regenerated plant derived from protoplast culture or a single colony derived from protoplasts in culture.
- **Protocol:** The step by step experiments proposed to describe or solve a scientific problem or the defined steps of a specific procedure.
- **Protocorm:** In orchids, seeds contain an unorganized embryo comprising only a few hundred cells. During seed germination this embryo forms a tuberous structure called a protocorm, from which develops a complete plant.
- **Protoderm:** A primarily meristem tissue that gives rise to epidermis.
- **Protogyny:** The condition in which the female reproductive organs (carpels) of a flower mature before the male ones (stamens), thereby ensuring that self fertilisation does not occur.

- **Proto-oncogenes:** The normal counterparts in the eukaryotic genome to the oncogenes carried by some retroviruses. They are given names of the form *c-onc*.
- **Protoplasm:** Coined by J.E Purkinje in 1840, it is a general term referring to the entire contents of a living cell; living substance.
- **Protoplast:** A unit consisting of the living parts of a cell, including the protoplasm and cell membrane but not the vacuoles or (in plants) the cell wall.
- **Protoplast culture:** The isolation and culture of plant protoplasts by mechanical means or by enzymatic digestion of plant tissues or organs or cultures derived from these.
- **Protoplast fusion:** The coalescence of the plasmalemma and cytoplasm of two or more protoplasts in contact with one another. Initial adhesion of two protoplasts is a random process but coalescence can be induced.
- **Prototroph:** An organism such as a bacterium, that grows on a minimal medium.
- **Protoxin:** A chemical compound that only becomes a toxin after it is altered in some way. For example, the *B.t.* protoxins (Cry9C, Cry1A (b), Cry1A (c), etc.) only become toxic after they are chemically altered by the alkaline environment inside the gut of certain insects.
- **Protozoa:** A microscopic, single-celled animal form. A unicellular organism without a true cell wall, that obtains its food phagotropically.
- **Provirus:** A duplex DNA in the eukaryotic chromosome corresponding to the genome of an RNA retrovirus.
- **PrP:** The protein that is than active component of the prion that causes scrapie and related diseases. The form involved in the disease is called PrPSc.
- **P-Selectin:** Formerly known as GMP-140 and PADGEM, it is a selectin molecule that is synthesized by endothelial cells before (adjacent) tissues are infected. Thus "stored in advance", the endothelial cells can present P-selectin molecules on the internal surface of the endothelium within minutes after an infection (of adjacent tissue) begins. This presentation of P-selectin molecules attracts leukocytes to the site of the infection, and draws them out of the bloodstream (the leukocytes "squeeze" between adjacent endothelial cells).

- **Pseudoautosomal region:** A section at one end of the X and Y chromosomes for which there is sufficient homology and there is pairing during meiosis I.
- **Pseudocarp false fruit:** A fruit that incorporates in addition to the ovary wall, other parts of the flower such as the receptable (e.g. strawberry).
- **Pseudodominance:** Expression of a recessive trait due to absence of a dominant allele.
- **Pseudogenes:** Inactivate but stable components of the genome derived by mutation of an ancestral active gene.
- **Pseudomonas fluorescens:** A normally harmless soil micro-organism (bacteria) that colonizes the roots of certain plants. At least one company has incorporated the gene for a protein that is toxic to insects (taken from *Bacillus thuringiensis*) into a *Pseudomonas fluorescens*. This was done in order to confer insect resistance to the plants, the roots of which are genetically engineered and *Pseudomonas fluorescens* has colonized.
- **Psoralene:** A toxic chemical (e.g. to ward off insects) that is naturally produced by (wild type) plants related to the domesticated celery plant.
- **Psychrophile:** An organism that requires 0°C (32°F) for growth.
- **Puc:** A widely used expression for denoting plasmid containing a galactosidase gene.
- **Puff:** An expansion of a band of a polytene chromosome associated with the synthesis of RNA at some locus in the band.
- **Pulse field gel electrophoresis (PFGE):** A procedure used to separate large DNA molecules by alternating the direction of electric current in a pulsed manner across a gel.
- **Pulse-chase:** Pulse-chase experiments are performed by incubating cells very briefly with a radioactively labeled precursor (of some pathway or macrmolecule); then the fate of the label is followed during a subsequent incubation with a nonlabeled precursor.
- **Punctuated equilibrium:** The occurrence of speciation events in bursts separated by long intervals of species stability.
- **Pure culture:** A culture containing only one species of micro-organism.
- **Pure line:** A pure line is a population that breeds truly for the particular character being studied; that is all offspring produced

by selfing or crossing within the population show the same form for the character.

- **Purine:** A basic nitrogenous heterocyclic compound found in nucleotides and nucleic acids; it contains fused pyrimidine and imidazole rings. Adenine and guanine are examples (Fig. 15).

Adenine **Guanine**

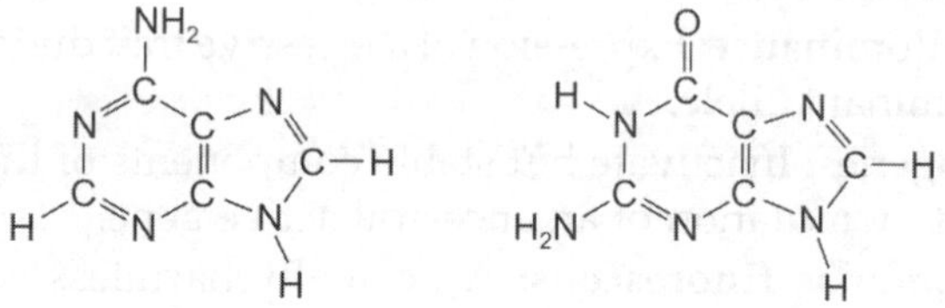

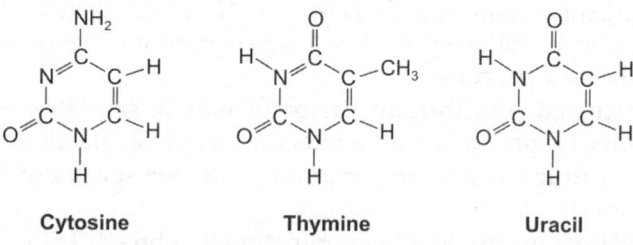

Fig. 15: Purine

- **Puromycin:** Is an antibiotic that terminates protein synthesis by mimicking a tRNA and becoming linked to the nascent protein chain.
- **Pyralis:** An insect that is also known as the European corn borer (*Ostrinia nubialis*).
- **Pyranose:** The six-membered ring forms of sugars are called pyranoses. This is because they are derivatives of the heterocyclic compound pyran.
- **Pyrethrins:** Active constituents of pyrethrum (*Tanacetum cinerariifolium*) flowers used as insecticides.
- **Pyrexia:** Fever; elevation of the body temperature above normal.
- **Pyrimidine:** A heterocyclic organic compound containing nitrogen atoms at (ring) positions 1 and 3. Naturally occurring derivatives are components of nucleic acids and coenzymes, uracil, thymine, and cytosine (Fig. 16). A six-membered single ringed nitrogenous base in DNA or RNA.

Cytosine **Thymine** **Uracil**

Fig. 16: Pyrimidine

- **Pyrimidine dimer:** Two adjacent pyrimidines are covalently joined by chemical bonds.
- **Pyrogen:** A substance capable of producing pyrexia (i.e. fever).
- **Pyrophosphate cleavage:** The enzymatic removal of two phosphate groups (designated as PPi) from ATP in one piece leaving AMP as another product. This cleavage releases more energy, which can be used in certain reactions that require more of a "push" to get them going.
- **Pyrrolizidine alkaloids:** A class of toxic chemical compounds which are produced naturally by certain plants, as a defense mechanism (against predators). One of the pyrrolizidine alkaloids, monocrotaline is consumed (preferentially) by the larvae (caterpillars) of the moth *Utetheisa ornatrix*. That moth subsequently utilizes the monocrotaline content of its body as a defense mechanism itself, against spiders that would otherwise eat that mouth.

P

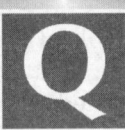

- **Q-beta replicase:** A viral RNA polymerase secreted by a bacteriophage that infects *Escherichia coli* bacteria. Q-beta replicase can copy a naturally occurring RNA (molecule) sequence (e.g. from bacteria, viruses, fungi, or tumor cells) at a geometric (very fast) rate.

- **Q-beta replicase technique:** An RNA assay (test) that amplifies RNA probes, a researcher is seeking. For instance, by using the Q-beta replicase technique to assay for the presence of RNA specific to the AIDS virus, it is possible to detect an AIDS infection in a patient's blood sample long before that infection has progressed to the point where antibodies would appear in the blood.

- **QCM:** Acronym for quartz crystal microbalances.

- **QPCR:** Acronym for quantitative polymerase chain reaction. Uses include gene expression analysis (i.e. quantitatively determine the amounts of each protein being expressed by a cell), genotyping, DNA quantification, etc.

- **Qualitative character:** A character showing a limited number of distinct classes, governed by one or few oligogenes, and relatively little affected by the environment.

- **Quantitative genetics:** A branch of genetics, which deals with inheritance and genetic analysis of quantitative or polygenic characters.

- **Quantitative inheritance:** Inheritance concerned with the inheritance of continuously varying traits. Most practical improvement programs involve the application of quantitative genetics.

- **Quantitative structure-activity relationship (QSAR):** A computer modeling technique that enables researchers (e.g. drug development chemists) to predict the likely activity (e.g. effect on tissue) of a new compound before that compound is actually created. QSAR is based on data from decades of research investigating the impact on activity of the chemical structures of thousands of thoroughly studied molecules. For example, the biological activity (i.e. bacteria-killing effectiveness) of most antibiotics correlates with their tendency to dimerize (i.e. link two molecules into a single molecular unit).

- **Quantitative structure-property relationship (QSPR):** A computer modeling technique that enables scientists to predict the likely properties of a new chemical compound before that chemical compound is actually created.

- **Quantitative trait loci (QTL):** Individual specific DNA sequences that are related to known traits (litter size in animals, egg production in birds, and yield in crop plants.).

- **Quantitative trait locus:** A locus that affects a quantitative trait.

- **Quantum:** An elemental unit of energy. Its energy value is hv, where h is Planck's constant is 6.62×10^{-27} erg second, and v is the frequency of the vibrations or waves with which the energy is associated.

- **Quantum dot:** A molecular structure that is between 1 nm and 100 nm in size, so it is midway between molecular and solid states. Quantum dots have been constructed of semiconductor materials, crystallites (grown via molecular beam epitaxy), etc. Quantum dots could conceivably be constructed to act as receptors (e.g. on biochips) for specific ligands (e.g. a blood component that is only present in a diseased patient), in a way that would signal the presence of disease when a (blood) sample was passed over the quantum dot. That signal might be electronic, emission of specific-wavelength light, etc.

- **Quantum speciation:** The rapid formation of new species primarily by genetic drift.

- **Quantum wire:** A strip or wire of (electricity) conducting material that is ten nanometers (nm) or less in its thickness or width. Indications from some research show that some forms of DNA molecules might be used as quantum wires.

- **Quarantine:** Originally keeping a person or living organism in isolation for a period (originally 40 days) after arrival, to allow disease symptoms to appear if there was any disease present. Now used for regulations restricting the sale or shipment of living organisms usually to prevent disease or pest invasion of an area.

- **Quartz crystal microbalances (QCM):** Refers to biosensors consisting of small quartz crystals (to which are attached a source of appropriate electric current), with sensitive measurement devices utilized to detect when the attachment of specific molecules (e.g. viruses, DNA sequences, antigens) to the quartz or to layers of certain materials previously deposited on the quartz surface, causes the specific oscillation frequency of that quartz crystal to change in a way that enables (electronic) identification of the specific molecule(s) that attached themselves to the QCM.

- **Quaternary structure:** The three-dimensional structure of an oligomeric protein; particularly the manner in which the subunit chains fit together.

- **Quercetin:** A phytochemical naturally produced in apples, onions, and some other plants. Research indicates that human consumption of quercitin helps prevent prostate and some other cancers.

- **Quick-stop mutant:** A type of DNA replication temperature-sensitive mutant (*dnd*) in *E. coli* that immediately stops DNA replication when the temperature is increased to 42°C.

- **Quick-stop:** The term used to describe how DNA mutants of *Escherichia coli* cease replication immediately when temperature increases to 42°C (108°F).

- **Quiescent:** Quiet at rest but not necessarily dormant, and have the potential for resumed activity; can apply to non meristematic cells.

Q

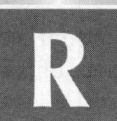

- **45S RNA:** A precursor that contains the sequences of both major ribosomal RNAs (28S and 18S rRNAs).
- **5.8S RNA:** An independent small RNA present on the large subunit of eukaryotic ribosomes. It is homologous to the 5′ end of bacterial 23 S rRNA.
- **5S RNA:** A 120 base RNA that is a component of the large subunit of the ribosome.
- **R genes:** Refers to genes within some plants that confer resistance (to certain plant diseases) through common signaling pathways involved in (surveillance and activation of) natural plant defense responses (e.g. SAR). For example, the gene that codes for (causes the manufacture of) harpin protein is only present in few bacteria (e.g. *Erwinia amylovora*), but R genes (i.e. those responsible for surveillance and activation of plant defense responses) which respond to the presence of harpin are present within the genomes of numerous species of plants. Thus, the spraying of man-made harpin protein onto any of those numerous species of (crop) plants causes those particular plants to initiate a protective/defensive response (cascade) against pathogenic bacteria, viruses, fungi, and even some insects.
- **R loop:** The structure formed when an RNA strand hybridizes with its complementary strand in a DNA duplex, thereby displacing the original strand of DNA in the form of a loop extending over the region of hybridization.
- **R segments:** The sequences that are repeated at the ends of a retroviral RNA. They are called R-U5 and U3-R.
- **Rab:** Proteins make-up a family of about 30 small Ras-like GTPases. Different Rabs are required for protein trafficking in different membrane systems. Although their exact role is not clear, Rabs appear to regulate membrane targeting and fusion.
- **Race:** Distinguishable group of organisms of a particular species that are geographically, ecologically, physiologically, physically

and/or chromosomically distinct from other members of the species.

- **Racemate:** An equimolar (equal number of molecules) mixture of the D and L stereoisomers of an optically active compound. A solution of dextrorotary (D) isomer (enantiomer) will rotate the plane in which the light was polarized to a specific number of degrees to the right (dextro) while a solution containing the same number of levorotary (L) isomer molecules will rotate the plane in which the light was polarized the same number of degrees to the left (levo). The difference between D and L enantiomers is that the rotations of the plane of plane-polarized light are equal in magnitude, but opposite in sign. Hence, a 50:50 mixture of both enantiomers (known as a racemic mixture) shows no optical activity. That is, a solution containing a 50:50 mixture of enantiomers will not rotate the plane of plane polarized light when it is passed through the solution.

- **Raceme:** An inflorescence in which the main axis is elongated but the flowers are borne on pedicels that are about equal in length.

- **Rachilia:** Shortened axis of a spikelet.

- **Rachis:** Main axis of a spike; axis of fern leaf (frond) from which pinnate arise; in compound leaves the extension of the petiole corresponding to the midrib of an entire leaf.

- **Radicle:** That portion of the plant embryo which develops into the primary or seed root.

- **Radioactive isotope:** An isotope with an unstable (atomic) nucleus that spontaneously emits radiation. The radiation emitted includes alpha particles, nucleons, electrons and gamma rays.

- **Radioimmunoassay:** A very sensitive method of quantitating a specific antigen using a specific radiolabeled antibody. Functionally, the antibody is made radioactive by the covalent incorporation of radioactive iodine. The radioimmuno probe thus prepared is exposed to its antigen (which may be a protein, or a receptor, etc.) in excess (the exact amount will have to be determined). The radiolabeled probe then binds to the antigen and the unbound, free probe is washed away. The radioactivity is then determined (counted) and by comparison to a standard plot which has been constructed previously, the amount of antigen (binding) is determined.

R

- **Radioimmunotechnique:** A method of using a radiolabeled antibody to quantify a known antigen.
- **Radiolabeled:** From the Latin *radiare*, to emit beams.
- **Ramet:** An individual member of a clone of ortet.
- **Random amplified polymorphic DNA (RAPD) technique:** A genetic mapping methodology that utilizes the fact that specific DNA sequences (polymorphic DNA) are repeated (i.e. appear in sequence) with the gene of interest. Thus, the polymorphic DNA sequences are linked to that specific gene. Their linked presence serves to facilitate genetic mapping (i.e. location of specific gene(s) on an organism's genome).
- **Random drift:** Describes the chance fluctuation (without selective pressure) of the levels of two alleles in a population.
- **Random mutagenesis:** A non-directed change of one or more nucleotide pairs in a DNA molecule.
- **Rapid lysis (r) mutants:** Display a change in the pattern of lysis of *E. coli* at the end of an infection by a T-even phage.
- **Rapid microbial detection (RMD):** A broad term used to describe the various testing products and technologies that can be utilized to quickly detect the presence of microorganisms (e.g. pathogenic bacteria in a food processing plant). These testing products are based on immunoassay, DNA probe, electrical conductance and/ or impedance, bioluminescence, and enzyme-induced reactions (e.g. which produce fluorescence or a color change to indicate the presence of specific microorganism).
- **ras Gene:** Discovered in 1978 by Edward Scolnick, who named it ras for rat sarcoma (the particular diseased tissue in which he found it). The ras gene is also present in the human genome, and it is an oncogene that is believed to be responsible for upto 90% of all human pancreatic cancer, 50% of human colon cancers, 40% of lung cancers, and 30% of leukemias. The ras gene codes for the production (manufacture) of ras proteins, which help to signal each cell to divide and grow at appropriate time(s), e.g. when free EGF attaches to relevant cell receptor on the plasma membrane. When the ras gene has been damaged or mutated (e.g. via exposure to cigarette smoke or ultraviolet light, etc.), it codes for (causes to be manufactured in the cell's ribosome) a mutated version of the ras protein that can cause the cell to become cancerous (i.e. divide and grow uncontrollably).

- **ras protein:** A transmembrane (i.e. through the cell membrane) protein for which the ras gene codes. The ras protein end outside the cell membrane acts as a receptor for applicable growth factors (e.g. fibroblast growth factor), and conveys that signal (to divide/grow) into the cell when that chemical signal (i.e. the growth factor) touches the receptor end of the ras protein. When the ras gene has been damaged or mutated (e.g. via exposure to cigarette smoke or ultraviolet light), that gene causes excess ras proteins to be manufactured, which causes oversignaling of the cell to divide and grow (i.e. cell becomes cancerous).

- **Rational drug design:** The engineering (building) of chemically synthesized drugs based on knowledge of receptor modeling and drug/target interaction(s) with the aid of supercomputers/interactive graphics/etc.; the educated, creative design of the three dimensional structure of a drug atom by atom, i.e. from the ground up. This approach represents a major advance over the prior practice of first synthesizing large number of compounds (or finding them in nature), followed by thousands of tedious screenings to test for efficacy against a given disease (target). The approach of rational drug design has, however, not yet been perfected and optimized due, in part, to gaps in our knowledge of drug/receptor interaction and to gaps our knowledge in general.

- **RBS1 gene:** A gene that confers to any soybean plant (possessing that gene in its DNA) resistance to the adverse effects of the soil born fungus *Phialophora gregata*, which can cause the plant disease brown stem rot (BSR) in soybean plants.

- **RBS3 gene:** See RBS1 gene.

- **Reading frame:** One of the three possible ways of reading a nucleotide sequence. Each reading frame divides the sequence into a series of successive triplets. There are three possible reading frames in any sequence, depending on the starting point. If the first frame starts at position 1, the second frame starts at position 2, and the third frame starts at position 3.

- **Read through:** At transcription or translation occurs when RNA polymerase or the ribosome, respectively, ignores a termination signal because of a mutation of the template or the behavior of an accessory factor.

- **Reassociation of DNA:** The pairing of complementary single strands to form a double helix.
- *rec:* mutations of E. *coli* cannot undertake general recombination.
- **RecA:** The product of the *recA* locus of E. *coli*; a protein with dual activities, activating proteases and also able to exchange single strands of DNA molecules. The protease-activating activity controls the SOS response; the nucleic acid handling facility is involved in recombination-repair pathways.
- **Recalcitrant:** Of seeds unable to survive drying and subsequent storage at low temperature.
- **Receding:** Events occur when the meaning of a codon or series of codons is changed from that predicted by the genetic code. It may involve altered interactions between aminoacyl-tRNA and mRNA that are influenced by the ribosome.
- **Receptacle:** Enlarged end of the pedicel or peduncle to which other flower parts are attached.
- **Receptor gene:** In operon model of eukaryotes, the gene located very neat to producer gene and activates the producer gene for initiation of transcription.
- **Receptor fitting (RF):** A research method used to determine the macromolecular structure that a chemical compound (e.g. an inhibitor) must have in order to fit (in a lock and key fashion) into a receptor. For example, a pain inhibitor compound blocking a pain receptor on the surface of a cell.
- **Receptor mapping (RM):** A method used to guess at (determine) the three-dimensional structure of a receptor binding site extrapolating from the known structure of the molecule binding to it. This approach can be carried out because of the complementary shape of the receptor and the binding molecule. Functionally, the researcher projects the (guessed-at) properties of the receptor ligands into a mathematical model in which the profile of the receptor is predicted by complementarity (to known chemical molecular structures). The receptor mapping process requires repetitive refinement of the mathematical model to fit properties continually being discovered via the use/interaction of chemical reagents bearing the known molecular structures.
- **Receptor:** A transmembrane protein, located in the plasma membrane, that binds a ligand in a domain on the extracellular

side, and as a result has a change in activity of the cytoplasmic domain. The same term is sometimes used also for the steroid receptors, which are transcription factors that are activated by binding ligands that are steroids or other small molecules.

- **Recessive allele:** Discovered by Gregor Mendel in the 1860s, this refers to an allelic gene whose existence is obscured in the phenotype of a heterozygote by the dominant allele. In a heterozygote, the recessive allele does not produce a polypeptide; it is "switched off". In this case, the dominant allele is the one producing the polypeptide chain (via cell's ribosome).
- **Recessive lethal:** An allele that is lethal when the cell is homozygous for it.
- **Recessive trait:** The opposite of dominant. A trait that is preferentially masked. A mutation or other genetic marker that does not exert its phenotype due to the presence of corresponding wild type marker in a diploid organism. A recessive allele is obscured in the phenotype of a heterozygote by the dominant allele, often due to inactivity or absence of the product of the recessive allele.
- **Recessive allele:** An allele that produces its characteristics phenotype only when its paired allele is identical.
- **Reciprocal cross:** Using male and female gametes for two different traits, alternating the source of gametes ($♀A × ♂B$) ($♀B × ♂A$).
- **Reciprocal recombination:** The production of new genotypes with the reverse arrangements of alleles according to maternal and paternal origin.
- **Reciprocal translocation:** Exchanges part of new genotypes with part of another chromosome.
- **Reciprocating shaker:** A platform shaker used for agitating culture flasks with a back and forth action at variable speeds.
- **Recognition helix:** The one of the two helices of the helix–turn–helix motif that makes contacts with DNA that are specific for particular bases. This determines the specificity of the DNA sequence that is bound.
- **Recognition site:** A nucleotide sequence composed of typically 4, 6 or 8 nucleotides that is recognized and to which a restriction endonuclease binds.
- **Recombinant DNA (rDNA):** DNA formed by the joining of genes (genetic material) into a new combination.

- **Recombinant DNA advisory committee (RAC):** The former standing US National Committee setup in 1974 by the US National Institutes of Health (NIH) to advise the NIH director on matters regarding policy and safety issues of recombinant DNA research and development. Over time, it had evolved to become part of the American government's regulatory process for recombinant DNA research and product approval. The RAC was terminated by the director of the NIH in 1996 because the "human health and environmental safety concerns expressed at the inception (of genetic engineering/biotechnology) had not materialized".

- **Recombinant DNA technology:** Procedure used to join together DNA segments in a cell-free system (an environment outside a cell or organism). Under appropriate conditions, a recombinant DNA molecule can enter a cell and replicate there, either autonomously or after it has become integrated into a cellular chromosome.

- **Recombinant genotype:** The genotype that consists of a new combination of genes produced by crossing over.

- **Recombinant joint:** The point at which two recombining molecules of duplex DNA are connencted (the edge of the heteroduplex region).

- **Recombinant:** Progeny have a different genotype from that of either parent.

- **Recombinant protein:** A protein whose amino acid sequence is encoded by a cloned gene.

- **Recombinant RNA:** A term used to describe RNA molecules joined *in vitro* by T4 RNA ligase.

- **Recombinant toxin:** A single multifunctional toxic protein that has been created by combining the coding regions of various genes.

- **Recombinant vaccine:** A vaccine produced from a cloned gene.

- **Recombinase:** An enzyme that acts to cut open the strand of DNA within a cell (e.g. to splice-out or splice-in) a given gene. During 2000, Nam-Hai Chua and and Jianru Zuo showed that activation of the gene for recombinase (via β-estradiol transcription factor) could be done to cause expression of recombinase in a manner that spliced out (removed) antibiotic-resistance marker genes from genetically enginee-red plants.

- **Recombination:** The process of crossing-over which occurs during meiosis I. It involves breakage in the same position of each of a pair of non-sister chromatids from homologous chromosomes followed by joining of non-sister fragments resulting in a reciprocal exchange of DNA between non-sister chromatids within an homologous pair of chromosomes (Fig. 1).

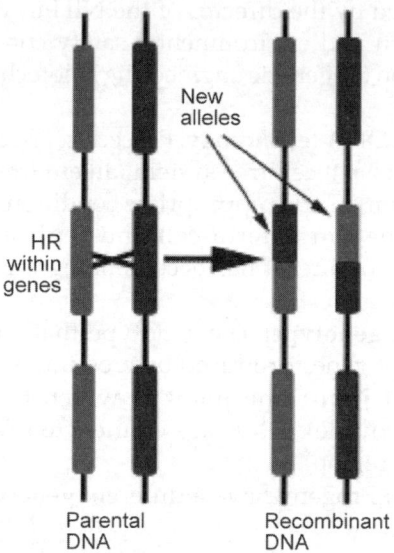

Fig. 1: Recombination

- **Recombination fraction:** The proportion of gametes that have arisen from recombination between two loci. It is estimated as the number of recombinant individuals among a set of offspring of a particular mating divided by the total number of offspring from the mating. Represented by the Greek letter theta (θ).
- **Recombination nodules (nodes):** Dense objects present on the synaptonemal complex, could be involved in crossing-over.
- **Recombination:** The joining of genes, sets of genes, or parts of genes, into new combinations, either biologically or through laboratory manipulation (genetic engineering).
- **Recombination-repair:** A mode of filling a gap in one-strand of duplex DNA by retrieving a homologous single-strand from another duplex.

- **Recon:** Smallest genetic unit between which recombination can occur.
- **Reconstructed cell:** A viable transformed cell resulting from genetic engineering.
- **Redement napole (RN) gene:** A swine gene that causes animals (possessing at least one negative allele of this gene) to produce meat which is more acidic than average, and thus that meat has a lower water-holding capacity. The RN gene was first identified in the Hampshire breed of swine in France. Since the 1960s, the Hampshire breed has been known to produce meat that is more acidic than average.
- **Redifferentiation:** Cell or tissue reversal from one differentiated type to another differentiated type of cell or tissue.
- **Reduction (biological):** The decomposition of complex compounds and cellular structures by heterotrophic organisms. In a given ecological system, this heterotrophic decomposition serves the valuable function of recycling organic materials. This occurs because the heterotrophs absorb some of the decomposition products (for nourishment) and leave the balance of the (decomposed) substances for consumption (recycling) by other organisms. For example, bacteria breakdown fallen leaves on the floor of a forest, thus releasing some nutrients to be utilized by plants.
- **Reduction (in a chemical reaction):** The gain of (negatively charged) electrons by a chemical substance. When one substance is reduced by another, the other compound is oxidized (loses electrons) and is called the reducing agent.
- **Redundancy:** A term used to describe the fact that some amino acids have more than one codon (that codes for production of that amino acid). There are approximately 64 possible codons available to code for 20 amino acids. Therefore, some amino acids will be specified by more than one codon. These (extra) codons are redundant.
- **Refractile bodies (RB):** Dense, insoluble (not easily dissolved) protein bodies (clumps) produced within the cells of certain microorganisms. The refractile bodies function as a sort of natural storage device for the microorganism. They are called refractile bodies because their greater density (than the rest of the microorganism's body mass) causes light to be refracted (bent) when it is passed through them. This bending of light

R

causes the appearance of very bright and dark areas around the refractile body and makes them visible under a microscope.

- **Regeneration:** Development of new organs or plantlets from a tissue, callus culture or from a bud.
- **Regulator:** Substance regulating growth and development of cells, organs etc.
- **Regulator gene:** That codes for a product, typically protein that controls the expression of other genes, usually at the level of transcription.
- **Regulatory enzyme:** An enzyme in a biochemical pathway which, through its responses to the presence of certain other biomolecules, regulates the pathway's act. This is usually done for pathways whose products may be needed in different amounts at different times, such as hormone production.
- **Regulatory genes:** Genes whose primary function is to control the state of synthesis of the products of other genes.
- **Regulatory sequence:** A DNA sequence involved in regulating the expression of a gene, e.g. a promoter or operator region (in the DNA molecule).
- **Rejuvenation:** Reversion from adult to juvenile.
- **Relaxase:** An enzyme that cuts one strand of DNA, and binds to the free 5′ end.
- **Relaxed mutants:** Relaxed mutants of *E. coli* do not display the stringent response to starvation for amino acids (or other nutritional deprivation).
- **Relaxed plasmid:** A plasmid that replicates independently of the main bacterial chromosome and is present in 10–500 copies per cell.
- **Relaxed replication control:** The ability of some plasmids to continue replicating after bacteria cease dividing.
- **Release (termination) factors:** It respond to termination codons to cause release of the completed polypeptide chain and the ribosome from mRNA.
- **Remediation:** The clean-up or containment (if chemicals are moving) of a hazardous waste disposal site to the satisfaction of the applicable regulatory agency [environmental protection agency (EPA)]. Such clean-up can sometimes be accomplished via use of microorganisms that have been adapted (naturally or via genetic engineering) to consume those chemical wastes present the disposal site.

- **Renaturation:** The return to the natural structure of a protein or nucleic acid from a denatured (more random coil) state. For example, a protein may be denatured [lose its native (natural) structure] by exposure to surfactants such as SDS or changes in the pH of the medium. If the surfactant is slowly removed, or the pH is slowly readjusted to the optimum for the protein, it will refold (snap) back into its original (native) form.
- **Renin:** A proteolytic enzyme secreted by the juxtaglomerular cells of the kidney. Its release is stimulated by decreased arterial pressure and renal blood flow resulting from decreased extracellular fluid volume. It catalyzes the formation of angiotensin I from hypertensinogen. Angiotensin I is converted to angiotensin II by another enzyme located in the endothelial cells of the lungs. Angiotensin II then causes the increase in the force of the heartbeat and constricts the arterioles. This scenario causes a rise in the blood pressure and is thus a cause of hypertension (high blood pressure).
- **Renin inhibitors:** Those chemicals that act to block the hypertensive (i.e. high blood pressure-inducing) effect of the enzyme, renin.
- **Reovirus:** A virus containing double-stranded RNA (Fig. 2). It is isolated from the respiratory and intestinal tracts of humans and other mammals. The prefix "reo" is an acronym for respiratory enteric orphan.

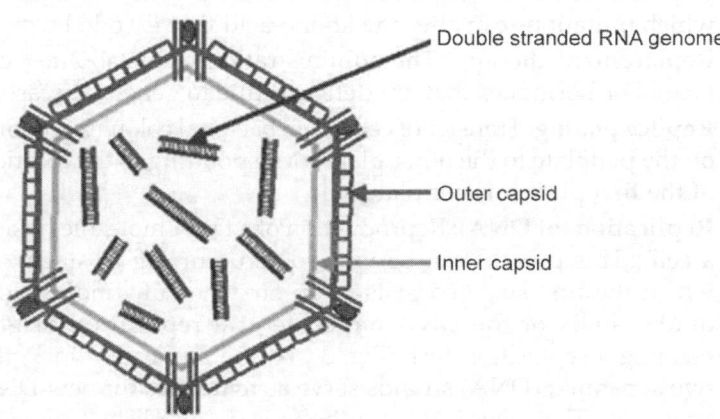

Fig. 2: Reovirus

- **Repair:** Repair of damaged DNA can take place by repair synthesis, when a strand that has been damaged is excised and replaced by the synthesis of a new stretch. It can also take place by recombination reactions, when the duplex region containing the damaged is replaced by an undamaged region from another copy of the genome.

- **Repeat unit:** A sequence of bases that occurs repeatedly in the genome often end-to-end, i.e. tandem.

- **Repeated DNA sequence:** A sequence of nucleotides which occurs more than once in a genome. It may be present in a few to many millions of copies. The length of individual repeated sequence may be a few nucleotides to several kb.

- **Repeating:** Unit in a tandem cluster is the length of the sequence that is repeated; appears circular on a restriction map.

- **Reperfusion:** The restoration of blood flow to an occluded (blocked) blood vessel. May be done biochemically (e.g. via tissue plasminogen activator) or via surgery.

- **Repetition frequency:** The (integral) number of copies of a given sequence present in the haploid genome; equals 1 for non-repetitive DNA, <2 for repetitive DNA.

- **Repetitive DNA:** It behaves in a reassociation reaction as though many (related or identical) sequences are present in a component, allowing many pair of complementary sequences to reassociate.

- **Replacement sites:** Replacement sites in a gene are those at which mutations can alter the amino acid that is coded.

- **Replacement therapy:** The administration of metabolites, co-factors or hormones that are deficient due to genetic disease.

- **Replica plating:** Transfer of cells from bacterial colonies growing on the petiplate to the other plate corresponding to the location of the first plate (master plate).

- **Replication (of DNA):** Reproduction of a DNA molecule (inside a cell). This process can be viewed as occurring in stages, in which the first stage consists of an enzyme "unwinding" the double helix of the DNA molecule at a replication origin, forming a replication fork (Fig. 3). At the replication fork, the two separated (DNA) strands serve as templates for new DNA synthesis. That new DNA synthesis is accomplished on each strand via enzymes known as DNA polymerase, which travel

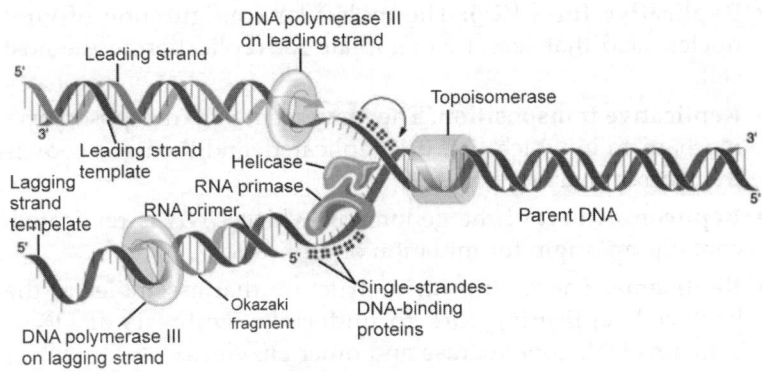

Fig. 3: Replication

along each (single) strand making a second complementary strand by catalyzing the addition of DNA bases (to the new, growing strands). The end result is two new double helices (DNA molecules), each of which has one chain from the original DNA molecule and one chain is newly synthesized by the DNA polymerase enzymes.

- **Replication (of virus):** Reproduction of the original virus. This process can be viewed as occurring in stages, in which the first stage consists of the adsorption of the virus to the host cell; penetration of the virus (or its nucleic acid) into the cell, the taking over of the cell's biomachinery and harnessing of it to replicate viral nucleic acid alongwith the synthesis of other virus constituents; the correct assembly of the nucleic acids and other constituents into a functional virus; followed finally by release of the virus from the confines of the cell.

- **Replication eye:** A region in which DNA has been replicated within a longer, unreplicated region.

- **Replication fork:** The point at which strands of parental duplex DNA are separated so that replication can proceed.

- **Replication:** Replication of duplex DNA takes place by synthesis of two new strands that are complementary to the parental strands. The parental duplex is replaced by two identical daughter duplexes, each of which has one parental strand and one newly synthesized strand. It is called semiconservative because the conserved units are the single strands of the parental duplex.

- **Replication-defective virus:** Loss one or more gene essential for completing the infective cycle.

- **Replicative form (RF):** The molecular configuration of viral nucleic acid that server as template for replication in the host cell.

- **Replicative transposition:** The movement of a transposon by a mechanism in which first it is replicated, and then one copy is transferred to a new site.

- **Replicon:** A unit of the genome in which DNA is replicated; contains an origin for initiation of replication.

- **Replisome:** The multiprotein structure that assembles at the bacterial replicating fork to undertake synthesis of DNA; Contains DNA polymerase and other enzymes.

- **Reporter gene:** A coding unit whose product is easily assayed (such as chloramphenicol transacetylase); it may be connected to any promoter of interest so that expression of the gene can be used to assay promoter function.

- **Repressible enzyme:** An enzyme whose production is generally continuous but can be halted if a particular substance is present in concentrations greater than normal.

- **Repressible:** Operon is expressed unless the small molecule co-repressor is present.

- **Repression (of an enzyme):** The prevention of synthesis of certain enzymes when their reaction products are present.

- **Repression (of gene transcription/translation):** The inhibition of transcription (or translation) by the binding of a repressor protein to a specific site on the DNA (or RNA) molecule. The repressor molecule is the product of a repressor gene.

- **Repression:** The ability of bacteria to prevent synthesis of certain enzymes when their products are present; more generally, refers to inhibition of transcription (or translation) by binding or repressor protein to a specific site on DNA (or mRNA).

- **Repressor (protein):** The product of a regulatory gene, it is a protein that combines with both an inducer (or corepressor) and an operator region (e.g. of DNA).

- **Repressor:** An active protein binds to operator sequences nearby to promoter of an operon and prevents transcription of the operon. It exerts a negative control.

- **Reproduction:** The production of an organism, cell or organelle like itself (self-propagation).

- **Repulsion:** The phase state in which a dominant (or wild type) allele at one locus and a recessive (or mutant) allele at a second locus occur on the same chromosome. Also called trans configuration.
- **Research foundation for microbiological diseases:** (includes Institute of physical and chemical research) Also known as Riken. A Japanese institution that performs research on infectious diseases, apart from other research.
- **Residues:** The components of macromolecules, e.g. amino acids, nucleotides.
- **Resistance:** Term commonly used to describe the ability of an organism to withstand a stress, a force or an effect of a disease or its agent or a toxic substance.
- **Resistance factor:** A plasmid that confers antibiotic resistance to a bacterium.
- **Resolution:** Occurs by a homologous recombination reaction between the two copies of the transposon cointegrated. The reaction generates the donor and target replicons, each with a copy of the transposon.
- **Resolvase:** Enzyme activity involved in site-specific recombination between two transposons present as direct repeats in a cointegrated structure.
- **Respiration:** Oxidative process in living cells in which oxygen or an inorganic compound serves as the terminal (final, ultimate) electron acceptor. Aerobic organisms obtain most of their energy from the oxidation of organic fuels. This process is known as respiration.
- **Response element:** A sequence in a eukaryotic promoter that is recognized by a specific transcription factor.
- **Rest period:** An endogenous physiological condition of viable seeds, buds or bulbs that prevents growth even in the presence of otherwise favourable environmental conditions. By some seed physiologists, this is referred dormancy.
- **Restitution nucleus:** A nucleus with introduced or doubled chromosome number that results from the failure of a meiotic or mitotic division.
- **Restorer gene:** A gene, usually dominant, that effectively overcome the effect of male sterile cytoplasm on male fertility, i.e. produces functional male gametes even in the presence of the male sterile cytoplasm.

- **Restriction endoglycosidases:** A class of enzymes, each of which cleaves (cuts) oligosaccharides (the side chains on glycoprotein molecules) at a specific location within the chain. They are important tools in carbohydrate engineering, enabling the carbohydrate engineer to sequence (i.e. determine the structure of) existing oligosaccharides, to create different oligosaccharides, and to create different glycoproteins via removal/addition/change of the oligosaccharide chains on glycoprotein molecules.
- **Restriction endonuclease (Type II):** An enzyme that recognizes a specific duplex DNA and phosphodiester bonds on both the strands between specific nucleotides.
- **Restriction enzymes:** Recognize specific short sequences of DNA and cleave the duplex (sometimes at target site, or elsewhere, depending on type).
- **Restriction fragment:** A fragment of DNA produced by cleaving (digesting, cutting) a DNA molecule with one or more restriction endonucleases.
- **Restriction fragment length polymorphism (RFLP):** A difference in the size of restriction fragment obtained by cutting DNA from two different strains with the same restriction endonuclease.
- **Restriction map:** A pictorial representation of the specific restriction sites (nucleotide sequences that are cleaved by given restriction endonucleases) in a DNA molecule (plasmid or chromosome).
- **Restriction site:** The sequence of nucleotide pairs of double stranded DNA that is recognized by a type II restriction endonuclease.
- **Resveratrol:** Also known as 3, 5, 4 trihydroxy stilbene, it is a naturally occurring (in grapes) anti-fungal agent (e.g. against grape fungus). Resveratrol is thought to be responsible for the fact that consumption of red wine by humans helps in lowering humans' blood fat (triglycerides) levels and blood cholesterol levels; thereby reducing the risk of cardiovascular disease. Resveratrol is a phytochemical produced by certain plants in response to wounding (e.g. by fungal growth on plant) or other stress. Plants that produce resveratrol include red grapes, mulberries, soybeans, and peanuts. Resveratrol inhibits cell mutations, stimulates at least one enzyme that can inactivate

certain carcinogens, and (when consumed by humans) lowers blood cholesterol and blood fat levels.

- **Retention signal:** The part of a protein that prevents it from leaving a compartment. An example is the transmembrane domain of Golgi resident proteins.

- **Retention time:** The time that has elapsed from the injection of the sample into the chromatographic system to the recording of the peak, maximum of the component in the chromatogram.

- **Reticulocyte:** A young red blood cell.

- **Retinoids:** A group of biologically active compounds that are chemical derivatives of vitamin A. Among other effects on living cells, some of the retinoid compounds act to deprive cancerous cells of their ability to proliferate endlessly, so these (formerly cancerous) cells then progress to a natural death (after exposure to an applicable retinoid).

- **Retroelement:** Any of the integrated retroviruses or transposable elements that resemble them.

- **Retrograde translocation (Reverse translocation):** The translocation of a protein from the lumen of the ER to the cytoplasm. It usually occurs to allow misfolded or damaged proteins to be degraded by the proteasome.

- **Retrograde transport:** Describes movement of proteins in the reverse direction in the reticuloendothelial system, typically from Golgi to endoplasmic reticulum.

- **Retroposon:** A transposon that mobilizes via RNA form; the DNA element is transcribed into RNA, and the reverse-transcribed into DNA, which is inserted at a new site in the genome.

- **Retroviral vectors:** Certain retroviruses used by genetic engineers to carry new genes into cells. These molecules become part of that cell's protoplasm.

- **Retroviruses:** (From the Latin word *retrovir*, which means backward man) Oncogenic (cancer-producing), single-stranded, diploid RNA (ribonucleic acid) viruses that contain (+) RNA in their virions and propagate through a double-helical DNA intermediate. They are known as retroviruses because their genetic information flows from RNA to DNA (reverse of normal). That is, the viruses contain an enzyme that allows the production of DNA using RNA as a template. Retroviruses can only infect cells in which DNA is replicating, such as tumor cells (since they are constantly replicating) or cells comprising the lining of the stomach (since that lining replace itself every few days).

- **Reversal transfer:** Transfer of a culture from a callus supporting medium to a shoot induced medium.

- **Reverse genetics:** Using linkage analysis and polymorphic markers to isolate a disease gene in the absence of a known metabolic defect, and then using the DNA sequence of the cloned gene to predict the amino acid sequence of its encoded protein.

- **Reverse micelle (RM):** Also known as reversed micelle or inverted micelle. A spheroidal structure formed by the association of a number of amphipathic (i.e. bearing both polar and nonpolar domains) surfactant molecules dissolved in organic, nonpolar solvents such as benzene, hexane, iso-octane, and oils such as corn and sesame. The structure of an RM is the reverse of that of a micelle. Reverse micelles may be characterized by a structure in which the polar groups of the surfactant and any water present are centrally located with the surfactant hydrocarbon chains pointing outward into the surrounding hydrocarbon medium. Reverse micelles may be used to solubilize polar molecules (i.e. water, enzymes) in organic nonpolar solvents and oils.

- **Reverse phase chromatography (RPC):** A method of separating a mixture of proteins or nucleic acids or other molecules by specific interactions of the molecules with a hydrophobic (water hating) immobilized phase (stationary substrate) which interacts with hydrophobic regions of the protein (or nucleic acid) molecules to achieve (preferential) separation of the mixture.

- **Reverse transcriptases:** Also known as RNA directed DNA polymerases. A class of enzymes first discovered to be present in RNA tumor virus, which allows the synthesis of DNA (complementary to the RNA) using the RNA present in the virus as a template. This is the reverse of what normally happens and hence the name. Reverse transcriptases closely resemble the DNA directed DNA polymerases in that they require the same materials and conditions as the DNA polymerases (e.g. for RT-PCR).

- **Reverse transcription:** Synthesis of DNA on a template of RNA; accomplished by reverse transcriptase enzyme.

- **Reverse translation:** A technique for isolating genes (or mRNAs) by their ability to hybridize with a short oligonucleotide sequence, prepared by predicting the nucleic acid sequence from the known protein sequence.
- **Reversed phase:** A chromatographic mode in which the mobile phase is more polar than the stationary phase.
- **Reversion:** Reversion of a mutation is a change in DNA that either reverses the original alteration (true reversion) or compensates for it (second site reversion in the same gene).
- **Revertants:** Derived by reversion of a mutant cell or organism.
- **Rf:** The distance traveled by the compound divided by the distance traveled by the solvent.
- **RF1:** The bacterial release factor that recognizes UAA and UAG as signals to terminate protein synthesis.
- **RF2:** The bacterial release factor that recognizes UAA and UGA as signals to terminate protein synthesis.
- **RF3:** A protein synthesis termination factor related to the elongation factor EF-G. It functions to release the factors RF1 or RF2 from the ribosome when they act to terminate protein synthesis.
- **rh:** Used to denote compounds (human molecules) made through the use of recombinant DNA technology [Recombinant (r) human (h)].
- *Rhizobium* **(bacteria):** Refers to strains of bacteria that live in the soil and colonize the roots of certain plants (i.e. legumes) symbiotically to thereby fix nitrogen from the air (i.e. change gaseous nitrogen into the chemical form that can be used by plants). For the legume known as the soybean plant (*Glycine max* L.), the relevant strain of the bacteria is *Rhizobium japonicum*. For the legume known as the alfalfa plant, the relevant strain of the bacteria is *Sinorhizobium meliloti*.
- **Rhizosphere:** The zone of immediate vicinity of growing plant roots that harbours increased microbial population.
- **Rho factor:** A protein involved in assisting *E.coli* RNA polymerase to terminate transcription at certain (rho-dependent) sites.
- **Rho-dependent terminators:** The sequences that terminate transcription by bacterial RNA polymerase in the presence of the rho factor.
- **Rho-independent terminators:** Sequences of DNA that cause *E. coli* RNA polymerase to terminate *in vitro* in the absence of rho factor.

R

- **rhTNF:** Recombinant human TNF.
- **Ri plasmids:** These are found in *Agrobacterium tumefaciens*. Like Ti plasmids, they carry genes that cause disease in infected plants. The disease may take the form of either hairy root disease or crown gall disease.
- **Ribonuclease:** An enzyme that hydrolyses RNA.
- **Ribonucleases (RNAases):** Enzymes that cleave RNA. They may be specific for single-stranded or for double-stranded RNA, and may be either endonuclease or exonuclease in nature.
- **Ribonucleic acid (RNA):** A long-chain, usually single-stranded nucleic acid consisting of repeating nucleotide units containing four kinds of heterocyclic, organic bases: adenine, cytosine, guanine, and uracil. These bases are conjugated to the pentose sugar ribose and held in sequence by phosphodiester (chemical) bonds. The primary function of RNA is protein synthesis within a cell. However, RNA is involved in various ways in the processes of expression and repression of hereditary information. The three main functionally distinct varieties of RNA molecules are: (1) messenger RNA (mRNA), which is involved in the transmission of DNA information, (2) ribosomal RNA (rRNA), which makes up the physical machinery of the synthetic process, and (3) transfer RNA (tRNA), which also constitutes another functional part of the machinery of protein synthesis.
- **Ribonucleoprotein:** A complex of RNA with proteins.
- **Ribonucleoside triphosphate:** A nitrogenous base (A, G, C, or U) attached to a ribose sugar with three phosphate groups attached in a tandem to the 5′ carbon of the sugar.
- **Ribose:** D-Ribose sugar, a five-carbon-atom monosaccharide. It is important to life because it and the closely allied compound deoxyribose form a part of the molecules that constitutes the backbone of nucleic acids.
- **Ribosomal binding site:** A nucleotide sequence near 5′ end of mRNA that facilitates the binding of the mRNA to the small ribosomal sub unit. It is also called Shine-Dalgarno sequence.
- **Ribosomal DNA (rDNA):** A tandemly repeated series of genes, coding for a precursor of the two large rRNAs.
- **Ribosomal RNA (rRNA):** A major component of the ribosome. Each of the two subunits of the ribosome has a major rRNA as well as many proteins.

R

- **Ribosome:** A large assembly of RNA and proteins that synthesizes proteins under direction from an mRNA template. Bacterial ribosomes sediment at 70S, eukaryotic ribosomes at 80S. A ribosome can be dissociated into two subunits (Fig. 4).

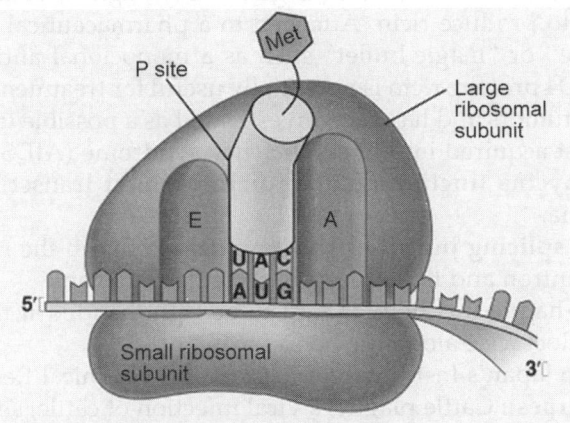

Fig. 4: Ribosome

- **Ribosome stalling:** Describes the inhibition of movement, that occurs when a ribosome reaches a codon for which there is no corresponding charged aminoacyl-tRNA.
- **Ribosome-binding site:** A sequence on bacterial mRNA that includes an initiation codon that is bound by a 30S subunit in the initiation phase of protein synthesis.
- **Ribozyme:** An RNA that has catalytic activity.
- **Ribozymes:** Discovered by Thomas Cech and Sidney Altman, they are RNA molecules that act as enzymes; possess catalytic activity and can specifically cleave (cut) other RNA molecules. The ribozyme (RNA) molecule and the other RNA molecule come together, whereupon the ribozyme molecule cuts the other RNA molecule at a specific defined (three-base) site. Because the ribozyme molecule acts as an enzyme in this reaction, the ribozyme molecule is not consumed or destroyed, but goes on to similarly cut other RNA molecules. During 2000, Thomas Steitz et al. proved that ribosomes (i.e. the cell's internal protein-synthesis machinery) are functionally ribozymes.
- **Ribulose:** A keto pentose sugar ($C_5H_{11}O_5$) that is involved in carbon dioxide fixation in photosynthesis.

- **Ribulose bisphosphate (rubp):** A five-carbon sugar that is combined with carbon dioxide to form a six-carbon intermediate in the first stage of the dark reaction of photosynthesis.
- **Ricin:** A lethal-to-cells protein naturally produced in castor beans. In 1994, Robert J et al. genetically engineered a tobacco plant to produce ricin. Attached to a pharmaceutical "guided missile" or "magic bullet" such as a monoclonal antibody or the CD4 protein, ricin is potentially useful for treatment against some tumors and has been investigated as a possible treatment against acquired immune deficiency syndrome (AIDS).
- **Rifamycins (including rifampicin):** Inhibit transcription in bacteria.
- **Right splicing junction:** The boundary between the right end of an intron and the left end of the adjacent exon.
- **Right-handed:** A helix is said to be right-handed if the turns runs clockwise along the helical axis.
- **Riken:** Japan's Institute for Physical and Chemical Research.
- **Rinderpest:** Cattle plague; a viral infection of cattle, sheep and goats.
- **Ribonuclease (RNAse):** A group of enzymes that catalyse the cleavage of nucleotides in RNA.
- **RNA editing:** Information that is contained in the DNA is not always found in the RNA products used to make proteins. Mitochondria and chloroplasts contain the biochemical machinery to alter the sequence of the final transcription product. For example, majority of the events involve C to U transition. So editing can convert a tryptophan codon to a arginine codon (CGG to UGG). Stop codons can be created by editing CAG, CAA and CGA codons.
- **RNA interference:** A biological process in which RNA molecules inhibit gene expression typically by causing the destruction of specific mRNA molecule.
- **RNA ligase:** An enzyme that functions in tRNA splicing to make a phosphodiester bond between the two exon sequences, are generated by cleavage of the intron.
- **RNA polymerase:** An enzyme that catalyzes the synthesis of a complementary mRNA (messenger RNA) molecule from a deoxyribonucleic acid (DNA) template in the presence of a mixture of the four ribonucleotides (ATP, UTP, GTP, and CTP). Also called transcriptase.

R

- **RNA replicase:** An enzyme that synthesizes RNA using an RNA template (used for replication by RNA viruses).

- **RNA splicing:** The process of excising the sequences in RNA that correspond to introns, so that the sequences corresponding to exons are connected into a continuous mRNA.

- **RNA vectors:** Ribonucleic acid (RNA) vehicle for transferring genetic information from one cell to another.

- **RNase:** An enzyme whose substrate is RNA.

- **RNA-driven hybridization reactions:** Use an excess of RNA to react with all complementary sequences in a single-stranded preparation of DNA.

- **Roentgen:** Obsolute unit of ionizing radiation. The SI unit is the Sievert (symbol: Sv1 Sv >> 8.4 r).

- **Rolling circle:** A mode of replication in which a replication fork proceeds around a circular template for an indefinite number of revolutions; the DNA strand newly synthesized in each revolution displaces the strand synthesized in the previous revolution, giving a tail containing a linear series of sequences complementary to the circular template strand.

- **Root:** The descending axis of a plant normally below ground which in serves anchoring the plant and absorbing, conducting water and mineral nutrients.

- **Root apex:** The apical meristem of a root very similar to the shoot spical meristem in that it forms the three meristematic areas: the protoderm (developing into the epidermis) the procambium (which develops into the stele) and the growth meristem (which forms the cortex).

- **Root cap:** A thimble like mass of cells covering and protecting the apical meristem of a root.

- **Root culture:** The culture of isolated root tips of apical or lateral origin to produce *in vitro* root system with indeterminate growth habits.

- **Root cutting:** Cutting made from sections of roots alone.

- **Root hairs:** Outgrowths from epidermal cell walls of the root specialized for water and nutrient absorption.

- **Root nodule:** A small round mass of cells that is located on the roots of plants and contains nitrogen fixing bacteria.

- **Root tuber:** Thickened root that stores carbohydrates.

- **Root zone:** The volume of soil or growing medium containing the roots of a plant. In soil science, the depth of the soil profile in which roots are normally found.
- **Root stock:** The trunk or root materials to which buds or scions are inserted in grafting.
- **ROS:** Acronym for Reactive Oxygen Species.
- **Rosemarinic acid:** A phenolic compound (naturally found in some plants) that acts as an antioxidant in the body's tissues when consumed by humans. For example, rosemarinic acid is naturally produced in the edible herbs *Origanum vulgare* and *Salvia officinalis*.
- **Rot:** The product of RNA concentration and time of incubation in an RNA-driven hybridization reaction.
- **Rotary shaker:** Rotating apparatus with a platform on which containers can be shaken such as Erlenmeyer flasks containing cells in liquid nutrient medium (Fig. 5).

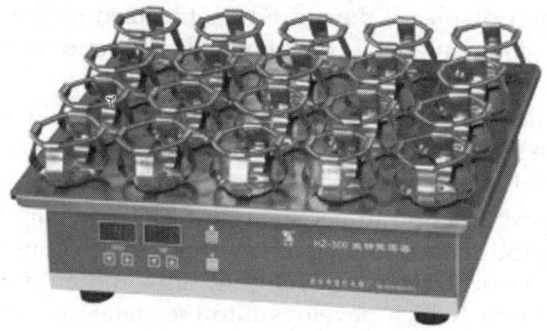

Fig. 5: Rotary shaker

R

- **Rotational positioning:** Describes the location of the histone octamer related to turns of the double helix, which determines which face of DNA is exposed on the nucleosome surface.
- **Rough endoplasmic reticulum (rough ER):** Refers to the region of the endoplasmic reticulum to which ribosomes are bound. It is the site of synthesis of membrane proteins and secretory proteins.
- **r-loops:** Single-stranded DNA regions in RNA-DNA hybrids formed *in vitro* under conditions where RNA-DNA duplexes are more stable than DNA-DNA duplexes.
- **r-protein:** One of the proteins of the ribosome.

- **Rps1c gene:** A gene that confers to any soybean plant (possessing that gene in its DNA) resistance to several strains/races of *phytophthora* root rot (PRR) disease.
- **Rps1k gene:** A gene that confers to any soybean plant (possessing that gene in its DNA) resistance to as many as 21 strains/races of *phytophthora* root rot (PRR) disease.
- **Rps6 gene:** A gene that confers to any soybean plant (possessing that gene in its DNA) resistance to some strains/races of PRR disease.
- **rRNA (ribosomal RNA):** The nucleic acid component of ribosomes, making up approximately two-thirds of the mass of the bacteria *Escherichia coli* ribosome, and approximately one-half of the mass of mammalian ribosomes. Ribosomal RNA accounts for nearly 80% of the RNA content of the bacterial cell.
- **RTK:** Abbreviation for "receptor tyrosine kinase". These kinases are membrane-bound proteins with large cytoplasmic and extracellular domains. Specific binding of a ligand, such as a growth factor, to the extracellular domain causes the cytoplasmic domain to phosphorylate other proteins on tyrosine residues.
- **RT-PCR:** Acronym for reverse transcriptase polymerase chain reaction technique.
- **Rubitecan:** A pharmaceutical that either shrinks or halts the growth of pancreatic cancer tumors in humans. The pharmacophore (i.e. active portion of molecule) in rubitecan was derived from a Chinese flowering tree *Camptotheca acuminata*; thus that "family" of drugs is known as camptothecins. Camptothecins inhibit a critical enzyme required for cell division to occur, thus inhibits rapidly growing tumors.
- **Rusts:** Various fungal diseases (*Puccinia* spp.) that attack small grain plants such as wheat, corn/maize, sorghum, oats, barley and rye. Its visual appearance is like that of rust on the surfaces of those plants.

S

- **"Stacked" genes:** Refers to the insertion of two or more (synthetic) genes into the genome of an organism. One example would be of a plant into which a gene from *Bacillus thuringiensis* (*Bt*) and a gene for resistance to a specific herbicide have been inserted.
- **10 sequence:** The consensus sequence centered about 10 bp before the start point of a bacterial gene. It is involved in melting DNA during the initiation reaction.
- **35 sequence:** The consensus sequence centered about 35 bp before the start point of a bacterial gene. It is involved in initial recognition by RNA polymerase.
- **S domain:** The sequence of 7S RNA of the SRP that is not related to Alu RNA.
- **S phase activator:** The cdk-cyclin complex that is responsible for initiating S phase.
- **S phage:** The restricted part of the eukaryotic cell cycle during which synthesis of DNA occurs.
- **S region:** An intron sequence involved in immunoglobulin class switching. S regions consist of repetitive sequences at the 5′ end of gene segments encoding the heavy chain constant regions.
- **S1 nuclease:** An enzyme that specifically degrades (destroys) single-stranded sequences of DNA.
- **SAAND:** Acronym for Selective Apoptotic Antineoplastic Drug.
- **Saccharification:** Enzymatic hydrolysis (by glucoamylase) of polysaccharides resulting in maltose and glucose.
- **SAGB:** Senior Advisory Group on Biotechnology.
- **Salicylic acid (SA):** SA is a signaling molecule in systemic acquired resistance (SAR) when SAR is triggered in plants (e.g. via spray application of COBRA (R) herbicide to soybean plants, harpin protein to various plants, via chewing by insects on the leaves of tomato plants, and/or via entry into plant of certain pathogenic bacteria/fungi, etc.).

- *Salmonella*: A genus of bacteria, consisting of more than 2,400 serovars (strains/types) classified within two species (*Salmonella enterica* and *S. bongori*). All of these serovars are potentially pathogenic (disease-causing) to humans. For example, some variants of *S. typhimurium* can cause typhoid fever. The non-typhoid strains of *Salmonella* generally cause enterocolitis; although that enterocolitis can lead to more serious systemic infections. *S. enteritidis* and *S. typhimurium* are increasingly causing outbreaks of foodborne illnesses (e.g. when foods are not washed or cooked thoroughly enough prior to consumption by humans).

- *Salmonella enteritidis* (Se): A pathogenic strain of *Salmonella* bacteria that can cause fatal infections in poultry and humans (when undercooked eggs are eaten by humans).

- *Salmonella typhimurium*: A pathogenic strain of *Salmonella* bacteria, which can cause disease in humans (when contaminated food is not washed and cooked enough prior to consumption).

- **Salt tolerance:** Refers to the trait (of a plant) that enables a plant to grow/survive in soil that contains a high level of salt. For example, during 2001, Eduardo Blumwald and Hong-Xia Zhang inserted a salt-tolerance gene from *Arabidopsis thaliana* into a tomato plant (*Lycopersicon esculentum*) and thereby made that tomato plant resistant to salt concentrations upto 200 mM (far higher than it could previously survive). The (*Arabidopsis* origin) gene enables the tomato plant to extract salt from the soil, and then sequester and store the salt in vacuoles (small compartments) within its leaf cells.

- **Saltatory replication:** A sudden lateral amplification to produce a large number of copies of some sequence.

- **Salting out:** A technique used for forcing (dissolved) proteins out of a solution by increasing the concentration of salt in the solution. The Na^+ and Cl^- ions derived from the salt compete for and "tie up" water molecules that are solubilizing the protein molecules, thereby rendering them insoluble or more insoluble.

- **Sam-K gene:** A gene naturally present within the *E. coli* bacteriophage T3. If the sam-K gene is inserted via genetic engineering into a plant's (fruit crop) genome, that causes greatly reduced production of the chemical compound S-adenosylmethionine (SAM) in that plant's fruit. Because the SAM is normally converted (chemically) into l-aminocyclopropane- 1-carboxylic acid (ACC) in the fruits of traditional vaieties of (fruit crop) plants, such sam-K gene-containing plants produce fruits which ripen/soften far slower than fruit from traditional varieties of those plants; which can reduce spoilage/loss in the harvest and transport of such fruit. That is because ACC is required for fruits to produce ethylene, the plant hormone which triggers (over) ripening/softening of fruit.

- **Sanitary and phytosanitary (SPS) agreement:** The agreement to GATT/WTO via which WTO member nations agreed to their technical barriers (regarding some imports, designed for the protection of human health or the control of animal and plant pests/diseases) only on an assessment of actual risks posed by the particular import in question, and to utilize only scientific methods in assessing those risks.

- **Saponification:** Alkaline hydrolysis of tri-acyl glycerols to yield fatty acid salts. The molecules thus produced are known as surfactants (surface active agents), commonly called soap. The process of soap-making.

- **Saponins:** A group of phytochemicals (i.e. sugars linked to a triterpene or a steroid molecular subunit) produced by certain plants (that of soybean, spinach, tomatoes, potatoes, ginseng plant, etc.). Evidence suggests that human consumption of saponins (e.g. produced in soybeans) can help to lower a person's blood content of low-density lipoproteins (LDLP) and can help prevent certain types of cancer.

- **SAR:** Acronym for Systemic Acquired Resistance.

- **SARS (Severe acute respiratory syndrome):** It is caused by a virus thought to be a combination of the Coronavirus family (cause of the common cold) and the paramyxovirus family (cause measles and mumps). The syndrome includes fever and coughing or difficulty in breathing, and can be fatal. It is thought to have originated in Mainland, China in 2003 and has spread to other countries.

- **Satellite DNA:** Consists of many tandem repeats (identical or related) of a short basic repeating unit.

- **Saturated fatty acids (SAFA):** Fatty acids containing fully saturated alkyl chains (on their molecules). This means that the carbon atoms comprising the chains are held together by one carbon-to-carbon bond and not two or three. High levels of dietary SAFA have been related to increased blood cholesterol levels, which tends to lead to coronary heart disease (CHD) in humans. The sole exception is stearic acid (also known as stearate), which on research has shown no impact on the blood cholesterol levels of humans, that consume it. Beef fat typically contains approximately 54% saturated fatty acids; sheep fat contains approximately 58%, pork contains approximately 45%, and chicken fat contains approximately 32% saturated fatty acids. In general, fats possessing the highest levels of saturated fatty acids tend to be solid at room temperature, while fats possessing highest levels of unsaturated fatty acids tend to be liquid at room temperature. That rule of thumb was the original "dividing line" between the terms "fats" and "oils," respectively.

- **Saturation density:** The density to which cultured eukaryotic cells grow *in vitro* before division is inhibited by cell-cell contact.
- **Saturation hybridization:** An *in vitro* reaction in which one polynucleotide component is in great excess, causing all complementary sequences in the other polynucleotide component to enter a duplex form.
- **Saxitoxins:** Paralytic poisons produced by certain shellfish.
- **Scaffold:** A proteinaceous structure in the shape of a sister chromatid pair, generated when chromosomes are depleted of histones.
- **Scale-Up:** The transition step in moving a (chemical) process from experimental (e.g. "test tube", small, bench) scale to a larger scale producing more or much more product than the bench scale (e.g. production of tons/year in a chemical plant). A process may require number of scale-ups, each producing more product than the earlier one.
- **Scarec (complex) mRNA:** Consists of a large number of individual mRNA species, each present in very few copies per cell.
- **Scrapie:** A infective agent made of protein.
- **scRNPs:** Small cytoplasmic ribonucleoproteins (scRNAs associated with proteins).
- **SDM:** Site-directed mutagenesis.
- **SDS (Sodium dodecyl sulfate):** Also known as sodium lauryl sulfate (SLS). A surfactant commonly used in biochemical and biotechnological applications for the solubilization of membrane components and hard-to-solubilize (dissolve) molecules. For example, it is often utilized at high concentration in water solution (along with potassium acetate) to dissolve plant DNA samples (when a scientist wants to sequence that sample of plant

DNA). The SDS/PA in water solution helps the scientist to separate out contaminants commonly present in samples from plant tissues (polysaccharides, proteins, etc.) because DNA molecules are much more soluble in SDS/PA solution than in contaminant molecules. Above a critical concentration (CMC), SDS forms micelles in water which are thought to be responsible for its solubilizing action. SDS is also used in such items as shampoo adhesion molecules. A class of molecular structure related to lectins that mediate (control, cause, etc.) the contacts between a variety of cells (leukocytes and endothelial cells), and function as cellular adhesion receptors.

- **Second messenger gated channel:** An ion channel whose activity is controlled by small signaling molecules inside the cell.
- **Second messenger:** A small molecule that is generated when a signal transduction pathway is activated. The classic second messenger is cyclic AMP, which is generated when adenylate cyclase is activated by a G protein (the G protein itself activated by a transmembrane receptor).
- **Secondary attachment site:** A locus on the bacterial chromosome into which phage lambda integrate inefficiently because the site resembles the *att* site.
- **Secondary immune response:** An organism's immune response upon a second exposure to a given antigen. This second exposure is also referred to as a "booster". The secondary immune response is characterized by a more rapid induction, greater magnitude, and higher affinity antibodies than the primary immune response.
- **Secondary metabolite:** The metabolite that is not required by a cell for its growth or metabolism but produce as a byproduct for protection against microorganisms during stationary phase of growth.
- **Second-site reversion:** Describes the occurrence of a second mutation that suppresses the effect of a first mutation.
- **Secretory granule:** A membrane-bounded compartment that contains molecules to be released from cells by regulated exocytosis (that is, the molecules are concentrated and stored in secretory granules, and are released only in response to a signal). It is also called a secretory vesicle.
- **Secretory vesicle:** A membrane-bounded compartment that contains molecules to be released from cells by regulated

exocytosis (that is, the molecules are concentrated in secretory vesicles and are released only in response to a signal). It is also called a secretory granule.

- **Sector:** A patch of cells made up of single altered cell and its progeny.
- **Securins:** A class of proteins that prevent the initiation of anaphase by binding to and inhibiting separin, a protease which cleaves the structural component required for holding sister chromatids together. Inhibition of separin by securin ends when securin itself proteolyzed as a result of activation of the anaphase promoting complex (APC). Many organisms have a segmented body plan that divides the body into a number of repeating units, called segments, along the anterior-posterior axis.
- **Segment polarity:** In *Drosophila*, segment polarity genes are a set of genes that help in setting up the segmentation of the embryo. They are expressed in a striped pattern with one stripe in every future segment. Each stripe indicates the posterior margin of a segment.
- **Segmentation genes:** Concerned with controlling the number or polarity of body segments in insects.
- **Segregation disorder:** A gene or some other genetic element, which alters the ratio of segregating alleles recovered in the gametes; in *Drosophila*, the SD+ cells are eliminated during gametogenesis.
- **Selectable:** Having a gene product that enables to identify and propogate a particular cell type.
- **Selectable marker:** A gene, usually encoding resistance to an antibiotic, added to a vector constructed to allow easy selection of cells that contain the construction from the large majority of cells that do not.
- **Selection:** A method to isolate and identify a specific organisms in a mixed culture. The use of particular conditions to allow survival only of cells with a particular phenotype to obtain the desired strain.
- **Selective apoptotic antineoplastic drug (SAAND):** A category of pharmaceuticals that acts to prevent neoplastic growth (cancer) by allowing normal cell apoptosis to occur again (by blocking an enzyme that is hindering normal apoptosis) in abnormal precancerous cells and cancerous cells. Examples of SAANDs include sulindac, which blocks phosphodiesterases (enzymes).

- **Selective breeding:** A process in which new or improved strains of plants or animals are developed, mainly through controlled mating or crossing and selection of progeny for desired traits.
- **Selective estrogen effect:** A term used to describe how certain phytochemicals (flavones, flavonols, isoflavones, etc.) and pharmaceuticals (evista/raloxifene, tamoxifen, etc.) possessing molecular structures that are similar to estrogen (a hormone) impart some beneficial effect on the human body when consumed by humans, without any of the adverse impacts of estrogen (promotion of the growth of certain tumors by estrogen).
- **Selective estrogen receptor modulators:** Abbreviated SERM. This term refers to chemical compounds (isoflavones, the pharmaceuticals Evista/raloxifene and tamoxifen, etc.) which impart some beneficial effect on the human body when consumed by humans, without any of the adverse impacts of estrogen (e.g. promotion of the growth of certain tumors by estrogen).
- **Selectivity:** The ratios of the capacity factors for two substances measured under identical chromatographic conditions; sometimes termed separation factor.
- **Self-assembly:** Refers to the ability of a protein (or of a complex of proteins) to form its final structure without the intervention of any additional components (such as chaperones). The term can also refer to the spontaneous formation of any biological structure that occurs when molecules collide and bind to each other.
- **Selfish DNA:** Describes sequences that do not contribute to the genotype of the organism but have self-perpetuation within the genome as their sole function.
- **Selfish gene:** Those genes, which propagate themselves despite being detrimental to the organisms that carry them.
- **Semiconservative replication:** A type of DNA replication in which the daughter DNA strands is composed of one old and one newly synthesized strand.
- **Semiconserved:** (Semi-invariant) position is one where comparison of many individual sequences finds the same type of base (pyrimidine or purine) always present.
- **Senescent:** Cells show visible changes in the appearance of a culture as the result of limitations posed by telomere shortening on the number of chromosomal replications that can occur.

- **Semidiscontinuous replication:** The mode in which one new strand is synthesized continuously while the other is synthesized discontinuously.
- **Semisynthetic catalytic antibody:** An antibody produced (e.g. via monoclonal antibody techniques) in response to a carefully selected antigen (i.e. one of the molecules involved in the chemical reaction that you are trying to catalyze). Such an antibody is then made to be catalytic by "attaching" a (molecular) group that is known to catalyze the desired chemical reaction. This attaching is done either via chemical modification of the antibody, or via genetic engineering of the cell (DNA) that produces that antibody.
- **Senior advisory group on biotechnology (SAGB):** An association of approximately 35 of the largest European companies that are engaged in at least some form of genetic engineering research or production. Similar to America's biotechnology industry organization (BIO), the SAGB works with governments and the public to promote safe and rational advancement of genetic engineering and biotechnology. It was formed in 1989 and is based in Brussels, Belgium.
- **Sense:** Normal (forward) orientation of DNA sequence (gene) in genome.
- **Separins:** Proteins which play a direct role in initiating anaphase by cleaving and inactivating a component (a cohesin) that holds sister chromatids together.
- **Sepsis:** Also known as systemic inflammatory response syndrome, this life-threatening condition ("septic shock") occurs when the body's immune system over-responds to infection (e.g. by Gram-negative bacteria) in which release of bacterial endotoxin [(lipopolysaccharide (LPS)] occurs. Those immune system cells (macrophages, etc.) overproduce numerous inflammatory agents (cytokines), which induce fever, shock, and sometimes organ failure.
- **Septal ring (Z-ring):** A complex of several proteins coded by *fis* genes of *E. coli*, form at the mid-point of the cell. It gives rise to the septum at cell division. The first proteins to be incorporated is FtsZ, which gave rise to the original name of the Z-ring.
- **Septum:** The material that forms in the center of a bacterium to divide it into two daughter cells at the end of a division cycle.
- **Sequence (of a DNA molecule):** The specific nucleic acids that comprise a given segment of a DNA molecule.

- **Sequence (of a protein molecule):** The specific amino acids (and the order in which they are coupled together) that comprise a given segment of a protein molecule.
- **Sequence characterized amplified regions (SCARs):** A fragment of genomic DNA present at a single locus, identified by PCR amplification using a pair of specific oligonucleotide primers.
- **Sequence map:** A pictorial representation of the sequence of amino acids in a protein molecule, the sequence of nucleic acids in a DNA molecule, or the sequence of oligosaccharide components in a glycoprotein/carbohydrate molecule.
- **Sequon:** A (potential) site on a protein molecule's "backbone" where a sugar molecule (or a chain of sugar molecules, i.e. an oligosaccharide) may be attached.
- **Serine (ser):** A non-essential amino acid; a biosynthetic precursor of several metabolites, including cysteine, glycine, and choline. In 1999, Solomon H Snyder, et al. conducted research that showed that some mammals synthesize (manufacture) D-serine within their brains, and it functions as a neurotransmitter there.
- **Seroconversion:** The development of antibodies (specific to that disease-causing microorganism) in response to vaccination or natural exposure to a disease-causing microorganism.
- **Serology:** A subdiscipline of immunology, concerned with the properties and reactions of blood sera. It includes the diverse techniques used for the "test tube" measurement of antibody-antigen reactions, including blood typing (e.g. for transfusions).
- **Seronegative:** Refers to negative results of a serology test.
- **Serotonin:** A compound that occurs in the brain, intestines, and blood platelets and acts as a neurotransmitter, as well as inducing vasoconstriction and contraction of smooth muscle; 5-hydroxytryptamine (5HT).
- **Serotypes:** A variety (sub-strain) of a microorganism that is distinguished from others (in the strain) via its serological effects (within immune system of the host organism it inhabits).
- **Serpentine:** Receptor has seven transmembrane segments. Typically, it activates a trimeric G protein.
- **Serum:** Blood plasma that has its clotting factor removed.
- **Serum dependence:** The need of eukaryotic cells for factors contained in serum in order to grow in culture.

- **Serum lifetime:** The average length of time that a molecule circulates in an organism's bloodstream before it is cleared from the bloodstream.
- **Serum response element (SRE):** A sequence in a promoter or enhancer that is activated by transcription factor(s) induced by treatment with serum. This activates the genes that stimulate cell growth.
- **Sessile:** Microorganisms that are attached to a (support) substrate directly by their base; not attached via an intervening peduncle (i.e. stalk); can also refer to fruit or leaves that are attached directly to the main stem or branch of a plant.
- **Sex chromosomes:** A chromosome that is inherited differently in the two sexes, that is concerned directly with the inheritance of sex, and that is the seat of factors governing the inheritance of various sex-linked and sex-limited characters.
- **Sex linkage:** The pattern of inheritance shown by genes carried on a sex chromosome (usually the X).
- **Sex plasmid:** An episome; it is able to initiate the process of conjugation, by which chromosomal material is transferred from one bacterium to another.
- **Sex-linked:** A gene coded on a sex chromosome, such as the X-chromosome linked genes of flies and man.
- **Sexual conjugation:** An infrequent occurrence, in which two adjacent bacteria stretch out portions of their (cell) membranes to touch one another, fuses, and then passes transposons, jumping genes, or plasmids to each other.
- **SH2:** Domain (named originally as the *Src*/omology domain because it was identified in the Src product of the Rous sarcoma virus) is a region of ~100 amino acids that is bound by the SH2-binding domain of the protein upstream in a signal transduction cascade.
- **SH2-binding site:** An area on a protein that interacts with the SH2 domain of another protein.
- **SH3:** Domain is used by some proteins that contain SH2 domains to enable them to bind to the next component downstream in a signal transduction cascade.
- **Shine-dalgarno sequence:** A sequence (AGGAGG) about 10 bp before the AUG initiation codon in 5' end of bacterial mRNA is complementary to 3' end of 16S rRNA and helps in the positioning of ribosome for initiation of translation.

- **Short-period interpersion:** A pattern in a genome in which moderately repetitive DNA sequences of ~300 bp alternate with non-repititive sequences of ~1,000 bp.
- **Shotgun cloning method:** A technique for obtaining the desired gene that involves "chopping up" the entire genetic complement of a cell using restriction enzymes, then attaching each (resultant) DNA fragment to a vector and transferring it into a bacterium, and finally screening those (engineered) bacteria to locate the bacteria that are producing the desired product (a protein).
- **Shotgun experiment:** A crude but effective method used to identify a specific gene associated with a disease, based on hybridization of shotgun sequencing.
- **Shotgun sequencing:** Sometimes called Wholegenome shotgun sequencing. A technology for rapid sequencing of DNA, in which an organism's genome (DNA) is first fragmented ("broken up"), and then randomly selected pieces of the DNA are individually sequenced. Those individual pieces' sequences must subsequently be "bridged" ("assembled" in an over-lapping end-by-end pattern) in order to assemble a complete map (e.g. of an organism's chromosome or genome).
- **Shuttle vector:** A plasmid constructed to have origins for replication for two hosts (*E. coli* and *S. cerevisiae*) so that it can be used to carry a foreign sequence in either prokaryotes or eukaryotes (Fig. 1).

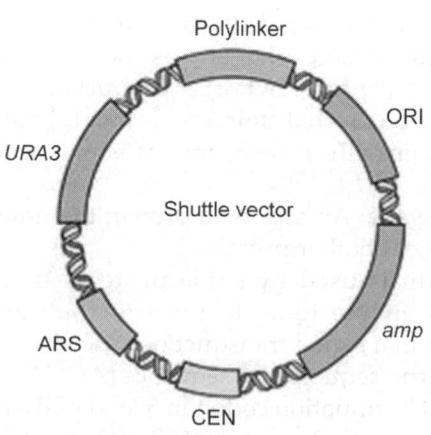

Fig. 1: Shuttle vector

- **SI nuclease:** An enzyme that degrades single stranded DNA.
- **Sickle cell anemia:** A hereditary human disease controlled by a recessive gene characterized by sickle cell shape of RBC and anaemic condition.
- **Siderophore:** A low molecular weight Fe-chelating protein synthesized by several soil microorganisms.
- **Sigma factor:** The subunit of bacterial RNA polymerase needed for initiation; the major influence on selection of binding sets (promoters).
- **Sign inversion:** Model describes the mechanism of DNA gyrase. DNA gyrase binds a positive supercoil (inducing a compensatory negative supercoil elsewhere on the closed circular DNA), breaks both strands in one duplex, passes the other duplex through, and reseals the strands.
- **Signal end:** Produced during recombination of immunoglobulin and T cell receptor genes. The signal ends are at the termini of the cleaved fragment containing the recombination signal sequences. The subsequent joining of the signal ends yields a signal joint.
- **Signal hypothesis:** The role of the N-terminal sequence of a secreted protein in attaching nascent polypeptide to membrane; that is, mRNA and ribosome are attached to membrane via the N-terminal end of the protein under synthesis.
- **Signal peptidase:** An enzyme within the membrane of the ER that specifically removes the signal sequences from proteins as they are translocated. Analogous activities are present in bacteria, archaebacteria, and in each organelle in a eukaryotic cell into which proteins are targeted and translocated by means of removable targeting sequences. Signal peptidase is a component of a large protein complex.
- **Signal recognition particle (SRP):** A ribonucleoprotein complex that recognizes signal sequences during translation and guides the ribosome to the translocation channel. SRPs from different organisms may have different compositions, but all contain related proteins and RNAs.
- **Signal sequence:** A segment of about 15 to 30 amino acids at the n' terminus of a protein that enables the protein to be secreted. The signal sequence is removed as the protein secreted through the membrane. It is also called signal peptide and leader peptide.

- **Signal transducers and activators of transcription (STATs):** Molecules that cause signal transduction to occur (when a hormone or other chemical "binds" to it), or molecules that cause transcription to occur (when transcription factor(s) "bind" to it). STATs can be attached to solid surfaces (in a bioassay or biosensor) for use in such research applications as high-throughput screening.
- **Signal transduction:** The process by which a receptor interacts with a ligand at the surface of the cell and then transmits a signal to trigger a pathway within the cell.
- **Signaling molecule:** A molecule utilized to "signal" (communicate) with cells, or to deliver a signal to other organisms (e.g. a signal by the soybean plant to attract beneficial *Rhizobium* bacteria to colonize the roots of plant). For example, the young offspring of fleas can remain immature (larvae) for upto 2 years in the absence of a food source, until carbon dioxide molecules and heat from a nearby mammal (potential host/food source) signal them to mature into adults in order to prey on the mammal. Another example: the larvae of North American tree frogs are signaled by chemicals released into a pond's water when the first such frog larva is killed by a (predatory) dragonfly nymph (i.e. when those dragonflies first arrive each year at a given pond, to prey on the frog larvae). That chemical "signal" causes all of the North American tree frog larvae in that pond to subsequently grow tails that are twice as large as were grown by them prior to that chemical signal, to facilitate their escape from the dragonfly nymphs.
- **Signaling:** The "communication" that occurs between and within cells of an organism, e.g. via hormones, nitric acid, etc. Such signaling "tells" certain cells to grow, change, or produce specific proteins at specific times.
- **Silencer:** A short sequence of DNA that can inactivate expression of a gene in its vicinity.
- **Silencing:** Describes the repression of gene expression in a localized region, usually as the result of a structural change in chromatin.
- **Silent mutation:** A mutation in a gene that causes no detectable change in the biological characteristics of that gene's product (e.g. protein).

- **Silent site:** A *in situ* coding region where mutation does not change the sequence of the protein.
- **Silk:** A natural, protein polymer with a predominance of alanine and glycine amino acids. Silk is produced by silkworms that have fed on mulberry tree leaves. The body of a silkworm can retain proteins (raw material for silk) amounting to as much as 20% of its body weight. It is thought that silk may be altered, via genetic engineering of silkworms, to produce fibers of very high strength.
- **Simple protein:** A protein that yields only amino acids on hydrolysis (cleavage of the protein molecule into fragments), and does not have other molecular constituents such as lipids or polysaccharide attachments.
- **Simple sequence repeat (SSR) DNA marker technique:** A "genetic mapping" technique which utilizes the fact that microsatellite sequences "repeat" (appear repeatedly in sequence within the DNA molecule) in a manner enabling them to be used as "markers".
- **Simple-sequence DNA:** Equals satellite DNA.
- **SINES:** A class of retroposons found as short interspersed repeats in mammalian genomes; derived from transcripts of RNA polymerase III.
- **Single cell protein (SCP):** Cells or protein extracts of microorganisms produced in large quantities for use as human or animal protein supplements.
- **Single copy:** Plasmid replicates under a control system analogous to the bacterial chromosome that allows only one copy to exist in an individual bacterial cell.
- **Single nucleotide polymorphism (SNP):** Describes polymorphism (variation in sequence between individuals) caused by a change in a single nucleotide. This is responsible for most of the genetic variation between individuals.
- **Single X hypothesis:** The inactivation of one X chromosome in mammals female.
- **Single-cell protein (SCP):** Protein derived from single-celled organisms with a high protein content, used as a food supplement or substitute.
- **Single-copy plasmids:** Maintained in bacteria at a ratio of one plasmid for every host chromosome.

S

- **Single-nucleotide polymorphisms (SNPs):** Variation between two DNA sequences consisting in the difference of a single nucleotide, frequently the substitution of thymine for cytosine.
- **Single-strand assimilation:** (single-strand uptake) describes the ability of RecA protein to cause a single strand of DNA to displace its homologous strand in a duplex; that is, the single strand is assimilated into the duplex.
- **Single-strand binding protein (SSB):** Attaches to single stranded DNA, thereby preventing the DNA from forming a duplex.
- **Single-strand exchange:** A reaction in which one of the strands of a duplex of DNA leaves its former partner and instead pairs with the complementary strand in another molecule, displacing its homolog in the second duplex.
- **Single-strand passage:** The type of reaction catalyzed by type I topoisomerase in which one section of single-stranded DNA is passed through another strand.
- **Sister chromatids:** The copies of a chromosome produced by its replication.
- **Site directed mutagenesis:** The process of nucleotide changes in cloned genes by site specific mutagenesis.
- **Site-directed mutagenesis (SDM):** A technique that can be used to make a protein that differs slightly in its structure from the protein normally produced (by an organism or cell). A single mutation (in the cell's DNA) is caused by hybridizing the region in a codon to be mutated with a short, synthetic oligonucleotide. This causes the codon to code for a different specific amino acid in the protein gene product. Site-directed mutagenesis holds the potential to enable man to create modified (engineered) proteins that have desirable properties not currently available in the proteins produced by existing organisms.
- **Site-specific recombination:** It occurs between two specific (not necessarily homologous) sequences, as in phage integration/excision or resolution of cointegrate structure during transpositions.
- **Sitostanol:** A chemical (ester) derived from sitosterol (a sterol present in pine trees), and fibers (the hull or seed coat) of corn/maize (*Zea mays*) or soybeans (*Glycine max* L.). When sitostanol is consumed by humans in sufficient quantities, it causes their total serum cholesterol and their low density lipoprotein (LDLP)

S

levels to be lowered by approximately 10%, via inhibition (the sitostanol is preferentially absorbed by the gastrointestinal system instead of cholesterol). During 2000, the US Food and Drug Administration approved a (label) health claim that associates consumption of sitostanols with reduced blood cholesterol content and reduced coronary heart disease (CHD).

- **Sitosterol:** A phytosterol that is naturally produced in fibers within soybean (*Glycine max* L.) hulls, pumpkin seeds, pine trees, fibers of corn/maize (*Zea mays*) seed coats, etc. Sitosterol can exist in several different molecular forms (known as alpha a, beta b, etc.). A human diet containing large amounts of sitosterol and/or certain other phytosterols (campesterol, stigmasterol, etc.) has been shown to lower total serum (blood) cholesterol and low-density lipoprotein (LDLP) levels; and thereby lower the risk of coronary heart disease (CHD). Evidence indicates that certain phytosterols (including sitosterol) interfere with absorption of cholesterol by the intestines, and decrease the body's recovery and reuse of cholesterol-containing bile salts, which causes more cholesterol to be excreted from the body than previously. During 2000, the US Food and Drug Administration (US-FDA) approved a (label) health claim that associates consumption of sitosterols with reduced blood cholesterol content and with reduced coronary heart disease (CHD).

- **SL RNA (spliced leader RNA):** The small RNA which provide spliced leader sequences, SL1, SL2, SL3, SL4 and SL5 (short sequences which are joined to the 5′ ends of pre-mRNAs, by trans-splicing). They are found primarily in primitive eukaryotes (protozoans and nematodes).

- **Slime:** An extracellular (i.e. outside of the cell) material produced by some (micro)organisms and characterized by a slimy consistency. The slime is of varied chemical composition. However, usual components are polysaccharides (polysugars) and specific protein molecules.

- **Slow component:** Of a reassociation reaction is the last to reassociate; usually consists of nonrepetitive DNA.

- **Slow-stop:** *dna* mutants of *E. coli* complete the current round of bacterial replication but cannot initiate another at 42°C.

- **Small cytoplasmic RNAs (scRNAs):** Found in the cytoplasm and are sometimes also found in the nucleus.

- **Small nuclear RNA (snRNA):** One of many small RNA species confined to the nucleus; several of the snRNAs are involved in splicing or other RNA processing reactions.
- **Small subunit:** Part of the ribosome (30S in bacteria, 40S in eukaryotes) that binds the mRNA.
- **Smooth ER:** A region of endoplasmic reticulum devoid of ribosomes.
- **SNARE hypothesis:** Proposes that the specificity of a transport vesicle for its target membrane is mediated by the interaction of SNARE proteins. In this hypothesis, a SNARE on the vesicle (v-SNARE) binds specifically to its cognate SNARE on the target membrane (t-SNARE).
- **snoRNA:** A small nuclear RNA that is localized in the nucleolus.
- **SNP MAP:** A group of known/detailed SNPs (single-nucleotide polymorphisms), superimposed onto the genome map of an organism (e.g. to facilitate genetic/population studies, such as of genetically related disease susceptibility).
- **snRNPs (Snurps):** Are small nuclear ribonucleoproteins (snRNAs associated with proteins).
- **Solanine:** A glycoside neurotoxin naturally present at low levels within potatoes. As a result, solanine is present at detectable levels in the bloodstream of humans who consume potatoes. The US-FDA prohibits the sale of potatoes in US which contain more (than a very low level of solanine); e.g. the naturally present level in potatoes can unfortunately increase in potatoes that are exposed to direct sunlight.
- **Soluble CD4:** A synthetic version of the CD4 protein that may interfere with the ability of HIV (i.e. AIDS) viruse to infect human immune system cells with the acquired immune deficiency syndrome (AIDS) virus.
- **Somaclonal variation:** The genetic variation (new traits) that results from the growing of entire new plants from plant cells or tissues (maintained in culture). Frequently encountered when plants are regenerated (grown) from plant cells that have been altered via genetic engineering. However, somaclonal variation (new genetic traits) can occur even when plants are regenerated from cells that were part of the same original plant.
- **Somaclone:** Plants derived from any form of cell culture involving the use of somatic plant cells.

- **Somatic cell gene therapy:** Gene delivery to a tissue other than reproductive cells of an individual to correct gene defect.
- **Somatic cells:** All eukaryote body cells, except the gametes and the cells from which they develop.
- **Somatic embryogenesis:** In plant culture, the process of embryo initiation and development for vegetative or non-gametic cells.
- **Somatic hybridization:** A technique of fusing protopasts from two contrasting genotypes for production of hybrids or cybrids which contain various mixtures of nuclear and/or cytoplasmic genomes, respectively.
- **Somatic mutation:** A type of mutation occurring in a somatic cell, and therefore affecting only its daughter cells; it is not inherited by descendants of the organism. Somatic mutations are generally spontaneous, but a case of directed mutation occurs in the immune system where more diversity is generated in rearranged immunoglobulin genes by somatic mutation.
- **Somatic recombination:** Describes the process of joining a C gene to a C gene in a lymphocyte to generate an immunoglobulin or T cell receptor.
- **Somatic variants:** Regenerated plants (clones) derived (produced) from cells that originally came from the same plant, but are not genetically identical. Such plants (clones) are called "sports" or somatic variants because they vary (genetically) from the "parent" plant. Sometimes such somatic variants are developed by man to become a new plant variety the nectarine.
- **Somatomedins:** A family of peptides that mediates the action of growth hormone on skeletal tissue, and stimulates bone formation.
- **Somatostatin:** A 14 amino acid peptide that inhibits the release of growth hormone.
- **Somatotropin:** Category of hormone that is produced naturally in the bodies of all mammals, including man.
- **Sorting signal:** A motif in a protein (either a short sequence of amino acids or a covalent modification) that is required for it to be incorporated into vesicles that carry it to a specific destination.
- **SOS box:** The DNA sequence (operator) of ~20 bp recognized by LexA repressor protein.
- **SOS response:** The coordinate induction of many enzymes, including repair activities, in response to irradiation or other

damage to DNA; results from activation of protease activity by RecA to cleave LexA repressor (in *E. coli*).

- **Southern blot analysis:** A test that is performed on biological samples such as plant DNA (e.g. to ascertain if "inserted" DNA is present in particular plant cells). Gel electrophoresis is used to separate the DNA fragments according to size, and then those fragments are transferred to a filter (blot). Radiolabeled DNA probes or RNA probes are added, and the one which are complementary to each of the (separated, on blot) fragments will hybridize to those respective DNA fragments. The location (on the blot) and "radioactive label" of those hybridized probes can then be utilized to determine the nature of the DNA that was in those plant cells.

- **Southern blotting:** The procedure for transferring denatured DNA from an agarose gel to a nitrocellulose filter where it can be hybridized with a complementary nucleic acid (Fig. 2).

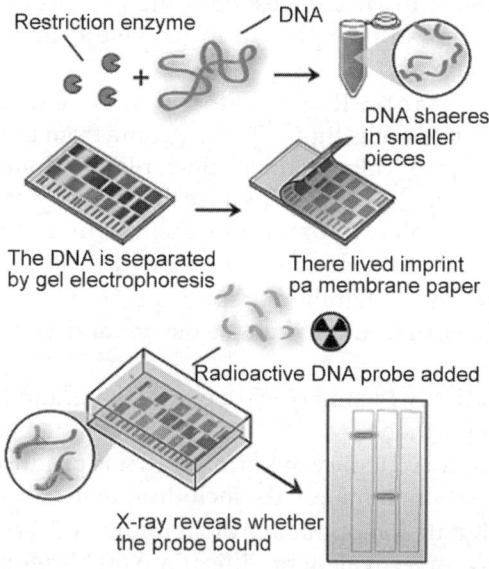

Fig. 2: Southern blotting

- **Southern corn rootworm:** Latin name *Diabrotica undecimpunctata hawardii*.

- **Southwestern blot:** The molecules transferred are protein and the probe is DNA.

- **Soy protein:** An edible protein (after heat processing) produced within its beans (seeds) by the soybean plant (botanical name *Glycine max* (L.) Merrill). When removed from soybeans via crushing, extrusion, or other process(es) involving adequate heat treatment, soy protein is (historical average) composed of 2.5% cysteine, 3.4% histidine, 5.2% isoleucine, 8.2% leucine, 6.8% lysine, 1.1% methionine, 5.6% phenylalanine, 4.2% threonine, 1.3% tryptophan, 4.2% tyrosine, 5.4% valine, 4% alanine, 7.7% arginine, 6.9% aspartic acid, 19% glutamic acid, 3.7% glycine, 0.1% 4-hydroxyproline, 5.3% proline and 5.4% serine. Soy protein (concentrate) is a complete ("ideal") protein (i.e. it provides all essential amino acids) for humans. It is a good dietary source of calcium, with an absorption rate equivalent to milk. In its initial form (following crushing/extrusion from soybeans as described above), the soy protein is known as soybean meal, and contains a bit less than half protein by weight.

- **Soybean aphid:** An aphid (*Aphis glycines*) native to China, but accidentally introduced into the US during the 1990s (apparently via aphid eggs adhering to an ornamental plant). It feeds on the sap of the soybean plant (*Glycine max* L.).

- **Soybean cyst nematodes (SCN):** A plant-parasitic nematode and a devastating pest of the soybean worldwide. The nematode infects the roots of soybean, and the female nematode eventually becomes a cyst.

- **Soybean oil:** An edible oil that is produced within its beans (seeds) by the soybean plant (*Glycine max* (L.) Merrill). When removed from soybeans via crushing and refining processes, soybean oil is (historical average) composed of 60.8% polyunsaturated fatty acids (PUFA), 24.5% monounsaturated fatty acids, and 15.1% saturated fatty acids. However, soybean varieties have recently been created that possess as little as 7% saturated fatty acids.

- **Soybean plant:** [*Glycine max* (L.) Merrill]. A green, bushy legume that is the world's single largest provider of protein and edible oil for mankind's use. This summer annual plant varies in height from less than a foot (0.3 meter) to more than three feet (one meter) tall. The seeds (soybeans) are borne in pods, and historically have contained 13–26% oil and 38–45% protein (on a moisture-free basis). Its leaves contain some carotenoids. The soybean plant has approximately 80,000 genes. It is a self-pollinating plant (i.e. there are male and female reproductive structures on the same plant so it is monoecious). Soybean oil contains a total of 327 mg/100 g of the plant sterols (phytosterols) campesterol, stigmasterol, and beta-sitosterol (β-sitosterol). Soybeans contain the highest amount of isoflavones of any plant (seeds) i.e. up to 0.3% of each soybean's dry weight. The traditional soybean, possessing (average) 20% oil content, contains an average of 3% stachyose within its meal (i.e. the solids remaining after the soybean oil is removed) (Fig. 3).

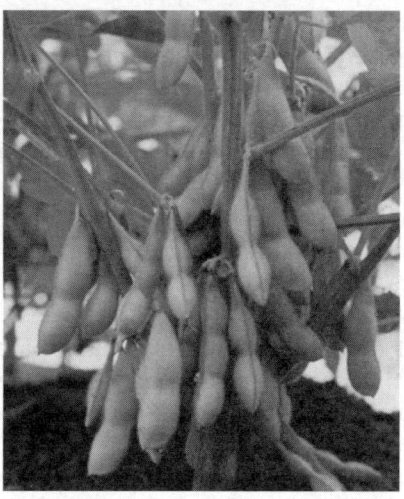

Fig. 3: Soybean plant

S

- **Spacer:** A sequence in a gene cluster that separates the repeated copies of the transcription unit.
- **Specialized transduction:** Transfer of only specific host gene with the help of transducing phages.
- **Species:** A single type (taxonomic group) or organism as determined by the distinguishing characteristics used for the particular group of life forms (the horse is one species among the mammals). While the horse is easily distinguished from other, obviously nonsimilar mammals, such as humans (due to the horse's four legs vs. the human's two legs and two arms), it is less easy to distinguish a horse from a more closely related animal such as a donkey or a zebra. The so called "boundary between different species" is determined by human assessment/

categorization (whether systematics or cladistics are utilized by those doing the species categorizations and definitions), and sometimes changes when more information becomes known at a later date (if new 2D electrophoresis tests reveal certain types to be genetically related or not).

- **Species specific:** Refers to a compound (a protein) or a disease (a viral infection) or some other effect that only acts in/on one specific species of organism. For example, the antibiotic penicillin kills bacteria by blocking an enzyme that is critical for growth and repair of the bacterial cell wall (peptidoglycan layer), but penicillin does not harm other species (man). Bovine somatotropin is a protein hormone that increases the growth rate of young cattle and also increases the efficiency of mature cows in converting their feed into milk. Bovine somatotropin has no effect on humans, and (if eaten) is simply digested like any other food protein. It appears that most growth hormones are species specific.

- **Specific activity:** An enzyme unit defined as the number of moles of substrate converted to product by an enzyme preparation per unit time under specified conditions of pH, substrate concentration, temperature, etc. Specific enzyme activity units may be expressed as: moles of product produced/minute/mg of protein used (or mole of enzyme used if the preparation is pure).

- **Spectrophotometer:** An instrument that measures the concentration of a compound that has been dissolved in a solvent (water, alcohol, etc.). The instrument shines a light through the solution, measures the fraction of the light that is absorbed by the solution, and calculates the concentration from that absorbance value (Fig. 4).

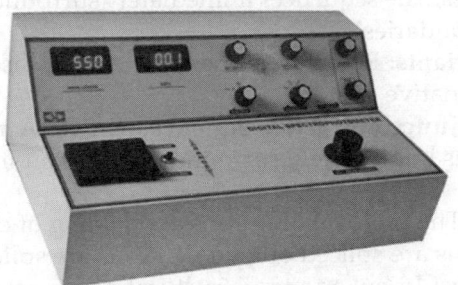

Fig. 4: Spectrophotometer

- **Spheroplast:** A bacterial or yeast cell whose wall has been largely or entirely removed.
- **Spindle:** A slender mass of microtubules formed when a cell divides. At metaphase the chromosomes become attached to it by their centromeres before being pulled towards its ends (Fig. 5).

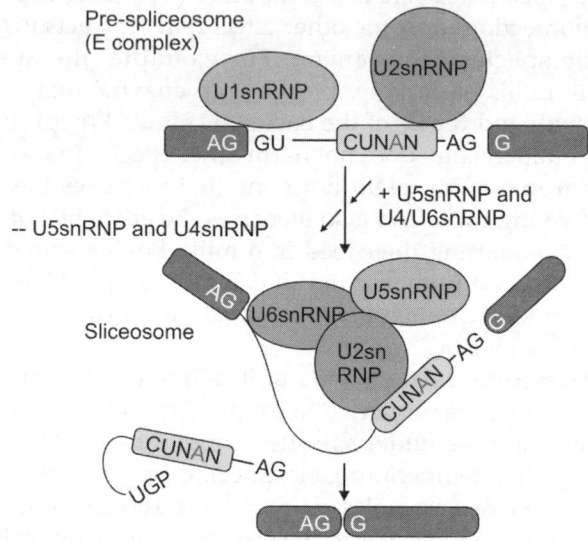

Fig. 5: Splicing

- **Splice recombinant:** DNA results from a Holliday junction being resolved by cutting the non-exchanged strands. Both strands of DNA before the exchange point come from one chromosome; the DNA after the exchange point come from the homologous chromosome.
- **Splice sites:** The sequences immediately surrounding the exon-intron boundaries.
- **Splice variants:** Refers to all possible gene transcripts (arising from alternative splicing).
- **Splicing junctions:** The sequences (in RNA molecules) of nucleotides immediately surrounding the exon-intron boundaries.
- **Splicing:** The removal of introns and joining of exons in RNA; thus introns are spliced out, while exons are spliced together.
- **Split genes:** In eukaryotes, structural genes are split up by a number of non-coding regions called introns.

S

- **Spliceosome:** A complex formed by the snRNPs that are required for splicing together with additional protein factors.
- **Spontaneous mutation:** Mutations that occur in the absence of any added mutagen to increase the mutation rate, as a result of errors in replication.
- **Sporulation:** The generation of a spore by a bacterium (by morphological conversion) or by a yeast (as the product of meiosis).
- **SPS:** Acronym for the Sanitary and Phytosanitary Standards Agreement of the World Trade Organization (WTO), a multinational trading agreement that "sets the rules" governing international trade. Sanitary (human and animal) and phytosanitary (i.e. plant) standards are important in preventing the transfer of diseases from one nation to another via international trade. SPS standards are designed to protect animal, plant, and human life/health (within WTO member countries) from: 1. Entry of pests (insects, weeds, etc.) 2. Entry of disease-carrying organisms (European Corn Borer) 3. Entry of disease-causing organisms (*Aspergillus flavus*) 4. Toxins, contaminants, or disease-causing organisms in foods, beverages, or feedstuffs WTO member nations are required to base their SPS standards as much as possible on existing (e.g. Codex Alimentarius, IPPC, and OIE) international sanitary/phytosanitary standards and practices.
- **Squalamine:** A potent antimicrobial agent (steroid, antibiotic) discovered in the tissues of the dogfish shark in 1992. It has been found to be active against a broad spectrum of bacteria, protozoa, and fungi. Squalamine was chemically synthesized by man in 1993.
- **Squalene:** A sterol that is produced in some plants.
- **SR protein:** It has a variable length of n Arg-Ser-rich region and is involved in splicing.
- **SRB (sulfate reducing bacterium):** Any organism that metabolically reduces sulfate to H_2S (hydrogen sulfide). This includes a variety of microorganisms.
- **sRNA:** A small bacterial RNA that functions as a regulator of gene expression.
- **SSB:** The single-strand protein of *E. coli*, a protein that binds to single-stranded DNA.
- **Stachyose:** A carbohydrate (oligosaccharide) naturally produced in soybeans (and some other plants), relatively

insoluble in water, and much less available for digestion by monogastric animals (swine, poultry) than the other carbohydrate components within soybeans.

- **Stacking:** Ordering or arranging and concentrating macromolecules according to their effective mobilities.

- **Staggered cuts:** The cleavage of two opposite strands of duplex DNA at points near one another.

- **Starch:** A polymer of glucose molecules (a polysaccharide) used by plants to store energy. Plants produce starch in two different molecular forms, amylopectin and amylose. For example, the starch content in traditional corn (maize) kernels averages 72–76% amylopectin and 24–28% amylose. Starch is broken down by enzymes (amylases) to yield glucose, which can be used as an energy source. The analogous polymer used by mammalian systems is called glycogen or, in old usage, "animal starch".

- **START (restriction point):** It is the point during Gl phase at which a cell becomes committed to division.

- **Startpoint (startsite):** The position on DNA corresponding to the first base incorporated into RNA.

- **Stationary phase:** The portion of separation system that is immobilized in the column.

- **Stearate (stearic acid):** A saturated fatty acid, containing 18 carbon atoms in its molecular "backbone", that is essentially neutral in effect on coronary heart disease in humans (i.e. doesn't appreciably increase low-density lipoproteins in the bloodstream). Because of the heart disease neutrality, stearate-containing oils (high-stearate soybean oil) are an acceptable cooking oil choice, with resistance to oxidation/breakdown of a saturated fatty acid, but no bloodstream-cholesterol increasing effect. In mid-1990s, the American Cocoa Research Institute/ Chocolate Manufacturers Association filed a petition with the US-FDA to differentiate stearate (on food product labels) from the other saturated long-chain fatty acids used as food ingredients. In order to make milk, dairy cows require more stearic acid than a conventional digestive system, alone could be provided from the cow's (mainly carbohydrate) diet. Therefore, cows utilize microorganisms living in their rumen (a special sort of pre-stomach) to convert carbohydrate (grass) to stearic acid. Thus, high-performance dairy cows might benefit from a diet that contains high-stearate soybeans, if their milk output is limited by dietary stearate availability.

- **Stearoyl-ACP desaturase:** A "family" of enzymes that is naturally produced in oilseed plants. They play the central role in determining the ratio of saturated to unsaturated fatty acids (in the vegetable oils produced from such plants).
- **Stem cell growth factor (SCF):** A growth factor (glycoprotein hormone) that acts upon stem cells in a wide variety of ways to increase growth, proliferation, and maturity (into red blood cells or white blood cells).
- **Stem cell:** The single stem cell in the bone marrow of a fetus from which every immune system cell in the adult is subsequently derived. The primordial stem cell is stimulated to develop into the mature immune system's differentiated, specialized cells by interleukin-7.
- **Stem cell:** A precursor cell that undergoes division and gives rise to different lineages of differentiated cells.
- **Stem:** The base-paired segment of a hairpin.
- **Stereoisomers:** Molecules that have the same structural formula but different spatial arrangements of dissimilar groups (of atoms) bonded to a common atom (in the molecule). Many of the physical and chemical properties of stereoisomers are the same, but there are differences in the crystal structures, in the direction in which they rotate polarized light (which has been passed through a solution of the stereoisomer), and in their use in an enzyme-catalyzed (biological) reaction.
- **Steric hindrance:** Refers to the compression that a group (chemical entity) suffers by being too close to its non-bonded neighbors. If an enzyme and a substrate try to come together in order to react, but the substrate has on it a bulky group that disallows close contact between the two (because the group bumps into the enzyme), then the reaction will not occur because of steric hindrance. Seen another way, two chemical groups bump into each other and cannot get by each other because they are held in place by the bonds binding them to other atoms. Hindrance of movement or activity occurs because chemical groups bump into each other and cannot occupy the same space.
- **Sterile (environment):** One that is free of any living organisms or spores. For example, a hypodermic needle that has been

sterilized (by heating it) and is free of living microorganisms is said to be sterile.

- **Sterile (organism):** One that is unable to reproduce. For example, a bull that has been castrated is rendered sterile.
- **Sterilization:** The process for elimination of microorganisms.
- **Steroid:** A chemical compound composed of a series of four carbon rings joined together to form a (molecular) structural unit called cyclopentanoperhydrophenanthrene. A group of naturally occurring, fat-soluble substances essential to life, usually classed as lipids. Steroids of importance to the body are the sterols, which are bile acids (produced by the liver, characterized by the presence of a carboxyl group in the molecule's side chain), and the hormones of the sex glands and the adrenal cortex. In addition, the plant kingdom possesses a wide variety of steroid glycosides.
- **Steroid receptors:** Transcription factors that are activated by binding of a steroid ligand.
- **Sterol:** A compound containing a planar steroid ring.
- **Sticky ends:** Complementary single strands of DNA (deoxyribonucleic acid) that protrude from opposite ends of a DNA duplex or from ends of different DNA duplex molecules. They can be generated by staggered cuts in DNA. They are called "sticky" because the exposed single strands can bind (stick) to complementary single strands on another DNA molecule. A hybrid piece of DNA is hence produced (by that binding).
- **Stigmasterol:** A phytosterol produced within the seeds of the soybean plant (*Glycine max* L.), among others. Evidence indicates that human consumption of stigmasterol helps reduce levels of total serum cholesterol and low-density lipoproteins (LDLP); thereby lowering risk of coronary heart disease (CHD). Evidence indicates that certain phytosterols (including stigmasterol) interfere with absorption of cholesterol by the intestines, and decreases the body's recovery and reuse of cholesterol-containing bile salts; which causes more cholesterol to be excreted from the body.
- **Stirred tank fermentor:** A bioreactor in which cells or microorganisms are mixed by mechanically driven impellers.
- **Stop codon (termination codon):** One of three triplets (UAG, UAA, UGA) that causes protein synthesis to terminate. They are also known historically as *nonsense codons*. The UAA codon

is called ochre, and the UAA codon as called amber, after the names of the nonsense mutations by which they were originally identified.

- **Strain:** A group or organisms of the same species that possess(es) distinctive genetic characteristics that set it apart from others within the same species, but whose differences are not "severe" enough for it to be considered a different breed or variety (of that species). The basic taxonomic unit of microbiology. Can also be used to designate a population of cells derived from a single cell.

- **Strand displacement:** A mode of replication of some viruses in which a new DNA strand grows by displacing the previous (homologus) strand of the duplex.

- *Streptococcus mutants:* The strain of *Streptococcus* bacteria that grows on the surface of teeth and can contribute to causing tooth "decay" .

- *Streptococcus:* A bacterium of a genus *Streptococcus* that icludes the agents of souring of milk and dental decay, and haemolytic pathogens causing various infections such as fever and pneumonia.

- **Streptolydigins:** Inhibit the elongation of transcription by bacterial RNA polymerase.

- **Stress proteins:** Discovered by Italian biologist Ferruchio Ritossa in the 1960s, these molecules are also called heat-shock proteins. Proteins made by many organisms' (plant, bacteria and mammal) cells when those cells are stressed by environmental conditions such as certain chemicals, pathogens, or heat. When corn/maize (*Zea mays* L.) is stressed during its growing season by high night-time temperatures, than plant switches from its normal production of ("immune system" defense) chitinase to production of heat-shock (i.e. stress) proteins, instead. Stress proteins are also produced by tuberculosis and leprosy bacteria after these bacteria have invaded (infected) cells in the human body, in an attempt by those bacteria to mimic the stress proteins that (mammal) cells would normally manufacture to repair damage done to the (mammal) cells. This mimicry makes it more difficult for the immune system to recognize and attack those pathogenic bacteria (and/or repair mis-shaped protein molecules in the body's cells). Similarly, production of stress proteins helps some types of cancer cells to avoid being attacked by the immune system. Because consumption of genistein by humans causes a reduction in the production of stress proteins, genistein may thereby help the human immune system in destroying cancerous cells. In 1996, Richard I. Morimoto discovered that two stress proteins known as HSP 90 and HSP 70 help ensure that certain crucial proteins in cells are folded into the configuration/conformation needed by that cell.

- **Stringency:** Of a hybridization describes the effect of conditions on the degree of complementarity that is required for reaction. At the most stringent conditions, only exact complements can hybridize. As the stringency is lowered, an increasing number of mismatches can be tolerated between the two strands that are hybridizing.

- **Stringent factor:** It is the protein RelA, which is associated with ribosomes. It synthesizes ppGpp and pppGpp when uncharged aminoacyl-tRNA enters the A site.

- **Stringent replication:** The limitation of single-copy plasmids to replicate *pari passu* with the bacterial chromosome.

- **Stringent response:** The ability of a bacterium to shut down synthesis of tRNA and ribosomes in a poor-growth medium.

- **Stromelysin (MMP-3):** A collagenase (enzyme) that "clears a path" through living tissue, ahead of tumor cells, thereby enabling a cancer to spread within the body.

- **Structural distortion:** A change in the shape of a molecule.

- **Structural gene:** A gene that codes for any ribonucleic acid (RNA) or protein product other than a regulator molecule. It determines the primary sequences (the amino acid sequences) of a polypeptide (protein).

- **Structural genomics:** Study of, or discovery of, where (gene) sequences are located within the genome, and which (DNA) subunits comprise those sequences.

- **Structural maintenance of chromosomes (SMC):** It describes a group of proteins that include the cohesins, which hold sister chromatids together, and the condensins, which are involved in chromosome condensation.

- **Structural periodicity:** The number of base pairs per turn of the double helix of DNA.

- **STR (short tandem repeats):** Short DNA sequences that are repeated in a head-to-tail manner. They are useful in DNA profiling.

- **STS sulfonylurea (herbicide)-tolerant soybeans:** These are soybeans that have been bred (via insertion of ALS gene by traditional breeding methods) to resist the (weed killing) effects of sulfonylurea-based herbicides. The ALS gene was discovered by Scott Sebastian in 1986.

- **Sub-culture:** Sub-division of a culture and its transfer to a fresh medium.

- **Substance P:** A neuropeptide (peptide produced by cells of the nervous system) which is involved in activation of the immune system, pain sensation, and (when in excess) some psychiatric disorders. In the case of chronic, intractable pain (hypersensitivity), approximately 1% of the nerve cells in the human spine processes substance P (thereby "transmitting" its pain message via signal transduction). In 1997, Patrick Mantyh showed that killing those (1%) cells relieved chronic pain hypersensitivity without impairing sense of touch or normal (beneficial) pain sensation, in humans.

- **Substrate (chemical):** The substance acted upon by an enzyme. For example, the enzyme amylase catalyzes the breakdown of starch molecules into glucose polysaccharide molecules; starch is the substrate (of the enzyme amylase).

- **Substrate (in chromatography):** The (usually solid or gel) substance that attracts and noncovalently binds (interacts) with one or more of the molecules in a solution that is passed over that substrate (in a chromatography column). This preferential binding (interaction with the substrate) enables one or more of the solution's molecular ingredients to be separated from the other(s).

- **Substrate (structural):** The substance (support) to which the agent of interest (a molecule) is attached. For example, some catalyst molecules are chemically attached to nonreactive solids to preserve the catalyst from being flushed away when the chemical substrate (the molecule to be converted by the catalyst) is washed by the catalyst immobilized on the structural substrate.

- **Subviral pathogen:** An infectious agent that is smaller than a virus, such as a virusoid.

- **Sudden death syndrome:** A plant disease caused by the *Fusarium solani* fungus, that sometimes afflicts soybean plants.

- **Suicide gene:** A gene that codes for an antibiotic that can kill the host bacterial cell. It is genetically modified into the bacterium along with a molecular switch that is controlled by a nutrient in the environment. When the nutrient disappears the suicide gene is switched on and the bacterium dies.
- **Sulforaphane:** A compound naturally produced within cruciferous plants such as broccoli and cabbage. Research indicates that human consumption of significant amounts of sulforaphane helps lower the risk of several cancers.
- **Sulfosate:** An active ingredient in some herbicides, it kills plants (weeds) by inhibiting the crucial plant enzyme EPSP synthase. Chemically, sulfosate is a trimethylsulfonium salt of the same organic acid as glyphosate, so sulfosate can be applied over crops (soybeans) that have been genetically engineered to be tolerant to glyphosate- based herbicides.
- **Superantigens:** Certain types of antigens that activate a large proportion of an organism's immune system T cells. These superantigens, which thus over activates the organism's immune system, are thought to be responsible for some auto-immune diseases (in which T cells attack and destroy the organism's own, healthy tissues).
- **Superbug:** A recombinant *Pseudomonas putida* prepared by Dr AM Chakrabarty.
- **Supercoiling:** Also known as superhelicity. The coiling of a closed duplex DNA (deoxyribonucleic acid) in space so that it crosses over its own axis (Fig. 6).
- **Supercritical carbon dioxide:** A solvent that, when combined with water and an appropriate surfactant (fluoroethers), forms

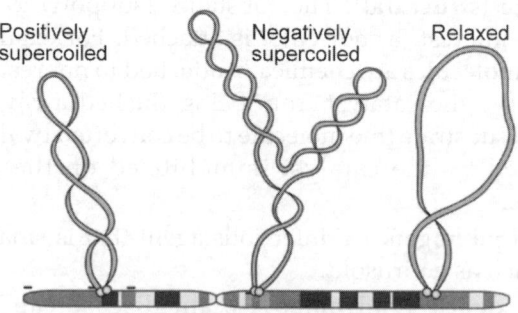

Fig. 6: Supercoiling

a solvent system that can effectively dissolve large biological molecules without causing those molecules to lose biological activity. Carbon dioxide is a gas at normal (atmospheric) pressure and ambient temperature, but in its supercritical state— temperature above 31.3°C (88°F) and pressure greater than 72.9 atmospheres—carbon dioxide becomes a dense (sort of) liquid. Some coffee processors have used supercritical carbon dioxide as a solvent to remove caffeine from coffee. In 1995, Keith Johnston added the surfactant ammonium carboxylate perfluoropolyether to a supercritical carbon dioxide system containing water and proved that the large biological molecule bovine serum albumin, dissolved inside the micelles, that form via water droplet surrounded by fluoroether molecules. Subsequent to that, Eric Beckman proved that the protease subtilisin Carlsberg can be extracted from crude (impure) cell broth because that protease preferentially dissolves in a supercritical carbon dioxide/water system containing fluoroether amphiphiles as surfactants.

- **Supercritical fluid:** Refers to a material that has been heated to a temperature above its (normal atmospheric pressure) boiling point, but which is kept in a state that resembles a liquid via the application of high pressure. Less commonly, refers to a liquid that has been cooled to a temperature below its normal freezing point, but which is kept in a liquid state by various means. For example, water will remain "liquid" upto a temperature of 375°C (617°F) if it is placed under enough pressure. Ammonia will remain "liquid" upto a temperature of 133°C (271°F) if it is placed under enough pressure, despite the fact that ammonia normally becomes a gas (at standard atmospheric pressure) whenever the temperature is higher than –33.35°C (–30°F). One predatory mite (*Alaskozetes antarcticus*) living in Antarctica is able to survive subfreezing temperatures by preventing ice crystals from (supercritical water) inside its body, even when the environmental temperature is below the freezing point (supercritical). Most supercritical fluids have unique physical properties (they are often better solvents than their true liquid forms). Some supercritical fluids (supercritical carbon dioxide) can be used to extract biological molecules (chlorophyll) from mixtures (ground-up plant leaves). After the biological molecule has dissolved out of the mixture, the biological molecule is recovered by releasing pressure so the carbon dioxide returns to gaseous form, and drifts away.

- *Superfamify:* A set of genes a related by presumed descent from a common ancestor, but now showing considerable variation.
- **Superrepressed:** The occurrence of changes that eliminate the effects of a mutation, without reversing the original change in DNA.
- **Support:** The particles on which the stationary phase is held.
- **Suppression:** Describes the occurrence of changes that eliminate the effects of a mutation without reversing the original change in DNA.
- **Suppressor (extragenic):** Usually a gene coding a mutant tRNA that reads the mutated codon either in the sense of the original codon or to give an acceptable substitute for the original meaning.
- **Suppressor (intragenic):** A compensating mutation that restores the original reading frame after a frameshift.
- **Suppressor gene:** A gene that can reverse the effect of a specific type of mutation in other genes, such as a premature termination sequence.
- **Suppressor mutation:** A mutation that totally or partially restores a function lost by a primary mutation. It is located at a site in the gene different from the site of the primary mutation.
- **Suppressor T cells:** Those T cells (thymus derived lymphocytes) that are triggered (after other types of T cells and other immune system cells have successfully fought-off an infection) to slow down gradually and halt the body's immune response (to the now-conquered pathogen). Discovered by Tomio Tada in 1971, suppressor T cells inhibit B cell activity. Failure to halt the immune response in time could lead to harm to the body by its own immune system. The B and T lymphocytes are indistinguishable in size and general morphology. Only the existence or nonexistence of certain proteins on their cell surface distinguishes the two classes of lymphocytes.
- **Supramolecular assembly:** Refers to a very large molecular structure.
- **Surfactant:** Acronym for surface active agent. Amphipathic molecules (i.e. molecules that contain both a polar and nonpolar domain) due to their unique properties, position themselves at interfacial regions (surfaces) such as an oil/water interface.

S

When surfactants are dissolved above a certain critical concentration in either water or nonpolar solvents, they may form micelles or reverse micelles, respectively. Surfactants are commonly used to solubilize cell membrane components and other hard-to-solubilize molecules.

- **Surrogate:** A person or animal that functions as a substitute for another. In the case of a surrogate mother, a woman or female animal carries an embryo and ultimately gives birth to a baby that was formed from the egg of another female.

- **Surveillance:** The systems check nucleic acids for errors. The term is used in several different contexts. One example is the system that degrades mRNAs that have nonsense mutations. Another is the set of systems that react to damage in the double helix. The common feature is that the system recognizes an invalid sequence or structure and triggers a response.

- **Suspension culture:** A culture consisting of cell aggregates initiated by placing callus tissue or sometimes seedling in an agitated liquid medium.

- **Sustainable development:** Defined in 1987 United Nations report "our common future" to be development (e.g. economic development) that meets the needs of the present without compromising the ability of future generations to meet their own needs.

- **SWI/SNF:** A chromatin remodeling complex; it uses hydrolysis of ATP to change the organization of nucleosomes.

- **Switch proteins:** Refers to certain protein molecules that signal a plant when environmental conditions are so dry (or cold, etc.) that the plant needs to protect itself (via extreme measures) to survive.

- **Symbiosis:** A symbiotic relationship between two organisms for mutual benefits.

- **Symbiotic:** Refers to the mutually beneficial living together of organisms, in an intimate association or union. For example, lichen are a life form consisting of algae and a fungus growing together as a unit on a solid surface (e.g. a tree trunk or a rock). Each helps the other to survive and grow.

- **Symporter:** A type of carrier protein that moves two different solutes across the plasma membrane in the same direction. The two solutes can be transported simultaneously or sequentially.

- **Synapse:** A connection between a neuron and a target cell at which chemical information or electrical impulses may be transmitted.
- **Synapsis:** The association of the two pairs of sister chromatids representing homologous chromosomes that occurs at the start of meiosis; the resulting structure is called a bivalent (Fig. 7) .

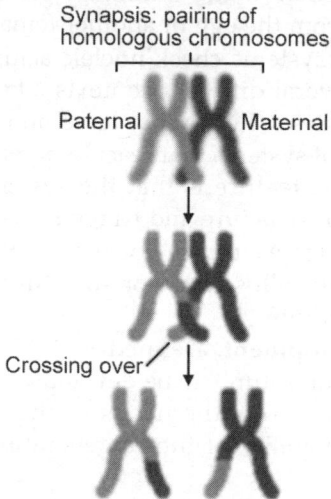

Synapsis: pairing of homologous chromosomes

Paternal   Maternal

Crossing over

Fig. 7: Synapsis

- **Synaptonemal complex:** The morphological structure of synapsed chromosomes.
- **Synchronous culture:** A symbiotic in which a specified proportion of the cells are at the same phase of the cell cycle, enters the same indicated phase of the cell cycle simultaneously, and/or exhibit approximately the same duration of cell cycle.
- **Synonym:** Codons haves the same meaning in the genetic code.
- **Synonym tRNAs:** Bear the same amino acid and responds to the same codon.
- **Syntenic:** Genetic loci lie on the same chromosome.
- **Synteny:** Describes a relationship between chromosomal regions of different species where homologous genes occur in the same order.

- **Synthesizing (of DNA molecules):** The building (i.e. polymerization) of a known sequence of nucleotides into a chain called an oligonucleotide (of which genes are made) or DNA (deoxyribonucleic acid). Invented by Har Gobind Khurana and his colleagues at the University of Wisconsin, Madison, in 1968, this process enables scientists to create genes or gene fragments for use in research. In 1973, Robert Bruce Merrifield developed a means to partially automate the oligonucleotide assembly process. This led to automated machines that can now rapidly manufacture a gene fragment, gene, or DNA probe.
- **Synthesizing (of oligosaccharides):** Chemical synthesis (manufacture) of a known oligosaccharide (structure). For example, a synthesis of a defined-sequence oligosaccharide (molecular) "branch" at a specific site on a glycoprotein in order to "cover up" an antigenic site on that glycoprotein molecule (e.g. so the glycoprotein can be used as a pharmaceutical).
- **Synthesizing (of proteins):** Chemical synthesis (manufacture) of a known protein molecule. Devised based upon the solid phase synthesis methodology developed by Robert Bruce Merrifield in 1963, the desired proteins are assembled by repetitive coupling of the constituent amino acids to a growing polypeptide backbone, which itself is attached to a polymeric support (substrate). This procedure has been automated, so it is now possible to make proteins via automated synthesizers.
- **Systematics:** An extension of taxonomy, it is the scientific classification of living organisms.
- **Systemic acquired resistance (SAR):** Discovered in 1992 (applicable to harpin induced SAR) and in 1996 by J.A. Ryals, U.H. Neuenschwander, M.G. Willits, A. Molina, H.Y. Steiner, and M.D. Hunt, SAR is a sort of "immune (cascade) response" by a plant, against infection (by bacteria, fungus, etc.). One example of this is the production of stress proteins or pathogenesis related proteins when certain plants are attacked by certain pathogens. Via such SAR response triggered by low-level fungal or viral infection, many plants successfully resist fungal/bacterial/viral attacks. In 1998, the U.S. Environmental Protection Agency (EPA) approved one herbicide (COBRAR owned by Valent Corp.), whose active ingredient is the chemical

lactofin, to be applied to soybean plants "at or near bloom stage" in order to trigger SAR against white mold disease. In 2000, the U.S. EPA approved harpin protein to be applied to some crops in order to trigger SAR against certain plant diseases.

- **Systems biology:** A hypothesis driven field of research that creates predictive mathematical models of complex biological processes or organ systems.

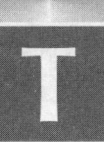

- **"Treatment" IND regulations:** Food and drug administration (FDA) regulations promulgated in 1987, to provide a more rapid formal pharmaceutical approval mechanism than the usual Investigational New Drug (IND) regulatory approval process. Its purpose is to enable drug developers to provide promising experimental drugs to patients suffering from immediately life-threatening diseases or certain serious conditions e.g. acquired immune deficiency syndrome (AIDS), or before complete data on that drug's efficacy or toxicity are available.
- **T – DNA:** A fragment of Ti-plasmid of *Agrobacterium tumifaciens* that is transferred and integrated into chromosome of plant cells.
- **T cell growth factor (TCGF):** Also known as Interleukin-2.
- **T cell modulating peptide (TCMP):** A short protein chain that is thought to restrain certain types of T cells from attacking an (arthritis) afflicted patient's tissues (mainly cartilage). Arthritis is caused by the sufferer's own immune system attacking the body's cartilage tissues.
- **T cell receptor (TCR):** The antigen receptor on T lymphocytes. It is clonally expressed and binds to a complex of MHC class I or class II protein, and antigen-derived peptide.
- **T cells:** Lymphocytes of the T (thymic) lineage; may be subdivided into several functional types. They carry a TCR (T-cell receptor) and are involved in the cell-mediated immune response (Fig. 1).
- **T4 bacteriophage:** A bacteriophage is a virus which infects bacteria. It contains about 168.800 base pairs of double stranded DNA.
- **T4 DNA ligase:** An enzyme produced by *E. coli* after infection by T4 bacteriophage. It catalyses the joining of DNA duplex and repairs nick in DNA molecules. It uses ATP as source of energy.

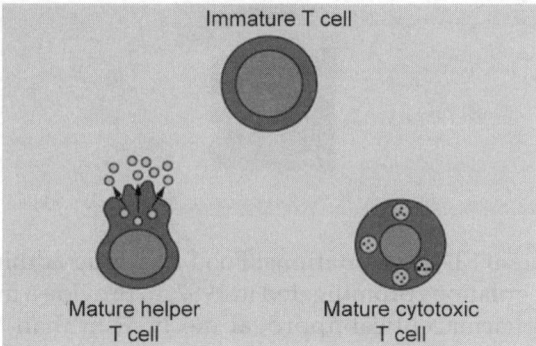

Fig. 1: T cells

- **Tachykinins:** A class of neuropeptides (peptides produced by cells of the nervous system; neurons) that includes neurokinin A, neurokinin B, eledoisin, physalaemin, kassinin, substance P, and substance K. Some of these neuropeptides (e.g. substance P) are picked up by mast cells, lymphocytes, and/or monocytes; and cause those three types of immune system cells to release certain lymphokines (tumor necrosis factor, interleukin-1, etc.), thus activating the immune system.

- **TBP-associated factors (TAFs):** The subunits of transcription factor (TFnD) that assist TATA binding protein (TBP) in binding to DNA. They also provide points of contact for other components of the transcription apparatus.

- **Tailing:** Addition of some nucleotides *in vitro* by the enzyme terminal transferase to 3'-OH ends of a duplex DNA molecule. It is also called homopolymer tailing.

- **Tandem array:** A DNA molecule containing two or more identical sequences in series.

- **Tandem repeats:** Multiple copies of the same sequence lying in series.

- *Taq* **DNA polymerase:** A 94 kilodalton DNA polymerase, which was originally isolated from the thermophilic bacteria *Thermus aquaticus*. Commonly utilized to catalyze PCR reactions due to its heat resistance (needed for thermal cycles utilized in the PCR technique).

- **Target (of a herbicide or insecticide):** The molecule (receptor, enzyme, etc.) within a weed plant or a pest insect, a given herbicide or insecticide is "aimed" at (e.g. when scientists are conducting research aimed at creating that herbicide or insecticide). For example, glyphosate-containing herbicides act on the (target) crucial plant enzyme EPSP synthase. For example, insect resistant transgenic plants containing "*Bt* gene(s)" act on (target) receptors inside the digestive system of specific insect species via the *Bt* protoxin.

- **Target (of a therapeutic agent):** The molecule (receptor) or moiety that a given drug or therapeutic regimen (e.g. gene delivery) is "aimed" at (when scientists are working to create/discover that drug or regimen). Targets can normally be occurring constituents of the body (receptors, enzymes, factors, hormones, ion channels, nuclear receptors, DNA, etc.), non abnormal constituents of the body (tumors, antigens on tumor surfaces, etc.), or pathogenic (external, invading) agents (microorganisms, viruses, parasites, etc.).

- **Target-ligand interaction screening:** A methodology of high-throughput screening (HTS) that is utilized to screen a large number of candidates (e.g. compounds) based upon their interaction (e.g. chemical "binding") to a preselected "target" (e.g. molecule present within a cell membrane, molecule placed on a biochip or other bioassay to facilitate HTS, molecule present on the surface of a nematode utilized in HTS, etc.).

- **Target-site duplication:** A sequence of DNA that is duplicated when a transposable element inserts, usually found at the end of insertion.

- **TAT:** The name of a protein that helps the HIV ("AIDS virus") to cross the human cell plasma membrane, thereby enabling infection to those cells by human immunodeficiency virus (HIV). TAT is the main activator of HIV gene expression in cells; it is a protein which complexes with TAR (a 60-nucleotide sequence found in all viral messenger ribonucleic acid) to mediate synthesis of proteins (in an infected cell) necessary for HIV to reproduce.

- **TATA box:** A conserved A-T-rich septamer found about 25 bp before the startpoint of each eukaryotic RNA polymerase II transcription unit; may be involved in positioning the enzyme for correct initiation.

- **TATA homology:** An adenine-thymidine-rich (gene) sequence present 20–30 nucleotides "upstream" of the transcription start site on most eukaryotic protein coding genes; it is required for correct expression. Recent research indicates that blocking this portion of the (gene) sequence may inhibit ability of the AIDS virus to reproduce.

- **TATA-binding protein (TBP):** The subunit of transcription factor TFTID that binds to DNA.
- **TATA-less promoter:** Does not have a TATA box in the sequence upstream of its start point.
- **Tautomerization:** The process of shifting of hydrogen atoms from one position to another in a purine or in a pyrimidine base. Product of this process is known as tautomer.
- **Taxol:** A phytochemical that is naturally produced in some plants and functions to protect those plants from the plant pathogen known as water mold. Coined during the 1960s by Monroe E Wall when it was originally isolated from the Pacific yew tree (genus *Taxus*), Taxol™ is now a trademark of the Bristol-Myers Squibb Co. refering to the antitumor pharmaceutical sold by the company. The active compound from Pacific yew tree is now known as paclitaxel. Both Taxol™ and paclitaxel act by binding and stabilizing microtubules in cells (thereby halting/preventing the uncontrolled cell growth/proliferation that is cancer).
- **Tay-sachs disease:** A lethal hereditary disease. The progressive accumulation of a substance called ganglioside in the brain causes paralysis, mental deterioration and blindness. Death usually occurs before the age of four.
- **TBT:** Acronym for the technical barriers to trade (TBT) agreement to WTO.
- **T-DNA:** The segment of the Ti plasmid of *Agrobacterium tumefaciens* that is transferred to the plant cell nucleus during infection. It carries genes that transform the plant cell.
- **Technical barriers to trade (TBT) agreement:** The agreement to GATT/WTO, via which WTO member nations agreed to base their import (restrictive) regulations and standards (e.g. mandatory packaging, package marking, testing, certification, labeling requirements, etc.)—known as TBT measures—only on scientific assessments of actual risks (i.e. for those TBT measures intended to protect human health, animal and plant health, or the environment) and to require only those TBT measures that do not create unnecessary obstacles to international trade.

- **Technical barriers to trade (TBT) measures:** These are (restrictive) import regulations and standards (e.g. mandatory packaging, package marking, testing, certification and labeling requirements, etc.). Some of them are designed to protect human health, animal and plant health, and/or the environment. In the Technical Barriers to Trade (TBT) Agreement to GATT/WTO, the WTO member nations agreed to base their TBT measures only on requirements that do not create unnecessary obstacles to international trade.

- **Technology transfer:** The process of transferring discoveries made by basic research institutions such as universities and government laboratories to the commercial sector for development into useful products and services.

- **Telethia controversia koon smut:** A fungal disease that sometimes afflicts wheat (*Triticum aestivum*) plants.

- **Telomerase:** An enzyme that enables the "repair" of telomeres (thereby stabilizing their length, and preventing "shortening" of the telomeres). The telomerase enzyme is only present in cancerous cells (thereby enabling the "immortality" of cancerous cells). Human telomerase contains an RNA component and a catalytic-protein component (a member of the reverse transcriptase "family" of enzymes).

- **Telomeres:** DNA sequences, that do not code for proteins, which are located at the (end) tips of chromosomes. Telomeres consist of the sequence GGGGTT repeated many times. With the exception of certain types of cells (zygotes, cancerous cells, "immortal" hybridoma cells), portions of each telomere "breaks off" each time the cell containing that chromosome divides. This "shortening" process serves to limit the lifetime (number of replications) of those (noncancerous, nonzygote, nonhybridoma, etc.) cells.

- **Telomeric silencing:** Describes the repression of gene activity that occurs in the vicinity of a telomere.

- **Temperate bacteriophage:** A bacteriophage having a lysogenic life cycle and capable of inserting its DNA into that of the host bacterium.

- **Temperature-sensitive mutation:** Creates a gene product that is functional at low temperature but inactive at higher temperature (the reverse relationship is usually called cold-sensitive).

- **Template:** In general terms, it is a mold or pattern that can be copied or its shape reproduced. When used with reference to molecular dimensions, it is a macromolecular mold or pattern for the synthesis of another macromolecule. An RNA or single stranded DNA molecules on which a complementary strand is synthesized. It is also called antisense strand.

- **Template strand:** The polynucleotide strand being used by DNA polymerase for determining nucleotide sequence during synthesis of a new strand.

- **Teosinte:** A wild plant (*Zea diploperennis*), native to the country of Mexico, which is related to (domesticated) corn/maize (*Zea mays* L.).

- **Teratoma:** A growth in which many differentiated cell types including skin, teeth, bone and others grow in disorganized manner after an early embryo is transplanted into one of the tissues of an adult animal.

- **Terminal protein:** Allows replication of a linear phage genome to start at the end. The protein attaches to the 5' end of the genome through a covalent bond, is associated with a DNA polymerase, and contains a cytosine residue that serves as a primer.

- **Terminal redundancy:** The repetition of the same sequence at both ends of a phage genome.

- **Terminal region:** The part of an N-linked oligosaccharide that consists of all the sugar residues added subsequent to formation of the inner core.

- **Terminal system:** In *Drosophila*, the terminal system is one of the maternal systems that establishes the polarity of the oocyte. The set of genes in the terminal system play a role in the proper formation of the terminal structures at both ends of the fly.

- **Terminal transferase:** An enzyme that adds nucleotides to the 43 kd N-terminus of DNA molecules.

- **Terminalization:** Repelling movement of the centromeres of bivalents in the diplotene stage of the meiotic prophase that tends to move the visible chiasmata towards the ends of the bivalents.

- **Terminase:** Enzyme cleaves multimers of a viral genome and then uses hydrolysis of ATP to provide the energy to translocate the DNA into an empty viral capsid starting with the cleaved end.

- **Termination codon:** Also known as terminator sequence. One of three triplet sequences (U-A-G, U-A-A, or U-G-A) found in DNA molecules (genes) that cause termination of protein synthesis;

they are also called nonsense codons. The sequences cause the termination of the peptide chain and its release in free form.

- **Termination:** A separate reaction that ends a macromolecular synthesis reaction (replication, transcription, or translation), by stopping the addition of subunits, and (typically) causing dissolution of the synthetic apparatus.
- **Terminator:** A sequence of DNA, represented at the end of the transcript, that causes RNA polymerase to terminate transcription.
- **Terminus:** A segment of DNA at which replication ends.
- **Ternary complex:** In initiation of transcription consists of RNA polymerase and DNA and a dinucleotide that represents the first two bases in the RNA product.
- **Tertiary structure:** The three-dimensional folding of the polypeptide (i.e. protein) molecular chains that characterizes a protein molecule in its native state.
- **Test cross:** A cross between a heterozygous individual or one of the unknown genotype and an individual homozygous recessive for the gene in question. When a single trait is being studied, a test cross is a cross between an individual with the dominant phenotype but of unknown genotype (homozygous or heterozygous) with a homozygous recessive individual. If the unknown is heterozygous (Yy), then approximately 50% of the offspring should display the recessive phenotype (Yy × yy gives 1:1 ratio).
- **Testosterone:** An androgen (steroid hormone) that is biochemically synthesized (made) from androstenedione, which is itself synthesized from progesterone. Testosterone is responsible for the development of male secondary sex characteristics in humans such as greater strength, larger body size, facial hair, a deeper voice, etc.
- **Tetrahydrofolic acid:** The reduced, active coenzyme form of the vitamin folic acid; involved in C1 transfers. Tetrahydrofolate (also known as FH4) serves as an intermediate carrier (molecule) of methyl, hydroxymethyl, or formyl groups (all containing one carbon atom) in a relatively large number of enzymatic reactions in which such one-carbon groups are transferred from one metabolite to another.
- **TFnD:** The transcription factor that binds to the TATA sequence upstream of the start-point of promoters for RNA polymerase

II. It consists of TBP (TATA binding protein) and the TAF subunits that bind to TBP.

- **TGA:** The government regulatory agency charged with approving all pharmaceutical products sold within Australia.
- **Thalassemia:** Disease of red blood cells resulting from lack of either α or β globin.
- **Thale cress:** Common name for *Arabidopsis thaliana*.
- **Thawing:** A slight melting of precooled specimen before long-term storage at −196°C.
- **Theoretical plate number:** A number defining the efficiency of the chromatographic column.
- **Therapeutic agent:** A chemical compound used for treatment of disease. It is also called as drug.
- **Therapeutic cloning:** Generally refered to as somatic cell nuclear transfer technology. It involves replacing the nucleus of an egg cell with the nucleus from a cell from a patient's body and allowing it to develop to form a blastocyst. The embryonic stem cells from the inner cell mass, are then harvested and used to establish a cell line that has the same genetic makeup of the patient. These cells can then be directed to develop into the tissue needed for transplant.
- **Thermoduric:** An organism that can survive high temperatures but does not necessarily grow at such temperatures.
- **Thermophile:** An organism whose optimum temperature for growth is close to, or exceeds, the boiling point of water (100°C, 212°F).
- **Thermophilic bacteria:** Literally "heat loving" bacteria. They are a category of thermophiles generally found near geothermal vents beneath bodies of water.
- **Thioesterase:** A "family" of enzymes naturally produced within some plants, such as the California bay tree (*Umbellularia californica*). Thioesterase catalyzes those plants' production of the fatty acid laurate.
- **Thiol group:** Refers to a specific chemical entity (on a molecule).
- **Third base degeneracy:** Describes the lesser effect on codon meaning of the nucleotide present at the third codon position.
- **Threonine (thr):** A crystalline, α-amino acid considered essential for normal growth of animals. It is biosynthesized (made) from aspartic acid and is a precursor of isoleucine in microorganisms.

T

- **Thrombin:** The key to thrombus (blood clot) formation. Thrombin is a proteolytic enzyme that cleaves fibrinogen into (molecular) pieces, which then spontaneously assemble themselves into fibrin, which forms a clot.
- **Thrombolytic agents:** Blood-borne compounds (such as tissue plasminogen activator) that work to disintegrate (breakup or lyse) blood clots.
- **Thrombomodulin:** A cell surface protein found on endothelial cells that plays a key role in modulating the final step in the coagulation process. After thrombin binds to thrombomodulin, thrombin loses its ability to cleave fibrinogen to form fibrin. In addition, once thrombin binds to thrombomodulin, thrombin's activation of protein C is increased 200-fold and this activated protein C then degrades factors Va and VIIIa which are both required for the production of thrombin from prothrombin. Hence, thrombomodulin modulates the activity of the enzyme thrombin causing a cessation of full-blown clotting activity.
- **Thrombosis:** The intravascular (i.e. inside of blood vessel) formation of a blood clot.
- **Thrombus:** The blood clot itself. The mass of blood coagulated *in situ* in the heart or other blood vessel. For example, such a clot causes a heart attack when the coagulation occurs in the vessels feeding the heart.
- **Thymine (thy):** A pyrimidine component of nucleic acid first isolated from the thymus. Its hydrogen-bonding counterpart in RNA is uracil (Fig. 2).

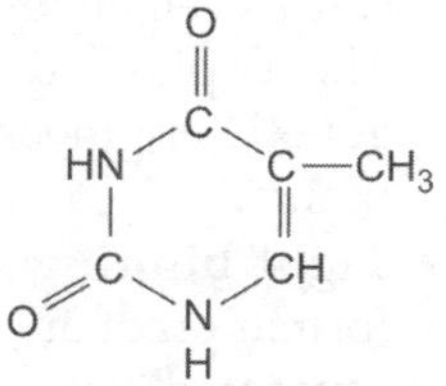

Thymine (T) in DNA

Fig. 2: Thymine

- **Thymine dimer:** A chemically cross-linked pair of adjacent thymine residues in DNA, a result of damage induced by ultraviolet irradiation.
- **Thymoleptics:** A class of drugs that primarily exerts its effect on the brain influencing feeling and behavior.
- **Thymus:** A gland that enables cells of the immune system of mammals to mature. In humans, it lies behind the breast bone and extends upward as far as the thyroid gland. The thymus is the place in the body where T lymphocytes are "taught" to distinguish foreign (e.g. pathogen) antigens from "self" cell antigens, to avoid immune responses in which the body's

immune system attacks organs and other cells within the body (resulting in autoimmune diesease). Any T lymphocytes that remain "autoreactive" (i.e. would tend to attack "self" cells, such as organs in the body) are destroyed by the thymus via a cytotoxic mechanism. An example of an autoimmune disease is multiple sclerosis (MS), where the body's acetylcholine receptors are attacked by the body's immune system. Since acetylcholine is crucial in the transmission of nerve impulses to the body's muscles, such destruction of acetylcholine receptors results in loss of control of the body's muscles.

- **Thyroid gland:** A gland that is found on both sides of the trachea ("windpipe") in humans. This gland secretes the hormone thyroxine, which increases the rate of metabolism.

- **Thyroid stimulating hormone (TSH):** A hormone that causes the thyroid gland to secrete additional amount of thyroxine.

- **Ti plasmid:** Abbreviation for tumor-inducing plasmid or tumor induction plasmid. It is the plasmid of *Agrobacterium tumefaciens* bacteria that naturally has part of its DNA transferred to a plant when *Agrobacterium tumefaciens* infects that plant (e.g. via a wound in the plant). After it has been transferred into the plant, that Ti plasmid DNA segment (now known as T-DNA or transferred DNA) inserts itself into the plant's DNA, where it causes cells to grow into tumor-like structures known as galls. The Ti plasmid can be modified so that it can be utilized (by genetic engineers) to insert genes from other organisms into plants.

- **Tight binding:** Of RNA polymerase to DNA describes the formation of an open complex (when the strands of DNA have separated).

- **TIM complex:** Resides in the inner membrane of mitochondria and is responsible for transporting proteins from the intermembrane space into the interior of the organelle.

- **t-IND treatment:** Investigational New Drug Application to the US Food and Drug Administration (US-FDA).

- **Tissue culture:** The growth and maintenance (by researchers) of cells from higher organisms *in vitro*, i.e. in a sterile test tube or petri dish environment which contains the nutrients necessary for cell growth. One use of tissue culture is to produce disease free offspring from certain (valuable, high quality) crop plants. Another use of tissue culture methods is for "embryo rescue" to enable "wide crosses" between two different species of plants. In that procedure, pollen from one plant species (e.g. a wild plant possessing disease resistance) is induced to fertilize a plant from another species (e.g. a domesticated crop). The resultant fertilized plant embryo, which would not grow on its own, is "rescued" via tissue culture methods. Following maturation, that wide cross (i.e. a hybrid plant from two species that normally would not cross) produces fertile seeds on its own without any need for further intervention by man.

- **Tissue plasminogen activator (tPA):** A glycoprotein that possesses thrombolytic (blood clot-dissolving) activity. It is used as a drug to dissolve clots and acts by first binding to fibrin (clots). It then activates (proteolytically cleaves) plasminogen (molecules) to yield plasmin, a blood-borne enzyme that itself cleaves molecular bonds in the fibrin clot. The plasmin molecules diffuse through the fibrin clot and cause the clot to dissolve rapidly. With the dissolution of the clot, blood flow to the formerly blocked blood vessel (e.g. the heart) is restored.

- **T_m:** The abbreviation for melting temperature.

- **TME (N):** Abbreviation for "true metabolizable energy (corrected for nitrogen)"; a measure of the amount of energy that a given animal (e.g. chicken) can extract from a given feed ration.

- **Tn:** Bacterial transposons that contain markers that are not related to their function, e.g. drug resistance, are named as Tn followed by a number.

- **Tobacco hornworm:** Caterpillars (pupae) of the Lepidopteran insect *Manduca sexta*. Tobacco Hornworm is susceptible to Cry1A(b) protein (e.g. they are killed if they eat plants genetically engineered to contain Cry1A(b) protein).

- **Tobacco mosaic virus (TMV):** One of the smallest viruses, consisting of some 2,200 chains of identical polypeptides and a molecule of RNA. All of the genetic/heredity information of the Tobacco Mosaic Virus is contained in its RNA. The first discovery of a self-assembling, active biological structure occurred in 1955, when Heinz Frankel et el. showed that TMV will reassemble into functioning, infectious virus particles (after the TMV has been dissociated into its components via immersion in concentrated acetic acid). The TMV virus infects the leaves of tomato and tobacco plants, causing disease. Tobacco plants can be genetically engineered to resist TMV infection. A tomato plant, genetically engineered to resist TMV infection, has been commercially available since 1992 (Fig. 3).

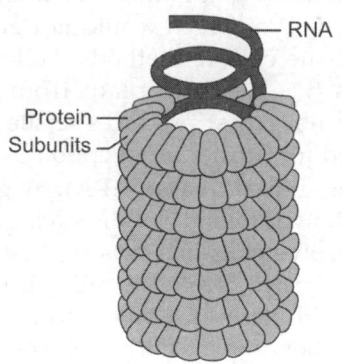

Fig. 3: Tobacco mosaic virus

- **Tocopherols:** A family of different molecular forms of vitamin E each of which has a saturated phytyl "tail" attached (to the "backbone" of the molecule). Commercial tocopherols are extracted from soybeans, although some are also naturally present in canola and sunflower.
- **Tocotrienols:** A family of different molecular forms of vitamin E each of which has an unsaturated isoprenoid "side chain" attached (to the "backbone" of the molecule). Tocotrienols are naturally present in cereal grains (oats, barley, rye, and rice bran).
- **Tolerance:** The lack of an immune response to an antigen (either self antigen or foreign antigen) due to clonal deletion.
- **Toll-like receptor (TLR):** A plasma membrane receptor that is expressed on phagocytes and other cells and is involved in signaling during the innate immune response. TLRs are related to IL-1 receptors.
- **TOM complex:** Resides in the outer membrane of the mitochondrion and is responsible for importing proteins from the cytosol into the space between the membranes.
- **Tomato:** A green bushy plant, botanical name *Lycopersicon esculentum*. The wild type is native to South America, but the (domesticated) tomato is grown worldwide today. Its fruit, known as tomatoes, are a natural source of the antioxidant

carotenoid lycopene, a phytochemical whose consumption has been linked to a reduction in coronary heart disease and some cancers (prostate cancer).

- **Topoisomerase:** An enzyme that can alter the topology of a DNA molecule by cutting one or both strands of DNA.
- **Topological isomers:** Molecules of DNA that are identical except for a difference in linking number.
- **Totipotency:** A property of normal cells that they have the genetic potential to give rise to a complete individual, except terminally specialized cells.
- **Totipotent stem cells:** Bone marrow cells that (when signaled) mature into both red blood cells and white blood cells. Receptors on the surface of totipotent stem cells "grasp" passing blood cell growth factors (e.g. interleukin- 7, stem cell growth factor, etc.), bringing them inside these stem cells and thus causing the maturation and differentiation into red and white blood cells. These receptors are called FLK-Z receptors.
- **Totipotent:** The ability of a cell to respond according to environmental stimuli and divide to form differentiated cell types.
- **Toxic:** Poisonous.
- **Toxic substances control act (TSCA):** A 1976 American Federal Law under which the US Environmental Protection Agency (EPA) has regulated the release of genetically engineered organisms (bacteria or plants) that produce natural insecticides. This is based on legal analogy to synthetic chemical insecticides, which are clearly regulated under TSCA.
- **Toxicogenomics:** A branch of toxicology that deals with the reactions between toxins and the specific differences in response to different organisms due to their different genomes/DNA (of the different individuals that consume the same toxin). For example, some rare humans can tolerate eating certain poisonous mushrooms (which sicken or kill all other humans that consume those particular mushroom species). During 2001, Fred Gould et al. showed that a rare, recessive gene (allele) known as BtR-4 could confer (to tobacco budworms possessing two copies of that particular gene) resistance to at least some of the "cry" proteins (which kill all other tobacco budworms that consume those "cry proteins"). The subgroup of all those individuals whose DNA (genome) causes their bodies to resist the effects of a given toxin, is known as a haplotype. A haplotype

could (theoretically) be as small as one individual, because the particular resistance-to-toxin could result from one single nucleotide polymorphism (SNP).

- **Toxin:** A substance (e.g. produced in some cases by fungi, weeds, ants, or disease-causing microorganisms) which is poisonous to certain other living organisms.

- **Tracer (Radioactive isotopic method):** A metabolite that is labeled by incorporation of an isotopic atom into its structure. The metabolic fate of the labeled metabolite can then be traced in intact organisms. That is, one is able to ascertain where (in what kind of structure) the metabolite ends up, as well as the transformation products (intermediate molecules) that were involved in its formation. Certain atoms of a given metabolite are labeled. This is done by substituting radioactive isotopes for the atom in question. Because an atom is replaced by an isotope, the metabolite as a whole is chemically and biologically indistinguishable from its normal analog. The presence of the isotope allows the metabolite and its transformation products to be detected and measured. Without this technique, many aspects of metabolism could not have been studied. These include: the process of photosynthesis, metabolic turnover rates, and the biosynthesis of proteins and nucleic acids.

- **Traditional breeding methods:** A phrase utilized by some people to refer to some or most techniques/technologies utilzed by crop plant breeders prior to some arbitrarily chosen date (after which some people feel that "genetic engineering" arrived abruptly). For example, in 1992 Tim Croughan discovered a single rice (*Oryza sativa*) plant that had survived (what should have been a lethal dose of) an imidazolinone-based herbicide, due to a (mutated) gene in its DNA that made it resistant to imidazolinones. That plant was then propagated via straight-forward breeding to yield seeds still sown today. Many years ago, some other crops similarly were given new traits (herbicide tolerance, compositional improvements, etc.) via mutation breeding (soaking seeds or pollen in mutation-causing chemicals, or bombarding seeds with ionizing radiation to cause random genetic mutations, followed by grow-out and selection of the particular mutation desired such as herbicide tolerance, as described above). Other crops were given new traits via crossing them with related wild plants, which occasionally resulted in extremely high levels of natural toxicants in those plants/seeds (solanine, psoralene, etc.). Still others were given new traits via wide-crossing them with other domesticated species (e.g. the tangelo is a hybrid of the grapefruit and the tangerine). The US-FDA regulates all new crop plants similarly (also requires testing of plants produced via "traditional breeding methods" for the potential presence of introduced or increased natural toxicants).

- **Trailer (3′ UTR):** A nontranslated sequence at the 3′ end of mRNA following the termination codon.
- **Trait:** A characteristic of an organism, which manifests itself in the phenotype (physically). Many traits are the result of the expression of a single gene, but some are polygenic (result from simultaneous expression of more than one gene). For example, the level of protein content in soybeans is controlled by five genes.
- *Trans* **configuration:** Of two sites refers to their presence on two different molecules of DNA (chromosomes).
- *Trans* **face:** Face of a golgi stack at which material leaves the organelle for the cell surface or another cell compartment. It is adjacent to the trans Golgi network.
- *Trans* **fatty acids:** One of the two isomeric forms that fatty acids can exist in. *Trans* fatty acids are naturally present in some meat and dairy products (which constitutes approximately 5% of the average American diet).
- *Trans***:** Configuration of two sites refers to their presence on two different molecules of DNA (chromosomes).
- *Trans***-acting protein:** A *trans*-acting protein has the exceptional property of acting (having an effect) only on the molecule of DNA (deoxyribonucleic acid) from which it was expressed.
- **Transaminase:** A large group of enzymes that catalyze the transfer of the amino group from any one of at least 12 amino acids to a keto acid to form another amino acid. Also known as aminotransferases.
- **Transamination:** The reaction of the enzymatic removal and transfer of an amino group from one specific compound to another.
- **Transcribed spacer:** The part of an rRNA transcription unit that is transcribed but discarded during maturation, that is, it does not give rise to part of rRNA.

- **Transcript:** The RNA product produced by copying one strand of DNA. It may require processing to generate a mature RNA.
- **Transcription factor:** It is required for RNA polymerase to initiate transcription at specific promoter(s), but is not itself part of the enzyme.
- **Transcription:** The enzyme-catalyzed process whereby the genetic information contained in one strand of DNA (deoxyribonucleic acid) is used as a template to specify and produce a complementary mRNA strand. Transcription may be thought of as a rewriting of the information contained in DNA into RNA. The language, however, is the same — both are nucleic acid-based. This is in contrast to translation, in which the information is translated from one language (RNA, nucleic acid-based) into another language (protein, amino acid-based).
- **Transcription unit:** A group of genes that code for functionally related RNA molecules or protein molecules. This group of genes is expressed (transcribed) together (as a unit, thus the name).
- **Transcriptome:** The complete set of RNAs present in a cell, tissue, or organism. Its complexity is due to mostly mRNAs, but it also includes noncoding RNAs.
- **Transcytosis:** The transport of molecules from one type of plasma membrane domain to another in polarized cells, such as neurons and epithelial cells.
- **Transdifferentiation:** The process whereby a specialized cell de-differentiates and re-differentiates into different cell type or the process whereby an adult stem cell from a specific tissue type becomes a cell type from a very different tissue (for example a nerve stem cell differentiates into a kidney cell).
- **Transducing phage:** Bacterial DNA instead of viral genetic material is incorporated into viral protein coat.
- **Transducing virus:** Carries part of the host genome in place of part of its own sequence. The best known examples are retroviruses in eukaryotes and DNA phages in *E. coli.*
- **Transduction (gene):** The transfer of bacterial genes (DNA) from one bacterium to another by means of a (temperature or defective) bacterial virus (bacteriophage). There exist two kinds of transduction: specialized and general. In the case of specialized transduction, a restricted group of host genes becomes integrated into the virus genome. These "guest" genes

usually replace some of the virus genes and are subsequently transferred to a second bacterium. In the case of generalized transduction, host genes become part of the mature virus particle in place of, or in addition to, the virus DNA. However, in this case, genes can come from virtually any portion of the host genome and this material does not become directly integrated into the virus genome. In the case of plants, the vector can be *Agrobacterium tumefaciens*.

- **Transduction:** Virus mediated gene transfer from one bacterium to another.

- **Transesterification:** Reaction breaks and makes chemical bonds in a coordinated transfer so that no energy is required.

- **Transfection:** This term has several different meanings, depending on the context in which it is used: A word utilized generally to refer to insertion of DNA segments (genes) into cells (via electroporation, endocytosis, etc.); a special case of transformation in which an appropriate recipient strain of bacteria is exposed to (free) DNA isolated from a transducing phage with the "take up" of that DNA by some of the bacteria and consequent production and release of complete virus particles. The process involves the direct transfer of genetic material from donor to recipient.

- **Transfer region:** A segment on the F plasmid that is required for bacterial conjugation.

- **Transfer RNA (tRNA):** A class of relatively small RNA (ribonucleic acid) molecules of molecular weight 23,000 to about 30,000. tRNA molecules act as carriers of specific amino acids during the process of protein synthesis. Each of the 20 amino acids found in proteins has at least one specific corresponding tRNA. The tRNA binds covalently with its specific amino acid and "leads" it to the ribosome for incorporation into the growing peptide chain (Fig. 4).

- **Transferases:** Enzymes that catalyze the transfer of functional groups to molecules (from other molecules).

- **Transferrin receptor:** The receptor molecule (located on the surface of cells throughout the body) responsible for binding to transferring molecules, then bringing those iron rich transferrin molecules into the cell, where iron is released to be used by the cell.

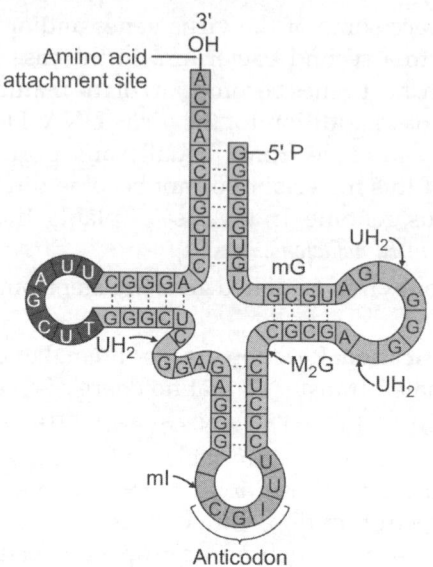

Fig. 4: tRNA

- **Transferrin:** The protein molecule responsible for transporting iron (molecules) to tissues throughout the body, via the circulatory system.
- **Transformation (of bacteria):** The acquisition of new genetic markers by incorporation of added DNA.
- **Transformation (of eukaryotic cells):** Their conversion to a state of unrestrained growth in culture, resembling or identical with the tumorigenic condition.
- **Transformed:** The cultured cells that have acquired many of the properties of cancer cells.
- **Transforming growth factor-alpha (TGF-alpha):** An angiogenic growth factor produced by tumor cells. It is able to induce specific malignant characteristics in normal cells (such as fibroblasts), thereby "transforming" those cells. TGF-alpha appears to possess a variety of potentially useful pharmaceutical properties, such as powerful stimulation of scar tissue formation following wounding of a tissue, as indicated by preliminary research.
- **Transforming growth factor-beta (TGF-beta):** An angiogenic growth factor produced by tumor cells, able to induce specific

malignant characteristics in normal cells (such as fibroblasts), thereby "transforming" those cells. TGF-beta stimulates blood vessel growth, even though it inhibits the division of endothelial cells. TGF-beta is a strong "attracting agent" for macrophages (i.e. TGF-beta is chemotactic), and appears to be responsible for the high concentrations of macrophages often found in tumors. TGFbeta has shown immunosuppressive activity (i.e. it suppresses the immune system). For example, transforming growth factor-beta works together with osteoinductive factor (OIF) to promote bone-formation by causing connective tissue cells to grow together to form a matrix of cartilage (e.g. across a bone break); bone cells slowly replace that cartilage.

- **Transforming principle:** DNA that is taken up by a bacterium and whose expression then changes the properties of the recipient cell.
- **Transformylase:** The enzyme that transfers a formyl (–CHO) group to the amino group of methionine to make formylmethionine.
- **Transgalacto-oligosaccharides:** A "family" of oligosaccharides (produced via enzymatic conversion of lactose, using β-glucosidase enzyme), some of which help to foster the growth of beneficial bifidobacteria in the lower colon of monogastric animals (humans, swine, etc.).
- **Transgene:** A "package" of genetic material (DNA) that is inserted into the genome of a cell via gene splicing techniques. May include promoter(s), leader sequence, termination codon, etc.
- **Transgenesis:** Introduction of gene into animal or plant cells that is successively transmitted to onward generations.
- **Transgenic:** An organism whose gamete cells (sperm/egg) contain genetic material originally derived from an organism other than the parents, or in addition to the parental genetic material.
- **Transgenic plant:** A fertile plant consisting of a foreign gene in its germ line.
- **Transgenics organisms:** Plants, microorganisms or animals in which novel DNA has been incorporated into their germ line cells.
- **Transgressive segregation:** A plant breeding (propagation) technique, in which genetically very different members of the same

species are mated with each other. The offspring of that mating can be more healthy, productive (e.g. fast growing), and uniform than their parents, a phenomenon known as "hybrid vigor."

- **Transient transfectants:** These have foreign DNA in an unstable, i.e. extrachromosomal form.
- **Transient:** Of short duration.
- **Transit peptide:** A peptide that, when fused to a protein, acts to transport that protein between compartments within eukaryotic cells. Once inside the "destination compartment," the transit peptide is cleaved off the protein and that protein is then free (to do its designed task).
- **Transition:** A mutation in which one pyrimidine is substituted by the other or in which one purine is substituted for the other.
- **Transition state (in a chemical reaction):** That point in the chemical reaction at which the reactants (i.e. chemical entities about to react with each other) have been "brought to the brink." It is a point in the chemical reaction process in which an "activated condition" is reached. From this point the probability of the reaction going to completion and producing a product is very high. The transition state separates (energetically) products from reactants. It is viewed as being at the top of the energy barrier separating reactants and products. The reacting species in the transition state can, because of their location at the "top" of the energy barrier, "fall" to either products or reactants.
- **Transition vesicle:** A small membrane-bounded compartment that mediates transport between organelles, especially the rough endoplasmic reticulum and Golgi complex. It is also known as a transport vesicle. COPI- and COPII-coated vesicles are transition vesicles.
- **Translation:** The process whereby the genetic information present in an mRNA molecule directs the order of incorporation of specific amino acids, and hence the growth of the polypeptide chain during protein synthesis. One can think of translation as the process of translating one language into another. In this particular case the nucleic acid-based language represented by mRNA is translated into the amino acid-based language of proteins.
- **Translational positioning:** Describes the location of a histone octamer at successive turns of the double helix, that determines which sequences are located in linker regions.

- **Translocation (of gene):** The appearance of a new copy at location in the genome elsewhere from the original copy.
- **Translocation (of protein):** Its movements across a membrane.
- **Translocation (of ribosome):** Its movement as one codon along mRNA after the addition of each amino acid to the polypeptide chain.
- **Translocon:** A discrete structure in a membrane that forms a channel through which (hydrophilic) proteins may pass.
- **Transmembrane protein (integral membrane protein):** Extends across a lipid bilayer. A hydrophobic region (typically consisting of a stretch of 20–25 hydrophobic and/or uncharged amino acids) or regions of the protein resides in the membrane. Hydrophilic regions are exposed on one or both sides of the membrane.
- **Transmembrane region (transmembrane domain):** The part of a protein that spans the membrane bilayer. It is hydrophobic and in many cases contains approximately 20 amino acids that form an α-helix. It is also called the transmembrane domain.
- **Transplantation antigen:** Protein coded by a major histo-compatibility locus, present on all mammalian cells, involved in interactions between lymphocytes.
- **Transport signal:** The part of a cargo molecule that is recognized by coat proteins or cargo receptors for incorporation into budding transport vesicles. Examples of transport signals are short amino acid sequences, secondary structure, and a protein modification such as phosphorylation.
- **Transporter:** A type of receptor that moves small molecules across the plasma membrane. It binds the molecules on its extracellular surface, and releases them into the cytoplasm.
- **Transposition immunity:** The ability of certain transposons to prevent others of the same type from transposing to the same DNA molecule.
- **Transposition:** The movement of a transposon to a new site in the genome. (*See also* nonreplicative transposition, replicative transposition and conservative transposition.)
- **Transposon tagging:** Insertion of transposable element into nearby gene, thereby making that gene with a known DNA sequence.

- **Transposon:** A DNA sequence able to insert itself at a new location in the genome (without any sequence relationship with the target locus).
- **Transposase:** An enzyme that catalyzes the movement of a DNA sequence to a different site in a DNA molecule.
- **Transvection:** The ability of a locus to influence activity of an allele on the other homolog only when two chromosomes are synapsed.
- **Transversion:** A mutation in which a purine is replaced by a pyrimidine or vice versa.
- **Transwitch®:** A "sense" technology used to "turn off " (suppress) a gene (e.g. the one that causes tomato to ripen) that causes an unwanted effect (e.g. premature softening of tomato). Transwitch® and its registered trademark are owned by DNA Plant Technology Corp.
- **Trehalose:** A disaccharide (simple sugar) that is naturally synthesized (manufactured) by many plants and animals in response to the stresses by freezing, heating, or drying.
- **Tremorgenic indole alkaloids:** A family of toxic alkaloids (chemical compounds) that are naturally produced (within some plants) by certain fungi (which sometimes grow in those plants). For example, the alkaloid known as Penitrem D is produced by certain fungi which grow in some grass species. It causes tremors, weakness, lack of coordination, and convulsions in animals that consume those fungus-infested grasses.
- *Trichoderma harzianum*: A microorganism that possesses (natural) fungicide activity.
- **Trichosanthin:** An enzyme extracted from a specific Chinese plant. It has been discovered to "cut apart" the ribosomes in some cells infected with the HIV (AIDS) virus, thus potentially stopping the virus and preventing infection of additional cells.
- **Triglycerides:** The primary constituent of fats or oils. Triglycerides are molecules that consist of three fatty acids attached to a glycerol "molecular backbone". More accurately called triacylglycerols, although long-term historical usage of "triglycerides" has made the latter term more common. Similarly, the term "diglyceride" is often used to refer to those molecules which consist of two fatty acids attached to a glycerol "molecular backbone". "Diglycerides" (more accurately called diacylglycerols) can result from the splitting-off (i.e. hydrolysis)

of one fatty acid from a triacylglycerol ("triglyceride") molecule (e.g. during fat breakdown/oxidation); or from the combination of two fatty acids with glycerol (e.g. during synthesis of fats). The "triglyceride level" in human bloodstream refers to the blood's content of noncholesterol total fats. Research during the 1990s provided evidence that high blood levels of triglycerides in humans (e.g. immediately after meals) contribute to thrombosis.

- **Triploid:** Refers to organisms that possess three sets of chromosomes, instead of the normal two sets. Conversion of a diploid (two sets of chromosomes) organism to triploid can be done by man (certain fish, "seedless" grapes, etc.). For example, fish are ordinarily diploid. By exposing fish eggs to certain specific combinations of temperature and pressure, immediately after fertilization of those eggs, scientists can cause the resultant fish to become triploid. Triploid fish are unable to reproduce. This sterility is desired by man, in order to prevent certain fish (e.g. those that have been genetically engineered) from mating with wild fish. Such induced (triploid) sterility also prevents the (genetically engineered) fish from wasting energy on the act of reproduction, so they grow faster and larger. That transfer (of energy use from reproduction to growth) also holds true for "seedless" grapes, watermelons, etc.

- **Triploidy:** The condition in which a cell or organism possesses three haploid sets of chromosomes.

- **Triskelion:** Is formed by the interaction of three heavy chains and three light chains of clathrin.

- **Trisomy:** When an individual has three particular type of chromosome. Monosomy and trisomy occur in plants and animals; in autosomes of animals, it is generally lethal. Non-lethal human monosomics and trisomics include Turner syndrome: monosomy where the individual has single X chromosome; Down syndrome is most common occurs due to trisomy among humans; it involves chromosome 21.

- **tRNAf Met:** The special RNA that initiate protein synthesis in bacteria. It mostly uses AUG, but can also respond to GUG and CUG.

- **tRNAiMl!t:** The special tRNA used to respond to initiation codons in eukaryotes.

- **tRNAm Met:** Insert methionine at internal AUG codons.

- **Tropism:** Orientation movement of a sessile organism in response to a stimulus. Movement of curvature due to an external stimulus that determines the direction of movement. Also known as topotaxis.
- **True reversion:** A mutation type that restores the original sequence of the DNA.
- **True-breeding:** Organisms are homozygous for the trait under consideration.
- **Trypsin:** A proteolytic (protein molecular chain-cutting) enzyme produced by the pancreas, to facilitate digestion within certain animals. Trypsin cleaves polypeptide (protein) molecular chains on the carboxyl (group) side of arginine and lysine units (residues); and it is often utilized by man to break apart protein molecules (e.g. to enable scientists to study that protein's constituent peptides).
- **Trypsin inhibitors:** A type of serine protease inhibitor that reduces the biological activity of trypsin. Trypsin is an enzyme involved in the breakdown of many different protein, including as part of digestion in humans and other animals.
- **Tryptophan (trp):** An essential amino acid, it is a precursor of the important biochemical molecules indoleacetic acid, serotonin, and nicotinic acid. L-tryptophan is used as a common feed additive for livestock to ensure that their diet includes an adequate amount of this essential amino acid (Fig. 5).

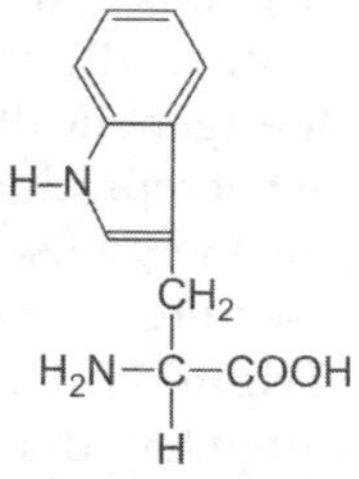

Tryptophan

Fig. 5: Tryptophan

- **Tubulin:** A cell protein required for cell mitosis (i.e. the cell-reproduction process in which a cell divides into two identical cells). When the drugs paclitaxel or Taxol™ are administered to the body (e.g. in chemotherapy), they bind tubulin; which halts cell division and causes apoptosis in the affected cells (e.g. tumor cells) by binding Bc1-2 (a protein that prevents apoptosis in cells).
- **Tumor:** A mass of abnormal tissue that resembles normal tissues in structure, but which fulfills no useful function (to the organism) and grows at the expense of the body. Tumors may be malignant or benign. Malignant tumors (which infiltrate adjacent healthy tissues) can result from oncogenes and/or carcinogens. They can eventually kill their host if unchecked.

Epidermal growth factor encourages rapid cell growth in more than 50% of human tumors.

- **Tumor necrosis factor (TNF):** Literally, tumor death factor. A cytokine (protein that helps regulate the immune system) that has shown potential to combat (kill) malignant (cancer) tumors. Tumor necrosis factor was discovered to be 10,000 times more toxic in humans than in rodents, where it had been tested for toxicity prior to human clinical tests. This example illustrates one potential pitfall of non-target animal testing in that sometimes animal testing does not accurately reflect or foretell what will happen in humans. Another drawback to using TNF as a drug to combat human tumors is the fact that it is one of the substances released (in the disease rheumatoid arthritis) that destroys tissue in the joints. When released as part of the AIDS (disease), TNF causes cachexia, which is "wasting away" of the body due to the body's inability to process nutrients received via digestion.

- **Tumor suppressor:** It is identified by a loss-of-function mutation that contributes to cancer formation. They usually function to prevent cell division or to cause death of abnormal cells. The two most important are p53 and RB.

- **Tumor virus:** A cell-free filtrate held to be a virus responsible for a specific neoplasm.

- **Tumor-associated antigens:** Discovered by Thierry Boon in 1991, these are distinctive protein molecules that are produced in the surface membrane of tumor cells. These protein molecules are used by the body's cytotoxic T cells to recognize (and destroy) tumor cells, so such proteins hold promise for use in vaccines.

- **Tumor-infiltrating lymphocytes (TIL cells):** The white blood cells of a cancer patient which have been: 1. Taken from that patient's tumor (where those white blood cells had been attempting to combat the cancer, albeit unsuccessfully). 2. Stimulated with doses of interleukin-2 (to make the lymphocytes more effective against the cancer). 3. Multiplied *in vitro* (i.e. outside of the patient's body) to make them more numerous (and thus more likely to successfully combat the cancer). When these "souped up" lymphocytes (white blood cells) are reintroduced into that same patient's body, the lymphocytes (now called TIL cells because they have been "souped up") attack the cancer tumor (malignant growth) more vigorously than before.

- **Tumor-suppressor genes:** Also called anticancer genes. Genes within a cell's DNA that code for (cause to be manufactured in cell's ribosomes) proteins that hold the cell's growth in check. If these genes are damaged (e.g. by radiation, by a carcinogen, or by chance accident in normal cell division), they no longer hold cell growth in check—and the cell becomes malignant (if the cell's DNA also contains a gene called an oncogene). Oncogenes must be present for the cell to become malignant, but oncogenes cannot cause a cell to become malignant until a tumor-suppressor gene is damaged. As with all genes, tumor-suppressor genes are inherited in two copies (alleles, one from each parent) and either copy can code for the proteins necessary for cell growth control. However, an organism born with one defective copy of a tumor-suppressor gene (or in whom one copy is damaged early in life) is especially prone to cancer (malignancy).

- **Tumor-suppressor proteins:** Proteins that are coded (caused to be manufactured in the cell's ribosomes) by tumor-suppressor genes (e.g. the p53 gene). Such proteins (e.g. the p53 protein) then act upon the cell's DNA in order to prevent uncontrolled cell growth and division (i.e. cancer).

- **Turbidostat:** An open continuous culture into which fresh medium flows in response to an increase in the turbidity of culture.

- **Turner's syndrome:** In human beings, individuals having XO chromosome constitution, being phenotyically female but having rudimentary sexual organs and mammary glands.

- **Turnover number:** The number of molecules of a product produced per minute by a single- enzyme molecule when that enzyme is working at its maximum rate. That is, the number of substrate molecules converted into a product by one enzyme molecule per minute, when that enzyme is "going (catalyzing) as fast as it can".

- **Twisting number (of DNA):** The number of base pairs divided by the number of base pairs per turn of the double helix.

- **Two hybrid:** Assay detects interaction between two proteins by means of their ability to bring together a DNA-binding domain and a transcription-activating domain. The assay is performed in yeast using a reporter gene that responds to the interaction.

- **Two-dimensional (2D) gel electrophoresis:** A technology/ methodology developed during the 1970s to separate the various proteins within a given biological sample, prior to their analysis. The proteins are moved by applying an electrical field. The sample is moved through two different gels (i.e. two different dimensions). The initial gel has a pH gradient that separates the different proteins based on their respective isoelectric points. The second gel (dimension) sample is moved through a gel that separates the protein molecules based on their individual molecular weights. That gel acts as a "molecular sieve" (i.e. smaller proteins move faster—and farther—than larger proteins do through this gel, in a fixed amount of time). A fixed-time gel run (i.e. with appropriate gel and the appropriate electrical field applied to the gel) leaves a scientist with approximately 1,000 "spots" (of protein molecules) on the gel. Each "spot" is a collection of the molecules of one protein (or of several proteins with similar molecular weights) from the original sample (mixture). To identify the protein(s) in the "spots," the scientist stains them, then assesses the entire gel with an electronic image scanner (or he assesses it visually). From the pattern (coupled with intensity) of the "spots," two such gels could be utilized to confirm if two organisms were of the same species/strain/ variety, or to determine the differences (in gene expression) between samples of diseased vs. healthy tissues.
- **Ty:** Stands for transposon yeast, the first transposable element to be identified in yeast.
- **Type I diabetes:** The form of diabetes disease that usually strikes young people (thus, it was formerly known as juvenile or insulin dependent diabetes). This disease is characterized by the body's immune system destroying the insulin-producing cells (Beta cells) of the pancreas. If not treated in time (i.e. via insulin injections), the person can die suddenly. Even when treated, the person is at increased risk of blindness, atherosclerosis, coronary heart disease, heart attack, stroke, and kidney disease.
- **Type I topoisomerase:** An enzyme that changes the topology of DNA by nicking and resealing one strand of DNA.
- **Type II diabetes:** The form of diabetes disease that usually strikes people who are more than 40 years old. Also known as

adult-onset diabetes, this disease is characterized by the body's tissues becoming insensitive to insulin. Effects on the body include increased likelihood of blindness, atherosclerosis, coronary heart disease, heart attack, stroke, and kidney disease.

- **Type II topoisomerase:** An enzyme that changes the topology of DNA by nicking and resealing both strands of DNA.
- **Type specimen:** The actual physical specimen (e.g. a stuffed lizard or a dried insect) that a scientist (who describes and names a previously unknown species) must place in a museum (or other recognized repository) in order to have the right to name that newly discovered species. This "officially deposited specimen" is required for three purposes: 1. Comparisons can later be made if there is ever a doubt whether another "new" species is simply a member of this same species (and thus already named) 2. Taxonomists (who determine and keep the official scientific names by which scientists must refer to each of the world's organisms) can name each of the newly discovered species in accordance with the complex rules of the International Codes for Nomenclature. Examples of such names in this glossary are *Arabidopsis thaliana*, *Escherichia coli*, and *Agrobacterium tumefaciens*. 3. Patent claims for genetically engineered organisms can later be enforced.
- **Tyrosine (tyr):** An aromatic nonessential amino acid; a component of proteins. It is a metabolic precursor of thyroxine, the pigment melanine, and other biologically important compounds (Fig. 6).

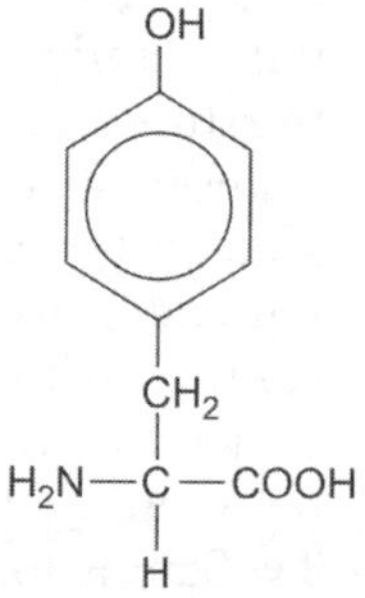

Fig. 6: Tyrosine

- **Tyrosine kinase inhibitors (TKI):** Refers to various chemical compounds that inhibit the activity of tyrosine kinase enzyme (inside the body). One example of TKI is genistein. Because the activity of tyrosine kinase helps cancerous (tumor) cells to metastasize (spread/grow), consumption by humans of relevant TKI acts to help prevent (spreading of) certain cancers.
- **Tyrosinosis:** A human disease controlled by a recessive gene and characterized by excretion of p-hydroxyl phenyl pyruvic acid and tyrosine into urine.

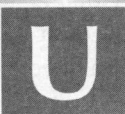

- **US patent and trademark office (USPTO):** The Washington, DC-based American Government agency responsible for common patent protection matters for all of America's 50 states and its territorial possessions. The USPTO allows the patenting of new and unique microbes, plants, and animals, as well as the new and unique methods to produce such biotechnology advances.
- **U3:** The repeated sequence at the 3' end of a retroviral RNA.
- **U5:** The repeated sequence at the 5' end of a retroviral RNA.
- **Ubiquitin:** A small protein present in all eukaryotic cells (ubiquitous) that plays an important role in "tagging" other proteins destined (marked) for destruction (via proteolytic cleavage). Such proteins are then broken down and removed because they are damaged or no longer needed by the body. Such "tagged" protein molecules are said to have been ubiquitinated.
- **Ultracentrifuge:** A high-speed centrifuge that can attain revolving speeds upto 85,000 rpm and centrifugal field upto 500,000 times gravity. The machine is used to sediment (i.e. cause to settle out) and hence separate macromolecules (large molecules) and macromolecular structures in a mixture/solution. In general, a centrifuge is a machine that whirls test tubes around rapidly, like a merry-go-round, to force the heavier suspended materials (in the solutions in the test tubes) to the bottom of those test tubes before the lighter material.
- **Ultrafiltration:** A mixture separation methodology that uses the ability of synthetic semipermeable membranes (possessing appropriate physical and chemical natures) to discriminate between molecules in the mixture, primarily on the basis of the molecules' size and shape. Invented and developed by Dr Roy J Taylor in the 1950s and 1960s, ultrafiltration is typically utilized for the separation of relatively high-molecular-weight solutes

(e.g. proteins, gums, polymers, and other complex organic molecules) and colloidally dispersed substances (e.g. minerals, microorganisms, etc.) from their solvents (e.g., water).

- **Ultrasonication:** Disruption of cells or DNA molecules by high frequency sound waves.
- **Umber codon (opal codon):** The UGA codon, one of the three termination codons that end protein synthesis.
- **Underwinding (of DNA):** The effect of negative supercoiling on a structure of DNA.
- **Underwound:** A stretch of underwound DNA has fewer base pairs per turn than the usual average (10 bp = 1 turn). This means that the two strands of DNA are less tightly wound around each other, ultimately this can lead to strand separation.
- **Unequal crossing-over:** A recombination event in which the two recombining sites lie at non-identical locations in the two parental DNA molecules.
- **Unidirectional replication:** The movement of a single replication fork from a given origin.
- **Uninducible:** The mutant where the affected gene(s) cannot be expressed.
- **Union for protection of new varieties of plants (UPOV):** A group of countries the world's that have jointly agreed to mutually protect the intellectual property (of owners, breeders) that is inherent in new plant varieties developed by man. These intellectual property protections are often collectively referred to as "Breeder's Rights". Established in 1961, the secretariat for this union (UPOV) is in Geneva, Switzerland.
- **Uniporter:** A type of carrier protein that moves only one type of solute across the plasma membrane.
- **Unit cell:** Describes the state of an *E. coli* bacterium generated by a new division. It is 1.7 m long and has a single replication origin.
- **Units (U):** A measure (quantitation) of biological activity of a substance, as defined by various standardized assays (tests).
- **Univalent shift:** The phenomenon of some of the progeny of an aneuploid plant would become aneuploid for a different chromosome as compared to the parent plant. This shift generally occurs in monosomic lines and is a result of univalent formation in a chromosome other than that for which they are monosomic.

- **Unsaturated r fatty acid:** A fatty acid containing one or more double bonds (between individual atoms of the molecule).
- **Unscheduled DNA synthesis:** Any DNA synthesis occurring outside the S phase of the eukaryotic cell.
- **Up promoter mutations:** Increase the frequency of initiation of transcription.
- **Upstream activator sequence (UAS):** Is the equivalent in yeast of the enhancer in higher eukaryotes.
- **Upstream:** Identifies sequences proceeding in the opposite direction from expression; for example, the bacterial promoter is upstream of the transcription unit, the initiation codon is upstream of the coding region.
- **Uracil:** An important pyrimidine base, a component of ribonucleic acid (RNA). Its hydrogen- bonding counterpart in DNA is thymine (Fig. 1).

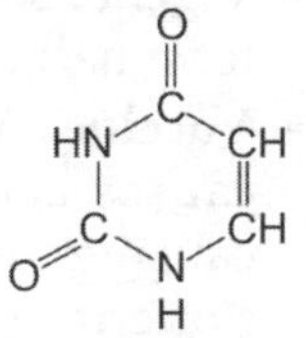

Uracil (U)
(in RNA)

Fig. 1: Uracil

- **URF:** An open (unidentified) reading frame, presumed to code for protein, but for which no product has been found.
- **Urokinase:** A thrombolytic (clot-dissolving) enzyme used as a biopharmaceutical.

U

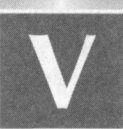

- **V gene:** Sequence coding for the major part of the variable (N-terminal) region of an immunoglobulin chain.
- **Vaccine:** Any substance, bearing antigens on its surface, that causes activation of an animal's immune system without causing actual disease. The animal's immune system components (e.g. antibodies) are then prepared to quickly vanquish those particular pathogens when they later enter the body.
- **Vaccinia:** A nonpathogenic virus believed to be a (modified) form of the virus that causes cowpox. *Vaccinia* readily accepts genes (inserted into its genome via genetic engineering) from pathogenic viruses, so it can be used to make vaccines that do not possess the risk inherent in attenuated-virus vaccines (i.e. that the attenuated virus "revives" and causes disease). Such genetically engineered *vaccinia* codes for (presents) the proteins of the pathogenic virus on its surface, which activates the immune system (of vaccinated animal) to produce antibodies against that pathogenic virus.
- **Vacuoles:** A membrane-bound sac within a cell, within which water, food, waste, or salt, etc. are temporarily stored. Also pigments, in certain plant cells.
- **VAD:** Acronym for vitamin A deficiency.
- **Vagile:** Wandering or roaming (a microorganism that is not attached to a solid support tends to "wander" through its environment as it gets pushed about by currents of air or liquid).
- **Vagility:** The ability of organisms to disseminate (e.g. spread throughout a given habitat).
- **Vaginosis:** The process whereby a cell internalizes an entity (such as a virus or a protein) that has bound to the cell's outer membrane. Once that "bound entity" is inside the cell, the cell membrane together fuses again.

- **Valine (val):** An amino acid considered essential for normal growth of animals. It is biosynthesized (made) from pyruvic acid (Fig. 1).

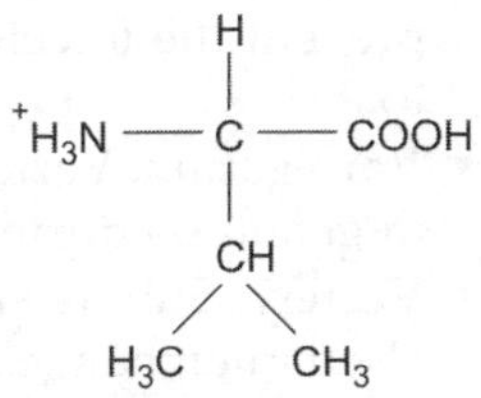

$$^+H_3N — \overset{\displaystyle H}{\underset{\displaystyle CH}{C}} — COOH$$

$$\overset{}{\underset{H_3C \quad CH_3}{}}$$

Fig. 1: Valine

- **Value-added traits:** Modified crops produced with traits such as improved taste, nutritional value, or utility to provide value for the consumer.

- **Value-enhanced grains:** Those grains that possess novel traits that are economically valuable (e.g. higher-than-normal protein content, better quality protein, higher-than normal oil content, etc.). For example, high oil corn (maize) possesses a kernel oil content of 5.8% or greater, vs. oil content of 3.5% or less for traditional No. 2 yellow corn. Glutamate dehydrogenase (GDH) corn (maize) possesses a kernel protein content that tends to be approximately 10% greater than the protein content of traditional corn (maize) varieties. High-amylose corn possesses a kernel amylose content of 50% or more of the total kernel starch, etc.

- **van der Waals forces:** The relatively weak forces of attraction between molecules that contribute to intermolecular bonding (i.e. binding together two or more adjacent molecules). Historically, it was thought that van der Waals forces were always weaker than the hydrogen bond forces responsible for intramolecular bonding. However, in 1995, Dr. Alfred French discovered that van der Waals forces are primarily responsible for holding together a mass of cellulose molecules, with hydrogen bonding playing a lesser role. During 2000, Kellar Autumn discovered that van der Waals forces (acting between foot skin hairs and the surface climbed) are responsible for enabling the Tokay gecko (*Gecko gecko*) to climb vertical surfaces and also to hang upside down. These forces work (to "adhere" a gecko's foot) even underwater or in a vacuum.

- **Variable region:** An immunoglobulin chain is coded by the V gene and varies extensively when different chains are compared, as the result of multiple (different) genomic copies and changes introduced during construction of an active immunoglobulin.

- **Variable surface glycoprotein (VSG):** The protein on the surface of a trypanosome that changes during an infection so as to prevent the infected host from mounting an immune reaction to it.

- **Variegation:** Variegation of phenotype is produced by a change in genotype during somatic development.
- **Variety:** Subdivision of a species for taxonomic classification. Used interchangeably with the term cultivar, to denote a group of individual that is distinct genetically from other groups of individuals in the species. An agricultural variety is a group of similar plants that by structural features and performance can be identified from other varieties within the same species.
- **Vascular endothelial growth factor (VEGF):** A human growth factor (GF) that causes growth/proliferation of blood vessels/ endothelium and endothelial cells.
- **Vector:** The agent used (by researchers) to carry new genes into cells. Plasmids currently are the biological vectors of choice; though viruses and other biological vectors such as *Agrobacterium tumefaciens* bacteria or BACs are increasingly being used for this purpose. Non-biological vectors include the metal microparticles (coated with genes) which are "shot" into cells by the Biolistic® gene gun.
- **Vegetative phase:** The period of normal growth and division of a bacterium. For a bacterium that can sporulate, this contrasts with the sporulation phase, when spores are being formed.
- **Vegetative propagation:** Reproduction of plants using a non-sexual process, involves the culture of plant parts such as stem and leaf cuttings.
- **Very low-density lipoproteins (VLDL):** VLDLs and LDLPs are the specific lipoproteins that are most likely to deposit cholesterol on artery walls inside the human body, which increases the risk of coronary heart disease (CHD).
- **Vesicles:** Small bodies bounded by membrane, derived by budding from one membrane, often able to fuse with another membrane.
- **Vesicular transport (of a protein):** One of three means for a protein molecule to pass between compartments within eukaryotic cells. The compartment wall (membrane) possesses a sensor (receptor) that detects the presence of correct protein (e.g. after that protein has been synthesized in the cell's ribosomes), then bulges outward alongwith that protein molecule. The membrane bulge containing protein then breaks

V

off and carries (transports) the protein to its destination in another compartment in the cell.

- *vir* **gene:** A set of genes present on Ti-plasmid which facilitate the transfer of T-DNA segment into a plant cell.
- **Viral superfamily:** Comprises of transposons that are related to retroviruses. They are defined by sequences that code for reverse transcriptase or integrase.
- **Viral transactivating protein:** The specific protein used by a lytic virus to "switch on" the cascade of gene regulation by which that virus "takes over" a healthy cell and subverts its molecular processes (machinery) to produce virus components. This (transactivating) protein is key to the whole lytic cycle of the virus and therefore a potential target for therapeutic intervention.
- **Virion:** The complete, infective form of a virus outside a host cell, with a care of RNA and a capsid (Fig. 2).

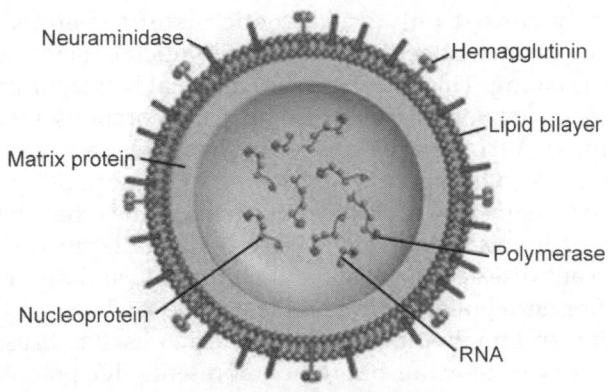

Fig. 2: Virion

- **Viroid:** Small infectious nucleic acid that does not have a protein coat.
- **Virology:** Study of viruses.
- **Virulence:** Ability to infect or cause disease.
- **Virulent:** Virulent phage mutants are unable to establish lysogeny.
- **Virus:** A simple, noncellular particle (entity) that can reproduce only inside living cells (of other organisms), which was first proved to exist in 1892 by Dimitry Ivanovsky (Fig. 3). The simple

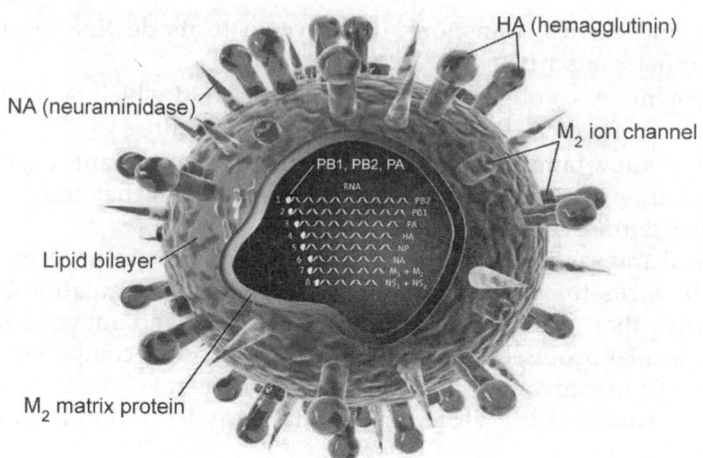

Fig. 3: Virus

structure of virus is their most important characteristic. Virus generally consist only of a genetic material—either DNA (deoxyribonucleic acid) or RNA (ribonucleic acid)—and a protein coating. This (combination) material is categorized as a nucleoprotein. Some viruses also have membranous envelopes (coatings). Viruses are "alive" in that they can reproduce themselves—although only by taking over a cell's "synthetic genetic machinery"—but they have none of the other characteristics of living organisms. Viruses cause a large variety of significant diseases in plants and animals, including humans. They present a philosophical problem to those who would speak of living and nonliving systems because in itself a virus is not "alive" as we know life, but rather represents "life potential" or "symbiotic life".

- **Virusoid (satellite RNA):** A small infectious nucleic acid that is encapsidated by a plant virus together with its own genome.
- **Viscosity:** A measure of a liquid's resistance to flow, as expressed in units called poise (P; grams per cm per sec). The degree of "thickness" or "syrupiness" of a liquid.
- **Vitamin E:** Refers to a group of related, naturally occurring compounds consisting of tocopherol and tocotrienol "families". It is a fat-soluble vitamin with antioxidant properties (helps to prevent lipids in the body from breaking down). Vitamin E is especially effective at preventing oxidation of low-density

lipoproteins (so-called "bad cholesterol"), whose oxidation products (beta-hydroxycholesterol) can be deposited onto the interior walls of blood vessels (arteries) in the form of plaque—which can result in the disease atherosclerosis—and/or adversely increasing blood platelet aggregation (clotting). Vitamin E occurs naturally in soybeans, cereal grains, etc., so it can be considered a phytochemical. In 2000, the Institute of Medicine of the US National Academy of Sciences issued a report that called for an increase in the amount of vitamin E consumed each day, to improve citizens' health.

- **Vitamin:** Any of a group of a unrelated organic substances occurring in many foods in small amounts and necessary in trace amounts for the normal metabolic functioning of the body; they may be water-or fat-soluble (Fig. 4).

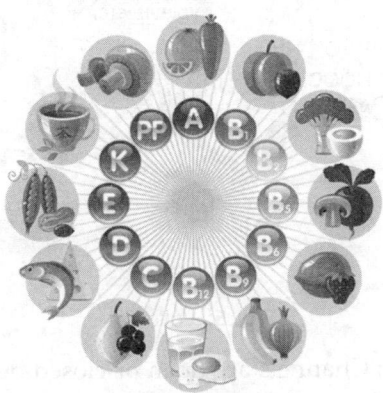

Fig. 4: Vitamins

- **Vitrification:** An undesirable condition of *in vitro* tissues characterized by succulence, brittleness and glassy appearance.
- **VNTR (variable number tandem repeat):** Regions which describe very short repeated sequences, including microsatellites and minisatellites.
- **VNTRs (Minisatellites):** Polygenic markers.
- **Void Volume:** The interstitial volume of the chromatographic column, that is the volume of mobile phase imbibed in the pores and around the stationary phase in a column.
- **Volicitin:** A chemical compound produced by Beet Armyworm caterpillars (*Spodoptera exigua*) after they have consumed some

linoleic acid (in plants they chew on, such as corn/maize). The body cells of Beet Armyworm caterpillars conjugate (i.e. chemically join together) the linoleic acid molecules onto glutamine molecules. The conjugated molecule, consisting of one linoleic acid (molecule) joined to one glutamine (molecule), is known as volicitin. When Beet Armyworm caterpillars subsequently chew on corn/maize plants, some volicitin is inadvertently inserted by those caterpillars into the tissue of the corn (maize). That volicitin causes the corn (maize) plant to emit certain volatile compounds that attract type(s) of wasps which are natural enemies of the Beet Armyworm; leading them to attack those Beet Armyworm caterpillars (which are feeding on the maize/corn) (Fig 5).

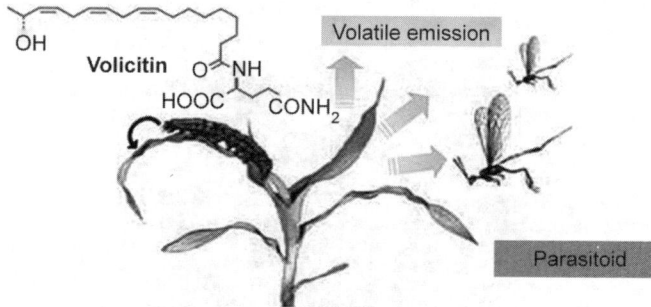

Fig. 5: Volicitin

- **Voltage-gated:** Channels are open or closed depending on the voltage across the membrane.

V

W

- **Water activity (*Aw*):** A measure of the "free" unbound water (e.g. in a processed food product) available to sustain the growth of microorganisms (spoilage) and/or to sustain undesired chemical reactions (e.g. "staling" of baked food products). Most bacteria are unable to grow in foods possessing a water activity below 0.90. Most yeasts and molds that cause spoilage cannot grow in foods possessing a water activity below 0.80. Sugarscan be added to certain foods in order to increase Aw, as they "bind up" the (formerly) free water present.
- **Water soluble fiber:** Food fiber (e.g. oat fiber, barley fiber, soybean fiber) that dissolves in water. It apparently absorbs low density lipoproteins (LDLP) in the intestine, before the fiber passes from the body; plus it inhibits absorption of LDLP by the body's intestinal walls due to increase in the viscosity of the intestine's contents. These two effects thus lower the amount of "bad" cholesterol (i.e. LDLP can lead to hardening/blockage of arteries) in the body and thereby coronary heart disease (CHD). Additional to those two effects, water soluble fiber also absorbs/binds bile acid and causes it to be excreted alongwith that water soluble fiber. That helps to lower cholesterol levels in the body (bloodstream), because the liver synthesizes (manufactures) more bile acids (to replace those absorbed and removed by the fiber) from cholesterol. Water soluble fiber from oat bran is a polysaccharide known as beta-glucan; composed entirely of glucose (molecular) units. US FDA regulations also include gums, pectins, mucilages, and certain hemicelluloses in the category of water soluble fiber. Soybean flour/meal is also a source of water soluble fiber. In 1997, the US FDA approved a (label) health claim that associates consumption of oat fiber with reduced blood cholesterol content and with reduced coronary heart disease (CHD). In 1998, the US FDA approved a (label) health claim that associates soluble fiber from psyllium husks with reduced risk of coronary heart disease (CHD).

- **Waxy corn:** Refers to corn (maize) hybrids that produce kernels in which the starch contained within those kernels is at least 99% amylopectin, versus the average of 72–76% amylopectin in traditional corn starch (Fig. 1).

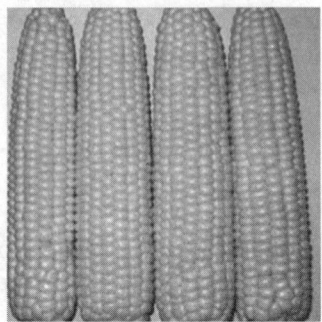

Fig. 1: Waxy corn

- **Waxy wheat:** Refers to varieties of wheat (*Triticum aestivum*) that produce a higher amylopectin content, and thus a lower amylase content in the starch within their seeds than traditional varieties of wheat. For example, bread flour made from waxy wheat would contain 0–3% amylose, vs. 24–27% amylose in bread flour made from traditional varieties of wheat. Because bread made from such waxy (i.e. lower amylose) wheat becomes firm at a much slower rate than bread made from traditional wheat varieties, bread made from waxy wheat would probably require less shortening (added to the flour) to keep that bread soft.

- **Weak interactions:** The forces between atoms that are less strong than the forces involved in a covalent (chemical) bond (between two atoms). Weak interactions include ionic (chemical) bonds, hydrogen bonds, and van der Waals forces.

- **Weed:** An undesirable plant.

- **Weediness:** Unwanted effects of a plant.

- **Weevils:** A term describing a number of insects that consume grains (grown and used by man) (Fig. 2). Many of the weevils consume (and proliferate in) stored grains, and stored grain products (e.g. flour). One example of a weevil is the insect known as the pea weevil, which lays its eggs on pea pods or dried peas. When the larvae hatch, they burrow into the pod and eat the peas inside. The insect *Theocolax elegans* attacks the larvae of maize weevils (*Sitophilus granarius*, *Triboleum castaneum*), rice weevils (*Sitophilus oryzae*), and the lesser grain borer. Thus, it

W

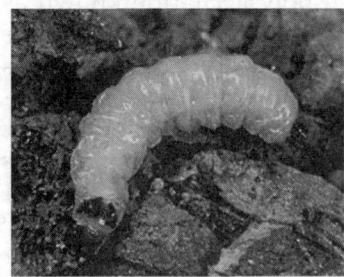

Fig. 2: Weevils

could potentially be added to grain storage bins (silos) as part of an Integrated Pest Management (IPM) program.

- **Western blot:** A technique in which protein is transferred from an electrophoretic gel to a cellulose or nylon support membrane following electrophoresis. A particular protein is then identified by probing the blot with a radiolabelled antibody which binds on the specific protein to which the antibody was prepared (Fig. 3).

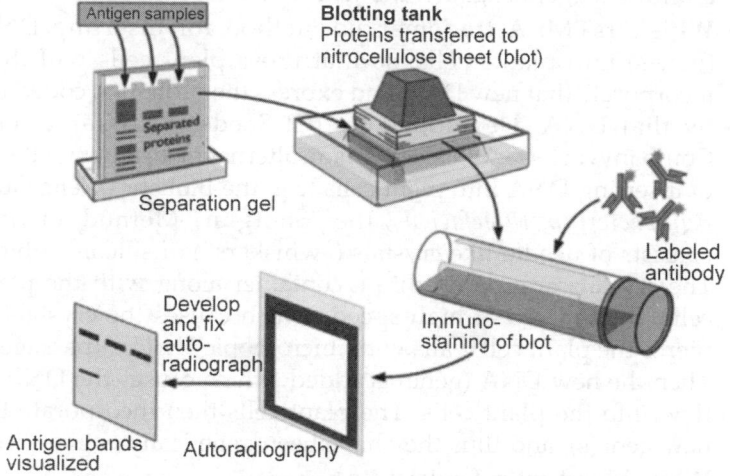

Fig. 3: Western blotting

- **Western corn rootworm:** Latin name *Diabrotica virgifera virgifera* LeConte.
- **Wheat:** Refers to a family of related small grains descended from the natural crossing of three Middle East grasses (*Triticum monococcum, Aegilops speltoids,* and *Triticum tauscii*) centuries ago (Fig. 4). As a result, wheat's genome is triploid (i.e. it incorporates three complete sets of deoxyribonucleic acid (DNA)), and contains approximately 17 billion base pairs (bp). Wheat is historically an annual plant that can attain a height of four feet (1.2 meters),

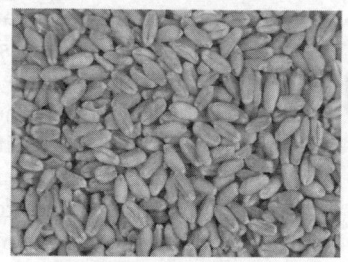

Fig. 4: Wheat

W

although variations (e.g. shorter) have been bred. The Latin name for traditional (bread) wheat is *Triticum aestivum*, and for durum (pasta) wheat is *Triticum durum* desf. Historically, wheat kernels have contained 15% or less protein. Most of the rest of the kernel is composed of starch (amylose and amylopectin).

- **Wheat take-all disease:** A fungal disease that attacks wheat (*Triticum aestivum*) plant roots, and causes dry rot and premature death of the plant. Certain strains of *Brassica* plants and *Pseudomonas* bacteria produce compounds that can act as natural antifungal agents against the wheat take-all fungus.

- **WhiskersTM:** A trademarked method for inserting DNA (genes) into plants cells, so that those plant cells will then incorporate that new DNA and express the protein(s) coded for by that DNA. Developed by ICI Seeds Inc. (Garst Seed Company) in 1993, Whiskers™ is an alternative to other methods of inserting DNA into plant cells (e.g. the Biolistic® Gene Gun, *Agrobacterium tumefaciens*, the "Shotgun" Method, etc.); it consists of needle-like crystals ("whiskers") of silicon carbide. The crystals are placed into a container along with the plant cells, then mixed at high speed, which causes the crystals to pierce the plant cell walls with microscopic "holes" (passages). Then the new DNA (gene) is added, which causes the DNA to flow into the plant cells. The plant cells then incorporate the new gene(s); and thus they have been genetically engineered.

- **White blood cells:** Leukocytes.

- **White mold disease:** The common name that refers to a plant disease caused under certain conditions (e.g. moist, humid, etc.) by *sclerotinia sclerotiorum* fungus. In 1998, the US Environmental Protection Agency (EPA) approved one herbicide (COBRA(R), owned by Valent Corporation), whose active ingredient is the chemical lactofin, to be applied to soybean plants "at or near bloom stage" in order to trigger systemic acquired resistance (SAR) a sort of "immune response" in those soybean plants against white mold disease. Use of no-tillage crop production (methodology) for some crops helps to reduce the incidence of white mold disease (Fig. 5).

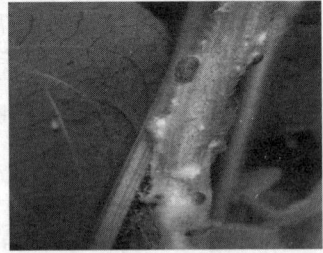

Fig. 5: White mold disease on plant

W

- **Wide cross:** Refers to the plant breeding technologies/techniques utilized to cross two plant species that would not normally cross in nature.
- **Wide hybridization:** When individuals from two different species of the same genus or from two different genera are crossed.
- **Wild type:** The traditional/historical form of an organism as it is ordinarily encountered in nature, in contrast to domesticated strains, natural mutant, or laboratory mutant individuals (organisms). One example of a measurable difference between the two types is that wild strains of animals respond to the presence of EMF fields (e.g. weak magnetic fields such as those generated near power transmission cables), but laboratory strains of the same animals do not. The organism as it was first isolated from nature. The normal type in a genetic experiment the strain from which the mutants were derived.
- **Wild-type allele:** The non-mutant form of a gene, encoding the normal genetic function. Generally, but not always a dominant allele.
- **Wobble hypothesis:** Accounts for the ability of a tRNA to recognize more than one codon by unusual (non-G-C, non-A-T) pairing with the third base of a codon (Fig. 6).

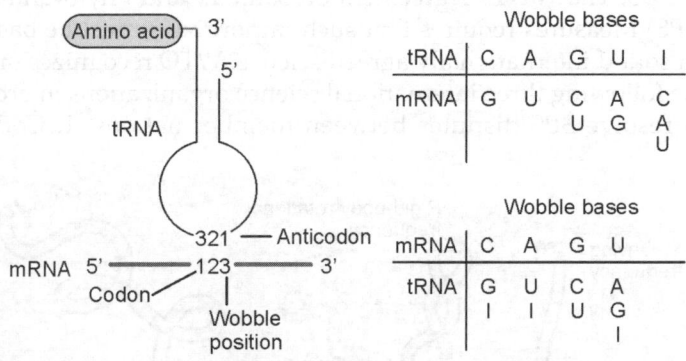

Fig. 6: Wobble hypothesis

- **Wobble:** Difference of codons of the same amino acid at the third base of mRNA. Wobble hypothesis accounts for the ability of a tRNA to recognize more than one codon by unusual (non-G.C, non-A.T) pairing with the third base of a codon (Fig. 7).

Wobble positions in anticodon and codon interactions

C	A	G	U	I
G	U	C	A	C
		U	G	U
				A

Wobble positions in codon and anticodon interactions

C	A	G	U
G	U	C	A
I	I	U	G
			I

Fig. 7: Wobble

- **World trade organization (WTO):** The international organization composed of more than 100 nations that signed the General Agreement on Tariffs and Trade (GATT), which contain 38 Articles that lay out the rules and procedures, which signatory countries must observe in their conduct of international trade and trade policy. GATT was WTO's predecessor body. The WTO permits signatory countries to ban specific imports from other countries in order to protect the health of humans, animals, or plants. Such import bans are allowed based on the (GATT/ WTO) Agreement on Sanitary and Phytosanitary Measures, or the Agreement on Technical Barriers to Trade; which were approved in 1994 by GATT. WTO was established on January 1, 1995. The WTO's Agreement on Sanitary and Phytosanitary (SPS) Measures requires that such import bans must be based on sound internationally agreed science. WTO recognizes only the following three international science organizations in order to resolve SPS disputes between member nations: 1. Codex

(a) Axial-spinning (b) Solid-body rotation (c) Plectoneme-creation

Fig. 8a to c: Writhing number

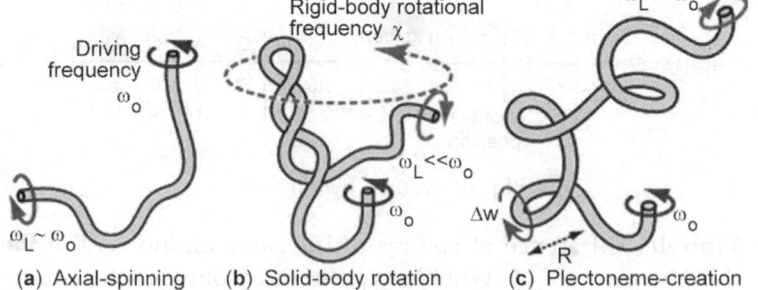

Alimentarius Commission for foods and food ingredients. 2.
International Plant Protection Convention (IPPC) for plants. 3.
International Office of Epizootics (OIE) for animal diseases.
- **Writhing number:** The number of times a duplex axis crosses
  over itself in space (Fig. 8a to c).

W

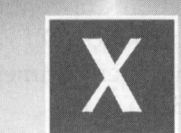

- **X Chromosome:** A sex chromosome that usually occurs in pair in each female cell, and single (unpaired) in each male cell in those species in which the male typically has two unlike sex chromosomes (humans).

- **Xanthine oxidase:** An enzyme responsible for production of free radicals in the body.

- **Xanthophylls:** A "family" of carotenoids (i.e. plant-produced pigments that act as protective antioxidants in photosynthetic plants, and in the bodies of animals that consume those cartenoids). Among other plants, xanthophylls are produced by yellow carrots. Consumption of xanthophylls by humans and animals assists development of healthy eye tissue. Research indicates that consumption of xanthophylls by humans helps in preventing lung cancer and some other cancers.

- **Xenia:** Hereditary influence from the pollen parent to the endosperm in the seed in certain plants.

- **Xenobiotic compounds:** Those compounds (veterinary drugs, agrochemical herbicides, etc.) designed for use in an ecosystem comprised of more than one species. For example, herbicides intended to kill weeds but leave commercial crops undamaged or veterinary drugs that are intended to kill parasitic worms but leave the host livestock unharmed.

- **Xenogeneic organs:** From the Greek word *xenos*, stranger. Xenogeneic literally means "strange genes." Refers to genetically engineered ("humanized") organs that have been grown within an animal of another species. For example, several companies are working to engineer and grow inside swine a number of organs to be transplanted into humans that need those organs (due to loss of their own organs via disease or accident). If successful, this would free human organ transplant recipients from having to use immunosuppressive drugs continually in order to keep their body from "rejecting" the new organ.

X

- **Xenogenesis:** The (theoretical) production of offspring that are genetically different from, and genotypically unrelated to, either of the parents.
- **Xenotransplant:** From the Greek word *xenos*, stranger. Xenotransplant is the implantation of an organ or limb from one species to another organism in a different species. When performed in animals, "rejection" of the transplant by the recipient's immune system is a common response.
- **Xenotransplantation:** The procedure that involves the transplantation of live cells, tissues, or organs from one species to another, including animal to human transplantation.
- **X-linked disease:** A genetic disease caused by a mutation on the X chromosome. In X-linked recessive condition, a normal female "carrier" passes on the mutated X chromosome to an affected son.
- **X-ray crystallography:** The use of diffraction patterns produced by X-ray scattering from crystals (of a given material's molecules) to determine the three-dimensional structure of the molecules (Fig. 1).

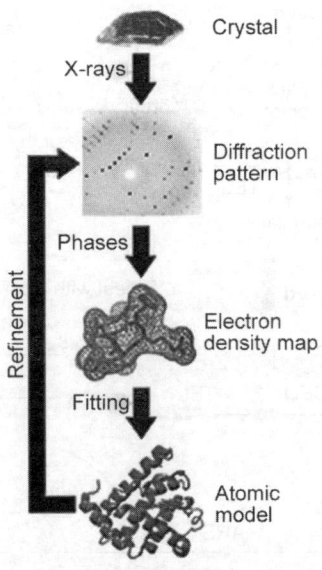

Fig. 1: X-ray crystallography

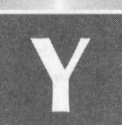

- **Y Chromosome:** A sex chromosome that is characteristic of male zygotes (and cells), in species in which the male typically has two unlike sex chromosomes.
- **Yeast:** A fungus of the family *Saccharomycetaceae* that is used by man especially in the making of alcoholic liquors and as a leavening agent in bread making. Some strains of yeast cells are also commonly used in bioprocesses, because they are relatively simple to genetically engineer (via recombinant DNA) and relatively easy to propagate (via fermentation) to yield desired products (proteins).
- **Yeast artificial chromosome (YAC):** It is a synthetic DNA molecule (for propagation of genes in yeast cells), with an origin

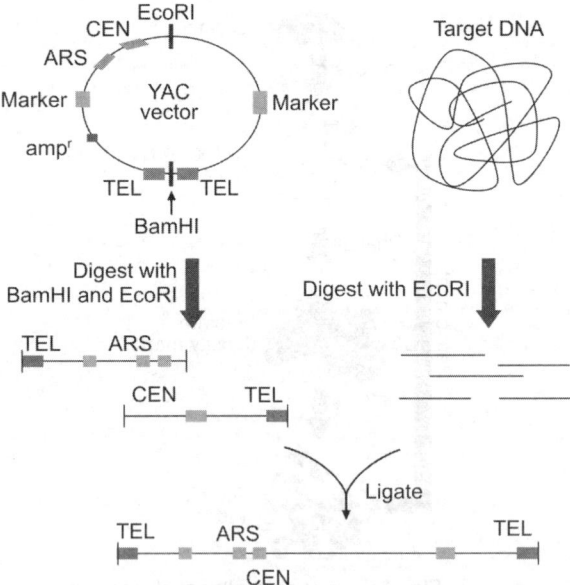

Fig. 1: Yeast artificial chromosome (YAC)

of replication, a centromere for segregation, telomeres to seal the ends, and also marker genes from yeast. YACs are used to clone long stretches of eukaryotic DNA (Fig. 1).

- **Yeast episomal plasmid (YEP):** A cloning vehicle used for introduction of constructions (i.e. genes and pieces of genetic material) into certain yeast strains at high copy number. YEP can replicate in both *Escherichia coli* and certain yeast strains.

Z

- **Z-DNA:** A left-handed helix (molecular structure) of DNA, in contrast to A-DNA and B-DNA which are right-handed helix structures. The difference is in the direction of the double-helix twist. Z-DNA has the most base pairs per turn (in the helix), and so has the least twisted structure; it is very "skinny" and its name is taken from the zigzag path that the sugar-phosphate "backbone" follows along the helix. This is quite different from the smoothly curving path of the backbone of B-DNA. The Z-form of DNA has been found in polymers that have an alternating purine-pyrimidine sequence. One possible biological importance of Z-DNA is that it is much more stable at lower salt concentrations, and there is a possibility that the

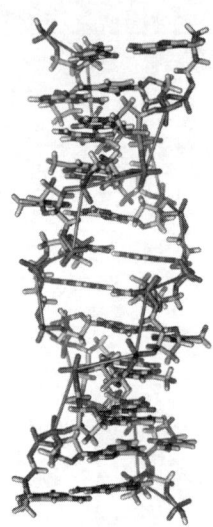

Fig. 1: Z-DNA

Z-DNA form (of DNA within cells) is the cause of certain diseases (certain cancers). During 2000, Jonathan Chaires, Waldemar Priebe, and John Trent showed that WP 900 (the enantiomer of daunorubicin, a natural chemical compound which inhibits cancer) binds tightly (and selectively) to a Z-DNA polymer (Fig. 1).

- **Zearalenone:** One of the mycotoxins (toxins produced by a fungus), it causes reproductive difficulties in swine (reduced sperm production, halting of estrus, etc.) when consumed by animals (in contaminated grain such as corn/maize). Zearalenone is produced by certain strains of *Fusarium* fungi when climate (moisture and temperature) conditions during the grain growing season, combined with entry points (holes chewed into the grain plants by insects) facilitate growth of those *Fusarium* strains in grain.

Z

- **Zeaxanthin:** A carotenoid ("light harvesting" compound utilized in photosynthesis) that is naturally produced in Brussels sprouts, summer squash, maize, avocado, green beans, and dark green leafy vegetables. Zeaxanthin is a phytochemical/ nutraceutical whose consumption by humans has been shown to reduce the risk of the disease age-related macular degeneration, a leading cause of blindness in elderly people (Fig. 2).

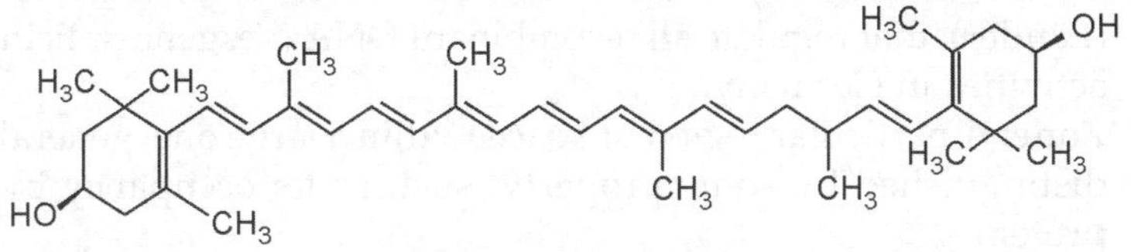

Fig. 2: Zeaxanthin

- **Zero time-binding DNA:** It enters the duplex form at the start of a reassociation reaction; results from intramolecular reassociation of inverted repeats.
- **Zeta potential:** The potential produced by the effective charge of a macromolecule, usually taken at the boundary between what is moving with the macromolecule and the rest of the solution.
- **Zinc finger:** A DNA-binding motif that typifies a class of transcription factor.
- **Zinc finger protein:** It has a repeated motif of amino acids with characteristic spacing of cysteines that may be involved in binding zinc; is characteristic of some proteins that bind DNA and/or RNA (Fig. 3).
- **ZKBS (central committee on biological safety):** The advisory body on safety in gene-splicing labs and plants for the German Government's Ministry of Health. It is the German counterpart

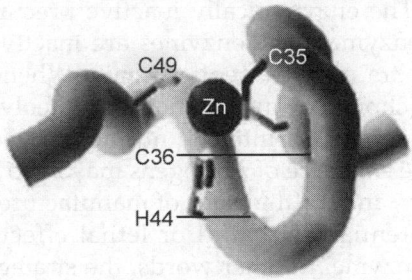

Fig. 3: Zinc finger protein

Z

of the American Government's Recombinant DNA Advisory Committee (RAC), Australia's Genetic Manipulation Advisory Committee (GMAC), Brazil's National Biosafety Commission (CTNBio), and the Kenya Biosafety Council. The ZKBS is composed of 10 experts from the biology and ecology sectors, trade union representatives, and representatives from the industrial sector and environmental pressure groups. The ZKBS advises the Ministry of Health and the individual German States (Länder), that regulate all recombinant DNA (i.e. gene-splicing) activities in Germany.

- **Zone:** A particular region or space within a large one, generally distinguished by some property, such as its occupancy by a protein.
- **Zoo blot:** The use of Southern blotting to test the ability of a DNA probe from one species to hybridize with the DNA from the genomes of a variety of other species.
- **Zoonoses:** Diseases that are communicable from animals to humans.
- **Zygote:** A fertilized egg formed as a result of the union of the male (sperm) and female (egg) sex cells. The zygote gives rise to the placenta (lining of the uterus) in addition to growing into the adult (organism) body (Fig. 4).

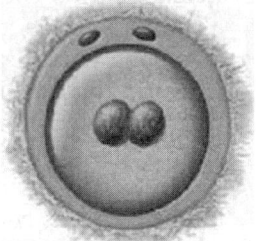

Fig. 4: Zygote

- **Zyme systems:** Chemical reactions characterized by the presence of an inactive precursor of an enzyme. The enzyme is activated via another enzyme that normally removes an extra piece of peptide chain at a physiologically appropriate time and place.
- **Zymogens:** The enzymatically inactive precursors of certain proteolytic enzymes. The enzymes are inactive because they contain an extra piece of peptide chain. When this peptide is hydrolyzed (clipped away) by another proteolytic enzyme, the zymogen is converted into the normal, active enzyme. The reason for the existence of zymogens may be to protect the cell, its machinery, and/or the place of manufacture within the cell from the potentially harmful or lethal effects of an active, proteolytic enzyme. In other words, the strategy is to activate the enzyme only when, and especially where, it is needed.

Z